Since psychiatry remains a descriptive discipline, it is essential for its practitioners to understand how the language of psychiatry came to be formed. This important book, written by a psychiatrist–historian, traces the genesis of the descriptive categories of psychopathology and examines their interaction with the psychological and philosophical context within which they arose.

Arguing that historical information should be available as freely to clinicians as are statistical and clinical data, the author explores particularly the language and ideas that have characterized descriptive psychopathology from the mid-nineteenth century to the present day. In the early chapters descriptive psychopathology is defined as the theoretical set of vocabularies and protocols created to depict mental symptoms, and it is suggested that these symptoms result from the interaction between a signal, expressing a neurobiological lesion, and prevailing personal and psychosocial codes. The author considers the implications for current research of this fragmentation of abnormal behaviour into a narrow repertoire of symptoms.

Following on from this introduction, this absorbing work consists of a masterful survey of the history of the main psychiatric symptoms, from the metaphysics of classical antiquity to the operational criteria of today. Tracing the evolution of concepts such as memory, consciousness, will and personality, and of symptoms ranging from catalepsy and aboulia to anxiety and self-harm, this part of the book provides fascinating insights into the subjective nature of mental illness, and into the ideas of British, Continental and American authorities who sought to clarify and define it. For all those attempting to understand or treat mental disorders, this is an essential account of the foundations of their discipline.

The history of mental symptoms

Descriptive psychopathology since the nineteenth century

The history of
mental symptoms

Descriptive psychopathology since
the nineteenth century

GERMAN E. BERRIOS

Department of Psychiatry

University of Cambridge, UK

Hist.
RC437.5
B468
1996

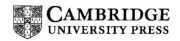

CAMBRIDGE
UNIVERSITY PRESS

Published by the Press Syndicate of the University of Cambridge

The Pitt Building, Trumpington Street, Cambridge CB2 1RP

40 West 20th Street, New York, NY 10011-4211, USA

10 Stamford Road, Oakleigh, Melbourne 3166, Australia

First published 1996

Printed in Great Britain at the University Press, Cambridge

A catalogue record for this book is available from the British Library

Library of congress cataloguing in publication data

Berrios, German E.

   The history of mental symptoms: descriptive psychopathology since the nineteenth century/
G. E. Berrios.

   p. cm.

   Includes bibliographical references and indexes.

   ISBN 0 521 43135 2 (hardback). ISBN 0 521 43736 9 (pbk.)

1. Psychology, Pathological – Philosophy. 2. Descriptive psychology. 3. Psychology, Pathological – History. 4. Mental illness – Terminology – History. 5. Mental illness – Classification –
History. 6. Mental illness – Classification – Social aspects.

I. Title.

   [DNLM: 1. Mental Disorders – history – nomenclature.

2. Psychopathology – history – nomenclature. 3. Nomenclature. WM 15

B533h 1995]

RC437.5.B468 1996

616.89′001–dc20   95–20315 CIP

DNLM/DLC

for Library of Congress

ISBN 0 521 43135 2 HARDBACK

ISBN 0 521 43736 9 PAPERBACK

WV

*Je crois vraiment que l'imprécision du terms n'est pas
due ici à autre chose qu'à l'imprecision des idées.*

La Psychiatrie est-elle une langue bien faite?
CHASLIN, 1914

to GERMAN ARNALDO BERRIOS

(1961–1977)

'For being dead, with him is beauty slain,
And, beauty dead, black chaos comes again.'

Contents

Preface

This book deals with the history of the main mental symptoms, i.e. of what is called *descriptive psychopathology*. Based on research carried out during the last 25 years, it covers about two centuries of French, German, Italian, Spanish, and British primary sources. Due to my ignorance of eastern European languages, the corresponding fields of inquiry have been left unexplored. The seriousness of this omission will depend on how important these psychiatric cultures have been to the development of western descriptive psychopathology.

The reader will notice that the book mainly examines the nineteenth century and after. The reason for having chosen this time span is ideological. During the 1960s, I was influenced by Gaston Bachelard and his notions of epistemological *rupture* and *refonte*. Preliminary research then suggested that something like a rupture and a 'recasting' had affected the discourse of insanity during the first half of the nineteenth century. Further work has provided reasonable evidence that such a change gave rise to the new language of mental symptoms.

Trying to identify the reasons that led nineteenth century alienists to select certain words and concepts to describe (and explain) the signs and symptoms of insanity is an awesome task. In addition to the pitfalls posed by interpreting subjective choice, there is the problem of documentary (both published and archival) unevenness caused no doubt by the bellic vicissitudes of Europe. Hence, the attentive reader will soon find out that more is known about some symptoms than others. I hope to correct this imbalance in the future.

The alienists whose work features in this book were great practitioners of the arts of medicine, and confronted clinical problems far worse than anything we will ever see in our own medical practice. For one, there was a high incidence of organic disorders, and death was a common occurrence amongst their patients. This provided them with the opportunity to undertake post-mortem diagnostic ascertainment. I have been, therefore, interested in exploring the interaction between their brain findings and the descriptive language itself which is, after all, the real (and only) basis for clinical reliability and validity. When possible, I have analysed the patient sample on which the 'first' descriptions were based. I am aware of the fact that history alone cannot solve this problem, and at the moment I am completing a companion volume in which a re-calibration of the language of description is suggested. Hopefully, this will help to redress the mismatch that now exists between symptom description and the information provided by the new neurobiological research techniques.

As social historians correctly remind us, the alienists of yester-year were also socially ambitious individuals, and their scientific views were often influenced by all manner of 'non-cognitive' factors. This perspective has been covered so well in the many social histories of psychiatry available that repetition would be out of place.

For this book, thanks are owed to my Oxford teachers: E. Anscombe, A. Crombie, M. Davidson, B. Farrell, R. Harré, G. Ryle, M. Teich, J.O. Urmson, and Ch. Webster, from whose varied and enduring research I first learned the power of conceptual and/or historical analysis; to Professor M. Gelder, from the Oxford University Department of Psychiatry, who about 26 years ago kindly suggested that I might want to fill a gap in the literature by writing a book on the history of psychopathology; to Professor E.S. Paykel, from the Cambridge University Department of Psychiatry for his gentle encouragement, and to my students for asking that I publish my historical lectures. I should also like to thank Dr Richard Barling and Dr Jocelyn Foster, both from Cambridge University Press, whose epistolary promptings flattered me into bursts of weekend writing. Thanks are also due to the editors of some learned journals for allowing the use of published material, and to colleagues and students for their help with some of the chapters (both are acknowledged in the appropriate sections of the book). I am also grateful to the brotherhood of psychiatric librarians for exercising on my behalf their uncanny power to locate the rarest of references; and to Doris, my wife, for organizing and keying in thousands of notes and references, and for having so gracefully eased for me the task of living. Lastly, the lion's share of my gratitude must surely go to whoever invented the photocopying machine, for without this gadget it would have been impossible to indulge in the disreputable trade of being a weekend 'historian'.

German E. Berrios, Cambridge

Acknowledgements

Thanks are due to the *British Journal of Psychiatry* (Royal College of Psychiatrists), *Comprehensive Psychiatry* (W.B. Saunders Company) and *Psychological Medicine* (Cambridge University Press) for granting permission to use material from papers of mine which appeared in their pages.

Introduction

Psychiatry is the branch of medicine that deals with mental disease. Almost universally, a language (*descriptive psychopathology*) (DP) is now used to record the symptoms of mental disease, and it consists of a vocabulary, a syntax, assumptions about the nature of behaviour, and some application rules. This language was composed in Europe during the first half of the nineteenth century, and has proved to be surprisingly stable. It is likely that both neurobiological and psychological and social factors are responsible for this stability which, at least in theory, depends on: a) the durability of the cognitive or social aims of the 'community of users'[1] or 'thought collective',[2] b) the permanency of the object of inquiry itself, namely the neurobiological signal,[3] and c) the dynamic matching between object and the language of description.[4] Descriptive psychopathology is thus a conceptual network meshing observer, patient and symptoms together.

Mental symptoms are (mostly) intermittent and quantitative variations in speech and human action. The latter, in turn, are complex, theory-bound states. It follows that attempts at producing 'atheoretical' or 'phenomenological' descriptions of mental signs and symptoms are misconceived.[5] Successful description in psychiatry consists in little more than the obtention of reliable morsels of behaviour which, hopefully, still contain enough of the biological signal which caused them in the first place and which provides the information for diagnosis, treatment, and research. Infelicitous descriptions, or descriptions 'manqué' are likely to be a common occurrence in the daily affairs of psychiatric practice. The rub here is that *prima facie* it is very difficult to tell. One obvious test might be treatment failure. However, the latter can result from so many imponderables that clinicians would rarely blame their original descriptions. And yet, what they originally described is all they have in the way of information.

It would seem, therefore, that the 'final description' of a symptom results from the interaction between a tenuous biological *signal* (originated in an affected brain site) and the layers of psychosocial codes (noise) partaking in the process of symptom formation. Some symptoms are likely to be mostly noise (e.g. manipulation),[6] others, predominantly signal (e.g. hallucination, disorientation, stupor, etc.).[7] The crucial point here is that clinical 'observation' is never a cognitively innocent activity. Indeed, its biases[8] will exercise philosophers for a long time to come.[9]

One important (yet often neglected) bias concerns regular shifts in 'episteme' or 'themata', i.e. in the way in which observers are instructed by their culture to perceive mental disorder.[10] The existence of such a changing perspective encourages the 'relativist' belief that mental symptoms (and diseases) are *only* 'cultural' constructs. Culture-related variations in symptom presentation, however, do not necessarily override the biological signal.[11] Furthermore, it has also been argued that, even in the behavioural sciences, 'facts' are 'partially interchangeable' between observers[12] thereby permitting some 'triangulation', and hopefully the teasing out of signal from noise. Lastly, the fact that, since its inception, western DP has remained stable suggests that, as proposed in their day by Kant and Levi–Strauss, cognitive categories for the description and organization of the world, which are actually wired into the human brain, may be in operation.

The term 'episteme' deserves some comment. It is here used to name (more or less) autonomous ideological domains contained within some temporal boundaries. These ideological systems feed, so to speak, meaning into historical events. Thus, individuals working within a given episteme are likely to share more conceptual frames than individuals from different epistemes. Such a commonality of concepts would constitute what Levy–Brühl has called a *mentalité*. However, this notion jars the empiricist mind, and has recently been criticized.[13] From the point of view of the history of psychopathology, the period stretching from the middle of the nineteenth century to the present will be here regarded as an 'episteme'.

The problem with the 'epistemic' view in its strongest interpretation is that events only have meaning and value within a given period and cannot be compared with events from a different episteme. This conclusion is perturbing to clinicians who believe that medicine and her progress are 'trans-epistemic'.[14] The onus of solving this apparent paradox is upon the shoulders of the historian–clinician who should search for psychological, anatomical, or physiological 'trans-epistemic' invariants. For example, a trans-epistemic history of delirium may have to be constructed on the basis of the history of the *behaviours* themselves.

To compound matters further, national differences exist in the definition of 'psychopathology': whilst in the USA it is tantamount to psychiatry; in Continental Europe it refers to the science of the symptoms of the mind (including *description* and *explanation*), and hence it is traditionally subdivided into descriptive, experimental and psychodynamic. *Descriptive* (or phenomenological) psychopathology focuses on the 'form' of the symptom (e.g. visions and hearing voices are *both* instances of hallucination). The *experimental* or numerical approach, on the other hand, attempts to capture and measure the phenomenon by objective means (e.g. by ascertaining hallucinatory experiences by analysis of scanning eye movements or PET scanning). Lastly, *psychodynamic* psychopathology focuses on the semantics of content, and to achieve this a machinery is required of the type developed by Janet or Freud. This book exclusively deals with the history of descriptions.

The prudent clinician wants to calibrate psychopathology from historical, clinical and numerical perspectives. For example, when dealing with 'delusion', he / she wants to know about the history of the 'equivalent' words in the relevant languages (*historical and comparative etymology*), of the behaviours and brain changes involved (*behavioural palaentology*), and of the theories and concepts (*conceptual history*). To complete this task, however, she / he should also want to know about the current presentations of the symptom, incidence and prevalence and structural features (clinical analysis), and lastly about measurements (psychometry). The combination of these strands of knowledge will occasion a veritable re-calibration of the language of psychiatry. In as much as its historical analysis will identify the conceptual circumstances in which symptoms were constructed, this book should be understood as a contribution to the process of calibration. For, as it will be shown, defective capacity to gather information often results from defects in symptom construction.

NOTES

1 Laudan, 1977.
2 Fleck, 1979.
3 Hare, 1974; Marchais, 1983.
4 Berrios and Marková, 1995.
5 Berrios, On phenomenology, psychopathology and Jaspers, 1992.
6 Mackenzie *et al.*, 1978.
7 Berrios, On delirium, 1981.
8 Blashfield, 1982; Sülz and Gigerenzer, 1982.
9 Hesse, 1966; Wartofsky, 1979.
10 Bachelard, 1938; Holton, 1973.
11 Rack, 1982.
12 Parain-Vial, 1966.
13 Lloyd, 1990.
14 For a discussion of issues pertaining to progress in science, see Laudan, 1977.

PART I

The object of inquiry

CHAPTER 1

Matters historical

That psychopathological understanding and creativity are enhanced by knowledge of history was well understood by nineteenth century alienists. Calmeil, Morel, Trélat, Semelaigne, Kirshoff, Winslow, Ireland, Mercier, Bucknill and Tuke wrote full-blown historical pieces; Pinel, Haslam, Heinroth, Guislain, Esquirol, Feuchsterleben, Prichard, Connolly, Griesinger, Lucas, Falret and Dagonet included historical chapters in their clinical textbooks.

Some, like Haslam, even emphasized historical semantics: 'Mad is therefore not a complex idea, as has been supposed, but a complex term for all the forms and varieties of this disease. Our language has been enriched with other terms expressive of this affection . . .'.[1] Inspired by eighteenth century German 'historicism',[2] others saw their role as that of rescuing lost insights from an obscure (and mythical) psychiatric past. Heinroth, for example, subscribed to a cyclical, Vico-inspired, conception according to which history consisted of the recurrence of few great themes: 'the development of mental forces in humanity is accompanied by an ever advancing, ever more degraded degeneration of these forces'.[3] For him, psychiatry followed a 'developmental' path: 'a study of the kind and degree of recognition and treatment of mental disturbances observed in early antiquity shows that these bear a striking imprint of the childhood of the human spirit'.[4]

Pinel made use of a more 'presentistic' approach (history was a preparation for what was happening now). Influenced by the optimistic historiography of the French revolution, he regarded the past of psychiatry as a museum of failed endeavours. Thus, men, ideas, and even books were criticized: 'English monographs on mental alienation during the second half of the eighteenth century promise a great deal in view of the avowed intention of their authors to concentrate on specific topics; but this promise is rarely fulfilled. Vague and repetitious argument, old fashioned clinical approach and lack of clinical facts and doctrine contribute to this failure.'[5]

Prichard utilized historical material in a more personal way. Having adopted Faculty Psychology, he attacked the 'intellectualistic' view of insanity (as primarily due to a disorder of intellectual functions): 'It has been supposed that the chief, if not the sole disorder of persons labouring under insanity consists in some particular false conviction, or in some erroneous notion indelibly impressed upon belief . . .

from Mr Locke's time it has been customary to observe the insane reason correctly from wrong premises . . . that this is by far too limited an account of insanity and only comprises one among various forms of mental derangement, every person must be aware.'[6]

In their *Manual*, Bucknill and Tuke[7] included historical chapters on themes such as 'lay descriptions' of insanity, the 'opinion of medical writers', the concept of insanity, aspects of treatment, and classification. Giné y Partagás, considered as one of the great Catalan alienists of the nineteenth century, believed that throughout the ages insanity had reflected social values: 'human knowledge reflects the moral and political development of the nations; the best example of this is that branch of medicine that deals with mental illness.'[8] Influenced by Comtean and Darwinian ideas, Giné saw psychiatry as progressing away from medicine and neurology.

Few nineteenth century alienists have made their historiographic tenets as explicit as the Austrian Feuchtersleben. He believed that only the 'empirical sciences' could afford to dismiss their past as just a 'history of errors'. The rest of the sciences, including medical psychology, had to contend with the fact that 'the history of the science [was] properly the science itself'. Psychiatry, interestingly, 'belonged to both spheres': 'That part of it which was philosophical contained an abstract of that state of philosophy in every age, while that which is empirical has by no means attained such precision and clearness as to render a knowledge of previous opinions superfluous . . .' On account of this, Feuchtersleben concluded: 'I am obliged to treat the history of our branch of the profession.'[9]

Current state of the art

The history of psychiatry (less so that of descriptive psychopathology)[10] is going through exciting times, and for this we should be grateful to many.[11] The revival was marked in 1967 on the occasion of the Yale Symposium on the History of Psychiatry[12] when an evaluation was made of the fruits of traditional historiography.[13] The same innovative spirit led Marx[14] to state that psychiatric history required 'a view of history, a definition of psychiatry and a precept of what psychiatry should be' and later on to develop a Lakatoshian view of history as a 'tentative construct'.[15] Similar views have been expressed with respect to the history of the behavioural sciences[16] and of medicine.[17]

Since the Yale symposium, the history of psychiatry has become a popular discipline and much progress has been made. This has resulted from a decline in the post-Foucaultian industry[18] and efforts to correct the generalizations of its mentor.[19] Great French historians such as Ey, Baruk, Lanteri-Laura, Trillat, Bercherie and Postel never fully subscribed to the Foucaultian creed and this led to first-rate independent work. Important publications by social historians[20] have also helped to counterbalance earlier distortions caused by an excessively 'medical' approach; the social perspective, however, is more relevant to the history of asylums than to descriptive psychopathology.[21] In relation to the latter, there seems to be a 'legitimate' need[22] for studies that ask questions about the genesis of the categories of psychopathology and their interaction with the psychological and philosophical context.

The historiography of descriptive psychopathology

The young psychiatrist venturing for the first time into this field may be confused by the various (albeit) complementary approaches to the history of psychopathology. Biographical, anthological, narrative, socio-political, institutional and conceptual techniques reflect different fashions and theoretical influences. The history of psychopathology itself has been shaped by techniques created in the history of medicine. It is not surprising, therefore, that the biographical approach was used the earliest, followed by the anthological and narrative techniques. Intellectualistic approaches of the 'chain of being' type[23] came into fashion during the 1930s, and the Zilboorg volume is a good illustration of this.[24] These approaches encouraged an 'internalist', 'linear', or 'Whiggish'[25] type of historical explanation, until the time it was challenged by Michel Foucault.

In this regard, it should not be forgotten that the history of science herself went through a similar evolution and that the debate between 'naive realists' and 'social constructionists' has continued to this day.[26] The 'internalist' view is based on the belief that science consists of a piecemeal accumulation of observations and that theories emanate from these. Inductivism, the technical name for this mode of theory generation, makes assumptions about the nature of truth, the 'regularity' of nature, and the contexts of discovery and justification, all of which have come under attack. In this model there is little room for non-intellectual and contextual considerations. Incomplete as this approach may be, it gave rise to good scholarship in areas such as the history of physics, chemistry and astronomy. In the behavioural sciences (which includes the history of psychopathology) it was less successful because categories such as 'discovery', 'observation', 'replication', 'evidence', and 'experiment',[27] are far more difficult to define, and because their analysis depends on analogies and metaphors.[28]

During the 1950s, a similar crisis affected the history of the natural sciences culminating in the work of Toulmin[29] and Hanson[30] who proposed new models for scientific change. Following the lead of Gaston Bachelard, the much neglected French historian of science, these authors challenged the image of science as an exercise in pure rationality and suggested that historical accuracy had been sacrificed to superficial order and dubious progressivist views. Philosophers of science were also dissatisfied with the inductivist view already challenged by Popper in 1934.[31] Although Popper's notion of 'falsification' is not free from inductivist assumptions, the libertarian tones of his prose served as an exhortation against

non-cognitivism and irrationality. Popper also attacked psychoanalysis as
non-scientific, causing consternation amongst historians of psychiatry. Lakatos[32]
went on to propound a 'rational reconstruction of the past' and this view influenced
notable historians of psychiatry such as Otto Marx.[33] Since this time the philosophy
of science has moved back to a form of cautious realism.[34]

In his 'Structure of Scientific Revolutions'[35] Thomas Kuhn made use of a diluted
version of Bachelardian historiography (said to have been obtained via Alexandre
Koyré)[36] and proposed a view of science as a succession of superseding paradigms.
A 'paradigm' was a view of reality embodied in a theory. Once 'accepted' by a
'scientific community', it controlled the 'perceptions' and questions of its scientists.
Science thus practiced was called 'normal'. However, 'anomalies' (that is, non-
explained facts), gradually accumulated, eventually undermining normal science;
this led to a 'revolution', which consisted in the replacement of the old by a new
paradigm. The ensuing 'Gestalt shift' caused the scientific community to perceive
scientific fact in a different way. Kuhn's account proved surprisingly popular in the
1960s when some used his 'model' (originally created to deal with problems in the
history of physics) to let complex issues in psychology go untackled[37] on the excuse
that this discipline was 'backwards' (as compared to the natural sciences) because
it still inhabited a pre- (or multi-) paradigmatic limbo.[38] This view is likely to have
delayed the search for an epistemology of the inexact sciences[39] which, at least
since the time of Dilthey, Rickert and Weber has been a tantalizing possibility.

A problem with Kuhn's model was the ambiguity of the notion of 'paradigm'
(its central operative category), which in his original book was found to have more
than twenty meanings.[40] There is also the problem of historical evidence, i.e. the
fact that the history of some sciences (such as the behavioural disciplines) does not
follow a Kuhnian path. Lastly, as mentioned above, the facile application of Kuhnian notions to the history of the psychological sciences is likely to have caused the
neglect of continental writers such as Dilthey[41] and Politzer[42] or Bachelard who
offered superior solutions to the same problem.

Psychiatry is not a contemplative but a modificatory activity, and clinicians are
primarily interested in the capacity of psychopathological descriptions to diagnose
disease and predict clinical outcome; this capacity is assumed to reflect its truth
value, i.e. the extent to which it 'pictures' reality. To reach this state, symptom
descriptions must be unencumbered by semantic confusion and be based on multiple and reliable clinical observations. It is one of the objectives of the history of
psychopathology to ascertain the epistemological provenance of symptoms and any
changes of meaning that may result from their being transferred from one 'episteme' to the next (to answer questions such as does the term 'hallucination' mean
in 1995 the same as it did in 1814 when it was first operationalized?). This it
does, as mentioned above, by separately studying the words, concepts and putative
disorders of behaviour involved in the definition of a 'symptom'. Another objective
of historical psychopathology is to break the 'epistemological' codes that have

governed successive psychiatric discourses, and make explicit the assumptions that have inspired alienists throughout the ages (e.g. concepts of disease, and views on the nature of man).

Sources for a history of psychopathology

In historical research, techniques and questions may determine what counts as the 'object of inquiry' and what as 'supporting evidence'. Depending on how he defines his object of inquiry, the clinician interested, say, in the history of 'delusions' will find that earlier centuries offer either little or a plethora of information. Which it is will be determined by the nature of the 'invariant' he has chosen to postulate. An invariant is an entity (e.g. brain lesion or population of receptors) or concept (e.g. the unconscious) which acts as the 'referent' to a particular symptom and is robust enough (i.e. has sufficient ontology) to provide trans-epistemic continuity. To continue with the example, if there is a strong neurobiological basis for 'delusion', then the name under which it has travelled throughout history or the concepts used to explain it or whether or not it has been considered as a 'symptom' will matter little, for the behaviour will persistently re-appear in a recognizable form in successive historical periods. Conceptual invariants need not be only 'organic': the late George Devereux used psychodynamic structures for the same purpose in his work.[43]

The concept of 'invariant' may be challenged as a social construction. Indeed, the history of psychopathology is governed by two metaphors: one pictures the clinician as *cataloguing* plants in a garden (i.e. assuming ontological invariance); the other as a sculptor carving shapes out of formless matter, i.e. *creating* 'clinical forms' (constructionism). The 'garden' approach conceives of the 'discoverer' as an omnipotent eye that can see through misleading descriptions. The 'creationist' approach depends upon the depth of the 'contextualization' which ranges from hard 'social constructionism' that may even explain medical theory in terms of the personality of her practitioners[44] to milder forms which leave some room for invariants.[45] Whilst traditional medical history has followed the garden metaphor, current history of psychiatry has been influenced by the creationist view. In the case of the history of psychopathology, the clinician will have to decide which approach is more suitable to his own beliefs and the symptom under study.

A history for clinicians

Together with clinical research and quantitative analysis of clinical samples, the historical and conceptual analyses of descriptions form part of the periodic calibration of the language of psychiatry. Calibration here means re-adjustment of the descriptions to changes originating either in biology (caused, for example, by genetic mutations) or in psychology (new models of behaviour) or sociology (re-definitions of abnormal behaviour).

To effect such calibration, historical knowledge should be available to clinicians as freely as clinical or numerical data. Unfortunately, this is not the case at the moment for there has been little research into the history of psychiatric symptoms; indeed, it is not even known which research format or historiographical approach would be the most convenient for gaining the information needed for re-calibration. I believe that what is here called the 'conceptual' and 'statistical' formats will prove to be the most attractive to the clinician. They offer a separate account of the history of the term, concept and behaviour and make use of modern statistical techniques to corroborate the existence of putative clinical patterns in historical databases. In this sense, the historian does effectively contribute to current clinical knowledge. It is becoming clear that the use of psychotropic drugs may be attenuating or distorting the presentation of certain symptoms; if so, patient cohorts collected before such medication was available may contain important clinical information.[46] Likewise, based on the belief that mental symptoms are complex reflections of dysfunctional brain sites, the clinical historian should seek to determine which past 'symptoms' were just noise (the product of a cultural quirk, e.g. 'aural haematoma') and which described biological signals.

Throughout history, the language of psychiatry has shown periods of stability and change. Whereas change attracts much soul-searching, stability is taken for granted. The historian, however, should try and explain why descriptive psychopathology has remained in steady state for such a long time. He might then find that devices such as symbols, myths and other social constructions are as steadying a factor as the biological signal captured by the symptom. Their relative contribution, however, is yet unknown and should be of interest to the clinical historian.

Towards a history of psychopathology

Those whose business is the calibration of the language of psychiatry need the assistance of professional historians. The unenthusiastic response of the latter (who are, in general, interested in loftier issues) has led to the development amongst clinicians of a 'do-it-yourself' historical industry which often cannot overcome a lack of historical training, limited access to primary material, and linguistic obstacles. As a consequence, standards of research in the history of psychopathology, which should be as high as in any other area of medicine, have not been achieved. There is, therefore, a need for collaborative work between clinicians and historians, and in this book it is suggested that the first task should be the calibration of descriptive psychopathology. For example, an analysis should be carried out of its conceptual structure and historical origins.

To map such origins the clinical historian will need a historical model. One such is Braudel's,[47] according to which history is a harmonics of processes of short, medium and long duration. Psychiatric events can be placed at, and find explanation within, each of these 'durations'. For example, the accident that killed Wernicke (whose death, by the way, may have changed the direction of western psychiatry) can be considered as a short-process. On the other hand, the impact of Faculty Psychology on psychiatric classification and aetiological theory might be better understood as a medium-duration process. Lastly, changes in the understanding of madness which depend on medical and cultural changes are likely to be long-duration processes.

A detailed explanatory model is also needed. The one to be followed in this book is based on the analogy of the 'Chinese boxes', i.e. the 'inner' boxes containing philosophical–psychological explanations and the 'outer' ones socio-political accounts. The clinician has to decide at what level his efforts to explain a particular symptom formation must stop. On occasions, the 'inner boxes' should suffice as is often the case in 'conceptual history'. Not resorting to the 'outer boxes' is not necessarily a historiographic misdemeanour as there are no *a priori* rules to decide where to stop explaining. Each researcher should generate his own rules, and these may range from the clinically useful or intellectually satisfying to the fashionable and aesthetic.

Descriptive psychopathology and 'abnormal psychology' (as treated by clinical psychologists) are germane activities and the historian would expect much help from its historians. Surprisingly, however, it has been treated with reticence by conventional historians of psychology who have bothered little about topics such as the history of personality disorders, hallucinations, anxiety, etc.[48] In a way, this is not surprising for traditional psychological historiography has concentrated on loftier issues such as the philosophical sources of psychology, the historical mechanisms that led to its 'separation' from philosophy; and, of late, the origin and epistemological value of competing psychological theories and research techniques.

NOTES

1 p. 4, Haslam, 1809.
2 Engel-Janosi, 1944.
3 p. 40, Heinroth, 1975.
4 p. 41, Heinroth, 1975.
5 p. xix, Pinel, 1809.
6 p. 3, Prichard, 1835.
7 Bucknill and Tuke, 1858.
8 p. 1, Giné y Partagás, 1876.
9 p. 24, Feuchtersleben, 1847.
10 Berrios, Historiography of . . . 1994.
11 See *History of Psychiatry*, Vol. 2, Issue 3, 1991 which is fully dedicated to ongoing historical scholarship in various countries.
12 Mora and Brand, 1970.

13 Braceland, 1970.
14 p. 603, Marx, 1970; see also Marx, 1992.
15 Marx, 1977.
16 Young, 1966; also excellent book by Danziger, 1990.
17 Clarke, 1971.
18 Foucault, 1972.
19 Sedgwick, 1981; Castel, 1977; Swain, 1977; Gauchet and Swain, 1980.
20 Dörner, 1969; Jones, 1972; Scull, 1979; Scull, 1981; Alexander, 1976; Castel *et al.*, 1979; Blasius, 1980; Cooter, 1984; Digby, 1985; Alvarez-Uría, 1983; Comelles, 1988; Porter, 1987. More recently the excellent update by Micale and Porter, 1994.
21 Werlinder, 1978; Janzarik, 1979; Wallace and Pressley, 1980; Simon, 1978; Saurí, 1969; Roccatagliata, 1981; López Piñero, 1963; 1983; López Piñero and Morales Meseguer, 1970; Clarke, 1975; Dewhurst, 1982; Bercherie, 1980; Postel and Quetel, 1983.
22 Daumezón, 1980.
23 Lovejoy, 1936.
24 Zilboorg, 1941.
25 Butterfield, 1931; Hesse, 1973; Agassi, 1963.
26 Bloor, 1991; Jardine, 1986; 1991.
27 Danziger, 1990.
28 Sternberg, 1990; Leary, 1990.
29 Toulmin, 1953.
30 Hanson, 1958.
31 Popper, 1968.
32 Hacking, 1979; Lakatos and Musgrave, 1970.
33 Marx, 1977.
34 The literature in this area is enormous. The psychiatrist will find useful Suppe, 1977; Meyer, 1979; Smith, 1981; Jardine, 1986.
35 Popper, 1968; Stove, 1982; Hacking, 1981.
36 Lecourt, 1975; Tiles, 1984.
37 Kuhn, 1962.
38 Farrell, 1978; Warren, 1971; Lambie, 1991.
39 Helmer and Rescher, 1959.
40 Masterman, 1970.
41 Dilthey, 1883; Martin-Santos, 1955; López, 1990.
42 Roelens, 1962; Deleule, 1969; Politzer, 1967.
43 Devereux, 1980.
44 For an example of this debate see Barnes, 1972; Bury, 1986; Nicolson and McLaughlin, 1987; and Bury, 1987.
45 Jardine, 1991.
46 As examples of this see Berrios, Epilepsy and Insanity, 1984; Berrios, Depressive Pseudodementia, 1985; Berrios and Quemada 1990; Berrios, Affective disorders . . ., 1991.
47 Braudel, 1980.
48 See, for example, Boring, 1950; Murphy, 1949; Watson, 1978; Lowry, 1971; Klein, 1970; Hearnshaw, 1987.

CHAPTER 2

Descriptive psychopathology

The history of mental symptoms during the nineteenth century can be explored from four complementary perspectives: descriptive psychopathology (DP), aetiological theory, pathogenesis and taxonomy. DP refers to the language of description, aetiology to underlying causes, pathogenesis to the mechanisms that disrupt brain structure and /or function which, in turn, generate symptoms, and taxonomy to the clustering rules which govern symptom grouping. DP (also called 'psychiatric semiology' in Continental countries) owes much to eighteenth century theory of signs;[1] psychiatric aetiological theory and pathogenesis were moulded upon nineteenth century developments in general medicine;[2] and taxonomy grew out of metaphors of order and classificatory principles developed during the Enlightenment.[3] This book deals exclusively with the history of DP and enjoins historians to tackle the remainder, i.e. the history of psychiatric aetiological theory, pathogenesis and taxonomy during the nineteenth century on which, so far, near to nothing of substance has been written.

The development of DP

Inter alia, DP can be defined as a descriptive-cum-cognitive system designed to capture aspects of abnormal behaviour. This it does by applying words to segments of speech and action. To achieve its purpose, two components are needed: a lexicon and segments (symptoms or referents) which have to be 'outlined' or 'constructed'. Since the latter are not obviously delimited or tagged, the naming function of DP often entails fracturing the behaviour presented by mentally ill patients. Furthermore, since the resulting 'fragments' are not equally informational, only some need to be kept. The rules for such a decision are based on nosological and aetiological theories of mental illness.[4] But rules are also needed to decide at what level of severity, vividness or duration it is efficient to accept a 'symptom' as *present* (i.e. rules for 'caseness').[5] Although it is reasonable to assume that both sets of rules exist *de facto* (clinicians are, all in all, good at symptom recognition, at least for the purpose of everyday work), as far as this writer knows they have never been formulated in writing. This is why, to gain an idea of the size of inter-observer disagreement, researchers have developed objective estimations (e.g. kappa values) which indicate when it is safe to leave things as they are and when a tightening of definitions or more training to improve symptom recognition is required.[6]

It was otherwise during the nineteenth century.[7] When disputes arose, alienists appealed to the tribunal of 'common sense' and reference to the 'obvious' nature of disordered behaviour was often made. Likewise, one of the functions of the so-called psychiatric 'schools' (particularly on the Continent) was to standardize theory and observation. Disagreement arose, however, when opinions on the same case had to be provided by medical experts belonging to different schools or when one was not medically trained, as it happened in forensic psychiatry. The psychiatric profession agonized over these cases, for they were interpreted as a challenge to their knowledge.[8]

The absence of a veritable DP is, perhaps, the most striking feature of the psychiatric discourse *before* the nineteenth century. However rich in literary detail,[9] earlier references to insanity (and related terms such as dementia) were made in 'molar' terms. Indeed, since Greek times, the diagnosis of the great psychiatric categories (mania, melancholia, etc.) was of the 'all-or-none' type and revolved around the recognition of *behavioural* criteria[10] (signs) thus leaving little room for the nuance and chiaroscuro involved in subjective experience (symptoms).

The creation of DP took about 100 years to be completed. It started around the second decade of the nineteenth century and was ready just before the Great War. It has changed little since, which means that the success of current research depends on an instrument tooled a long time ago. Although DP has been refined during the twentieth century by statistical and decision-making routines, the historical question still remains: how did nineteenth century alienists manage, based on the longitudinal observation of what often were institutionalized patient cohorts (and hence biased and with high levels of social noise), to extract stable descriptions?

To throw light on this process, six factors need to be explored: a) the descriptive needs of the new asylum officers, and the new patient cohorts, b) the availability of psychological theories that might support stable descriptions, c) the changing notion of sign and symptom in medicine, d) the introduction of subjective symptomatology, e) the use of time as a contextual dimension, and f) the development of quantification.

During the early nineteenth century, the drive to build asylums for the insane appeared simultaneously in various countries.[11] These institutions rapidly accumulated patients within a confined physical space and created all manner of new medical, social and scientific needs: one was the presence of a physician to deal with (mainly infectious) diseases which often decimated the inmate population; another, that of recording medical events and ascertaining cause of death by postmortem. In England, medical practitioners were encouraged to work in asylums by the 1828 Act,[12] and brought with them the habit (and obligation) of documenting clinical change: as long as this related to physical state there was no problem as there already existed a well-recognized style for history taking.[13] But asylum patients were often physically healthy, and only needed recording of their mental state. Perusal of pre-1830s clinical log-books shows a poverty of description which is consonant with the absence of official 'symptom lists'. Early asylum doctors were thus forced to improvise and borrow: this activity was an important factor in the creation of a 'semiology' of mental illness. Consequently, after the 1850s, a change is noticed in the quality of case descriptions.

It can be argued that accounts of madness before the nineteenth century do occasionally include elegant descriptions of mental states;[14] this may be true but it never amounts to a common language of description, nor was it intended to be. Nineteenth century semiology is a *different conceptual enterprise*: it is analytical and pictorial throughout, dealing with symptoms as separate units of analysis, and assuming that the same symptom may be seen in different forms of madness.[15] The creation of such DP was a complex process and led to a major shift in the perception of madness. Changes in the 'semiology' of medicine are no doubt also important to this process, but a *sine qua non* was the availability of psychological theories which supported the construction of behavioural profiles.

In its current form DP emerged first in France and then Germany between the second and ninth decades of the nineteenth century. Books on insanity prior to this period were mostly concerned with molar descriptions; after the 1830s, however, they include clinical vignettes and often a short section on 'elementary' symptoms.[16] In this regard, there is a marked difference between the work of say, Pargeter, Arnold, Crichton, Haslam, Rush, Heinroth and Pinel, and that of Esquirol, Prichard, Georget, Guislain, Feuchtersleben, Griesinger, Morel, Falret, Baillarger and Bucknill and Tuke.

The main diagnostic groupings inherited by the nineteenth century were melancholia, mania, phrenitis, delirium, paranoia, lethargy, carus and dementia. By the 1850s, these categories had all been broken up in a process that Ey called the *'dissection de la vie psychique morbide'*.[17] Some of the fragments were kept and their recombination gave rise to the new nosology. Some old categories (e.g. delirium) emerged unchanged; others, such as melancholia and mania were totally refurbished with new clinical meaning; yet others such as *carus*, *phrenitis* or *catalepsy* were to disappear for good. The templates of the mind and of behaviour required by these recombinations were provided by Faculty Psychology and Associationism.

The psychological context

Faculty Psychology

Since antiquity 'some writers have been inclined to adopt the absolute unity or singleness of the mind of man'; others have considered it as a composite of faculties; [and] the 'number and names of these faculties have occasionally undergone change, in accordance with diverse theoretical systems.'[18] During those earlier periods, the word 'faculty' referred to 'operations' attributed to the soul; the theoretical basis for this being that the operations defined themselves in opposition to each other.[19]

During the eighteenth century, the notion of 'Faculty' (as an independent function) re-appeared in the work of Christian Wolff, called the 'father of faculty psychology.'[20] He regarded capacities such as attending, remembering, perceiving, etc. as more or less independent mental powers and based his own concept of mental faculty upon that of 'function'.[21] The 'feelings', however, only became accepted as an independent faculty towards the end of the eighteenth century for, in general, the passions (emotions) had until then 'oscillated between being reduced to either sensation – whether organic or not – or to an element of rational and contemplative life.'[22]

That DP developed in France earlier than elsewhere might be partially explained by the early arrival in that country of the version of Faculty Psychology espoused by Scottish Philosophy.[23] In their reaction against Condillacean associationism, men like Laromiguière, Royer-Collard, Cousin, and Jouffroy accepted a form of spiritualist 'functionalism' of the mind[24] based on the notion of 'inner experience' espoused by Maine de Biran.[25] During the early nineteenth century, Faculty Psychology inspired important intellectual movements amongst which the most famous was phrenology.[26] In this regard, it is not sufficiently emphasized that the conceptual basis of this discipline was an 'anatomized' form of Faculty Psychology.

Phrenology sought to establish correlations between the anatomical and psychological realms by stating that the magnitude of a personality trait (y) was a function of the size of an anatomical site (x), and that the relationship was governed by a rule (r). Anti-phrenology criticism has neglected to point out that Gall's weakness was not in trying to establish a link between (y) and (x), but in not offering an account of (r); and that he also confused the issue by establishing a vicarious correlation between (x) and the shape of the skull. Faculty Psychology declined towards the end of the nineteenth century as its 'scientific' analysis was made difficult by definitional ambiguities.

However, phrenology provided the first viable nineteenth century classification of mental disorders. Delusional, emotional and volitional insanities (as per Esquirol, Prichard, and Bucknill & Tuke) provided, in turn, the template for groupings that have lasted to this day: schizophrenia and delusional states, affective psychosis, and psychopathy, respectively. Of the three functional clusters, volition (the will) was the first to lose popularity.[27] This occurred towards the end of the century, and led to a terminological crisis, and terms such as 'motivation' and 'drive'[28] needed to be marshalled to replace it.

The emotional or orectic faculty has a different story. It was Kant who 'introduced in an explicit manner emotions and feelings as an autonomous category; they could act as an interface between reason and will.'[29] The Kantian tripartite concept of the mind was almost contemporary with the efforts by Scottish philosophers to develop Faculty Psychology.[30] Influenced by Wolff (his teacher at Königsberg), Knutzen, and Tetens, whose version of the tripartite view he followed,[31] Kant believed that mental illness resulted from a weakening of the mental faculties.[32] He did, however, rebel against the 'dogmatic rationalism' of Wolff,[33] and like Baumgarten,[34] he considered emotions as a *separate* faculty. For example, in the *Critique of Judgment* he put forward the view that the 'three faculties are irreducible and cannot be derived from a common root'.[35] Kant, however, over-emphasized the 'pathological' role played by 'feelings': emotions were for him disrupters of the rational life and potential causes of disease of the mind (*Krankheiten des Gemüts*).[36]

Jalley and Lefevre[37] have recently disinterred Kant's 1764 manuscript on the 'diseases of the mind', where he suggests a pathogenic mechanism: 'other diseases of the brain can, I believe, also be produced by changes in the intensity of the symptoms (I have already mentioned), or by particular associations between these symptoms or by disruptions caused by emotional states.'[38]

As Leibbrand and Wettley[39] have remarked, it must be remembered that Kant's contribution was not based on first-hand knowledge of clinical disorders.[40] Sauri has also noticed that the 'ideal schema' of the faculties used by Kant led him to classify delusional thinking no longer in terms of *content* but as a manifestation of a disorder of the intellectual function.[41] Evidence for the long-term influence of Kant's views on nineteenth century DP can be found, for example, in the acknowledgement by Magnan and Sérieux that he was one of the precursors of the concept of *délire chronique á évolution systematique*![42]

Associationism

Atomism provided the epistemological basis for the development of seventeenth and eighteenth centuries' science.[43] Lockean 'simple ideas' (the psychological counterpart of the atom) served as a 'unit of analysis' for the development of 'laws of association', a combinatorial algebra in terms of which the mind was reconstructed out of external sensations (e.g. Condillac's example of the statue).[44] The problem with this mechanistic approach was that it had perception as its model and led to a neglect of the emotions.[45] Hence Locke's 1690 view of madness: 'having joined together some *ideas* very wrongly, [madmen] mistake them for truths; and they err as men do that argue right from wrong principles.'[46]

A similar process unfolded in France where early in the nineteenth century associationism was confronted by Faculty Psychology, and by the anti-analytic views imported from Scotland by Royer-Collard and the alienist–philosophers of the period.[47] A version of the associationism of Condillac was adopted by Destutt de Tracy and the *ideologues*,[48] but soon after, it entered into conflict with the new Faculty Psychology whose direct psychological usefulness (as in its application to phrenology) had been obvious from the start.

In Germany, associationism also became psychologized during the first half of the nineteenth century,[49] a good example of this being the work of Herbart[50] who influenced Griesinger.[51] Through the work of this great physician, associationism

left its imprint on German abnormal psychology which, via Krafft-Ebing and Meynert, reached Wernicke (evident, for example, in the latter's 'connectionist' view
of aphasia).[52] Meynert also used associationistic principles[53] in his wiring diagrams;
Fechner's work, based on similar principles influenced Wundt[54] and Kraepelin[55]
who sought to establish experimental descriptions of insanity.

Locke's intellectualistic definition of insanity was challenged during the early
nineteenth century by Pinel who described cases with 'lesions of the function of
the will' 'whose symptoms appeared enigmatic upon the definitions of mania given
by Locke and Condillac.'[56] This quotation almost marks the instant when alienists
turned from associationism to Faculty Psychology.

Pre-nineteenth century, associationism had been more epistemological than
psychological. The work of Thomas Brown and James Mill,[57] however, marked a
change in emphasis, as these writers endeavoured to explain behaviour as a *separate
field of inquiry* as much as J.S. Mill and Bain were to do later.[58] Alienists liked the
analytical epistemology of associationism and applied the concept of 'unit of analysis' to abnormal behaviour. Indeed, symptoms such as obsessions, delusions and
hallucinations became the units of madness. In the event, this was consolidated in
the work of Chaslin[59] and Jaspers. Taxonomy, however, remained based on Faculty
Psychology; thus creating a tension between psychiatric nosology and semiology.

Form and content

The distinction between the 'form' and 'content' of a symptom is one of the enduring contributions of nineteenth century psychopathology. The Aristotelian 'eidos',
which referred to the 'essence or common character' of an object, is at the centre
of the DP notion of 'form'.[60] 'Eidos' held its semantic field well into the seventeenth
century when Francis Bacon proposed that 'form' might be considered as a synonym of 'figure': 'when we talk of forms, we understand nothing else than the
laws and types of action that govern and constitute any simple nature' and 'the
form of something is the very thing itself'.[61] Kant, in turn, suggested that form
should refer to the 'sense modality' in which a perception takes place in conjunction
with all its attending cognitive relationships.[62] Nineteenth century DP, and indeed
Jaspers at the beginning of the twentieth century, follow the Kantian definition:
'form must be kept distinct from content which may change from time to time,
e.g. the fact of a hallucination is to be distinguished from its content, whether this
is a man or a tree . . . Perceptions, ideas, judgments, feelings, drives, self-awareness,
are all forms of psychic phenomena; they denote the particular mode of existence
in which content is presented to us. It is true, in describing concrete psychic events,
we take into account the particular content of the individual psyche, but from the
phenomenological point of view it is only the form that interests us.'[63]

To this day, 'form' refers to those impersonal aspects of the mental symptom
that guarantee its stability in time and space; that is, its 'constancy' elements.
'Form' is easier to understand in physical medicine where colour, sound, surface,

solidity, smell and temperature may provide a context in relation to which the complaint achieves expression and stability.[64] The successful definition of signs and symptoms in medicine inspired nineteenth century alienists to seek, in their own realm, stable and public behavioural markers of disease. Emphasizing the 'form' of symptoms was one way of achieving this. In doing so, however, they committed nineteenth century DP to a metaphysics of 'natural kinds', defined by J.S. Mill as: 'every class which is a real kind, that is, which is distinguished from all other classes by an indeterminate multitude of properties not derivable from one another'.[65] Natural or essential kinds entailed a division *in re*, and this included behaviour. Thus, the stability of symptoms was due to their ontology and not the descriptive activity itself. The psychopathologist could, thus, not be accused of 'constructing' symptoms: he just carved out behaviour at the joints.

The physical signs of madness

A salient difference between pre- and post-1900 DP is that physical (somatic) signs played a far more important role in the former. Alienists had no problem in freely combining in the diagnosis of mental illness 'psychological' symptoms (e.g. delusions or hallucinations) with 'somatic' complaints (e.g. tremor, headache, tachycardia, pallor, blushing, cold hands, changes in bowel or urinary habit, general malaise). The latter were considered as *primary features* and as directly related to brain pathology as the typical manifestations of mental disorder. Conditions such as catatonia, obsessive insanity or neurasthenia were diagnosed on the basis of such somatic complaints and detailed studies were carried out of their neurobiological meaning. This approach only began to change at the turn of the century when psychiatric complaints began to be interpreted 'psychologically' and 'somatic' symptoms were *discarded* as non-specific. The work of Janet illustrates this well, particularly his book on psychasthenia[66] where patients are reported as having a plethora of physical signs which Janet considered as an *essential* part of the diagnosis. Even Eugen Bleuler considered discoloured complexion, greasy face, and cold, blue extremities as diagnostic of catatonic schizophrenia. The view that somatic complaints were primary symptoms of mental disorder did not decline as a result of empirical research but followed a shift in conceptual fashion.

Non-verbal behaviour

The great diagnostic categories of the past (e.g. mania, melancholia, phrensy, lethargy) relied on the observation of what the individual did, looked like, and said rather than on what he felt. This is particularly so in regard to mania and melancholia. The use of overt behaviour as the *métier* of psychopathological description was started by the Greeks.[67] But symptom mapping was influenced by their views on what constituted a 'harmonious behaviour'. The categories they created became the archetypal forms of insanity which, with little change, lasted well into the eighteenth century. Interest in the description of overt behaviour was renewed during this period,[68] particularly in the study of facial expression in the normal, in what came to be known as the science of Physiognomy.[69] Parsons, for example, attempted to establish correlations between emotions and gestures.[70] The application of these techniques to pathological states gave rise to a veritable 'iconography' of madness. This, in turn, influenced the way in which the mentally ill were perceived,[71] and exaggerated or distorted facial expressions were thought to indicate the intensity of the underlying derangement.

But, during the nineteenth century, a change occurred in the way in which the insane were depicted. After 1839, the old stereotypes of Hogarth and Tardieu gave way to a more 'realistic' approach made possible by the invention of the daguerreotype. This, in turn, introduced a bias in the type of photographic records kept for posterity as the early need for long exposure times selected in 'static' conditions such as stupor. Likewise, the view that there was a one-to-one correlation between inner state and gesture became less acceptable; indeed, it was believed that they often dissociated. This, in turn, gave rise to the idea that insanity could be concealed or simulated. To understand this further, Morison, Laurent and the great Pierret developed theories of 'mimia' and 'paramimia'.[72] Darwin's interest in this issue is also well known.[73]

Subjective experiences as symptoms

The incorporation of *subjective experiences* into the symptom-repertoire of DP is, perhaps, the single most important contribution of the nineteenth century. As mentioned above, pre-nineteenth century descriptions of insanity mostly relied on the observation of overt behaviour and psychosocial competence. During the early nineteenth century and particularly in France, changes in psychological theory made possible for the first time the acceptance of the 'inner experience' (as per Maine de Biran, see above) and the 'contents of consciousness' became a legitimate field of inquiry.[74] This was rapidly seized by alienists who were, at the time, searching for additional sources of clinical information.

Methods of eliciting and recording data were soon developed[75] and the *mental state assessment* – in its dialogical form – appeared during this period. At the basis of these methods was introspection, a method of psychological inquiry legitimated by nineteenth century psychology.[76] Introspection became an important method of information gathering until the time it was challenged by behaviourism early in the twentieth century.[77] After the Second World War, a form of introspection underwent a revival.[78]

In his *Psychologie Morbide*, the Frenchman Moreau de Tours[79] sought to legitimize the clinical value of subjective information[80] by offering a detailed analysis of drug-induced hallucinations, delusions, emotions and volitional experiences.[81] He also analysed the form of hallucinations by recording whether they were bilateral or unilateral, recognizable, single or multiple, etc.[82] Towards the second half of the same century, Brentano's[83] notion of intentionality drew attention to the 'content' of behaviour (including symptoms) culminating in the semantic focus of the psycho-dynamic doctrines.[84] In general, the nineteenth century emphasis on experience contributed to the psychologization of the old notion of consciousness which, since that time, has been central to psychiatry.[85]

Regarding subjective experiences as legitimate mental symptoms allowed for the re-definition of some mental disorders such as melancholia and mania whose meaning radically changed by making it depend upon the *quality* of the predominant mood states.[86] Likewise, paranoia re-appeared in the 1860s refurbished by the incorporation of pure delusional experiences,[87] and the stupors, until then lumped together, were teased out according to whether or not there was memory for the episode.[88] Subjective symptoms were also used to identify 'subtypes' of insanity which in the event led to a proliferation of forms (e.g. religious, metaphysical and erotic mania).

Time and descriptions

Until the early nineteenth century, the description and diagnosis of insanity occurred outside time, i.e. identification of certain symptoms on the cross-sectional assessments sufficed.[89] Furthermore, once made the diagnosis became connatural, for madness was regarded as timeless (i.e. once mad, always mad).[90] The fact that often enough mad subjects showed periods of 'normal behaviour' (what was then called the *lucid interval*) was not considered as a problem, for it was believed that they could 'stifle their disorder.'[91]

During the nineteenth century, asylum practice allowed for a longitudinal obser-vation of madness and this, in turn, forced a change in the descriptive framework. After the 1850s, 'time' was introduced as a dimension.[92] The longitudinal approach also encouraged changes in the very concept of mental illness which soon led to a distinction between acute and chronic insanity.[93] In 1863, Kahlbaum suggested that information from longitudinal observation might be used to *correct* diagnosis.[94] By the end of the century, 'duration' had become an important category in the analysis of disease. For example, Kraepelin considered 'evolution' and outcome the crucial criteria for diagnosis. In this regard, it has been suggested that he specially went to Dorpat to gain experience with chronic hospitalized cases.[95]

Psychopathology and numerical descriptions: the past

The mathematization of the natural world is said to have started in Europe during the seventeenth century[96] but the 'Newtonian paradigm' affected little psychological thinking. Likewise, both Descartes and Locke believed that numerical descriptions did not apply to behaviour.[97] The view that 'psychometry' (i.e. the measurement of psychological experience) was possible and desirable is attributed to Christian von Wolff who, when writing on the quantitative assessment of pleasure and dis-pleasure, stated: 'these theorems belong to 'psychometry' which conveys a math-ematical knowledge of the human mind and continues to remain a desideratum.'[98]

Also during the eighteenth century, Ramsay, Baumgarten, Crusius, de Maupertuis, Buck, Mendelssohn and Ploucquet agreed that measurement was possible in psychology although no one seems to have carried out experimental work.

The introduction of quantification into *medicine* followed a different path.[99] Numerical management of demographic information (e.g. bills of mortality) was well known to pre-nineteenth century government data collectors. Inferential analysis was, however, primitive[100] but during the nineteenth century, statistical analysis, based on probability theory, started in earnest.[101] This is clear in the work of Gavaret,[102] Louis,[103] Radicke,[104] Renaudin,[105] and also in that of Esquirol who made use of inferential percentages. Numerical descriptions extended gradually to psychopathology around the middle of the century.[106]

During the nineteenth century, the path to numerical description in psychology started by Wolff (and opposed by Kant and Comte) was continued by Herbart who even mentioned the possibility of a 'statistics' of the soul.[107] This conceptual change made easier the work of Johannes Müller and DuBois Reymond[108] and the instruments[109] they designed were to facilitate, in turn, the ideas of Weber and Fechner. On the other hand, there is little historical evidence before the 1850s that efforts were made to measure personality traits.[110] This is surprising, as Gall and Spurzheim made available to psychology a conception of *individual differences* susceptible to numerical description[111] (as has been mentioned above, phrenology sought to establish correlations between anatomical and psychological magnitudes).[112]

The measurement of psychological events started therefore, in areas other than psychopathology. For example, Fechner's work was not carried out on the insane nor are its conceptual origins to be found in Faculty Psychology. Fechner was a physicist with quaint ideas on the mind–body relationship. It was, in fact, his view on how 'sense data' related to the material world that provided him with the idea that there was a correlational link between stimulus intensity and its cognitive appraisal (as conveyed in verbal reporting). Because in his model the gap between stimulus and cognitive appraisal is wide, Fechner used as a 'metaphysical bridge' his belief that everything was interconnected in nature: 'Sensation depends on stimulation; a stronger sensation depends on a stronger stimulus; the stimulus however causes sensation only via the intermediate action of *some internal process of the body*. To the extent that lawful relationships between sensation and stimulus can be found they must include lawful relationships between the stimulus and this inner physical activity.'[113] Fechner believed that the sense datum was a function of the logarithm of the stimulus, and that the physiological excitation was proportional to such magnitude. Along the same lines, Wundt and Kraepelin developed techniques to measure symptoms such as fatigue and memory impairment. Based on their work, other alienists believed that physiological variables such as pulse and respiration might show characteristic changes in some insanities.[114] Interestingly enough, less research was done on perceptual parameters (e.g. 'just noticeable difference') and reaction times[115] in the mentally ill.

The fact that, during the nineteenth century, DP was not affected by the introduction of measurement into medicine and psychology requires explanation. Based
on Faculty Psychology, alienists concentrated on describing symptoms as natural
kinds. These 'packets' of disturbance were either present or absent and did not
allow for graded presentations. Stupor, confusion or delusion were monolithic
behaviours in relation to which measurement made little sense. This belief was
reinforced by the psychodynamic approach.

Units of analysis

Since the nineteenth century, the avowed task of DP has been the identification of
classes of abnormal mental acts; and in accordance with the theory of 'signs', each
needed a specific name.[116] Thus alienists proceeded to fractionate 'insane behaviour'
into discrete classes, concepts, kinds or 'units of analysis'. These Griesinger called
die Elementarstörungen (elementary disorders) of mental disease.[117] 'Units of analysis'
can be tested by ascertaining that they represent a meaningful and stable fragment
of abnormal behaviour (i.e. are valid), and that their utterance evokes the same
'form' or 'image' in the mind of trained observers (i.e. are reliable).

The latter part of the nineteenth century witnessed the accumulation of a fair
number of classifications of mental disorders which, in the main were based on
clinical presentation or speculative aetiology. The actual disorders, however,
consisted in little more than combinations and permutations of a relatively small
number of 'symptoms' (units of analysis). By the 1870s, alienists had realized
that symptom combinations per se had little discriminatory power. Thus, first
Kahlbaum and then Kraepelin proceeded to use diagnostic features such as age,
sex, duration, evolution and outcome, all of which went well beyond symptoms.
Likewise, speculative symptom groupings such as those put forward by Wernicke[118]
were less successful. Why was this the case has not yet been studied in any depth,
but it is likely that nineteenth century DP only allowed certain symptom
permutations.[119]

Descriptive psychopathology as a cognitive system

Lastly, DP can be considered as a mini- 'cognitive system'; i.e. a device to organize
knowledge of a particular kind. An early meaning of 'system' was 'collection of
objects'; another, started during the seventeenth century, was structure or organisation.[120] In this sense, a cognitive system is meant to capture information, and its
performance can be measured in terms of its capacity to do so. Because no rival
descriptive systems exist in western psychiatry, a degree of complacency may have
set in, and no attempt has yet been made to audit how good a cognitive system
DP is.

Since the eighteenth century, a number of features have been known as characteristic of a good system. Rescher lists 'wholeness, completeness, self-sufficiency,

cohesiveness, consonance, architectonic, functional unity, functional regularity, functional simplicity, mutual supportiveness and functional efficacy.'[121] Condillac,[122] whose influence on Pinel[123] and French psychiatry is well attested,[124] also distinguished 'speculative' and 'experimental' systems: the latter concerned the 'facts of observation' and hence generated knowledge about the world. There is little doubt that, during the nineteenth century, medical semiology in general, and DP in particular were considered as 'experimental systems'.

Systems can be considered as dynamic entities whose structure, compass and epistemological capacity vary according to subject matter. Rescher states that: 'Systematicity, has *vis-á-vis* its components, the character of a profile (rather than an average). Just as the health of a person is determined by a plurality of constituent factors so the systematicity of a body of knowledge is determined in terms of a wide variety of separable albeit inter-related considerations. And there will be trade-offs as between the various 'parameters of systematicity.'[125] In this regard, it is of interest to the clinical historian to find out what 'trade-offs' nineteenth century alienists had to accept to secure the survival of DP and meet the practical needs of their heterogeneous asylum population. For, if as Rescher has suggested, 'greater completeness may threaten consistency, greater connectedness may require the insertion of disuniform elements'[126] then, from the start, DP is likely to have been incomplete, i.e. blind to certain aspect of mental illness. This, it might have been felt at the time, was not too high a price to pay for a descriptive system that was otherwise simple, consistent and easy to apply. The problem, of course, is that needs change and that in the 1990s the new research techniques demand from DP information which it may simply not contain.[127]

Two complementary definitions of DP were formulated during the nineteenth century. Some writers (mainly psychologists and basic scientists) believed that *all morbid phenomena* were but quantitative variations of 'normal' mental functions. In support of the 'continuity' view Carpenter wrote: 'It may be unhesitatingly affirmed that there is nothing in the psychical phenomena of insanity which distinguishes this condition from states that may be temporarily induced in minds otherwise healthy'.[128] In this sense, psychopathology was a branch of normal psychology ('pathological psychology'). Alienists, on the other hand, believed that some symptoms were too bizarre to have a counterpart in normal behaviour. Griesinger put it thus: 'we find other psychological anomalies in the insane to which there is nothing analogous in the state of health'.[129] The 'discontinuity' view was also called 'psychological pathology'.

NOTES

1 For an early nineteenth century manifesto on the association between semiology and language see Landre-Beauvais, 1813; for general discussions, see Barthes, 1972; Lantéri-Laura, 1966; Bobes, 1973; and Juliard, 1970.
2 Laín-Entralgo, 1978; Albarracín, 1983; Canguilhem, 1966; Bynum, 1994.
3 Georgin, 1980; Larson, 1971; Whewell, 1857; Delasiauve, 1861; Boyer, 1873.
4 Kühne et al., 1985.
5 Wing et al., 1981; Vaillant and Schnurr, 1989.
6 This refers to a coefficient of inter-rater reliability that corrects for chance agreements; see Shrout et al., 1987.
7 Wilbush, 1984.
8 Smith, 1979.
9 Thanks to the pioneer work of Roy Porter, Michael McDonald and others, pre-1800 psychiatry, particularly the seventeenth and eighteenth centuries, is showing an unsuspected richness of clinical analysis, taxonomic preoccupation and aetiological debate. However, their research also confirms the hypothesis proposed in this book that no independent descriptive psychopathology seems to have existed before the nineteenth century.
10 Platt and Diamond, 1965.
11 Walk, 1964.
12 Jones, 1972.
13 Laín-Entralgo, 1961.
14 MacDonald, 1981; Battie, 1758; Burton, 1883; Diethelm and Heffernan, 1965; Hunter and Macalpine, 1963; Postel, 1984.
15 It could be claimed, of course, that it was the other way around (Foucault, 1972), i.e. that changes in the perception of madness (e.g. its medicalization) led to treating these phenomena as if they were brain lesions expressed in signs and symptoms. This might have been so at a general level, but the point made here is that, once the old molar notion of insanity was broken up into units of analysis, semantic interpretation concentrated on individual symptoms and on the way they clustered together. Consequently, the general semantics of insanity became unimportant.
16 See Feuchtersleben, 1847; Griesinger, 1867; Bucknill and Tuke, 1858; Falret, 1864.
17 Ey, Lé développement 'mechaniciste' . . ., 1952; Berrios, 1977.
18 p. 375 and p. 383, Blakey, 1850.
19 Abbagnano, 1961.
20 Müller-Freinfels, 1935.
21 p. 470, Klein, 1970.
22 Ferrater Mora, 1958.

23 Damirón, 1828; Dwelshauvers, 1920; Ravaisson, 1885; Boutroux, 1908;
    Grave, 1960.
24 Drevet, 1968; Moore, 1970; Swain, 1978; Ravaisson, 1885.
25 Royer-Collard, 1843; Losserand, 1967.
26 Lantéri-Laura, 1970; Cantor, 1975; Cooter, 1979.
27 See Chapter 14, this book.
28 Lorenz, 1950; Hinde, 1960. For origin of theories, see Arkes and Garske,
    1977.
29 Abbagnano, 1961.
30 Hilgard, 1980.
31 Windelband, 1948.
32 p. lix in Mora, 1975.
33 Brett, 1953.
34 Büchner, 1897.
35 Kant, 1914 (first edition 1790); Gardiner *et al.*, 1937.
36 Kant, 1974 (first edition, 1798). Little has been written on the influence
    of Kant on psychopathological thinking; Dr Chris Walker (Leicester) has
    carried out important work to support the view that the German
    philosopher was more influential on Jaspers than Husserl ever was.
37 Jalley, Lefebvre and Feline, 1977.
38 p. 221, Jalley, Lefebvre and Feline, 1977.
39 Leibbrand and Wettley, 1961.
40 However, one of Kant's most interesting writings in this field, 'On the
    organ of the mind (or soul)' was motivated by Sömmerring's dedication
    to him of a book of the same title (see Kant,1863). Thomas Sömmerring
    (1755–1830) was one of the great German anatomists of this period. He
    wrote a doctoral thesis on the origin of the cranal nerves and criticized
    the use of the guillotine on the grounds that it caused more pain than
    Dr Guillotin believed. He suggested that the soul was a gas-like substance
    trapped in the lateral ventricles. *Über das Organ der Seele*, the book he
    dedicated to Kant, was published in Königsberg in 1796 (Dureau 1881).
41 Saurí, 1969.
42 p. 607, Magnan and Sérieux, 1911.
43 Schofield, 1970; Hoeldtke, 1967.
44 Condillac, 1947 (first edition, 1754).
45 Meyering, 1989; also Gardiner *et al.*, 1937.
46 Locke, 1959. For a fuller analysis of Locke's views see Chapter 5, this
    book.
47 Swain, 1978; Benrubi, 1933.
48 Tracy, 1817 (first edition 1801); Mora, 1981.
49 Ribot, 1885.
50 Wolman, 1968.
51 Ackerknecht, 1957; Wahrig-Smith, 1985.
52 Wernicke, 1874; see also the excellent study by Lanczik, 1988.
53 Marshall, 1982; for a general account, see Boring, 1950.
54 Petersen, 1932.
55 Kraepelin went as far as starting a psychological journal in 1896,

published by Engelmann in Leipzig and entitled *Psychologische Arbeiten*. The first issue included his manifesto: Kraepelin, 1896; see also Kraepelin, 1983. His research mainly covered memory and fatigue; on these topics see, respectively, Chapters 9 and 15, this book.

56 p. 102, Pinel, 1809.
57 Brown, 1828.
58 Warren, 1921; Ribot, La psychologie anglaise . . ., 1896; Bain, 1859; Greenway, 1973.
59 Chaslin, 1912, and particularly his classical: Chaslin, 1914. On this great alienist see Daumezón, 1973; and the review of his 'Eléments' by Ritti, 1913.
60 Ferrater Mora, 1958.
61 (*Novum Organum*, Lib II, 13, 17; Bacon, 1858).
62 Abbagnano, 1961.
63 pp. 58–59, Jaspers, 1963.
64 Laín-Entralgo, 1982.
65 p. 81, Mill, 1898.
66 Janet, 1919.
67 Roccatagliata, 1973.
68 Bühler, 1968.
69 Lavater, 1891; Mantegazza, 1878; Caro Baroja, 1988.
70 Parsons, 1747.
71 Gilman, 1982.
72 pp. 116–118, Régis, 1906; Dromard, 1909.
73 Darwin, 1904; Browne, 1985.
74 Dwelshauvers, 1920; Royer-Collard, 1843.
75 Laín-Entralgo, 1961.
76 Boring, 1953; Danzinger, 1980; Lyons, 1986.
77 Danziger, 1990.
78 Pilkington and Glasgow, 1967; Lyons, 1986.
79 Bollote, 1973; Ey and Mignot, 1947.
80 pp. 193–243, Moreau (de Tours), 1859; Pigeaud, 1986. At the same time as French psychiatry was paying attention to mental contents, British psychiatrists were worrying about 'morbid introspections' as a potential cause of mental disorder (Clark, 1985).
81 Lantéri-Laura, La sémiologie . . . 1984.
82 Parish, 1897; Gurney, 1885.
83 Fancher, 1977.
84 Bercherie, 1983; 1988.
85 Burt, 1962; Bastian, 1870; Viziolo and Bietti, 1966; Ey, 1963; see also Chapter 11, this book.
86 Berrios, Psychopathology of Affectivity 1985; Berrios, Melancholia and Depression . . . 1988.
87 Lewis, 1970.
88 Berrios, Stupor: a conceptual history 1981.
89 Arnold, 1806.
90 This view reflected similar notions in the field of physical disease.

Referring to this period Charcot wrote 'disease was formerly considered as being independent of the organism, a kind of parasite attached to the economy', p. 4, Charcot, 1881. Diseases were not considered as contained within the temporal and spatial constraints of the body. For a discussion of this problem, King, 1982; Haas, 1864; and the important paper by Häfner, 1987.

91 Haslam, 1809.

92 Lantéri-Laura, 1972; 1986; Pistoia, 1971.

93 Kahlbaum, 1863; for a general discussion of this issue, see Berrios, Historical Aspects . . ., 1987.

94 Hoff, 1985; Berrios and Hauser, 1988; and the first-class thesis by Engstrom, 1990.

95 Marx, 1980. It has also been suggested that this introduced a bias in his description of dementia praecox for Dorpat patients spoke little German (and Kraepelin did not speak the local language) and hence he had to use 'objective' signs (Berrios and Hauser, 1988).

96 Dijksterhius, 1961.

97 Moravia, 1983.

98 Ramul, 1960.

99 Shryock, 1961; Murphy 1981; Underwood, 1951.

100 Perrot and Woolf, 1984.

101 Hilts, 1981; Porter, 1986; Pearson, 1978; Esquirol, 1838.

102 Wulff et al., 1986.

103 Ackerknecht, 1967.

104 Radicke, 1861.

105 Renaudin, 1856. In this paper Renaudin reported on the favourable view of statistics taken by the attenders to the Paris 1856 Statistics Symposium.

106 Parchappe, 1856.

107 Ribot, 1885.

108 Rothschuh, 1973.

109 Sokal et al., 1976.

110 Boring, 1961; Zupan, 1976; Bondy, 1974; Buss, 1976. For a good example of the use of mathematical and statistical reasoning in memory research, see Ebbinghaus, 1964 (first edition 1885).

111 Damirón, 1828; Spoerl, 1936; Lesky, 1970.

112 Lantéri-Laura, 1970.

113 p. 101, Fechner, 1966.

114 Whitwell, 1892; Ziehen, 1909.

115 Boring, 1942.

116 pp. 1608–1616, in Franck, 1875.

117 p. 60, Griesinger, 1861.

118 Burckard, 1931; Lanczik, 1988.

119 It may, of course, have also been due to factors extrinsic to their systems such as Wernicke's early death or his less powerful political network.

120 Meyering, 1989; Rescher, 1979; pp. 1703–1704, Franck, 1875.

121 Rescher, 1979.

122 pp. 121–217, Condillac, 1947.

123 Riese, 1968.

124 Leroy, 1927.

125 p. 11, Rescher, 1979.

126 p. 14, Rescher, 1979.

127 Berrios and Marková, 1995.

128 p. 658, Carpenter, 1879.

129 p. 62, Griesinger, 1867.

PART II

Cognition and consciousness

CHAPTER 3

Disorders of perception

There are excellent accounts of the history of hallucination and illusion but few in the English language.[1] Hallucination and illusion name reports of experiences ascribed to perception: illusion is defined as a perceptual distortion of a stimulus, and hallucination as a perceptual declaration, of varied degree of conviction, in the absence of a relevant external stimulus. The theoretical basis for this distinction was set during the nineteenth century,[2] although it had already been noticed by earlier writers.[3]

Before the nineteenth century

Experiences redolent of hallucinations and illusions are part of the common baggage of humanity.[4] Variously named, these experiences were in earlier times culturally integrated and semantically pregnant, i.e. their content was believed to carry a message for the individual or the world. That this feature of hallucinations has been mostly lost is a consequence of their 'medicalization' during the eighteenth century. During this period, hallucinations were considered as independent 'diseases'; indeed, the view that they were 'symptoms', i.e. fragments of behaviour common to various diseases is a nineteenth century invention. The absence of an entry for hallucination in the French Encyclopaedia suggests that, up to the 1750s, it had not yet reached the status of other 'psychiatric' terms. Hunter and McAlpine[5] have none the less shown that since the sixteenth century, hallucinatory *behaviours* were frequently mentioned; after 1700, Hartley and Battie added a further dimension by explaining these phenomena in terms of vibratory neurophysiology.[6]

In 1770, the French Dufour suggested that 'fallacies of the senses' might cause delusions: 'The false impression of the external senses, then, must necessarily create disorder and confusion in a person's conduct; because it happens most frequently, that they determine his actions. A person trusts to his former experience, which has taught him that bodies are present when they make an impression on him. Hence [there are] many fallacies of the senses, because objects are the causes of his perceptions. Hence it also arises, that we often consider things which are not present to our senses, as present, and as the causes of our perceptions: or if there be any thing wanting in an external object, imagination supplies the loss, and represents it as perfect'.[7] Commenting upon this, Crichton stated: 'that diseases of the external senses produce erroneous mental perceptions, must be allowed; but *it depends on the concurrence of other causes*, whether delusion follows.' (my italics)[8] This anticipates an important nineteenth century debate on whether hallucinations had peripheral or central origin.

Nicolaï versus Berbiguier

The writings of these men, one German and the other French, set the stage for the nineteenth century debate on whether or not hallucinations were a sign of insanity.[9] On 28th February 1799, a German bookseller called Nicolaï described his own hallucinatory experiences in a paper read before the Royal Society of Berlin entitled *Memoir on the Appearance of Spectres or Phantoms occasioned by Disease; with Psychological Remarks.*[10] One morning of 1790, and whilst under much stress, he 'suddenly observed, at the distance of ten paces, the figure of a deceased person. I pointed at it, and asked my wife whether she did not see it. She did not but being much alarmed, endeavoured to compose me, and sent for the physician. The figure remained some seven or eight minutes, and at length I became a little more calm . . . In the afternoon the figure which I had seen in the morning re-appeared. I was alone when this happened. I went therefore to the apartment of my wife, to whom I related it. But thither also the figure pursued me. Sometimes it was present, some-times it vanished; but it was always the same standing figure . . . The figure of the deceased person never appeared to me after the first dreadful day, but several other figures showed themselves afterwards very distinctly – sometimes such as I knew – mostly, however, of persons I did not know'.

Nicolaï tried to elicit his visions but they proved to be beyond his control. He learned, however, to differentiate them from real people and soon got used to them, feeling little anxiety even when the phantoms spoke to him. He sought medical help and after a few months he was free from these experiences. Nicolaï seemed to be describing episodes of hallucinosis with preservation of insight. Indeed, Brierre included his case under the category 'hallucinations compatible with reason'.[11]

In 1821, Alexis Vincent Charles Berbiguier de Terre-Neuve du Thym (1775–1841)[12] published a three-volume book entitled *Les Farfadets, or tous les demons ne sont pas de l'autre monde*[13] where he reported complex hallucinatory and delusional experiences. This work was to become the paradigm for insane hallucinations, and French alienists re-diagnose it at regular intervals. Berbiguier also recorded his interview with Pinel on 24th April 1816: 'After listening with great attention, this doctor told me that he knew of the type of disease affecting me, and that he had successfully treated people with it.'[14] He continued, however, feeling persecuted by monsters and bad spirits and accused Pinel of making false promises.

The nineteenth century

In 1817, Esquirol brought these phenomena under the common term 'hallucination' thereby introducing the false view that hallucinations affecting the various sense modalities were somehow symmetrical and uniform. Furthermore, by choosing a word whose etymology was, at the time, linked to *vision*, he generalized a restricted 'model' of perception (the one entailed by 'seeing' as the capture of a *public stimulus*) to other sense modalities.[15] Five of Esquirol's cases had visual hallucinations:[16] 'If a man has the intimate conviction of actually perceiving a sensation for which there is no external object, he is in a hallucinated state:[17] he is a visionary (*visionnaire*).'[18] 'Hallucinations of vision . . . have been called visions but this term is appropriate only for one perceptual mode. Who would want to talk about auditory visions, taste visions, olfactory visions? . . . However, the functional alterations, brain mechanisms and the clinical context involved in these three senses *is the same* as in visions. A generic term is needed. I propose the word hallucination.' (my italics)[19] This view, borrowed from Condillac,[20] assumed that olfaction, taste and touch also required a *public stimulus*.[21]

In regards to mechanisms, Esquirol wrote: 'there is a form of delusion (*une certaine forme de délire*) that makes subjects believe they are perceiving a sensation in one or more sense modalities when, in fact, there is no stimulus.'[22] 'In hallucinations there is no more sensation or perception than in dreaming or somnambulism, when no external object is stimulating the senses . . . In fact, hallucination is a cerebral or psychological phenomenon that takes place independently from the senses'.[23] 'The pretended sensations of the hallucinated are images and ideas reproduced by memory, improved by the imagination, and personified by habit'.[24] 'Hallucinations are not false sensations or illusions of sense or erroneous perceptions or errors of organic sensibility.'[25] 'The site of the hallucination is not in the peripheral organ of sensation, but in the central organ of sensitivity itself; in fact, the symptom cannot be conceived but as a result of something setting the brain itself in motion'.[26]

Esquirol's insistence on the 'central' origin of hallucinations was a departure from the peripheralist views that Hartley and others had made popular during the eighteenth century. More importantly, it was also an effort to 'internalize' the phenomenon, make it part of the psychological system, and bring it under the control of memory, imagination and *habitude*.[27] His claim that hallucination was a delusion differentiated it from mere sensory errors and brought it closer to the personality of the subject. This is why Ey believed that Esquirol 'brought psychiatry nearer the hallucinated individual'.[28]

Consistent with these views, Esquirol called illusions 'sensory errors': 'Earlier writers did not distinguish visions [i.e. hallucinations] from sensory illusions. Although still using the term hallucination to name both hallucinations and illusions, recent writers are beginning to distinguish between *mental* and *sensory* hallucinations. Nonetheless, they have not yet realized how different these two

phenomena are. In hallucinations it all happens in the brain: visionaries are dreaming whilst awake. Their brain activity is so marked that it confers body and actu-
ality upon images provided by memory. In the case of illusions, the sensibility of
the nerve endings is altered, exalted, or perverted, sense organs are over-active and
impressions are sent to the brain. In the insane, these [peripheral] impressions may
fall under the control of ideas and passions and lead to an erroneous interpretation
of the stimulus. Illusions are not rare in health but are dissipated by reason.[29]

Esquirol illustrated his point with 20 clinical vignettes, and concluded that
illusions: 'are provoked by internal and external sensations and result from an
interaction between peripheral stimulation and a central factor . . . are different
from hallucinations in that in the latter only the brain is excited . . . cause an
impairment of judgement on the nature of the sensation . . . are modified by sex,
education, profession, and habits . . . in the normal are dissipated by reason.'[30]

Lechner has suggested that, when writing on illusions, Esquirol tried also to
separate psychiatric from neurological hallucinations.[31] This is unlikely as some of
Esquirol's purported illusion cases are typical hallucinations; furthermore, he provides an aetiological rather than *clinical* criterion to differentiate the two phenomena. Esquirol was still alive when Honoré Aubanel argued against the separation of
illusions from hallucinations on the grounds that both phenomena often coexisted,
depended on a delusion, and that their nature (*nature intime*) was in fact the same.[32]

J. Baillarger (1809–1890)

In 1842, two years after Esquirol's death, Baillarger[33] read a paper before the Royal
Academy of Medicine in Paris on the relationship between hypnagogic states on
hallucinations, for which he was awarded the Civrieux Prize. Based on 30 cases,
he supported Esquirol's view on the analogy between dreams and hallucinations.
He went on to distinguish between dreams which were 'simple' or 'purely intellectual' and those which were 'accompanied by sensory hallucinations.'[34] Baillarger
believed that his cases also illustrated the view that all hallucinations were organic
(*symptôme puremente physique*).[35]

In 1844, the Royal Academy of Medicine called for papers on 'hallucinations,
their causes, and diseases', and entries were submitted by Baillarger, Claude
Michéa[36] and another nine candidates. In the event, the former was awarded first
prize and the latter a consolation medal. These authors had opposite views on the
nature of hallucinations and their debate re-opened a problem that Esquirol had
attempted to resolve. The abridged publication of Baillarger's manuscript covers
more than 200 pages and is divided into five chapters, the first and second being
on physiology and pathology; the third on a new disease, 'sensory madness' (*folie
sensoriale*), the fourth on the relationship of hallucinations and a number of diseases, and the fifth on medico-legal issues. By *physiologie* Baillarger understood clinical features, and the chapter includes sections on hallucinations of hearing, vision,
smell, taste and touch. Herein Baillarger described for the first time 'thought echo'.[37]

He summarized his view thus: 'The most frequent and complicated hallucinations affect hearing; invisible interlocutors address the patient in the third person,
so that he is the passive listener in a conversation; the number of voices varies,
they come from all directions, and can even be heard only in one ear. Sometimes
the voice is heard in the head, or throat, or chest; the insane-deaf is more prone to
hear voices. Visual hallucinations are however easier to study and understand.
Images vary a great deal in distinctness and duration and may occur during day
or night, with eyes open or shut. The blind may also have visual hallucinations. In
the case of smell and taste, hallucinations and illusions are difficult to separate, as
are their intellectual and sensory components. Subjects with touch hallucinations
often complain of insects crawling over their bodies. Genital hallucinations are more
common in women. Hallucinations affecting all sense modalities are more common
in acute diseases, and their connection can be explained on the basis of the theory
of association of ideas'.[38]

In the second chapter, dedicated to the nature of hallucinations, Baillarger asked:
are hallucinations psychological or psycho-sensory phenomena? Can they be
explained by alterations of brain or sensory organs? He proposed two types: psycho-
sensory (due to a double action of imagination and sense organs) and psychological
(independent from the organs of sense). The former referred to experiences where
an image was reported; the latter, to situations where there was no actual voice
for the 'communication came from mind to mind, or by intuition or magnetism.'[39]
It would seem that Baillarger was referring here to delusions of communication
rather than to hallucinations; in fact, his point was equally obscure to his
contemporaries.[40]

In the third chapter Baillarger explored mechanisms proposing that the initial
component in a hallucination had to be the 'intellect' 'because there were insur-
mountable objections to the view that it was an excitation of the sensory organ.
Furthermore, a central component was the only way to understand the frequent
co-existence of hallucinations in different sensory modalities' 'Hallucinations flowed
from within, i.e. exactly in the opposite direction to normal sensations'.[41]

Forty years later, Baillarger wrote a valedictory paper supporting the psychosensory view and acknowledging that, in the interim, the topic had been advanced by
men who had been but children or (like Ritti or Binet) not yet born when he first
wrote on hallucinations.[42]

Michéa (1815–1882)

In a shorter and less tidy entry, Michéa proposed a different view.[43] Based on the
philosophical eclecticism of Victor Cousin,[44] his over-theoretical definition glossed
over crucial issues:[45] 'hallucination consisted of a metamorphosis of thinking, was
neither a sensation nor a perception but intermediate between perception and pure
conception. It occupied the middle ground between these two facts of consciousness
and participates in both.'[46] Michéa divided hallucinations into idiopathic and

symptomatic, making the interesting clinical point that the latter diagnosis was more likely when only one sense modality was involved or when the experience was unilateral and short lasting, or unrelated to the objects in relation to which it appeared;[47] the converse was true of idiopathic hallucinations.[48] Michéa also believed that his groupings had prognostic value, e.g. symptomatic hallucinations were less serious.[49]

The work appeared in book form in 1846,[50] and two years later,[51] Laurent Cerise, an alienist of Italian origin, wrote a hostile review which even criticized the fact that Michéa had dedicated the book to Victor Cousin for his: ' praise [of Cousin] was exaggerated and undeserved';[52] the review was politically motivated and contributed little to the actual debate on hallucinations.[53]

The 1855 debate

As often happened in regards to other psychiatric themes, in 1855 an unplanned debate broke out at the *Société Médico-Psychologique* on the definition and theory of hallucinations.[54] In the session of the 26th February, Alfred Maury[55] challenged remarks by Delasiauve and Moreau on a putative association between hallucinations and mystic states. An untidy debate ensued including various issues which lingered on until April 1856. The theoretical nature of the topic encouraged the participation of non-clinicians such as Maury, Bouchez, Peisse, and Garnier.[56]

Three issues were debated: could hallucinations ever be considered as 'normal' experiences? Did sensation, image and hallucination form a continuum? Were hallucinations, dreams, and ecstatic trance similar states? A fourth issue (as Henri Ey noticed)[57] 'haunted everyone but was not made the base of the debate', namely, whether hallucinations had a 'psychological' origin. By the end of May 1856, the debate ended rather inconclusively in spite of efforts by Baillarger, Michéa, and Parchappe to draw some conclusions. This is not surprising as the issues in question were conceptual rather than empirical and at the time no appropriate methodology was available (indeed, none is available now) to solve them. Nineteenth century observers on this side of the channel also felt disillusioned and Gurney called the debate 'long and barren'.[58]

The second half of the century

Tamburini and the sensory hypothesis

During the 1870s, Tamburini[59] started his work on hallucinations, and in 1881 he suggested that they were not a 'psychiatric' problem.[60] This paper offered, as Ey aptly said, a 'neurological paraphrase', 'hallucinations stopped being a symptom [of insanity] and became a mechanical process.'[61] Jean Paulus, on the other hand, considered it as the 'start of a new research programme.'[62] The paper appeared at the time when cortical sensory physiology was becoming a credible option. For example, Soury[63] wrote: 'psychology, the science of the psychological aspects of life, will be (and perhaps it has already been) totally renewed by the modern doctrine of cortical and spinal localization'. Years later, Mourgue (not a follower of Tamburini's) remarked: 'what was most seductive in Tamburini's paper was that it offered solutions to all problems.'[64]

Writings on hallucinations between the beginning of the nineteenth century and Tamburini's time cannot be neatly classified. Alienists and philosophers were constrained by three dichotomies: Were hallucinations perceptual (sensations) or cognitive (images) events? Did they originate in the periphery (sensory organ irritations) or in the mind (psychical)? Were they always pathological? There was no common view, and a variety of answers were given by Esquirol, Lélut, Leuret, Moreau (de Tours), Griesinger, Baillarger, Michéa, Brierre de Boismont, Hagen, and Sigmond. The problem was not solved by the 1855–56 French debate.

Tamburini's 1881 French paper was based on an earlier Italian publication,[65] and appeared before his work on motor and visceral hallucinations.[66] The French view was challenged by the Italian's uncompromising 'organic' approach which opened the field to other Italian, British and German workers. Ey recognized that 'it was Tamburini who developed the first and most complete theory of hallucinations considered as the result of an excitation of the centres of images, as a sensory epilepsy.'[67] In 1890, Philippe Chaslin wrote: 'As far as the localization of hallucinations is concerned, I accept Tamburini's theory that relates hallucinations to the excitation of certain parts of the grey matter in the brain.'[68] And so did Parish, who followed Tamburini's typology[69] and Ducost who stated: 'Tamburini's theory is accepted by the majority of neurologists.'[70]

From a current perspective, Tamburini's paper: 1. brought under one explanation psychiatric and neurological hallucinations, 2. articulated a testable hypothesis (at least, in relation to hallucinations seen in neurological conditions), 3. legitimatized the use of the language and methods of neurophysiology in the field of insanity, and 4. simplified the old 'insanity' view of hallucinations by developing a mechanistic account of their genesis and doing away with preoccupations about meaning.

These four views have fared differently. The first three still govern research (mainly by neurologists) into hallucinations,[71] for example, Penfield[72] and later researchers[73] have endeavoured to identify the 'centre of images'. The psychiatric question, however, has remained: are the findings of cortical physiology relevant to the hallucinations of schizophrenia, mania or psychotic depression?

The fourth view has been opposed, and both psychoanalytic thinkers and conventional alienists have been loath to give up the semantic approach to hallucinations. Be that as it may, Tamburini's unitary approach broke down during the interbellum period, and by the late 1920s 'hallucinosis' was established as a compromise.[74] This category encompassed hallucinatory experiences related to neurological disorder and left out those considered as functional, psychiatric or psychotic.

Tamburini's paper marked the beginning of another 'neuropsychiatric' period in the history of psychiatry. As the doyen of a group of Italian neuroscientists, he wrote from a position of strength.[75] With him hallucinations become divorced from the patient's past history, for their content (imagery) is determined by random stimulation of brain sites. Even loss of insight (or the presence of an accompanying delusion) depended on whether or not a 'centre of ideation' was involved. But the introduction of the latter was too much for Soury: 'Tamburini has needlessly complicated the picture by invoking, in addition to the sensory centres, the so-called ideation centres'.[76]

Unfortunately, the neurologization of hallucinations caused a reactive over-emphasis on semantics and psychodynamics and between the time of Freud and of Ey, 'insane hallucinations'[77] and 'hallucinosis'[78] became very different phenomena which postponed the 'organic' approach to psychiatric hallucinations. On the other hand, and untrammelled by questions of meaning, neurologists were given *carte blanche* but their approach has been of limited value in the field of 'psychotic' hallucinations.[79] During the 1960s, hallucinogenic drugs offered an experimental model[80] which in the event led to nothing. Linguists[81] and psychologists[82] have offered new approaches but in the main these remain disconnected from neurobiology. Tamburini's work, however, rekindled interest in the question of hallucinations in the 'sane', of which the Charles Bonnet syndrome has become a fashionable example.

Charles Bonnet and his 'syndrome'

The Swiss philosopher Charles Bonnet (1720–1793)[83] in his *Essai Analytique sur les Facultés de L'Âmee* told of the bizarre experiences of his grandfather Charles Lullin, an 89 year-old magistrate (*syndic*) from Geneva, whom Bonnet described as 'healthy, sensible, and with no memory difficulties of any kind'. In 1758, Lullin had a bout of visual hallucinations lasting three months during which he saw 'without any external stimuli the image of men, women, birds, buildings that changed in shape, size and place but which he never accepted as real. The gentleman in question [having] had, at an advanced age, cataract operations on both eyes.'[84] It is not clear from the text whether the operations were performed *before* the hallucinatory episode. Bonnet concluded that these hallucinations 'had their seat in the part of the brain which contains the organ of vision.' Late in life, Charles Bonnet himself had similar experiences and saw, according to his biographer[85] 'a number of fantastic objects which he recognized as illusory'. In this respect, it is known that Bonnet had, since earlier in life, suffered from a marked reduction in visual acuity to the extent that he was forced to forfeit the use of the microscope.[86]

Early in the twentieth century, Fluornoy[87] located a manuscript by Lullin containing a self-description of his experiences, which does not tally with Bonnet's. Lullin stated that he had his visions only when standing up or sitting, but never when in the recumbent position and that the visions were clearer on his left visual field, disappearing when turning his eyes to the right.

In the 1880s, Bonnet's description was quoted (together with Nicolaï's) as an example of visual hallucinations in the sane.[88] In 1852, Guislain reported the case of an elderly lady without any cognitive impairment who could 'see' men with their elbows on the same table where she sat; she was aware of the falsity of her experience.[89] Naville described a similar case of visual hallucinations co-existing with reason,[90] and referred to similar experiences in Cabanis[91] who 'clearly saw people walking on a pathway at the distance'. Naville suggested that sane hallucinations occur in clear consciousness and do not deceive the subject and may be combined with normal perceptions. Such experiences were: exclusive to vision, unaccompanied by bizarre sensations, appeared and disappeared without obvious cause, and cause little anxiety. Some of these criteria are redolent of those suggested by Michéa (see above). Flournoy reported the case of an 89 year-old man with no intellectual impairment who after a cataract operation saw, even with his eyes closed, 'ravishing ladies elegantly attired coming out of a cloud (into his room) and disappearing through the window.'[92]

In 1936, Morsier coined the eponym 'Charles Bonnet syndrome',[93] and in a later paper reported a sample of 18 cases (11 males and 7 females) collected from the literature with a mean age of 81. He endeavoured to show that there was 'no correlation between onset of the visual hallucinations and eye pathology'. In five cases these had developed while the subject had normal vision.[94] He defined the syndrome as: 'visual hallucinations in elderly patients, without evidence of cognitive impairment and unrelated aetiologically to peripheral problems of vision'. He suggested that the cause was to be found in the brain itself.

Since Morsier's description, a wider definition has been proposed according to which any visual hallucination in the elderly, irrespective of accompanying symptomatology, might qualify for the Charles Bonnet syndrome such as those occurring in dementia,[95] ocular surgery,[96] and decreased visual acuity.[97] Such a wide definition depends to a large extent on the sensitivity of neurobiological investigations. In spite of recent efforts,[98] the Charles Bonnet syndrome has become a rag-bag for all manner of hallucinatory states in the elderly.

Parapsychology, statistics and hallucinations

By the second half of the nineteenth century, it was becoming clear that the approach of the French School, based on the description of samples of hallucinators collected in clinical venues might not solve the problem of whether there were hallucinations in the sane. In the event, help came from unlikely quarters in the shape of a survey organized by the *Society for Psychical Research*, founded in 1882 at Cambridge, England and whose leading lights became E. Gurney, F.W.H. Myers and H. Sidgwick.[99]

In 1885, Gurney[100] published a review on hallucinations fully based on continental sources and showing more theoretical eagerness than clinical sense.[101] The first 'statistical inquiry', as Parish called it, was carried out under the direction of Gurney, and the results reported in his book *Phantasms of the Living*.[102] A year after Gurney's tragic death, the 1889 Paris Congress of Psychophysiology approved a further inquiry to which the Society also contributed, and whose partial results appeared in its Proceedings.[103] Results were also reported to the 1892 London Congress for Experimental Psychology. Parallel surveys were carried out under the direction of W. James in the USA, L. Marillier[104] in France, and Von Schrenck-Notzing in Germany.

Analysis of the ideas and drive that led to the development of the Society is beyond the scope of this book.[105] Suffice it to say that, in order to accept the evidence that surveys provide, researchers must accept that probabilistic information has epistemological value.[106] The field was also primed by *Illusions. A psychological Study*,[107] where James Sully[108] defined illusions 'as the natural condition of mortals'[109] and discussed topics as wide as dreams, hallucinations, delusions and paramnesias.

About 400 'collectors' participated in the Society's survey but the original target of getting 50 000 answers was not achieved. The question put to (normal) persons was: 'Have you ever, when believing yourself to be completely awake, had a vivid impression of seeing or being touched by a living being or inanimate object, or of hearing a voice; which impression, so far as you could discover, was not due to any external physical cause?'. 17 000 answers were received, of which 2272 were positive but, once confusional and oniric states were discarded, the number was reduced to 1684.[110] Women reported a higher percentage. Parish compared these results with those obtained in Brazil, Russia, Germany, America and France and found that subjects in the first two countries offered more affirmative answers than subjects from English-speaking countries. Children seemed specially prone; visual hallucinations were more frequent than auditory ones and these more than the rest; combined hallucinations were the rarest. Only percentages and means were extracted from this enormous amount of data and hence it is difficult to make any real sense of the results.[111] The general conclusion of the surveys was that hallucinations were possible in subjects otherwise considered as normal.

Hallucinations: special types and issues

By the turn of the century, all that could be said on hallucinations within the conceptual and clinical constraints of the nineteenth century had already been said. Therefore, many issues remained unresolved: Were insane hallucinations of the same type as drug-induced or neurological ones? Was insight relevant to their classification? Were there hallucinations in the truly sane? Were visual hallucinations more common in organic states? Were the elderly more prone to hallucinations? Were some forms of auditory hallucination more frequent in the intellectual monomanias and delusional insanities (i.e. in schizophrenia)?

Not only had these questions found no answer but the clinical meaning of various subtypes (some of which are still with us) remained obscure. As in other areas of psychopathology, subtypes of hallucinations were started in clinical reports suggesting particular diagnostic meanings. Because only some subtypes have survived, it is not altogether misguided to assume that they captured some real differences in the world. However, there is little independent evidence to show that this is the case. For example, there is no controlled statistical evidence to show that pseudohallucinations (see below) or Lilliputian, peduncular, unilateral, or negative hallucinations have a specific diagnostic value.

Tactile hallucinations

The psychopathology of touch commands little diagnostic interest in current psychiatry. This may be due less to its infrequency than to uneasiness about its underlying concepts. Since Greek times, it has been a reluctant 'fifth sense'. Aristotle,[112] for example, considered touch as a primitive perceptual system and differentiated it from the 'distance' senses.[113] His view remained unchanged until the seventeenth century when British empiricism developed an interest in the epistemology of touch. Locke rejected the Cartesian view according to which extension constituted the essence of material substance; and he maintained that, in addition to extension, all bodies possessed the fundamental quality of 'solidity,' i.e. 'the idea most intimately connected with and essential to body, so as nowhere else to be found or imagined but only in matter'. This idea 'we receive by our touch: and it arises from the resistance which we find in body to the entrance of any other body into the place it possess, till it has left it.'[114]

The epistemological inquiry into what type of bodily information suggests the idea of solidity, identified 'feelings of resistance' and 'motor sensations', the second of which conveyed superior knowledge. Armstrong has expressed it thus: 'For all forms of sense perception beside seeing, hearing, tasting and smelling we employ the word feeling nevertheless it will be convenient to distinguish between at least two sorts of sense perception covered by the word 'feel': perception by touch and perception of our own bodily state'.[115] This distinction was introduced in psychology by Weber as *Tastsinn* (touch) and *Gemeingefühl* (common sensibility).[116] These two categories allowed late nineteenth century alienists to classify phenomena as diverse as tactile hallucinations, neurasthenia, coenesthopathy, and depersonalization.

Descriptions of 'imaginary itches' can be found in earlier literature. Darwin reported a case with imaginary diabetes who experienced 'a hallucinated idea (an itch) so powerfully excited that it was not to be changed suddenly by ocular sensation or reason.'[117] In a Lockean vein, Esquirol wrote 'touch, often appealed to by reason to correct the other senses may also deceive the insane. He may hallucinate rough surfaces or sharp ends hurting his skin, he may feel torn apart by cutting instruments.'[118] Sigmond observed that 'hallucinations of touch vary exceedingly; it is singular enough to find an individual who believes that he has rats crawling over him, that spiders infest him.'[119] Griesinger made the fundamental observation that in touch 'hallucinations and illusions cannot be distinguished from each other; or rather the phenomena which constitute them, so far as they do not depend on anaesthesia, are in every case to be considered as illusions because the specific anomaly consists in the false interpretation of certain sensations.'[120]

Brierre de Boismont stated 'it is said that hallucinations of touch are difficult to investigate because they are apt to be confounded with neurological affections' . . . 'there can be no question that there are some hallucinated persons quite capable of judging correctly of their sensations.'[121] Brierre believed that there was nothing neurologically wrong with patients experiencing tactile hallucinations. Tuke did not separate tactile from internal or corporal hallucinations and included under 'tactile hallucinatory experiences' 'electrical shock', 'delusion of being changed or Lycantropy' and 'sexual hallucinations'.[122] Störring included all these under 'hallucinations of the cutaneous sense': 'In delirium tremens patients often have hallucinatory sensations of spiders creeping over their skin, of ants running over them or of being covered by a fur.'[123] He also included more complex experiences 'they frequently complained of electrical currents traversing their bodies. Others feel as if they were being kissed, or as if someone were lying by their side'.

Classical writers knew of cocaine-induced tactile hallucinations.[124] Magnan and Saury described how their patients 'tried to remove bugs from under their skin'.[125] De Clérambault referred to these as 'hypodermic, distal and punctiform hallucinations', and believed that they were often accompanied by 'sensations of movement' and involvement of consciousness.[126] Tactile hallucinations following intoxication by *Atropa Belladonna* were described by Moreau de Tours who reported a case who felt 'that millions of insects were devouring his head.'[127] These states were likened to the feeling of ants crawling under the skin and termed *Psora Imaginaria* (imaginary itch)[128] and *formication*.[129]

In 1892, Dessoir developed the notion of 'Haptics', which was to be to touch what 'Optics' was to vision, and divided it into 'contact sense' and 'pselaphesia' (passive and active touch, respectively).[130] Movement and 'motor sensations' characterized active touch in Dessoir's classification.[131] As Régis wrote: 'hallucinations in active touch are rare . . . this is not so in passive touch where they manifest themselves as skin sensations such as formication, pinching, rubbing, crawling, etc.'[132] By this period the observation had already been made that paraesthesiae could be reported directly and obliquely. Direct reporting by 'normal' subjects was rarely seen by the alienist who had more experience with oblique or 'as if' reporting by the mentally ill in whom such feelings might lead to delusional interpretation. In a classic description of this transition, Griesinger wrote: 'the commencement of these delusions consists in certain painful sensations being merely fantastically compared by the patient to analogous phenomena. Therefore, hypochondriacs at first say only that it seems to them as if serpents crawled over their skin . . . but the prolongation of the sensations, the influence of unfavourable external circumstances, an increasing internal disharmony [may lead] patients to begin to consider the matter more earnestly, the comparison, at first imaginary, becomes a fully developed delusion.'[133]

Kraepelin included under 'morbid tactile sensations' formication, bizarre sexual feelings and experiences of movement. He stated that 'not frequently these imaginations, connected apparently with organic sensations, receive a very strange interpretation . . . as result of these hallucinations the conviction is often developed in the patients that they have become the sport of all sorts of influence.'[134] Bleuler separated bodily from tactile hallucinations, dedicated a long section to the former, and on the latter he wrote: 'tactile hallucinations are rare [in schizophrenia] occasionally patients complain of small animals, particularly snakes, crawling over their bodies.'[135]

The concept of cénesthopathie

This very French clinical notion[136] reflects the earlier German conceptual distinction between skin senses (*Tastsinn*) and common feeling (*Gemeingefühl*); the latter referring to sensations that are left after touch, temperature, pressure, and location sensations are separated off. Common feeling thus includes pain and 'objectless' sensations such as well-being, pleasure, fatigue, shudder, hunger, nausea, organic muscular feeling, etc. These sensations were also called the *coenesthesia*[137] and considered as providing a 'sense of existence'.[138] To explain bodily feelings of 'unity', two theories were put forward. Associationism stated that coenesthesia resulted from a *summation* of proprioceptive and interoceptive sensations;[139] Faculty Psychology postulated the existence of a hypothetical *brain centre* or function on which sensations converged. The same mechanism was also said to be involved in the generation of the 'body schema'.

The wide functional territory of coenesthesia was gradually eroded as feelings such as hunger, thirst, sexual pleasure, etc. began to be studied independently. In the end, what was left were indistinct sensations common to most organs such as deep pressure, pain, and unanalysable feelings such as 'tickling' or 'stuffiness'.[140]

It is at this stage that the term *cénesthopathie* entered into French psychiatry to refer to a 'local alteration of the common sensibility in the sphere of general sensation, corresponding to hallucinosis in the sphere of sensorium.'[141] Two groups of coenesthopathies – 'painful' and 'paraesthesic' – were recognized, and each in turn divided into cephalic, thoracic and abdominal. Patients in the 'painful' group felt their organs 'stretched, torn, twisted'; and in the 'paraesthesic' group experienced itching, hyperaesthesiae, paraesthesiae, etc. The independence of these syndromes was never recognized in Anglo-Saxon psychiatry where their clinical content was recatalogued as hypochondriasis, neurasthenia or dysmorphophobia.[142] In France itself, some coenesthapathies, for example *topalgie* (or cephalic coenestopathy), were reclassified as 'neurovegetative dystonias'[143] or psychosomatic syndromes.[144] Similar phenomena were also studied as 'disorders of the corporal scheme', and in other countries, classified as 'disorders of sensibility' or 'psychoneuroses'.[145] However, states, such as chronic tactile hallucinosis or delusional parasitosis became quasi-independent entities.

'Delusional' parasitosis

This complex clinical phenomenon consists of complaints of body infestation by insects or parasites occurring in clear consciousness; on occasions, visual hallucinations may complicate the picture. Historically, it has been considered as either a primary hallucinosis or a delusional state, and at the moment the latter is the predominant view. Early descriptions of 'itchy dermatoses',[146] 'acarophobia',[147] and 'parasitophobia'[148] have been anachronistically interpreted as meaning that once upon a time the syndrome was regarded as a phobia or a neurosis. This is not the case.[149] During the second half of the nineteenth century, 'phobia', 'obsession' and 'delusion' were all subtypes of the category 'fixed idea' whose semantic field was predominantly cognitive. For example, Perrin considered 'parasitophobia' as a hallucinatory state *unaccompanied* by anxiety or other affective disturbance![150] Perrin remained undecided as to whether the primary disorder was an 'alteration of intellectual faculties' (i.e. a delusion) or a hallucination thereby starting an ambiguity which has remained to the present day.[151]

Other types of hallucination

Donat in 1513, Calmet in 1751, and Baillarger in 1846 had already noticed the interesting phenomenon of *unilateral hallucinations* but interest in the topic only developed after 1880[152] probably encouraged by Tamburini's peripheralist hypothesis. This was, for example, the view of Robertson,[153] Régis[154] and Toulouse.[155] The fact that hallucinations can be reported as affecting only one eye or ear raises fascinating issues in regards to the epistemology, limits of language of description, and the mechanisms involved in their production. *Peduncular hallucinations*, on the other hand, were first described by L'Hermitte in 1922[156] who, according to van Bogaert, 'opened the new chapter of mesencephalic psychiatry.'[157] In two papers, L'Hermitte described florid visual hallucinations, without insight, which he put down to a disorder of dreaming caused by a lesion in the red nucleus and / or neighbouring areas: 'The hallucinated patient is therefore someone who is dreaming whilst awake, someone in whom the function of sleep is severely disordered.'[158] The hallucinations tended to get worse in the evening and it is likely that some of these subjects were in a delirious state. *Lilliputian hallucinations* consist in the 'vision of small people, men or women, of minute or slightly variable height. They are mobile, coloured, generally multiple. Sometimes it is a theatre of small marionettes, scenes in miniature ... the subject sometimes hears the small people talk, when the voice assumes a Lilliputian tone.'[159] The hallucinations have no diagnostic value and can be seen in both organic and functional disorders.

Hallucinations of smell and taste were also described by Baillarger and considered to be rare, on the basis that these sense modalities were less used in the human than vision and audition. This may explain why little attention was (and is) paid to these disorders; another explanation may have to do with the fact that, as Corbin has pointed out, there was, at least in France, a cultural and scientific ambivalence towards olfaction itself.[160] During the latter part of the nineteenth century, paroxysmal hallucinations of smell became known as a lesion marker in Jacksonian epilepsy.[161] In 1905, Leroy reported the case of a woman who smelt around her a terrible smell and also heard voices,[162] and Wedensky in 1912 reported that olfactory hallucinations might herald bouts of drinking in alcoholics.[163] Durand and others have offered a full historical review of these important phenomena.[164]

Although the phantom limb phenomenon was well described earlier in the nineteenth century (and indeed before), it only became of interest during its second half.[165] In 1861, Gueniot called the experience 'subjective heretotopia of the limbs' and a 'hallucination'.[166] Mitchell is credited with having coined the term 'phantom limb' ten years later.[167] By the end of century, major monographs had been published on the topic,[168] and William James was encouraged into carrying out a survey on its prevalence in the USA.[169]

Pseudohallucinations

It is unclear what the term pseudohallucination means: for example, it has been used to refer to real perceptions perceived as 'unreal',[170,171] isolated hallucinations which do not fit into favoured diagnoses,[172,173] side effect of drugs,[174,175,176] withdrawal hallucinations,[177] diabetic hallucinosis,[178] etc. Historical accounts are also confusing. For example, some German writers have (wrongly) considered pseudo-hallucinations as a German discovery;[179,180] and Jaspers[181] started the myth that Kandinsky originated the concept neglecting to notice that this sad man repeatedly acknowledged Baillarger, Michéa, Ball and others.[182,183] With the exception of Sedman,[184] British writers have followed the German view.[185,186] Historical error partly results from the fact that the history of the *word* pseudohallucination has been confused with the history of the *concepts* created to refer to 'false hallucinations' and with the history of some putative *experiential* phenomena.[187] In other words, the fact that the term pseudohallucination was coined in 1868 does not mean that the concept or the behaviour in question also appeared the same year.

MATTERS CONCEPTUAL Pseudohallucinations are still diagnosed in clinical practice in spite of an absence of agreed diagnostic criteria.[188] The conceptual obscurities besetting this notion may be framed as a series of dichotomous questions:

1. Are pseudohallucinations a form of perception or a form of imagery?
2. Are they voluntary or involuntary phenomena?
3. Are they only found in 'internal' subjective space?
4. Can they occur in any sensory modality, or are they restricted?
5. Are they continuous or discontinuous with hallucinations, or with normality?
6. Are they pale or particularly intense?
7. Do subjects have insight, or do they experience pseudohallucinations as 'real'? (The word 'reality' is also problematical, as it may refer to lack of insight but sometimes is applied to images perceived in external space.) Or is insight not important to diagnosis?
8. Are there subtypes of pseudohallucination, and if so how many?

In their effort to distinguish pseudohallucinations from other experiences, earlier authors have combined the above dichotomies in different ways. Hence, although in general terms it is possible to distinguish two sub-categories of pseudohallucination, namely, that of 'hallucination with insight' and of 'vivid internal imagery', no consistent operational definition has emerged. To make matters worse, it is unclear whether it is more heuristic to define pseudohallucinations 'positively' or 'negatively' and, in the event, both types have been used. 'Positive' definitions have attempted to capture the distinctive features of the pseudohallucinatory experience (e.g. the nature of its imagery) whilst 'negative' definitions have simply stated that they are experiences falling short of being hallucinations. Negative definitions are logically weaker because of their dependence on the validity and reliability of other concepts; for example, other 'pseudo-' terms have attracted criticism for this reason.[189]

Thus unrestrained, usage has strayed even wider, pseudohallucinations being sometimes applied to (i) phenomena which meet criteria for hallucinations or illusions, (ii) hallucinations in people without mental illnesses (e.g. the bereaved), (iii) the false perceptions of people recovering from psychotic illnesses, (iv) factitious hallucinations in malingerers, and (v) occasionally, normal but unusual perceptions which initially seem to be hallucinations (e.g. radio reception in dental amalgam[190] or intracranial shrapnel fragments).[191]

The latter part of this century saw three English language attempts to clarify matters[192–196] though only the first of these was an empirical study. Studying 72 patients, Sedman[197] found that both vivid imagery and pseudohallucinations were associated with 'insecure personalities' rather than psychotic illness, and concluded that the two phenomena were similar experiences. (Further to complicate the question of internal vs. external space, Sedman[198] argued that certain true hallucinations arising within the physical body are really in external space because they are 'ego-dystonic'.) In addition to Jaspers, the work of Sedman seems to have influenced the authors of the Present State Examination,[199] where pseudohallucinations are defined as being heard within the mind, not from the outside and not in objective space.

Hare suggested that the term pseudohallucination could be applied to 'subjective sensory experiences which are the consequences of functional psychiatric disorder and which are interpreted in a *non-morbid* way by the patient' (my italics).[200] However, he also commented on the broad concept of hallucination used in America, as a result of which there is little place for *pseudo*hallucinations. Kräupl Taylor postulated the existence of two distinct forms of pseudohallucination: *perceived* (hallucination with insight) and *imaged* (vivid internal imagery).[201] Taylor's 'perceived pseudohallucinations' and Hare's 'pseudohallucinations' are not fully coterminous as the former are not restricted to patients with psychiatric illness.

More recent literature contains few references to pseudohallucinations. For example, DSM-IV[202] only mentions the term once: as a possible presenting symptom of conversion disorder. This symptom is said to be a type of hallucination, putatively characterised by intact insight, the involvement of more than one sensory modality, naive/fantastic/childish content, and psychological meaning.

THE HISTORY OF THE CONCEPT The history of how the concept of pseudohallucination came to be formed is closely related to the history of the concept of hallucination itself. Indeed, most of the writers whose work is to be reviewed below used pseudohallucination as a *caput mortuum*, the boundaries of which changed according to how hallucination was defined.

French views Although hallucinations have been part of the experiential baggage of humanity, their medicalization only started during the eighteenth century.[203] At the time, one of the tasks was to ascertain their semantic and clinical extension, and to decide whether Nicolaï or Berbiguier exhibited the 'typical' form. This was a period of expansion for the concept of hallucination and not surprisingly little is heard on pseudohallucinations. None the less, experiences later to be considered as belonging to this category were already well known. For example, religious visionaries had since early been able to distinguish between 'sensory' and 'intellectual' visions, the latter being defined as free from sensory elements, occurring in an 'inner space' and being accompanied by insight.[204] It was believed that these experiences were instances of a supreme beatific vision, and the privilege of the blessed.[205]

A second task, undertaken by Esquirol, was to ascertain the clinical origin and meaning of 'the *conviction* [felt by the patient] of a sensation actually perceived' in the absence of an external object.[206] This opened a conceptual space for the possibility that hallucination-like experiences might exist in which conviction was shaky because 'sensoriality' was weak. Baillarger exploited this option by distinguishing between psychosensorial and psychical hallucinations. The ancillary status conferred by Baillarger upon the latter (and the clinical examples reported) strongly suggest that he was referring to pseudohallucinations.[207] Indeed, he wrote: 'books by mystics include precious evidence to illuminate the history of this phenomenon', 'their voices are intellectual, they occur within the soul', 'patients hear their thoughts by means of a sixth sense', etc.[208] (For an analysis of hallucinatory experiences in mystics, see Charbonnier-Debatty, 1875).[209] This problem remained alive in France until the early twentieth century[210] when Richet coined the term *crypt-esthésie* to refer to the 'intuitive' act[211] by means of which those visions were captured.[212]

However, Baillarger also included amongst his psychical hallucinations some of the experiences of chronic psychotic patients: 'apart from their delusions, the cognitive state of patients with psychical hallucinations differs little from those who talk to themselves', i.e. they have no real sensory experiences.[213] He believed that psychical hallucinations resulted from 'the involuntary exercise of memory and imagination and by the suppression of external impressions. The internal excitation of the sensorial system is not needed as *the phenomenon is not related to the activity of this system* (my italics).[214]

By the 1850s, a third problem appeared, namely, to decide whether hallucinations were compatible with reason. In practice, this was analysed in terms of *insight*: did the patient know that his/her images were false, that nothing external was causing them? J.P. Falret was one of the first to pose this question; but his answer was equivocal: 'if images are experienced without belief in their reality, then we must accept that there is no insanity. But is this sufficient to draw a line between reason and madness?'.[215] Falret's question was central to the 1855 debate at the *Société Médico-Psychologique*, and to later debates on hallucinations.[216] Not surprisingly, those against the view that true hallucinations could ever be present in the sane favoured the notion of pseudohallucination.

Michéa, who in 1844 had competed with Baillarger for the *Académie Royale de Medicine*'s award for the best 'essay on hallucinations', was as equivocal as Falret: 'hallucinations can be experienced when reason is normal; if he recognizes that there is no external object, the hallucinated cannot be considered as insane'. But later on he wrote: 'hallucinations are pathognomonic symptoms of mental alienation'.[217]

The fourth task was to deal with the view that psychic or false hallucinations (and some believed also true hallucinations) were related to dreaming.[218] Dreaming has been central to the analysis of 'reality' in western epistemology at least since Descartes.[219] However, views that dreaming and insanity may be related are even older.[220-224] During the nineteenth century, this association was given a medical interpretation. Thus, in 1805, Cabanis dedicated one of his *Memoires* to the relationship between dreaming and insanity: 'Cullen was the first to recognize the *constant and definitive relations between dreams and insanity*. Above all, it was he who showed that at the beginning of and throughout sleep the various organs may fall asleep only successively, or in a very unequal manner, and that the partial stimulation of the points of the brain that corresponds to them, by disturbing the harmony of its functions, must thus produce irregular and diffused images that have no basis in the reality of objects' (my italics).[225] In 1832, Dendy suggested that dreams and 'illusive representations' resulted from the same brain changes.[226] Winslow put it succinctly: 'dreaming and insanity are analogous in these two respects: in both, the mind's imaginings are mistaken for realities; and, in both, the thoughts succeed each other as suggested by associations, uncontrolled by the rational will'.[227] The same view was taken by Moreau de Tours.[228]

In 1881, Lasègue went further to claim that alcoholic psychosis was a form of dreaming;[229] and in 1900, Régis and Lalanne suggested that the same was the case for the psychoses of general paralysis of the insane.[230] Ey called dreams 'a primordial fact in psychopathology' and argued that their analysis suggested 'that the human mind had a hierarchical structure, and that there existed an imaginary world immanent to our very intellectual functioning, i.e. an unconscious contained in our consciousness'.[231]

The debate on whether all hallucinations are related to dream activity has petered out without reaching any conclusion. On the other hand, hallucinations occurring just before going to sleep (called *hypnagogic* by Maury)[232] have been considered both as psychosensory (i.e. real)[233] and as psychical hallucinations (i.e. as pseudohallucinations).[234] Steen considered them as 'hallucinations in the sane' and believed that they could be fully studied from 'a psychological point of view' and 'without mentioning the brain or nervous system'.[235] Such ambiguities provide another example of the pliable boundaries of the notion of pseudohallucination.

The 1855–56 SMP debate The *concept* of pseudohallucination was discussed in a famous debate at the *Société Médico-Psychologique* in Paris. It started on the 26th February 1855, when Buchez proposed that hallucinations should be divided into 'involuntary and voluntary'; and that the latter (as seen in painters and other artists) 'were not pathological'. Maury followed stating that the hallucinations seen in mystics, particularly after exhaustion and long fasts, were of the same 'normal type'. Then Baillarger intervened to remind the *Société* that since 1846 he had called these *psychical hallucinations*.[236]

Garnier then explained that hallucinations resulted from an over-exertion of the 'faculty of conception' leading to the generation of vivid inner representations; for him the crucial diagnostic criterion for pathological hallucinations was a 'belief in the exteriority of the image'.[237] (Garnier had fully discussed his theory in an early, monumental work on mental faculties.)[238] Peisse believed that Garnier's view was incomplete for, in addition to the 'faculty of conception', the generation of auditory hallucinations required the organs of phonation and language.

The session of 30th April, mostly dedicated to mechanisms, debated whether hallucinations were continuous or discontinuous with normal perception, and whether location in interior or exterior space was an important criterion. Sandras described his own hallucinatory experiences which he perceived not as a mere translation of a conception into a sensation but as a 'different, external event'.[239] Defending the 'continuity view' of hallucinations, Peisse renewed his attack on Garnier who 'had borrowed his view from the Scottish philosophers who used it to refer to general intellectual notions such as virtue, rights, etc. but not to *particular things such as noises or colours*' (my italics).[240]

The question of whether belief in the reality of hallucinations was compatible with normality occupied most of the session of 30th November. Castelnau, for example, believed that it was not.[241] Brierre de Boismont, then secretary of the SMP, and himself a specialist in hallucinations (his 1845 book went through three editions) spoke on the 31st of December rejecting the view that mystics and other visionaries were insane, and calling their special experiences 'physiological hallucinations' (this view is important to the later history of pseudohallucinations).[242] The debate, which continued until the 28th April of 1856, was on occasions a bitter one for by then the *Société* had become split along religious and political lines.[243]

It can be concluded therefore that, by the middle 1850s, the French had debated whether all hallucinations were abnormal; and whether location (internal versus external) and insight (present versus absent) were relevant factors to the definition of pathological hallucinations. These were the very same criteria that Jaspers was to attribute to Kandinsky. It also seems clear that these phenomena were well known to the French under the name 'psychical' or 'physiological' hallucinations and 'hallucination of mystics'. Indeed, even the tendency to define pseudohallucinations by default started during this period.

German-speaking psychiatry Pseudohallucinations have also been defined along a dimension of 'sensorial strength or vividness'. As early as 1861, Griesinger discussed this in detail: 'Doubtless there is still a difference between an hallucination and the internal excitation of the imagination . . . it may be asked, is this difference specific, or is it only an affair of degrees? . . . I have seen an interesting transformation of that obscure, pale, internal hallucination (*blassen Mithallucinirens der inneren Sinne*), which accompanies perception in ordinary states into hallucinations with real objective distinctness',[244] and on the issue of their relationship to madness, he wrote: 'hallucinations alone, even when considered as true, are not sufficient to constitute insanity. For this there must also exist a general profound perversion of the mind or fully developed insane ideas'.[245]

The coining of the word pseudohallucination In 1866, Kahlbaum published a major study on the anatomy, physiology and clinical aspects of hallucinations. Influenced by the then fashionable concept of 'apperception',[246] he proposed that there was an 'organ of apperception' which generated 'centrifugal' hallucinatory experiences;

these had little sensorial content, and were related to the spontaneous activity of memory.[247] Herbart had conceived of 'apperception' (a concept started with Leibniz) as an 'attentional and volitional process' by means of which 'new representations' were assimilated into older ones; and also as referring to the manner in which such material might be internally reproduced.[248] Like Griesinger, Kahlbaum was interested in sensory contents; his apperceptive or centrifugal hallucinations being but a form of pseudohallucination. Kahlbaum believed that the latter had little clinical value.

Hagen published his great paper on pseudohallucinations in 1868.[249] Therein, he referred to a book of his entitled *Die Sinnestäuchungen in Bezug auf Psychologie. Heilkunde und Rechspflege*, purportedly written 30 years earlier, and probably the one quoted by Griesinger.[250] (Unfortunately, I have been unable to trace a copy of this work.) Jaspers considered Hagen's 1868 paper as the *fons et origo* of the concept of pseudohallucination. This is inaccurate as Hagen freely acknowledged that he was simply following on the French debate and repeatedly quoted Esquirol, Baillarger, Michéa, Brierre de Boismont, Moreau, Falret, Marcé, and Lélut. Intriguingly, none of these authors is mentioned by Jaspers who, in his book on psychopathology, started the section on pseudohallucinations with the inaccurate statement: 'a certain class of phenomena were for a long time confused with hallucinations ...'[251]

Hagen separated illusions and delusions from hallucinations and considered the latter as a 'convulsion of the motor nerves'. For him all hallucinations were a manifestation of disease but, interestingly, not necessarily of mental illness. Hagen introduced the word 'pseudohallucination' to refer to what L. Mayer had called 'errors of the senses or illusions',[252] and agreed with Marcé that Baillarger's psychical hallucinations were not real hallucinations.[253] Hagen's paper starts the history of the *term* pseudohallucination.

Kandinsky Victor Kandinsky's first work on hallucinations included a detailed description of his own hallucinatory experiences. He also reported that whilst his physician had diagnosed him as having *Melancholie*, his own diagnosis was *primäre Verrucktheit* (which could be anachronistically translated as 'schizophrenia-like state');[254] nothing is yet said in this first paper on French views on the subject. Kandinsky's classical book on pseudohallucinations was published after moving from Moscow to St Petersburg.[255] He returned to hallucinations in a third work appended to his Russian translation of Wundt's book on physiological psychology. Kandinsky died in 1889, aged 40. At the time he was a patient at the Asylum of St Nicholas in St Petersburg, of which sadly he had once been superintendent.[256,257]

The reason why Kandinsky's book impresses the reader as a new start is his bold adoption of the term pseudohallucination as subtitle for the second and longest section (which actually includes a review of the work of Esquirol, Baillarger, Hagen, Ball, and Mayer), and his thorough exploration of the meaning of 'pseudohallucination'. He also dealt with the association between hallucinations and dreaming. The book ends with a chapter dedicated to Kahlbaum's 'apperceptive hallucinations'.

Well grounded in the associationism of Wundt, Kandinsky drew eight connectionist diagrams to represent 'errors of perception', dedicating two to pseudohallucinations. The first (*Eigentliche Pseudohallucination, Modus I*) followed the definition of Kahlbaum: images are generated in 'b' (centre for apperception) ('b': *Centrum der Apperception*); when 'read off' by 'A' consciousness (A: *das Centrum des klarbewussten Denkens*) they are not considered as having 'external objectivity' because of their reduced sensory fullness (*Leibhaftigkeit*). The second diagram (the only one referred to by Jaspers) (*Eigentliche Pseudohallucination, Modus II*) described experiences generated by 'a' (centre for abstract, unconscious Images) (*Centrum des abstracten, unbewussten Vortellens*); these images are sent both to 'A' (consciousness) and to 'b' ('centre for apperception'); 'b' then relays them to 'A', (consciousness). In this way, the sensory fullness of the images is *enhanced* as 'A' (consciousness) perceives them with great vividness. Interestingly, however, the images are not yet considered as having 'external objectivity'. Indeed, the latter feature is only achieved when the image originates in 's' ('perception centre') (*das subcorticale Sinnescentrum oder Centrum der Perception*). These images can be a real perception (i.e. the stimulus originates in the outside world) or a true hallucination (the stimulus is pathologically generated in the perception centre itself).[258]

Kandinsky considered the term pseudohallucination as confusing and preferred 'hallucination-like', 'hallucinoid', 'presentation', 'illustration', and 'illumination'. He defined the phenomena in question as: 'subjective perceptions which in vividness and character resemble real hallucinations except that they do not have objective reality ... my hallucinations are not just images generated by imagination or memory but are sensorially full and involuntary'.[259] In addition to vividness and involuntariness, pseudohallucinations were also 'forced' in character.[260] During the twentieth century this led some alienists, like de Clérambault and Ey, to suggest that the mechanism of 'mental automatism' might be responsible for the experience.[261]

Why did Kandinsky opt for his second model of pseudohallucination (i.e. the one with full-bodied image), in spite of the fact that the model represented in his first diagramme (the 'pale image' one) fitted in better with earlier French and German ideas? The answer is unclear. It could be speculated, however, that *his choice was determined by his own experiences*: 'Some of my hallucinations were vivid and diversified with the bright colours of the real objects of ordinary vision' ... 'there were hallucinations with the eyes open and the eyes closed' ... 'in time I became accustomed to the hallucinations of sight. They ceased to excite or overwhelm me, and at last simply amused me' ... 'my organs of sense were in a state of hyperaesthesia' ... ' this was expressed through noise in the ears, simple and coordinated sounds, through sparks in the eyes', etc.[262]

EARLY TWENTIETH CENTURY WRITERS

Lugaro In 1903 appeared one of the most important papers on pseudohallucinations ever. Ernesto Lugaro, the great alienist from Florence, wrote a full analysis of the concept which, with great historical sense, he identified with the psychical hallucinations of Baillarger.[263] After reviewing the French and German literature, Lugaro reported eight cases, exploring their incidence, specific features, differential diagnosis, relevance to schizophrenia, and pathogenesis. He concluded that pseudohallucinations:

1. were *pure representations*, having no objective character like hallucinations,
2. were ego-dystonic (*carattere di estraneità alla personalità*),
3. gave rise to secondary delusions,
4. resulted from cerebral irritation in the *associative* centres (and not in the *sensory centres* like hallucinations) (on this Lugaro followed Tamburini),[264] and
5. were seen in long-term psychotic states, such as chronic schizophrenia.

Petit During this period, two more writers made important contributions to the notion of pseudohallucination. George Petit presented a doctoral thesis at the University of Bordeaux entitled *Essai sur une variété de pseudo-hallucinations: les auto-représentations aperceptives*.[265] Pseudohallucinations constituted a group of left-over experiences (a veritable *caput mortuum*) whose only common feature was to have a similarity to hallucinations. Petit believed that their conceptual pedigree could be traced back to Baillarger and then to Kahlbaum, Kandinsky, and Séglas. The size of the original group was rapidly diminishing as authors separated off individual subtypes for specific treatment.

Petit described a subtype of phenomena which were automatic, i.e. emerged spontaneously and imposed their presence upon the subject, and in spite of this, were recognized as not originating from any sensory, motor or *cenésthesique* source for: 'the representation lacked in all the attributes of external sensation and was experienced directly in consciousness ... it was in this sense that they could be called apperceptive representations. Furthermore, the phenomena were perceived as ego-dystonic (*créations exogènes, étrangères par leur origine à son Moi conscient et créateur*).[266]

Petit then identified three clinical subgroups of 'automatic mental representations': (*a*) those consisting of a simple sensory image which the subject recognized as purely subjective, (*b*) those consisting of ideas formulated in a 'verbal' manner, like a voice, which the subject recognized as internal (these had been described by Séglas as *pseudo-hallucinations verbales*, see below), and (*c*) those consisting of tendencies, volitions or emotions which imposed themselves upon consciousness but which the subject recognized as foreign (Petit suggested that some of Kahlbaum's 'apperceptive hallucinations' fell into this category). His view that these phenomena were 'automatic' is theoretically related to the notion of psychological automatism resuscitated by Pierre Janet.[267]

Séglas Jules Séglas (1856–1939) was a great psychopathologist. For example, his long chapter on the *Séméiologie des affections mentales*[268] included in Ballet's *Traité* is a book within a book, and offers one of the most complete syntheses of what was then known on the symptoms of mental illness. In this work, Séglas dealt with the problem of pseudohallucinations. After tracing its origins to Michéa's notion of 'false hallucination', Baillarger's 'psychical hallucinations', Kahlbaum's 'appercep-tive hallucinations', and Kandinsky's 'pseudohallucination' (terms which Séglas described as 'not equivalent'), he recognized three types: one including phenomena which only have a gross similarity with hallucinations such as day-dreaming in chronic psychotics; a second including Kandinsky's second type, i.e. phenomena constituted by involuntary, vivid images, which none the less lack the feeling of 'exteriority'; and a third type, related to audition, which he had earlier called 'motor–verbal hallucinations'.[269]

Eleven years later, Séglas returned to pseudohallucinations.[270] After com-plaining of a bias in the literature in favour of German works, and of the fact that textbooks were not helpful (as examples, he quoted those by Kraepelin, Tanzi and Jaspers), he warned that pseudohallucinations meant different things for different people. Quoting the title of a paper just published by a great friend of his, Philippe Chaslin,[271] he explained that this confusion resulted from the fact that psychiatry was not a 'well-made language'. Taking into account Petit's work of a year earlier, Séglas proceeded to offer a new classification of pseudohal-lucinations: one group relating to vision of people and objects (such as those related by Kandinsky), and another subdivided into motor–verbal and pseudohal-lucinations proper.[272]

Jaspers Jaspers first wrote on pseudohallucinations in 1911: 'Kandinsky in the year 1885 separated from true hallucinations a group of phenomena which he explained as a pathological sub-category of the sensory representations of memory and imagination . . . these are different both from representations (*Vorstellungen*) and from true hallucinations in that they have far more sensory content than the former . . . and lack in the fullness, objectivity and exteriority of the latter'.[273] Jaspers criti-cised Goldstein for confusing the two criteria that Kandinsky had kept separate: objective character of an image, and judgment of reality. In this long article Jaspers completely ignored French writers who, for more than 60 years, had asked similar questions about insight and objectivity.

Jaspers returned to the topic the year after, in a didactic piece on false percep-tions. In a footnote, and for the first time, he referred to Baillarger, and warned against the use of Hagen's definition for he was referring to 'all phenomena which were not true hallucinations such as false memories'.[274]

In a short section on pseudohallucinations in *Allgemeine Psychopathologie*, Jaspers repeated his earlier views and included a table detailing theoretical differences between normal sense perceptions and images and ideas. Pseudohallucinations were different in that they were figurative, had a character of subjectivity, and occurred in an inner subjective space; they shared all other criteria with normal sense-perception.[275]

Claude and Ey In 1932, a youthful Henri Ey wrote with his teacher, Henri Claude, a long paper on hallucinations, pseudohallucinations and obsessions. Adding obsessions to the comparison was an important insight for, since the 1850s, it had been suspected that pseudohallucinatory experiences could have a compulsory character.[276]. In a surprising move, the authors resorted to a psychodynamic account, suggesting an interpretative view of the three phenomena and rejecting the 'mechanicist theory'. They attacked 'phenomenology' for encouraging over-description and showing 'false humility';[277] and made the fascinating point that 'the majority of symptoms called pseudohallucinations may simply be forms of obsessional behaviour'.[278] This is still of relevance to the present.

The work of Ey brings this section perilously close to the present. As mentioned above, the history of the word and concepts coined to capture so-called 'pseudohallucinatory' behaviour have never quite converged, and it is important to ask why. One possibility is that the definition of hallucination itself is unstable; another that the language of description is not refined enough to generate a stable difference; yet another that the concept of pseudohallucination is a total construct (i.e. there is no biological invariant attached to it) and hence its boundaries and usage will always be unbridled. This seems to be the case in current usage when clinical phenomena that have little to do with one another are all called pseudohallucinations. Thus, they seem to have the unpleasant role of being like 'jokers' in a poker game: by taking different clinical values pseudohallucinations occasionally allow clinicians to call into question the genuineness of true hallucinatory experiences which do not fit into a pre-conceived psychiatric diagnosis. Both the conceptual, historical, and 'usage' analyses of pseudohallucinations suggest that the term is unrescuable, and should be got rid of.

Summary

This chapter has outlined the history of one of the most important mental symptoms. For reasons of space, only important issue and subtypes have been touched upon. Basically, the phenomenon itself is as old as mankind. During the eighteenth century, it began to be conceptualized as a disease, and by the middle of the nineteenth century it had become a 'symptom'. Important historical changes have been the loss of semantic pregnancy, i.e. of the belief that their *content meant something*, that it was a portent. Hallucinations thus became but symptoms or markers of disease and what the patient saw or heard had no longer meaning in itself. The second change concerns the fact that by being all called 'hallucinations', these heterogeneous phenomena were lumped together under a common epistemological paradigm, that of the 'distant senses' (i.e. vision and audition). This has certainly caused the neglect of the tactile hallucinations which do not fit into that model.

In regards to aetiology, efforts were made to steer a middle course by dividing hallucinations into central and peripheral (i.e. resulting from irritation of the senses); the latter type being considered as less interesting from the psychiatric viewpoint. Insane hallucinations, on the other hand, were assumed to be generated at the highest central level. The history of hallucinations has oscillated between these two views. During the second half of the nineteenth century, Tamburini's hypothesis led to a predominance of the 'neurological' approach. This was followed by a reactive psychodynamic view of hallucinations (not treated here) which flourished in the work of Janet, the hypnosis tradition, and of Freud; according to this view, hallucinations, once again, told something about the subjects past and psychological structure. At the moment, an uneasy truce seems to exist, with the neurological and psychiatric views running parallel but with few researchers asking whether they are dealing, after all, with the same phenomena.

Lastly, and in regards to pseudohallucinations, it has been said that it is a term currently used to name imaginal experiences whose relationship to one another and to hallucinations 'proper' remains obscure. Clinicians, including specialists in psychopathology, disagree on how pseudohallucination must be defined and on its diagnostic role. Empirical research is unlikely to help as the term does not have a stable referent. Historical and conceptual analyses show that this has resulted from the fact that: (*a*) the history of the *word, concept(s)* and *putative behaviour*(s) have failed to 'converge' (i.e. there never has been a time when the three components have formed a stable complex), and (*b*) the concept of pseudohallucination is parasitical upon that of hallucination, and that the latter has proved to be far more unstable than what is usually recognized. It can be concluded that pseudohallucination is a vicarious construct (i.e. one created by a temporary conceptual need, and which is not associated with a biological invariant) and that it is used as the 'joker' in a poker game (i.e. made to take diagnostic values according to clinical need). This diagnostic complacency has retarded important decisions as to the nature and definition of hallucinations. Therefore, it looks as if the concept is irretrievably fuzzy and needs to be abandoned.[279]

ACKNOWLEDGEMENT Dr Tom Dening, from Fulbourn Hospital, Cambridge, greatly helped in the writing of the section on pseudohallucinations.

NOTES

1   Ey, 1973; Paulus, 1941; Quercy, 1930; Mourgue, 1932; James, 1986;
    Morsier, 1969; Sarbin and Juhasz, 1967.
2   Esquirol, 1838.
3   Quoted in Christian, 1886.
4   Quercy, Vol. 1, 1930.
5   Hunter and McAlpine, 1963.
6   For references and quotations, see Chapter 5, this book.
7   p. 146, Crichton, 1798. Jean François Dufour trained in Paris and his
    *Essai sur les opérations de l'entendement humain, et sur les maladies qui le
    dérangent*, from where the quotation was taken, was published in
    Amsterdam in 1770.
8   p. 143, Crichton, 1798.
9   p. 77, Ey, 1973.
10 Cited in pp. 33-35, Brierre de Boismont, 1862. This author took the
    quotation from p. 40, Ferriar, 1813; Ferriar, in turn, had taken it from
    Nicholson's Journal, 1803, 6: 161.
11 p. 33, Brierre de Boismont, 1862.
12 See excellent account by Lechner, 1983. Jacques Postel has written that
    'Berbiguier is our President Schreber of the beginning of the nineteenth
    century, to him Pinel was what Flechsig was to be the latter' (p. 697,
    Postel, 1984). Pinel examined Berbiguier in 1816 and soon became part
    of his delusional system.
13 A recent edition has appeared of this book with a preface by C.L. Combet,
    1990.
14 p. 98, Combet in Berbiguier, 1990.
15 Esquirol, 1817. In his philosophy of mind and theory of perception,
    Esquirol followed his teacher the philosopher Pierre Laromiguière whose
    lectures he attended in 1816 (p. 284, Morsier, 1969). At the beginning
    of the nineteenth century, the priest Laromiguière (1756–1837) became
    one of the beloved thinkers of France. A student of Condillac, he departed
    from the ideas of his teacher by emphasizing the activity of the mind in
    perception and other mental acts. The 'active' view of the mind is also
    found in Royer-Collard and Cousin and is important to the development
    of the central or imaginative theory of hallucination, of which, not
    surprisingly, Esquirol was a sponsor.
16 As instances of hallucinations Esquirol reported six cases (three males
    and three females): case one was a psychotic depressive who heard
    voices, four had combined auditory and visual, and case 5 visual alone;
    retrospective diagnosis is difficult, but cases 2 and 4 seemed
    schizophrenias.
17 Esquirol brought into circulation a term with an ambiguous etymology
    for which three origins have been suggested. Firstly, *hallucinatio* or
    hallucinari which means to err or to abuse; secondly the Greek 'alo'
    meaning 'uncertainty' or 'licentiousness of spirit'; and finally, *ad lucem*,

adlucinor, hallucinator, i.e. terms relating to light or illumination, and hence to a metaphor pertaining to vision (p. 77, Christian, 1886).

18 p. 159, Esquirol, 1838.

19 pp. 200–201, Esquirol, 1838.

20 Condillac, 1947.

21 Esquirol built into his definition of hallucination as a 'perception without object' the logical requirement that there should be 'an absence of an external and public object'. This has created problems for sensory modalities such as taste, touch and internal sensations where a public object criterion is not implementable. For example, the criterion cannot be used to distinguish between a real and a hallucinated itch.

22 p. 188, Esquirol, 1838.

23 *En effet, l'hallucination est un phénomène cérébral ou psychique, qui s'accomplit indépendamment des sens* in p. 191, Esquirol, 1838.

24 p. 192, Esquirol, 1838.

25 p. 195, Esquirol, 1838.

26 p. 196, Esquirol, 1838.

27 He borrowed this concept from Maine de Biran (Moore, 1970).

28 p. 40, Ey, 1939.

29 p. 203, Esquirol, 1838.

30 p. 223, Esquirol, 1838.

31 Lechner, 1983.

32 Aubanel, 1839.

33 One of the greatest alienist–neurologists of the nineteenth century, Baillarger contributed to areas as varied as language disorders, cortical neurohistology, hallucinations, epilepsy, general paralysis of the insane, etc. Ritti, 1892.

34 pp. 512–513, Baillarger, 1846.

35 p. 514, Baillarger, 1846.

36 Michéa was a polymath whose interests included history of medicine, the clinical aspect of depression, hypochondria, etc.

37 'On sait que les aliénés parlent souvent seuls; ils arrive alors qu'au lieu d'entendre exprimer tout haut leurs pensées, ils entendent répéter leurs paroles. Ces aliénés expliquent ce fait en disant qu'il y a autour d'eux comme une sort d'écho' (p. 282, Baillarger, 1846).

38 pp. 363–367, Baillarger, 1846.

39 p. 424, Baillarger, 1846.

40 pp. 86–87, Christian, 1886.

41 p. 474, Baillarger, 1846.

42 p. 38, Baillarger, 1886.

43 Michéa, 1846.

44 Under Louis-Philippe, Victor Cousin (1792–1867) was at once minister of education, director of *L'Ecole Normale Supérieure*, and arguably the most powerful philosophical figure in France. He lost everything after the 1851 *coup d'état*, and was forced into early retirement (pp. 174–175, Harvey and Heseltine, 1959).

45 Michéa's idea that hallucinations are complex and active states of mind

originates in Cousin's claim that 'There is one error [of John Locke's] which it is here necessary to expose – it is not true that we begin with simple ideas, and then proceed to complex ideas. On the contrary, we begin with complex ideas, and from then proceed to more simple; and the process of the mind in the acquisition of ideas is precisely the inverse of that which Locke assigns.' (p. 221, Cousin, 1856) and [there is yet another error in Locke, namely, that the] 'mind is passive in the acquisition of ideas [in fact] the mind is always active when it thinks.' p. 223, Cousin, 1856.

46 p. 243, Michéa, 1846.

47 p. 261, Michéa, 1846.

48 p. 263, Michéa, 1846.

49 p. 264, Michéa, 1846.

50 Michéa, 1846.

51 Cerise (1807–1869) was an alienist of Italian origin with Republican sympathies, and a friend of Bouchez.

52 p. 133, Cerise, 1848.

53 Like all his Republican friends, Cerise hated Cousin (who was a supporter of Louis-Phillipe) whom he considered as peddling 'philosophical whims and phantasies . . . who operated a reconciliation of four systems created in his own mind, and which no one, including himself really believed in' (p. 135, Cerise, 1848). One wonders whether Cousin had anything to do with Cerise's short imprisonment as an alleged Republican sympathizer during the *coup d'état* of 2nd December 1851!

54 Société Médico-Psychologique, 1855–1856.

55 Maury was a man of letters, influenced by the Scottish Philosophers, who wrote on sleep, dreams and hallucinations (Maury, 1878; and the excellent paper by Dowbiggin, 1990).

56 On Peisse, Buchez, and Maury see Dowbiggin, 1989. Adolphe Garnier was professor of Philosophy at the University of Paris and author of the *Traité des Facultés de L'Ame*, 1852; of which Paul Janet (uncle of Pierre) and a great philosopher in his own right said it was: *Le seul monument de la science psychologique de notre temps* (Franck, 1875).

57 p. 589, Ey, 1935.

58 p. 165, Gurney, 1885.

59 August Tamburini was born in Ancona on 18th August 1848 and studied at Bologna University. He worked under Carlo Livi at the psychiatric institute of San Lazzaro in Reggio and moved in 1876 to the Asylum for the Insane at Voghera where he was appointed to Lombroso's job (University of Pavia). The year after, he went back to Reggio to become director of the Asylum and professor of Psychiatry and Neurology. He made Reggio into one of the great centres for neuropsychiatric research in Italy and carried out important work with Luigi Luciani. He was invited in 1907 to take up the direction of the Psychiatric Institute in Rome, and died on 28th July 1919. His academic contribution included neurophysiology (cortical localization), clinical psychiatry (alcoholism, cretinism and pellagra), treatment and

management of the insane (book on treatment of the mentally ill in Italy), and scientific journalism (he started with Enrico Morselli *La Rivista Sperimentale de Freniatria e di Medicina Legale*). For biographic information see Anonymous, Tamburini, 1919; and for an excellent study of the Italian School, see Soury, 1891).

60 Tamburini, 1881.
61 p. 89, Ey, 1973.
62 p. 75, Paulus, 1941.
63 Jules Soury (1842–1915) was not a physician but a right-wing historian of religion and neurology (p. viii, Soury, 1891.)
64 p. 41, Mourgue, 1932.
65 Tamburini, 1880*a* (this was a reprint of: Tamburini, 1880*b*).
66 Tamburini, 1889; 1901.
67 p. 89, Ey, 1973.
68 p. 46, Chaslin, 1890.
69 Parish, 1897.
70 p. 171, Ducost, 1907.
71 Berrios, *Hallucinosis* 1985.
72 Penfield and Porot, 1963.
73 Gloor *et al.*, 1982; Halgren *et al.*, 1978; Hausser-Hauw and Bancaud, 1987.
74 Berrios, 1985.
75 The group included Bartomoleo Panizza (1785–1867) whose neglect Tamburini bemoaned in 1881. This great researcher trained in Padua under Caldani and Malacarne, and then at Bologna, Florence and Milan. As a military surgeon for the Napoleonic army he saw much action during the Russian campaign. He became professor of Anatomy at Pavia in 1815. His anatomical research included research on lymphatic vessels, teratology, and sensory cortical physiology (e.g. Osservazioni sul Nervo Ottico, *Giornale dell'Istituto Lombardo*, Vol. 5, 1855), the latter work was justly reclaimed by Tamburini as having anteceded that of Ferrier and others by about 20 years. (For further biographical information see Hahn, 1884.) Another neurophysiologist that deserves to be mentioned is Luigi Luciani (1840–1919) who was to achieve great reputation as a specialist in cerebellar neurophysiology. He trained under Ludwig at Leipzig whom he recognized as his teacher for the rest of his life. For further information, see Anonymous, Luciani, 1919; Ferraro, 1970. Other members of the group were Tanzi and Morelli.
76 p. 202, Soury, 1891.
77 Faure, 1965.
78 Ey, 1957.
79 Morsier, 1938; also Sutter, 1962.
80 West, 1962; Keup, 1970; and Siegel and West, 1975.
81 Castilla del Pino, 1984; Morenon and Morenon, 1991.
82 Slade and Bentall, 1988.
83 Charles Bonnet (1720–1793) was a Swiss naturalist and philosopher, and a follower of David Hartley's theory of association of ideas. For a

review on hallucinations in the elderly, including the Charles Bonnet syndrome, see Berrios, 1992.

84 pp. 176–177, Bonnet, 1769.

85 pp. 120–121, Levêque de Pouilly, 1794.

86 p. 21, Claparède, 1909.

87 Flournoy, 1902.

88 Ey, 1973; Christian, 1886. The earliest reference I have seen to this in the English language is on pp. 596-597, Sigmond, 1848.

89 p. 279, Guislain, 1852.

90 Naville, quoted in Morsier, 1967.

91 Pierre-Jean Cabanis (1757–1808) was a leading French philosopher, *idéologue*, and physician whose most important work is *Rapports du Physique et du Moral de l'Homme* (Cabanis, 1981).

92 Flournoy, 1923.

93 Morsier, 1936.

94 Morsier, 1967.

95 Burgermeister *et al.*, 1964.

96 Ajuriaguerra and Garrone, 1965.

97 Hécaen and Albert, 1978.

98 Podoll *et al.*, 1989; Fuchs and Lauter, 1992.

99 Gauld, 1968; Williams, 1985.

100 Edmund Gurney (1847–1888) was a fellow of Trinity College, Cambridge. A restless scholar, he studied classics, music, medicine, and the law, but stayed at none. One of the founders of the Society for Psychical Research, he participated in the survey on apparitions and extraordinary forms of human communication. He suffered from a cyclothymic personality, and died in Brighton after having taking an overdose of sleeping pills.

101 Gurney, 1885. He also published a major book: Gurney *et al.*, 1886.

102 Parish, 1897 (translation of improved version of Parish, 1894).

103 Sidgwick, 1889–1890; Sidgwick, 1894.

104 Translator into French of Gurney *et al.*'s *Phantasms of the Living* (*Les Hallucinations Télépathiques*, 1891). He also reported results to the Paris Congress: Marillier, 1890.

105 The great historian of psychology that was L.S. Hearnshaw has come as close as any to explaining this: 'Psychical research as an ostensibly scientific activity was born towards the end of the nineteenth century. It was a cross between the spiritualism, which we have already seen re-emerged after the hibernation of the age of reason in a new guise amid the table-turnings, rappings, and mediumistic trances of the 1850s, and the religious starvation of the scientific agnostic. For some highly intellectual members of the upper-middle classes, to whom the wordly utopias of the socialists for the most part made no appeal, it restored the hope of immortality and alleviated the fear of 'spiritual extinction' and 'spiritual solitude' . . . 'The movement began in a small way in the older universities [i.e. Oxford and Cambridge].' p. 157, Hearnshaw, 1964.

106 Ideological shifts of this nature were taking place in Europe at the time. For example, in 1883 Galton wrote 'The object of statistical science is to

discover methods of condensing information concerning large groups of allied facts into brief and compendious expressions suitable for discussion. The possibility of doing this is based on the constancy and continuity with which objects of the same species are found to vary' (p. 33, Galton, 1883). The same sentiment was being expressed by Ebbinghaus in relation to memory research when he argued that new psychological information could be obtained by looking at means and averages (see his superb Chapter II: *Möglichkeit der Erweiterung unseres Wissens über das Gedächnis:* pp. 9–29 in Ebbinghaus, 1885). A few decades earlier, Claude Bernard would not have approved of this statistical thinking; indeed, he had sarcastically referred to it as the theory of the 'average urine of the European man'. On the penetration of probability theory and statistics in biology *see* Gigerenzer *et al.*, 1989.

107 The book went through various editions, and was updated by Welby and Sully, 1895.

108 James Sully (1842–1923) was an English psychologist who became Grote professor of mind and logic at the University of London, and was more a communicator of knowledge than an original thinker.

109 'The phenomena of illusion have ordinarily been investigated by alienists, that is to say, physicians who are brought face to face with their most striking forms in the mentally deranged. While there are very good reasons for this treatment of illusion as a branch of mental pathology, it is by no means certain that it can be a complete and exhaustive one' ... [however] 'there is the view that all men habitually err, or that illusion is to be regarded as the natural condition of mortals', (p. 2, Sully, 1895).

110 p. 83, Parish, 1897.

111 In spite of obvious sampling biases, the present author is trying to trace the raw data from the original survey to carry out a computerized analysis.

112 Aristotle: *De Anima*, 1968.

113 'But there is a difference between the object of touch and those of sight and hearing, since we perceive them because the medium acts upon us while we perceive objects of touch not through the agency of the medium but simultaneously with the medium, like a man who is struck through his shield' (423.b.12, Aristotle, 1968).

114 Book II, Chapter IV, 1, Locke, 1959.

115 Armstrong, 1962.

116 Weber, 1846.

117 Darwin, 1796.

118 Esquirol, 1838.

119 Sigmond, 1848.

120 Griesinger, 1861.

121 Brierre de Boismont, 1862. For a history of the early evolution of these concepts in French psychiatry, see Azouvi, 1984.

122 Tuke, 1892.

123 Störring, 1907.

124 Maier, 1928.

125 Magnan and Saury, 1889.
126 de Clérambault, 1942.
127 Moreau de Tours, 1845.
128 Darwin, 1796.
129 Formication has been used in medicine since the time of Ambrosio Paré who described *pouls formicant* (formicant pulse) as 'a weak, frequent pulse that gives the sensation of crawling like an ant' (Littré, 1877). The earliest usage in dermatology dates back to 1707 (*Oxford English Dictionary*).
130 Titchener: in Baldwin, 1901.
131 Ziehen, 1909; Katz, 1930.
132 Régis, 1906.
133 Griesinger, 1861.
134 Kraepelin, 1919.
135 Bleuler, 1950.
136 Dupré, 1913.
137 Hamilton, 1859.
138 Gautheret, 1961.
139 Taine, 1890.
140 Titchener, 1901.
141 Dupré, 1913.
142 Reilly and Beard, 1976.
143 Bernard and Trouvé, 1977.
144 Ey, Hypocondrie 1950.
145 Ladee, 1966.
146 Brocq, 1892.
147 Thièbierge, 1894.
148 Perrin, 1896.
149 See Chapter 11, this book.
150 Perrin, 1896.
151 For a history of the vicissitudes of this concept, see Berrios, Tactile Hallucinations, 1982; Berrios, Delusional parasitosis 1985; and the excellent papers by Leon *et al.*, 1992 and Musalek *et al.* 1990.
152 For a review of this topic, see Ochoa and Berrios, 1996; Hammond, 1885; Higier, 1894; Lamy, 1895; Wormser, 1895; Féré, 1896; Joffroy, 1896; Lugaro, 1904.
153 Robertson, 1881; 1901.
154 Régis, 1881.
155 Toulouse, 1892.
156 L'Hermitte, 1922.
157 p. 608, Van Bogaert, 1927.
158 L'Hermitte, 1922 and p. 434, L'Hermitte, 1932.
159 p. 325, Leroy, 1922.
160 Corbin, 1986.
161 'She suddenly perceived a disagreeable smell, sometimes of smoke, sometimes of a fetid character, and quite uncomplicated by other sensory warnings. She compared it to the smell of burning rags or the smell of a match' (p. 411, Jackson, 1932).

162 Leroy, 1905.
163 Wedenski, 1912.
164 Bullen, 1899; Durand, 1955; Ey, 1973, Vol. 1.
165 Charles Bell wrote: 'The man whose arm has been amputated, has not merely the perception of pain being seated in the arm, but he has likewise a sense of its position. I have seen a young gentleman whose leg I amputated, making the motion of his hands to catch the leg and place it over the knee' in Bell, 1830 (see also Furukawa, 1990).
166 *Je pense, pour faire comprendre en quoi consiste, chez certains amputés, l'hallucination que nous proposons d'appeler hétérotopie subjective des extrémités.* (p. 423, Gueniot, 1861).
167 Mitchell, 1871.
168 Arondel, 1898; Culbetian, 1902. For a recent view, see Katz, 1992.
169 James asked 140 subjects who had lost a foot to feel it. He found a variety of responses from those who felt it to those who only 'fancy' their limb. p. 105 (footnote), James, 1890.
170 Wolinetz, 1980.
171 Boza and Liggett, 1981.
172 Heins et al., 1990.
173 Bacon, 1991.
174 Shaw et al., 1980.
175 Stobbia et al., 1980.
176 Nesse et al., 1983.
177 Neppe, 1988.
178 Kemperman and Hutter, 1989.
179 Grünbaum, 1917.
180 Glatzel, 1970.
181 Jaspers, 1948.
182 Kandinsky, 1881.
183 Kandinsky, 1885.
184 Sedman, 1966a.
185 Hare, 1973.
186 Taylor, 1981.
187 Berrios, Hallucinations . . ., 1994.
188 Dening and Berrios, 1995.
189 Bulbena and Berrios, 1986.
190 Wolinetz, 1980.
191 Boza and Liggett, 1981.
192 Sedman, 1966a.
193 Sedman, 1966b.
194 Sedman, 1966c.
195 Hare, 1973.
196 Taylor, 1981.
197 Sedman, 1966a.
198 Sedman, 1966b.
199 Wing et al., 1974.
200 Hare, 1973.

201 Taylor, 1981.
202 APA, DSM IV, 1994.
203 Berrios, Hallucinations . . ., 1994.
204 p. 290, Quercy, 1930.
205 Anonymous, 1930.
206 p. 80, Esquirol, 1838.
207 pp. 383–423; pp. 470–471, Baillarger, 1846.
208 pp. 384–389, Baillarger, 1846.
209 Charbonnier-Debatty, 1875.
210 Marie, 1907.
211 Chan and Berrios, 1996.
212 pp. 74–271, Richet, 1922.
213 p. 422, Baillarger, 1846.
214 p. 470, Baillarger, 1846.
215 p. 232, Falret, 1864.
216 Steen, 1917.
217 p. 267, Michéa, 1846.
218 Maury, 1878.
219 Malcolm, 1959.
220 Seafield, 1865.
221 Dechambre, 1881.
222 Delbœuf, 1885.
223 L'Hermitte, 1963.
224 Beauroy, 1973.
225 p. 602, Cabanis, 1981.
226 Dendy, 1832.
227 p. 338, Winslow, 1864.
228 Moreau de Tours, 1845; see also p. 588, Trillat, 1991.
229 Lasègue, 1971.
230 Vaschide and Piéron, 1902.
231 p. 277, Ey, Le rêve . . ., 1952.
232 Maury, 1848.
233 Schiller, 1985.
234 Ribstein, 1976.
235 p. 345, Steen, 1917.
236 pp. 526–538, SMP, 1855–56.
237 p. 537, SMP, 1855–56.
238 Vol 2, pp. 65–72, Garnier, 1852.
239 pp. 541–544, SMP, 1855–56.
240 pp. 545–546, SMP, 1855–56.
241 pp. 133–140, SMP, 1855–56.
242 Brierre de Boismont, 1862.
243 p. 85, Dowbiggin, 1991.
244 p. 91, Griesinger, 1861.
245 p. 93, Griesinger, 1861.
246 p. 24, Kahlbaum, 1866.
247 p. 41, Kahlbaum, 1866.

248 Lange, 1900.
249 Hagen, 1868.
250 p. 91, Griesinger, 1861.
251 p. 58, Jaspers, 1948.
252 p. 4, Hagen, 1868.
253 p. 27, Hagen, 1868.
254 p. 456, Kandinsky, 1881.
255 Kandinsky, 1885.
256 Rokhline, 1971.
257 Ireland, 1893.
258 Kandinsky, 1885.
259 p. 134, Kandinsky, 1885.
260 p. 49, Kandinsky, 1885.
261 p. 1215, Ey, 1973; on Ey's contribution to the understanding of hallucinations, see Clervoy *et al.*, 1993.
262 pp. 459–461, Kandinsky, 1881.
263 Lugaro, 1903.
264 Berrios, A Theory of Hallucinations, 1990.
265 Petit, 1913.
266 Petit, 1913.
267 Janet, 1889.
268 Séglas, 1903.
269 p. 216, Séglas, 1903.
270 Séglas, 1914.
271 Chaslin, 1914.
272 Séglas, 1914.
273 pp. 460–461, Jaspers, 1911.
274 p. 329, Jaspers, 1912.
275 p. 59, Jaspers, 1948.
276 Claude and Ey, 1932.
277 p. 286, footnote, Claude and Ey, 1932.
278 p. 310, Claude and Ey, 1932.
279 For a similar conclusion, but drawn from a different set of premisses, see Spitzer, 1987.

CHAPTER 4

Thought disorder

Reports of madmen talking nonsense or reaching weird conclusions are not difficult to find in the literature of the ages. These help if all that the historian wants is to show that the *behavioural phenomenon* existed before it was considered as a 'symptom'. It is, however, of less interest if the intention is to write on the history of the *concept* of thought disorder and on its association with particular diseases. In this regard, the historian must also decide whether 'thought disorder' is a *unitary construct* encompassing analogous forms of talking 'nonsense' or just a collection of dissimilar clinical states. Lastly, if a 'construct', he must identify the particular theory of thinking on which it has been based.

'Talking nonsense' or being 'thought disordered' has been predicated of patients making nonsensical *claims* (delusions), or showing weird usage of words (linguistic mannerisms) or fallacious ways of reaching conclusions (illogicality) or impaired articulation (dysarthria) or paraphrasing or fractured syntax or semantics (aphasia), etc. The clinical separation of these states occurred during the nineteenth century and was as much based on theory as it was on observation; and the most important theoretical frame concerned the relationship between thought and language.

This chapter uses as its search object the current definition of 'thought disorder', and accepts the claim that its prototype is seen in schizophrenia. It also accepts the view that clinicians can only 'observe' *disorganized speech* (as per DSM IV);[1] but it also notices that, for the strategy to work, a 1 to 1 correspondence between thought and speech must be assumed. Furthermore, it also notices that disorganized speech is no less a construct than 'thought disorder' and hence its validity will depend on a good theory of language and thought. Influential 'theories of thinking' have been available since Greek times and their creation had little to do with mental disorder. Hence, alienists have had to borrow and adapt these views to understand the speech of those of their patients who spoke nonsense.

If these points are accepted, then it is safe to say that 'thought disorder' was fully described as a *symptom* before the work of Kraepelin[2] or Bleuler.[3] In 1892, Séglas published a magisterial monograph on *Les Troubles du Langage chez les Aliénés*,[4] and in 1902 Renée Masselon his superb *Psychologie des Déments Précoces* including a chapter on thought disorder.[5] Although Kraepelin refers to Masselon in the eighth edition of his textbook, some have wrongly considered this work as the starting point in the history of thought disorder.[6] After the First World War, papers carrying the words 'language' or 'thought' disorder in schizophrenia began to appear: by the 1930s the trickle had become a flood[7] indicating that a new research industry had been born.

Ninteenth century theories of thinking

Two models of 'thinking' vied for supremacy during the nineteenth century:[8] the *associationistic*[9] approach was the legacy of British empiricism and started with Locke's description of simple and complex ideas: the former based on sensations, the latter resulting from 'reflection' (i.e. combinations of simple ideas). Thinking linked ideas together by means of laws of association. This model lasted well into the early twentieth century and influenced both Kraepelin and Bleuler. The second approach was based on Faculty Psychology. Since Greek times,[10] the view that the mind is a cluster of independent powers, capacities or faculties (one of them being the capacity to process information) has had great appeal. It re-appeared as a reaction against associationism (and its 'passive' view of the mind) in the work of Kant[11] and the Scottish philosophers of common sense.[12] The latter, in turn, inspired the phrenological view[13] that there was an independent 'intellectual faculty' comprising perceptive, reflective and germane functions all sited at the front of the brain.[14] For a time, alienists participated little in the debate between these two models and limited themselves to describing behaviours redolent of 'thought disorder'. It would be inaccurate to say, however, that their descriptions were theory free. Assumptions such as the belief that some mental functions *could not become diseased*; or that mental faculties could not be set asunder because the soul was a unitary entity can be found up to the 1920s.[15] The most important controlling principle, however, was their views on the relationship between thought and language.

The relationship between thought and language

The relationship between thought and language was discussed *in extenso* during the seventeenth century in relation to efforts to create a universal language. Whilst most of those involved in such an enterprise proposed systems *a posteriori*, i.e. based on components from known languages, philosophers such as Descartes commented that a truly universal language had to be based on the 'true philosophy', i.e. on the simple notions captured by the mind.[16]

But the version of the relationship that was to influence the nineteenth century was the result of a debate between Condillac and Rousseau. These writers reached the compromise solution that thought and language 'were interdependent in their development; one could not advance if the other ceased to progress. If, as the philosophers believed, the entire process of thought depends upon language, then it followed that to arrive at truths with any precision, language must be extremely accurate.'[17] Wilhelm Von Humbolt supported a similar view.[18] The interdependence hypothesis continued in the nineteenth century in the work of Max Müller[19] who also sponsored the view that, in practice, thought and language were inseparable. This explains why, up to the latter part of the century, alienists treated disorders of language and thought *together*, and why even after disorders such as aphasia, aphemia, and alalia had been described, cases were reported under these headings who suffered, in fact, from thought disorder and other 'nervous' and reversible pathology of language.[20] In the 1930s the Russian psychologist L.S. Vygotsky put forward the view that: 'the relation of thought to word is not a thing but a process, a continual movement back and forth from thought to word and from word to thought. In that process the relation of thought to word undergoes changes which themselves may be regarded as development in the functional sense. Thought is not merely expressed in words; it comes into existence through them.'[21] He also believed that speech was social in origin and that at first it was entirely used for emotional and social functions. At the time, Vygotsky's ideas were unknown and had little influence in western countries.[22]

Far more influential was the work of E. Sapir and B.L. Whorf who propounded that language had an absolute predominance: 'we cut nature up, organize it into concepts, and ascribe significances as we do, largely because we are parties to an agreement to organize it in this way – an agreement that holds throughout our speech community and is codified in the patterns of our language. The agreement is, of course, an implicit and unstated one, BUT ITS TERMS ARE ABSOLUTELY OBLIGATORY' (in capitals in original).[23] The strong version of this hypothesis is no longer popular, and its weaker version has influenced research into thought disorder in as much as the latter is considered as a primary disorder of speech production.[24]

Early descriptions of thought disorder

Esquirol distinguished between nonsense talk secondary to abnormal sensations (hallucinations) and *primary pathology* of the 'faculty that is in charge of coordinating ideas'. But his interest was not in detailed symptomatic description and he does not elaborate further. Furthermore, clinical vignettes illustrating such pathology show that he was, in fact, describing abnormal speech in patients with organic delirium.[25] Prichard, in turn, uses the term incoherence as a synonym for dementia which he subdivides into primary and secondary. (The term dementia referred in the 1830s to a clinical state very different from what it means today.)[26] Under both types, which he considered as syndromatic, Prichard includes clinical descriptions redolent of thought disorder: 'a want of sequence, or connection between the ideas, a failure of that aptitude in the mental constitution by which in the natural state one momentary condition of the mind follows in the train of its antecedents . . .'.[27]

But, up to the middle of the nineteenth century, no clear clinical criteria existed to differentiate between the nonsense uttered by the insane, the confused or the aphasic. Thus, Forbes Winslow reported under 'morbid phenomena of speech' patients with dysarthria, aphasia, obsessional utterances, mutism and thought disorder, e.g. 'the 20 year old man who was seized with a kind of cramp in the muscles of his mouth, accompanied with a sense of tickling upon the surface of his body, as if ants were creeping over it. After having experienced an attack of giddiness and mental confusion, a remarkable alteration in his speech was observed. He articulated easily and fluently, but made use of strange words which nobody could understand . . .'.[28]

That up to the 1840s 'thought disorder' (under whatever name) had not yet been fully described as a symptom is, in itself, an interesting historical issue. If, for a start, the facile explanation that it 'had not yet appeared' is discarded, one is still left with other possibilities. For example, that no theories of thinking were available at the time; this is unlikely as, for example, Feuchtersleben developed a detailed one in his work, and yet did not proceed to ask the question of whether there was a primary disorder of thinking.[29] More likely explanations are that most alienists still accepted the aprioristic Lockean belief that thought processes were *normal* in the insane, and that writers of textbooks often were in private practice and hence did not have experience with longitudinal cohorts; this is the case with Feuchtersleben whose book is long in theory but short in cases. And even those who did see chronic psychotics, may not have considered it necessary to bother about a primary disorder of thinking for 'taking non-sense' could easily be explained away as being secondary to delusions or hallucinations. One reason for the latter is that thought disorder is not a 'primary' (such as delusions or hallucinations) but a secondary symptom, i.e. one that is constructed by the observer and one for which the patient often has no direct insight.[30]

But, things started to move during the 1850s. Joseph Guislain's definition of *d' incoherence des idées* was one of the first to suggest a distinction between disorders of speech and thought : 'the madman responds with a series of disconnected phrases and words. The deficit seems to be in the mechanism that forms and combines words before these are confided to the tongue. Since there is no deviation of the latter nor the least difficulty in its movements it can be concluded that *there is nothing wrong with it* and that the disturbance *is higher up* in the brain . . . incoherence of ideas without delusions is rare . . . In the case of our patient, he believed he was the emperor' (my italics).[31] Guislain proposed a syndromatic view: 'incoherence of ideas can be seen in extreme old age, after stroke, after delusional mania, and in the defect state of mania.'[32]

Griesinger, in turn, divided the 'anomalies of thought' into 'formal deviations' (*formale Abweichungen*) and 'false contents' (*falscher Inhalt der Gedanken*, i.e. delusions and obsessions). He believed that 'too rapid succession of the ideas, extreme slowness in the course of thought, or disorder of the feelings accompanying them, might excite and promote morbid ideas.'[33] There also was 'incoherence of thought and speech (*verwirrte Incohärenz im Denken und Reden*) corresponding to projections of the thoughts and of the emotions, as anger' and 'still another which proceeds from incomplete abolition and deep destruction of the mental processes'. Griesinger proposed a mechanism, perhaps the first for formal thought disorder: 'The psychological mechanisms of this latter phenomenon is still obscure in its details; it appears that the incoherence depends on the fact that the perceptions are called forth, not only according to their (similar or contrasting) contents, but *specially according to external similarity of sounds in the words. Perhaps deficient recipro-cal action of the two halves of the brain* may have influence in producing incoherence'. (my italics)[34] Griesinger's psychopathological thoughts were influenced by Herbart's[35] model for information processing,[36] and Wigan's 'double brain' theory.[37]

The discovery of aphemia and aphasia

During the 1860s, two important events punctuate the history of the language disorders. One was the 'discovery' of aphemia,[38] the other the debate between Broca and Trousseau on the appropriateness of the terms *aphemia* and *aphasia*.[39] That this did not immediately bring about an improved definition of 'thought disorder' may be explained by the fact that the discovery of aphasia reflected a renegotiation of the brain localization of the language faculty[40] and not a change in the concepts governing the relationship between thought and language (this only came with Hughlings Jackson). Indeed, in the mind of the *alienists*, language and thought remained closely intertwined until the end of the century as shown in the work of Falret[41] and Séglas.[42]

Sèglas and language disorder in the insane

As mentioned earlier, Jules Séglas was one of the more imaginative 'semiologists' of his generation. He believed that, although language and gesture remained the media in which all the diagnostic symptoms of mental illness were conveyed, little interest had been shown to study them in detail. He proceeded to divide the language disorders according to whether there was a predominant defect in speech, writing, or mimic. Defects of speech, in turn, could result from a pathology of thought (*dyslogies*), language (*dysphasies*), and speech proper (*dyslalies*). Defects in writing were equally divided into those due to anomalies of thought, language and writing proper (graphia). Séglas analysed all these in detail but I shall only mention the *dyslogies*[43] which include typical cases of thought disorder.

Séglas wrote: 'When the problem is due to a disorder of thought, the function of language rests intact and speech shows, by its modifications, a fundamental intellectual disorder.'[44] According to whether the tempo, form, syntax, or content of language was disordered, Séglas described four types of dyslogia. *Tempo* could be increased (as in *logorrhée*, polyphrasie de Kussmaül, *fuite des idées*, *langage elliptique*, *lalomanie*) or decreased; in the latter case there was retardation which could end up in *mutisme vésanique*. Alterations in the *form* of language included changes in timbre, imitations of animal sounds, obscene or pompous terminology, verbiger-ation (as per Kahlbaum), and plaintiveness. Changes in *syntax* included referring to the self in the third person, using clumsy turns of phrase, and disintegration of sentence construction. Changes in *content* comprised fixation on certain themes (*paralogie thématique*), stereotypies, and neologisms classified as passive (resulting from automatic processes) and active (when the patient voluntarily invented new terms).[45]

Séglas also discussed two other *dyslogies*: emotional and reflex language disturb-ance; the former including flat, monotonous, vivacious or cadential language (in keeping with the subject's mood) and the latter resulting from certain stimuli included echolalia and (what Robertson in Britain, probably following William Warburton, had called) 'automatic speech'. Finally, disturbances of mimic were divided into those related or unrelated to thought disorder; the former including changes in expression, gestural mannerisms, etc.

It is difficult to imagine a more detailed description of thought disorder and cognate states.[46] Séglas refrained from quoting his theoretical sources nor did he venture any explanatory hypothesis. It is clear, however, that he considered these phenomena as 'symptoms' which could be present in diverse mental disorders;[47] only in few cases did he suggest that there was a special association between symp-tom and a particular disease.

J.H. Jackson

Jackson's views on language and its disturbances are only partially relevant to a history of thought disorder.[48] To understand his ideas on the affections of speech (as he called them), the reader must keep in mind that Jackson: (*a*) entertained a 'semantic' as opposed to a 'mechanistic' definition of speech, (*b*) opposed the concept of 'faculty' of language, as it was then popular in the French debate between Broca and others, (*c*) interpreted the affections of speech in terms of a hierarchical model (as he had done in the case of epilepsy and stroke), and (*d*) borrowed from Herbert Spencer the view that modes of expression in the human could be separated into intellectual and emotional.[49]

Jackson wrote: 'to speak is not only to utter words, it is to propositionize. A proposition is such a relation of words that it makes one new meaning',[50] therefore, 'loss of speech is loss of power to propositionize.'[51] He opposed the views (popular in his time) that there was a special faculty of language or that language was just a mechanical associations of words; and on this, he remained loyal to Locke and the empiricist tradition. His own solution, however, was not altogether clear: 'we do not mean by using the popular term power, that the speechless man has lost any 'faculty' of speech or propositioning; he has lost those words which serve in speech, the nervous arrangements for them being destroyed. There is no 'faculty' or 'power' of speech apart from words revived or revivable, any more than there is a faculty of 'co-ordination' of movements apart from movements represented in particular ways.'[52]

Jackson's view that the affections of speech reflected a phenomenon of 'dissolution' led him to identify both 'the patient's negative and positive condition'. Furthermore, automatic speech and other 'release' or positive phenomena were for him not the result of a brain lesion but the expression of a *healthy area* of the brain, and hence were still organized according to rules. It has been rightly suggested that this idea was influential on Freud's views on language[53] and on thought disorder which he considered not as 'noise' (resulting from the brain lesion) but the expression of lower but still meaningful mentations.[54]

Masselon and 'thought disorder'

A disciple of Paul Sérieux, Renée Masselon was only 28 years old when he published his study on the psychology of dementia praecox. In France, the Kraepelinian category had encountered much opposition. Marandon de Montyel, for example, claimed that 'Kraepelin's dementia praecox was neither a dementia nor was it praecox.'[55] Victor Parant argued against its putative age of onset, Protean symptomatology, and the fact that 'it did not lead to dementia.'[56] At the Le Puy Congress of French neurologists and alienists of 1913, Foville bemoaned the fact that the old Morelean term *démence précoce* had been commandeered by the Germans, and that in their hands it had gained over compliant boundaries.[57]

Other French-speaking alienists, like Soutzo,[58] took a more sympathetic attitude. But it was Sérieux who, by stating in the 1901 Gent Congress that 'his own research confirmed Kraepelin's results', threw his reputation behind the new disease.[59] He also inspired books[60] and doctoral theses, such as Monod's on the *Les Formes Frustres de la Démence Précoce*,[61] and Masselon's own. The latter includes measures of attention (by means of Ribot's model), reaction time both simple and choice (using Phillips chronometric paradigm), memory (both for recent and remote events), mood, and motor behaviour in 13 cases of dementia praecox. Thought disorder was assessed as 'coordination of ideas' and 'intellectual weakness and deterioration'. Masselon found that his subjects were distractible and often perceptually bound and concluded that this was caused by a 'marked impairment of attention', particularly of what he called 'voluntary attention'. Both reaction times were also prolonged, particularly choice reaction time. Memory was affected as was mood, all patients showing apathy, flatness, and aboulia.

Thought processes were particularly impaired. The commonest disorder involved judgement and synthesis of thoughts, with subjects showing 'fixation on few

themes, stereotypes, puerility, echolalia, tics of language', and marked reduction in
their capacity to monitor the environment. Masselon concluded that 'démence précoce was a disease that caused a primary impairment of the active faculties of the
mind, with apathy, aboulia, and loss of intellectual power being its symptomatic
triad. These primary impairments also led to affective disturbance.'[62]

Kraepelin, Bleuler, Jung and associationistic theories

To a large extent, Kraepelin replicated Masselon's findings and conceptualized
thought disorder in terms of associationistic psychology. Many of the 'psychic symptoms' of dementia praecox were, for him, manifestations of thought disorder. These
included injury of judgment, stereotypes, incoherence of the train of thought, derail-
ments in linguistic expression, paraphasias, neologisms, akataphasia (inability to
find the appropriate expression for a thought), impairment in the construction of
sentences, and speaking past the subject. Like Masselon, he also believed that these
symptoms were central to the diagnosis of dementia praecox.

Bleuler, with the help of the psychologist Gustav Jung, also viewed thought
disorder as the central symptom of schizophrenia, the name he coined for dementia
praecox.[63] According to Bleuler, the 'associations lose their continuity. Of the thousands of associative threads which guide our thinking, this disease seems to inter-
rupt, quite haphazardly, sometimes such single threads, sometimes a whole group,
and sometimes even large segments of them. In this way, thinking becomes illogical
and often bizarre.'[64] Bleuler tried to explain sub-symptoms as combinations and
permutations of such disconnections.

Jung's work on the psychology of dementia praecox was published in 1907,[65]
four years before Bleuler's. It has three parts: a review of the literature, a comparison of dementia praecox and hysteria, and a long report of the single case of a 62
year-old woman (first admission at age 42) with a putative diagnosis of dementia
praecox. The historical review, which mainly deals with the work of Gross,[66] Stransky,[67] Weygandt,[68] and Janet,[69] also dedicated critical space to Masselon's work.
Jung berated the French writer for not making up his mind as to what was the
central single defect of dementia praecox[70] and for using a 'concept of attention
which was too broad and comprehensive'.

Jung concluded that all earlier results 'converged towards the same goal . . .
the idea of a central disturbance which is called by various names: apperceptive
deterioration (Weygandt); dissociation, abaissement du niveau mental (Masselon,
Janet); disintegration of consciousness (Gross); disintegration of personality (Neisser
and others).'[71] Jung agreed that, as far as thought disorder was concerned, there
was a disturbance of associations but complained that little was known as to how
to separate abnormal from normal or unimpaired thinking: 'In dementia praecox,
where as a matter of fact countless normal associations still exist, we must expect
that until we get to know the very delicate processes which are really specific of

the disease the laws of the normal psyche will long continue to play their part').[72]

Jung believed that similar pathological processes operated in hysteria and dementia praecox: 'in dementia praecox, too, we find one or more complexes which have become permanently fixed and could not, therefore, be overcome. But whereas in persons predisposed to hysteria there is an unmistakable causal connection between the complexes and the illness, in dementia praecox it is not at all clear whether the complex caused or precipitated the illness.'[73] The crucial difference between the two, Jung thought, was the presence in dementia praecox of 'hypothetical X, a metabolic toxin, and its effect on the psyche.'[74]

The views of Jung, Bleuler, Janet, and Berze[75] reflect a move away from neurological explanations still common at the time.[76] Others, like Jaspers, steered a middle course by stating that speech disorders in the psychoses: 'include certain verbal performances which at present cannot be explained in terms of neurological mechanisms; nor can they be simply understood as a form of expression or as the communication of abnormal psychic contents. We have to deal with a territory of interest to both sides.'[77]

The return of the holistic approach

After the First World War, the stage was set for a major challenge to associationism and localizationism.[78] The new ideas emerged from different quarters but were all inspired by evolutionary theory. First, there were proposals for a return to 'holistic' approaches to human behaviour (following Jackson's views) such as Head's evolutionary neurophysiology,[79] Lashley's notion of 'equipotentiality' (in brain localisation),[80] Von Monakow's hierarchical views (in psychiatry),[81] and Koehler's[82] and Kofka's[83] Gestalt paradigms (in psychology).

Secondly, based on the assumption that there were *qualitative* differences between the mind or 'mentality' of the primitive races and that of civilized man,[84] the view developed that the thought processes of the insane were like those of the primitive man.[85]

Thirdly, in regards to the psychodynamic approach, Kasanin complained, 'After World War I, formal investigations in the field of schizophrenic thinking were stopped for almost two decades because of the extreme interest of the psychiatrist in the dynamic aspects of psychiatry as expressed in the teaching of Meyer, Freud, Jung and others. These investigators pointed out that schizophrenic speech utterances have a definite meaning and content even though they may be quite distorted and incomprehensible to the observer.'[86]

Lastly, Kurt Goldstein explored schizophrenic thinking from the point of view of Gestalt psychology, and compared it with thinking in brain-damaged subjects. In both, there was a fundamental change in the boundaries between figure and background (i.e. a 'disappearance of the normal boundaries between the ego and the world'). Although both organic and schizophrenic subjects showed 'concrete' thinking, the latter's performance showed intrusions related to delusional and other psychotic material.[87] Schilder took a similar view. In a classical paper on the psychology of general paralysis, he dealt with thought disorder from a gestaltic viewpoint, and reported that patients with thought disorder utilized: 'inexpedient methods in registration, elaboration and reproduction. The necessary anticipations and the integration of parts into wholes do not take place. The whole-apperceptions that do come about are not sufficiently structured. In the process of apperception,[88] concepts and situations are [freely] replaced by coordinate or superordinate concepts.'[89]

In 1927, Von Domarus published his classical paper on schizophrenic thinking.[90] Influenced by Vygotsky (see above) he suggested that schizophrenic patients differed from normal in that they were 'paralogical' i.e. did not require the 'identity of all predicates' to state that two objects were identical:[91] they might say that an orange and a house were the same simply because both shared one attribute (say the colour yellow). On occasions, the predicate may be something which was not even apparent to the observer (for example, that both were facing north). Domarus generalized from very few patients, and used no controls in his clinical analysis.

Summary

A history of the concept of thought disorder shows that the 'symptom' refers to a heterogeneous group of behaviours which, during the last 100 years, have been given uniformity and unity by the Procrustean device of applying to them successive theories of thinking. Whilst associationism held sway, emphasis was naturally given to 'connections' of ideas,[92] to the assumption that language and thought were closely associated, and that disturbances of the one always showed in the other. This theory inspired Griesinger, Séglas, and Masselon. Kraepelin, Jung and Bleuler added nothing new to these early insights, and their contribution was limited to claiming that such a symptom was *primary* to the diagnosis of schizophrenia.

With the decline of associationism, and the growth of holistic psychologies and evolutionary theory, 'thinking' was re-defined in terms of the recognition of wholes and of concept-making processes. This led to new ways of describing thought disorder which then became a disturbance of concept formation[93] due to a putative breakdown in the usage of logical rules.

One lesson to be learnt from this historical account is that 'thought disorder' is a secondary symptom, and a construct which remains parasitical upon theories of thinking. This means that, whether formulated in terms of association theory, information processing, attentional or computational models, or considered as a speech disorder, the actual 'behaviour' involved (i.e. talking weird or nonsense) is unlikely to be localizable on the brain in the way in which other symptoms (e.g. hallucination) might be.

NOTES

1   American Psychiatric Association, DSM IV, 1994.
2   Andreasen, 1982.
3   Harrow and Quinlan, 1977.
4   Séglas, 1892.
5   Masselon, 1902.
6   Kraepelin, 1919.
7   See the useful bibliography compiled by Lewis, 1936.
8   A good historical account of these ideas should be found in pp. 377–496, Porter, 1868; pp. 115-444, Garnier, 1852; Taine, 1901; Paulhan, 1889; and for a newer account, see Sternberg and Smith, 1988.
9   For a history of this theory, see Claparède, 1903; and Warren, 1921.
10 Blakey, pp. 375–410, 1850.
11 Hilgard, 1980.
12 Brooks, 1976.
13 Spoerl, 1936.
14 See, for example, Spurzheim, 1826; Combe, 1873.
15 For example, they constituted the main argument put forward by those who attacked the notion of monomania. A version of a *monade psychique* was still being defended by Mignard early this century (Mignard, 1928).
16 Slaughter, 1982.
17 pp. 45–46, Juliard, 1970; also pp. 13–43, Aarsleff, 1983.
18 p. 48, Von Humbolt, 1988. On Hegel's view on the relationship between thought and mind, see Simon, 1966.
19 Müller believed that language derived 'not from shrieks, but from roots, i.e. from general ideas' (p. xi, Müller, 1882). This view led him to clash with Darwin (see Knoll, 1986). For a good analysis of language and thought during the nineteenth century, see pp. 9–66, Dauzat, 1912.
20 See, p. 612, Falret, 1866.
21 p. 125, Vygotsky, 1962.
22 Wertsch, 1985; See also Alvarez and del Rio, 1991.
23 pp. 213–214, Carroll, 1956.
24 Chaika, 1982.
25 p. 5, Vol. 1, Esquirol, 1838.
26 Berrios and Freeman, 1991.
27 p. 86, Prichard, 1835.
28 For other similar cases, see pp. 471–510, Winslow, 1861.
29 p. 127, Feuchtersleben, 1847.
30 Berrios and Marková, 1995.
31 p. 316, Guislain, 1852.
32 p. 317, Guislain, 1852. By 'mania' Guislain meant delusional insanity (mainly schizophrenia-like states) rather than mania in the current sense of the term. Guislain put forward as an explanation for this *obscuration des facultés intellectuelles* a general mechanism of moral pain; see pp. 148-149, Guislain, 1852, Vol. 2.

33 p. 67, Griesinger, 1861.

34 p. 68, Griesinger, 1861.

35 Griesinger's psychopathology is largely the application to psychiatry of the psychology of the philosopher–mathematician J.F. Herbart (1776–1841) Ackerknecht, 1965; for a more critical view, see pp. 144-146, Wahrig-Schmidt, 1985.

36 On the model, see Fritzsch, 1932; and De Garmo, 1896.

37 Griesinger knew Wigan's 1844 book well (see p. 24, Griesinger, 1861) Wigan, 1844.

38 Moutier, 1908; Quercy, 1943; Hécaen and Dubois, 1969 (this is an anthology including important original publications).

39 Lefevre, 1988.

40 Ballet, 1886.

41 Falret, 1866.

42 Séglas, 1892.

43 Dyslogia was discussed at length in the 1930s by an American psychologist (see pp. 141–151, Stinchfield, 1933). For some reason, however, Andreasen has written: 'Dyslogia is a *new* term (*sic*), but one which derives from familiar roots, . . .' p. 297, Andreasen, 1982.

44 p. 16, Séglas, 1892.

45 Séglas also included here a lengthy discussion on neologisms (see pp. 46–66, Séglas, 1892). The only important work before Séglas was: Bartels, 1888; later works are Bobon, 1952; Cenac, 1925.

46 Surprisingly, recent authors have played down Séglas's contribution (see Pinard and Lecours, 1983); or ignored it altogether (see Boyer, 1981).

47 On Séglas's contribution, see Lantéri-Laura and Del Pistoia, 1980.

48 See Riese, 1955; 1965.

49 Also see monograph by López Piñero, 1973; and on the psychiatric aspects of Jackson's work see Dewhurst, 1982.

50 p. 159, Jackson, 1932, Vol. 2.

51 p. 160, Jackson, 1932, Vol. 2.

52 p. 160, Jackson, 1932, Vol. 2.

53 Freud, 1953 (first published in 1891).

54 Fullinwider, 1983.

55 p. 247, Marandon de Montyel, 1905.

56 Parant, 1905.

57 pp. 134–135, Chronique: Le XXXIIIe Congrès des Médecins Aliénists et Neurologistes de France et des Pays de Langue Française, 1913.

58 Soutzo, 1907.

59 p. 13, Masselon, 1902.

60 Deny and Roy, 1903.

61 Monod, 1905.

62 pp. 259–265, Masselon, 1902.

63 Berrios, 1987.

64 p. 10, Bleuler, 1911.

65 Jung, 1972 (first edition, 1907).

66 Gross, 1904.

67 Stransky, 1904.

68 Weygandt, 1904; although not quoted by Jung also see Weygandt, 1907.

69 Janet, 1903.

70 'In Masselon's work we find an assortment of views which he feels all go
    back to one root, but he cannot find this root without obscuring his work.'
    in p. 11, Jung, 1972.

71 p. 37, Jung, 1972.

72 p. 7, Jung, 1972.

73 p. 97, Jung, 1972.

74 p. 98, Jung, 1972.

75 Like Janet's, Berze proposed an 'energetist' hypothesis which he called
    'primary insufficiency' (see Berze, 1914). Italian writers like Rignano also
    supported a view of thought disorder based on a reduction of energy and
    in changes in the affective sphere (pp. 238–244, Rignano, 1922) (first
    Italian edition, 1920).

76 For example, Kleist claimed that 'I was able to isolate in 1914, from the
    many varieties of confused speech which one sees in that condition,
    several particular disturbances which could be regarded as based on
    cerebral pathology. In doing so I confirmed Kraepelin's hypothesis that
    some schizophrenic disorders of speech depend, like similar phenomena
    that are found in dream speech, on functional disturbances in the
    temporal speech area' (Kleist, 1930). For a good account of the role of
    neurology see Critchley, 1964; also Benson, 1973; Stengel, 1964.

77 p. 191, Jaspers, 1963 (first edition, 1913).

78 On 'imaginary localizations' see the excellent paper by Lantéri-Laura,
    1984.

79 On Head and the history of aphasia during the 1920s see pp. 167–215,
    Piéron, 1927.

80 Lashley, 1963 (first edition, 1929).

81 Monakow and Mourgue, 1928.

82 Peterman, 1932.

83 Koffka, 1928.

84 Lévy-Valensi, 1934, 92: 676–701; see also Lévy-Bruhl, 1928 (first edition,
    1910). Jung, for example, was influenced by Lévy-Bruhl's notion of
    'pre-logical' mentality. This idea was confronted by Leroy, 1927. For a
    recent attack on the notion of mentality in general see Lloyd, 1990. For a
    general history of the ideological background to Levy-Bruhl's work in this
    area, see Allier, 1929.

85 See Blondel, 1914. Blondel dedicated his book to Lévy-Bruhl and intimated
    that his own research programme had been inspired by the publication in
    1910 of Lévy-Bruhl's book.

86 p. 2, Kasanin and Lewis, 1944. The claim that research stopped for two
    decades was, perhaps, exaggerated. For an excellent study of schizophrenic
    language, see Piro, 1967; also Reed, 1970.

87 Goldstein, 1944. See also the excellent historical review by Payne et al.,
    1959.

88 On the concept of apperception in psychology, see Lange, 1900.

89 Schilder, 1930.
90 Domarus, 1927.
91 pp. 104–114, Kasanin and Lewis, 1944.
92 See Billod, 1855.
93 See historical account in Kasanin and Haufmann, 1938.

CHAPTER 5

Delusions

Historically, the concept of 'delusion' is intertwined with that of 'insanity' and depends upon contemporary theories of thinking and belief. On the continent, and up to the 1850s, *délire*[1] and *Wahn*[2] referred to either madness or delusion (the French term also named 'organic delirium'). Since the sixteenth century, the English word *delusion* has meant 'fixed false opinion or belief with regard to objective things' (*OED*, second edition). This intellectualist definition, albeit narrower, is easier to explore than its continental counterparts.

Delusions before the nineteenth century

Continental views

A good place to start is the French *Encyclopédie* where *délire*[3] is defined as 'an error of judgment by the spirit, during wakefulness, of things known to all.'[4] The author used the same word to refer to delusion and delirium and offered the same causal mechanism for both. Delusion and delirium were to be distinguished on the bases of aetiology, course, intensity, *presence or absence of fever*. All forms of *délire* were 'organic': 'the soul is always in the same state and is not susceptible to change. So, the error of judgment that is *délire* cannot be attributed to the soul but to the disposition of the bodily organs.'[5] Tension and relaxation of nerves led to manic or melancholic *délire*, respectively; and according to the number of nervous fibres involved,[6] *délire* was universal (organic delirium) or particular (delusion). Severity may range from mild to severe and was proportional to the 'strength of internal sensations'. In *délire* internal sensations are stronger than external ones. In a first stage, internal sensations impinge upon consciousness but no judgment is made (i.e. the subject remains insightful); in a second stage, erroneous judgments begin to appear as the subject loses insight; and in a third stage, emotions compound the picture. *Délire* can be manic or melancholic, with or without fever, habitual or accidental, and acute or chronic. D'Aumont, the author of the entry, did not fully distinguish between *délire* as a symptom and as a syndrome, but offered a mechanism for errors of judgment that worked for delusion, delirium, and in the event was to work for the psychoses. There is little doubt that the descriptive psychopathology of the latter is modelled upon that of 'phrensy' or 'delirium' (i.e. on the presence of hallucinations, delusions, insightlessness and the crossing of some notional 'reality' line).

VINCENZO CHIARUGI Working with a simplified version of Faculty Psychology[7] the Italian Chiarugi believed that reasoning and thought were the highest mental functions in the human. 'Delirium' was a dysfunction of thinking and the hallmark of insanity. This he defined as a combination of chronic delirium, primary impairment of perception, and absence of fever: 'sometimes it happens that through thought, ideas originating from internal causes are referred to external causes or they are united, or disunited, or understood improperly at variance from the common-sense of man. Consequently, movements, and the following actions, are the effect of ill-controlled will and of wrong judgment; hence, customs become perverted and the soul is influenced by unusual emotions. This condition of man, that is, this alteration of judgment and consequently of reasoning is what is called delirium'.

Chiarugi was aware of the ambiguities: 'it must be pointed out that this word, taken in its full meaning, deserves many distinctions, and it includes many differences, concerning particularly the source and nature of the cause, and concerning the pattern of the concomitant symptoms.' There were various types of delirium but: 'the main characteristic of the alterations of intellectual functions deserving of this name consists in the errors of judgment and reasoning.' Delirium was caused by organic changes for the soul cannot become diseased: 'How can delirium be called affection of the soul, in view of its [the soul's] unchangeable nature?' 'Where is the seat of delirium?' 'It is evident that true and basic errors of judgment and of reasoning, without any lesion in the organ of the external senses, must be due to a physical disease of the brain.'

Chiarugi offered a conceptual analysis of delusion: 'First of all, the wrong judgment consists of the relations of things, at variance with the proper opinion passed by man's common sense. Secondly, sometimes some false perception arises without there necessarily being a defect of the sensorium. Finally, there occurs in the mind of delirious persons certain unusual, extravagant and sudden associations of ideas.'[8] This analysis contains the very three criteria on which Jaspers was to base his own view on delusion in the twentieth century.

British views

THOMAS HOBBES Thomas Hobbes is an unlikely contributor to the history of delusions but his views on madness were to re-appear[9] in the work of John Locke. The great nonagenarian was intellectually a man of the late sixteenth century, and there is both freshness and simplicity in his views on madness. These can be found hidden in the first Part of *Leviathan*, when he deals with subversive behaviour in crowds.

Hobbes's psychology was influenced by mechanical and geometric analogies. His views on madness are interesting for in his time the question of whether madness resulted from passions or erroneous ideas had not yet been decided. He wrote: 'To have stronger and more vehement Passions for anything, than is ordinarily seen in others, is that which men call Madnesse . . . In summe, all Passions that produce strange and unusuall behaviour, are called by the generall name of Madnesse. But of the severall kinds of Madnesse, he that would take the paines, might enrowle a legion. And if the Excesses be Madnesse, there is no doubt but the Passions themselves, when they tend to Evill, are degrees of the same.'[10] Hobbes noticed, however, that excited or crazy behaviour was not a necessary feature of madness: 'though the effect of folly, in them that are possessed of an opinion of being inspired, be not visible alwayes in one man, by any very extravagant action, that proceedeth from such passion.'[11]

Instead, Hobbes suggested, delusions were a hallmark of madness: 'If some man in Bedlam should entertaine you with sober discourse; and you desire in taking leave, to know what he were, that you might another time requite his civility; and he should tell you, he were God the father; I think you need expect no extravagant action for argument of his Madnesse.'[12] Hobbes contrasted the old with the new: 'The opinions of the world, both in antient and later ages, concerning the cause of Madnesse, have been two. Some, deriving them from the Passions; some, from Dæmons,[13] or Spirits, either good, or bad, which they thought might enter into man, possesse him, and move his organs in such strange, and uncouth manner, as mad-men use to do.'[14] He was referring here to the controversy between 'emotive' and 'intellectualist' views of madness.[15]

JOHN LOCKE In his edition of the *Essay*, A.C. Fraser suggested that Locke showed ignorance of Hobbes's views on the association of ideas, and that: 'Locke, midway chronologically between Hobbes and Hartley introduces 'association' not, as they did, to explain human knowledge, but with the opposite intent of accounting for human errors.'[16] This is illustrated by Locke's view on madness.[17] When dealing with the 'abstract faculty' he asks: 'How far idiots are concerned in the want or weakness of any, or all of the foregoing faculties, an exact observation of their several ways of faltering would no doubt discover. For those who either perceive but dully, or retain the ideas that come into their minds but ill, who cannot readily excite or compound them, will have little matter to think on.'[18] Locke lists four causes of mental dysfunction: input, retention, reflection and retrieval, and suggests that 'naturals' are affected in all four: 'In fine, the defect of naturals seems to proceed from want of quickness, activity, and motion in the intellectual faculties, whereby they are deprived of reason.'[19] Whether or not Locke read Hobbes on madness is unknown. But when referring to the fact that madmen may look normal, he offers an example redolent of Hobbes:[20] 'Hence it comes to pass that a man who is very sober, and of a right understanding in all other things, may in one particular one be as frantic as any in Bedlam.'[21]

In an oft-quoted comparison, Locke wrote: 'whereas madmen, on the other side, seem to suffer by the other extreme. For they do not appear to me to have lost the faculty of reasoning, but having joined together some ideas very wrongly, they mistake them for truths; and they err as men do that argue right from wrong principles. For, by the violence of their imaginations, having taken their fancies for realities, they make right deductions from them.'[22] But why should madmen 'join together some ideas very wrongly'? Where did the defect lie? One writer has interpreted Locke as saying that madness consists 'in a failure to distinguish between imagining and remembering. The madman thinks that he is remembering when he is only imagining.'[23]

Locke suggested two mechanisms for the generation of delusions: 'if either by any sudden very strong impression, or long fixing his fancy upon one sort of thoughts, incoherent ideas have been cemented together so powerfully, so as to remain united.'[24] 'Thus you shall find a distracted man fancying himself a king, with a right inference require suitable attendance, respect, and obedience: others who have thought themselves made of glass, have used caution necessary to preserve such brittle bodies.'[25]

In a chapter inserted in the fourth edition of the *Essay*, Locke suggested what can be considered as a 'continuity view' of madness: 'There is scarce any one that does not observe something that seems odd to him, and is in itself really extravagant, in the opinions, reasonings, and actions of other men' 'this sort of unreasonableness is usually imputed to education and prejudice, and for the most part truly enough, though that reaches not the bottom of the disease, nor shows distinctly enough whence it rises, or wherein it lies' 'I shall be pardoned for calling it by so harsh a name as madness.'[26]

Locke also offered one of the earliest associationistic models of delusions: 'Some of our ideas have a natural correspondence and connection with one another: it is the office and excellency of our reason to trace these, and hold them together in that union and correspondence ... beside this there is another connection of ideas wholly owing to chance or custom. Ideas that in themselves are not all akin, come to be so united in some men's minds.'[27] This view was to hold sway until the middle of the nineteenth century.

DAVID HARTLEY One of the great eighteenth century associationists,[28] Hartley complemented Locke's view with a neurophysiological mechanism[29] and defined madness as an 'imperfection of the rational faculty'. He also supported the 'continuity view': 'it is impossible to fix precise limits, and to determine where soundness of mind ends, and madness begins.'[30] Examples of failures in the rational faculty were erroneous judgments in children and idiots, dotage, drunkenness, deliriums (organic), repetitive ideas, violent passions, melancholy and madness. Hartley suggested that: 'the causes of madness are of two kinds: bodily and mental. That which arises from bodily causes is nearly related to drunkenness, and to the deliriums attending distempers. That from mental causes is of the same kind with temporary alienation of the mind during violent passions, and with the prejudices of opinionativeness, which much application to one set of ideas only occasions.'[31] Both causes operated together and delusions were the central feature of true madness.

Hartley suggested a mechanism for the formation of delusions: 'thus suppose a person, whose nervous system is disordered, to turn his thoughts *accidentally* to some barely possible good or evil. If the nervous disorder falls in with this, it increases the vibrations[32] belonging to its ideas so much, as to give it a reality, a connection with self. For we distinguish the recollection and anticipation of things relating to ourselves, from those of things relating to other persons, chiefly by the difference of strength in the vibrations, and in their coalescences with each other' (my italics).[33]

WILLIAM BATTIE This eighteenth century physician[34] applied Hartley's vibratory mechanism to insanity. Battie rejected the view that the brain was a gland, that nerves were hollow, and that sensation was due to the circulation of a nervous fluid. His view was that the 'medullary substance' was *solid* and sensation occurred as the result of pressure on the nerves.[35] He defined madness in terms of sensory delusions: 'no one ever [doubts] whether the perception of objects not really existing or not really corresponding to the senses be a certain sign of madness. Therefore, deluded imagination is not only an indisputable but an essential character of madness' 'that man and that man alone is properly mad, who is fully and unalterably persuaded of the existence or of the appearance of any thing, which either does not exist or does not actually appear to him, and who behaves accordingly to such erroneous persuasion.'[36]

Insanity is preceded by 'nervous overexcitation' (Battie called it anxiety) and followed by 'nervous insensitivity'. Without any external stimulus, the subject may 'see' fire or 'hear' sounds (i.e. have hallucinations and refer them to an external cause): this was 'original' madness. Or an anomalous internal stimulus to his nerves could cause similar experiences: this was 'consequential' madness. The latter, posed a problem to Battie. Why only some 'pathological' stimuli caused delusions? He wrote: 'No external cause whatever can be supposed capable of exciting delusive any more than true perceptions, except such cause acts materially upon the nerve thereby disordered, and that *with force sufficient* to alter the former arrangements of its medullary particles. Which force necessarily implies impulse and pressure in delusive sensation, in the same manner and order as it does in the perception of objects really corresponding thereto.'[37] This meant that the anomalous stimulus had to be specific: 'every sort and degree of pressure does not always and unavoidably produce consequential madness. For the nerves may suffer external impulse, and yet the pressure thereby occasioned either may not have force sufficient to excite any idea at all; or may act with too great a force and in so shocking a manner as to dissolve or greatly disunite the medullary matter.'[38]

Battie did not specify: 'what this particular sort and degree of pressure is, which is capable of creating delusive sensation, we are not able to ascertain; because the *different circumstances of the unknown subject acted upon* will make the nervous effect variable' (my italics).[39] This is the nearest Battie got to including 'personality variables' in the development of delusions.

It has been suggested that: 'taking his cue from the physiology of sensation, [Battie] defined madness as deluded imagination, a view contrary to the one generally held that it was a manifestation of 'vitiated judgement.'[40] This is not altogether accurate: Battie believed that random *ideas* might set the nerves vibrating at a certain rate (i.e. cause particular sensations) which in turn lead to madness.

WILLIAM CULLEN William Cullen[41] narrowed down the boundaries of 'insanity', particularly those set by Sauvages and Sagar. The 'vesanias' included disorders characterized by 'erroneous judgments' and hallucinations. On delusions he wrote: 'another circumstance, commonly attending delirium, is a very unusual association of ideas. As, with respect to most of the affairs of common life, the ideas laid up in the memory are, in most men, associated in the same manner; so a very unusual association, in any individual must prevent his forming the ordinary judgment of those relations which are the most common foundation of association in the memory: and therefore this unusual and commonly hurried association of ideas, usually is, and may be considered as a part of delirium.'[42] 'In particular, it may be considered as a certain mark of a general morbid affection of the intellectual organs, it being an interruption or perversion of the ordinary operations of memory, the common and necessary foundation of the exercise of judgment' 'delirium, then, may be more shortly defined – in a person awake, a false judgment arising from perceptions of imagination, or from false recollection, and commonly producing disproportionate emotions.'[43] Cullen distinguished two kinds of delirium: 'as it is combined with pyrexia and comatous affections, or as it is entirely without such a combination. It is the latter case that we name insanity.'[44]

THOMAS ARNOLD The first edition of Arnold's *Observations* was published in 1782; the second, including his reply to critics, in 1806.[45] His debate with Alexander Crichton was less on nosology than on the interpretation of the Lockean distinction between 'idea of sensation' and 'idea of reflexion' and its application to delusion and insanity. Arnold introduced 'notion' for 'idea of reflection', and differentiated between 'notions' and 'ideas': 'the use of the term idea in the extensive sense in which it is used by the great Mr Locke, is unphilosophical' . . . 'is of too great a latitude; and is not consistent with its usual accuracy of discrimination: since idea seems, strictly speaking, to mean the internal representation, or mental perception, of an object of sense only: and that he ought to have distinguished the stores of the human mind into ideas images or phantasms, and mere notions; and to have given some common appellation to the aggregate of both; for though notions are derived from sensations, they certainly are not sensations, nor the direct representatives of sensations, and therefore not ideas.'[46]

Arnold had his own sources and influences: 'Cudworth[47] calls what I term ideas, passive ideas, and phantasms; and what I term notions, he calls noematical or intelligible ideas. The distinction is the same as mine' . . . 'he often calls the latter simply notions or intelligible notions, or conceptions of mind.' . . . 'Bolingbroke[48] uses the distinction of ideas and notions' . . . 'as we compound simple into complex ideas, so the compositions we make may be called more properly, and with less confusion and ambiguity, notions . . .'[49]

Based on such distinction, Arnold divided insanity into 'ideal' or 'notional'. The former is defined as: 'that state of mind in which a person imagines he sees, hears, or otherwise perceives, or converses with, persons or things, which either have no external existence to his senses at that time – or have no such external existence as they are then conceived to have – or, if he perceives external objects as they really exist, has yet erroneous and absurd ideas of his own form, and other sensible qualities – such a state of mind continuing for a considerable time; and being unaccompanied with any violent or adequate degree of fever.' The latter is defined as: 'that state of mind in which a person sees, hears, or otherwise perceives external objects as they really exist, as objects of sense; yet conceives such notions of the powers, properties, designs, state, designation, importance, manner of existence, or the like, of things and persons, of himself or others, as appear obviously, and often grossly erroneous, or unreasonable, to the sober and judicious part of mankind: it is of considerable duration; is never accompanied with any great degree of fever, and very often with no fever at all . . .'[50]

This distinction has been considered as an attempt to separate hallucinations from delusions.[51] Contextualized reading, however, indicates that Arnold unsuccessfully tried to distinguish between hallucination, illusion and delusion. His failure was entirely due to the limitations of empiricist epistemology; indeed, his clash with Crichton was about this very point.

ALEXANDRE CRICHTON Crichton followed, in odd combination, the philosophical ideas of Reid,[52] Moritz,[53] and Maimon;[54] and the physiological views of Unzer.[55] Moritz and Maimon were the editors of the *Magazine zum Erfahrungsseelenkunde* (started in 1783) from which Crichton borrowed much of the clinical material for his *Inquiry*.[56] On delusions,[57] Crichton wrote: 'all delirious people, no matter whether they be manics, or hypochondriacs, or people in the delirium of fever, or of hysteria, differ from those of a sound mind in this respect, that they have certain diseased perceptions and notions in the reality of which they firmly believed, and which consequently become motives of many actions and expression which appear unreasonable to the rest of mankind.'[58] This definition makes three points: that delirium [delusion] is present in both organic and 'functional disorders'; that perceptions and notions are 'diseased' rather than 'erroneous'; and that these symptoms control behaviour.

Crichton felt obliged to explain why he had abandoned the term 'erroneous':[59] 'The expression *diseased perceptions or notions* is here to be preferred to that of *false or erroneous* perceptions which is employed by other authors, first because the ideas in all kinds of delirium whatever, arise from a diseased state of the brain, or nerves, or both, . . . and secondly because the word erroneous does not describe anything peculiar to delirium; for every man, however sane or wise he may be, has some erroneous notions in which he firmly believes, and which often seriously affect his conduct . . .'[60]

Crichton divided 'diseased notions' into two groups which correspond to hallucinations and delusions: 'first, they are diseased perceptions, referred by the patient to some object of external sense; as when he believes he sees, hears, tastes and smells things which have no real existence . . . secondly, they are abstract notions, referrable to the qualities and conditions of persons and things, and his relation to them; as when he imagines that his friends have conspired to kill him; that he is reduced to beggary . . .'[61] Breaking away from Locke's view that erroneous perceptions necessarily lead to delusions, Crichton wrote: 'I presume to assert that the diseases of the external senses do not of necessity produce any aberration of mind. This is a point which must be settled before we proceed a step further; for a great deal of mistake, in regard to the nature of delirium [delusion], appears to have arisen from this source. That diseases of the external senses produce erroneous mental perception, must be allowed; but it *depends on the concurrence of other causes*, whether delirium [delusion] follows' (my italics).[62]

Crichton also distinguished between organic and psychotic hallucinations: 'In very many instances, the person is conscious of the error of the perception which is present in the mind; and in all such cases, therefore, no delirium [delusion] takes place. The lady of a very eminent surgeon, in town, had the muscles of her eyes so much weakened . . . that for some months afterwards could not direct them with the proper corresponding motions to the same object . . . the consequence of this was a number of very strange illusions of sight . . . yet no aberration of reason followed.'[63] 'from which it may be concluded, that although one of the most constant phenomena of insanity, and of all deliria, is erroneous perception, yet the cause or nature of the delirium is not to be sought for in that circumstance alone.'[64]

Crichton did not expand upon his view that hallucinations might lead to delusions if concurrent factors were present. The nearest he came to doing so is his section on aetiology where he resorts to the old hypothesis of changes in the level of nervous fluids and irritability. He suggested that delusions originating from internal sensations (when external ones are attenuated) were weaker and shorter lasting than those generated by external hallucinations.[65]

The first half of the nineteenth century

French-speaking psychiatry

The year 1800 is an artificial line of demarcation, for alienists like Pinel, Fodéré, and even Esquirol belong, in philosophical persuasion if not in age, to the Enlightenment. Around 1800, 'delirium' referred to insanity, organic delirium, and delusion proper. Their common mechanism was assumed to be a disorder of reasoning and judgment caused by an 'organic disease of the brain'. Organic delirium was different only in that it was accompanied by *fever and was transitory*; insanity was chronic and without fever; and delusion *was not yet recognized as a separate symptom*. Indeed, one of the objectives of this chapter is to describe when and how this recognition took place.

PHILIPPE PINEL[66] Pinel's views on delusions reflect the early reaction of French psychiatry against the intellectualistic ideas of Locke and Condillac.[67] During the earlier stages of his career Pinel was a follower of the 'sensationalism' of Condillac,[68] but later he came under the influence of the Scottish philosophy of Common Sense (via the French spiritualist philosophers of the beginning of the nineteenth century). From this new perspective, he found that both the views of Locke and Condillac were too narrow: 'I have seen at *Bicêtre* a manic patient whose symptoms would remain an enigma if Locke's and Condillac's views on insanity were to be followed.'[69]

Pinel also criticized Cullen's aetiological speculations on delusions: 'But the vain explanations and gratuitous theories that he [Cullen] offers after describing the facts, are they not in opposition to what should be a sober description of the facts? How is one to believe claims as to the movement of blood in the brain?'[70] And then he raised the fundamental point: 'We may justly admire the writings of Locke and none the less accept that his view on mania is wrong when he considers this condition as inseparable from delusions (*délire*) . . . I used to think likewise but I have been surprised to find patients without any impairment of the understanding who are victims of attacks of excitement as if only the affective faculties were involved (*comme si les facultés affectives avoient été seulement lésées*).'[71]

Pinel's concept of mental disorder was eighteenth century in style, i.e. monolithic and with little specification of individual symptoms.[72] He listed only four categories: mania, melancholia, dementia and idiocy, which he outlined by clinical example. In regard to delusions, and when forced to say something more specific, he repeated Locke's view that the faculty of judgment is normal in the insane and that 'any errors originate from the material on which the judgmental operation is performed.'[73] No wonder that Destutt de Tracy wrote that he had 'seen with great satisfaction that the phenomena which he [Pinel] described confirmed the manner in which I have conceived of thought, and are better explained in relation to ideology, by our way of considering our intellectual faculties.'[74]

AUGUSTINE JACOB LANDRÉ-BEAUVAIS Landré-Beauvais[75] believed that: 'as science makes progress, there should be a multiplication of the terms used to name
its various objects, that is, its language should adapt for, as Condillac said, the
perfection of a science is shown in the perfection of its language.'[76] He defined 'sign'
as: 'any phenomenon, any symptom by means of which one can get to know
hidden causes. It relates to the present, to that which has gone and to that which
will come. The sign is, therefore, an apparent effect that informs one of hidden
relationships which can be past, present or future. In summary, the sign is a conclusion drawn by the consciousness [of the physician] of the symptoms observed
by the senses. The sign belongs to the realm of judgment, the symptom to that of
the senses. Signs cannot exist without symptoms. The latter can be recognized by
everyone, the former only by the physician.'[77]

    Landré-Beauvais dealt with *délire* in the section of 'signs relating to the faculty
of understanding': 'the faculty of understanding, whose seat is in the brain, and
which relates to judgment, memory and imagination, is susceptible to lesions which
give rise to important signs of disease; it can be exalted, perverted, diminished or
abolished.' *Délire* was a form of perverted understanding: 'the perversion of the
functions of human understanding leads to: (*a*) the patient joining together ideas
which are incompatible, and taking these combinations as truths;[78] these constitute
diverse forms of *délire*; and (*b*) the patient developing false ideas in regard to one
or to a series of objects.'[79] Landre-Beauvais also described what he called *délire
symptomatique*, i.e. that which appears in the context of a number of brain diseases
(mainly delirious states).

JEAN ÉTIENNE DOMINIQUE ESQUIROL Esquirol's earliest conception of *délire*
included hallucinations and it is unclear whether he thought the latter a sub-type
or cause of *délire*. In his 1814 entry for the *Panckouke Dictionary* he wrote: 'A man
has a *délire* when his sensations are not in keeping with external objects, when his
ideas are not in keeping with his sensations, when his judgments and decisions
(*déterminations*) are not in keeping with his ideas, and when his ideas, judgments
and decisions are independent from his will.'[80] Delusions originated at any stage in
this causal cascade, including the first stage, which included the Esquirolean concept of hallucination: 'false sensations without sensory changes in the organs of
sensations – and hence depending on internal causes – present consciousness with
objects that do not exist and lead to *délire*: such is the state of someone who believes
he is perceiving an object in the external world . . . in fact he will be the sort of
person who, during *délire* will hear clocks ticking and guns firing . . . hallucinations
are the most frequent cause of *délire*'. Consistent with his definition, Esquirol analysed the way in which disorders of synthesis of ideas, memory, and judgment
caused *délire*.[81]

    Esquirol deals with the aetiology and clinical varieties of *délire* in the same old-
fashioned manner as d'Aumont. *Délire* can be febrile or vesanic, agitated or quiet,

original, symptomatic or sympathetic, and mono- and multi-ideational. It can affect self and personality, be related to sensations and ideas and lead to false judgments and bizarre actions; it may even appear as if resulting from a specific impairment of the will.[82]

Esquirol's all-encompassing view influenced French psychiatry for the rest of the century. *Délire* may involve all mental functions (i.e. intellect, emotions and will) and hence is a concept alien to the exclusively intellectualistic British definition of delusions.[83] Interestingly, it echoes the unconventional views of Crichton.[84] Esquirol's cascade model did not go unchallenged; for example, Falret noticed that it lacked the all-important criterion of awareness of illness.[85] Later nineteenth century writers agreed with this comment.[86]

It is also interesting to notice that, in contrast to the many other entries that Esquirol wrote for the *Panckoucke Dictionary* (dementia, demonomania, lypemania, erotomania, insanity, furor, idiocy, hallucinations, mania, monomania, suicide, and mental asylums), the one on *délire* was not included in his late book of 1838.[87] One can only speculate that this was because he no longer agreed with it. In his book Esquirol simply wrote: 'According to Locke, madmen behave like those who having normal reasoning draw false conclusions from false premisses.'[88] In general, he seemed to believe that hallucinations *were* a form of *délire*, but on occasions he also stated that they were different phenomena: 'hallucination is a cerebral or psychological phenomenon that takes shape independently from the senses. It may persist when *délire* has ceased, and vice versa'.[89] According to Ey, Esquirol's views actually 'oscillated' on this issue.[90]

ÉTIENNE GEORGET Georget[91] was, perhaps, the one writer of this period who captured more clearly than anyone else the difficulties involved in defining *délire*: 'the available definitions of *délire* are either vague, unintelligible or incomplete and nonspecific. This is because it is difficult, not to say impossible, fully to distinguish between groups or separate the normal from the pathological, or indeed place boundary stones between reason and *délire*, without feeling that some phenomena do not fit into the groups, that reasonable actions can be seen as *délire*, or *délire* as a reasonable action.'[92] He criticized excessive analytical approaches: 'this difficulty is made worse when these phenomena are studied in isolation, as if they had no connection with one another, instead of considering them as part of the totality of the brain.'

These claims are in sharp contrast with his youthful views of 1820: 'intellectual disorder is the essential and often only feature of insanity: there is no insanity without *délire*.'[93] Georget accepted the division of *délire* into acute (with fever and organic) and chronic (without fever and characteristic of insanity).[94]

JOSEPH GUISLAIN Guislain[95] dealt with *délire* (or *trouble des idées*) in lecture 12 of his *Leçons*. *Idées morbides* were a 'notable aberration of reason, a chronic error in the conceptions, and a disorder of ideas that the patient cannot fight or stop, and in which he regards as reality what are only phantoms of his imagination.'[96] Guislain classified *délire* according to scope and presentation. Delusions could be general (when they involved all ideas) and special (when affected only certain ideas – this he called *monodélire* and *monophrenic* delusion). According to presentation, *délire* could be essential (when it was isolated) and symptomatic (when it appeared with other symptoms and remitted with them).

There could also be situations: 'when reason and imagination were confused by error but the patient was aware that this was a figment of his imagination. This was not a delusion proper and he also called it 'delusion with insight' (*délire avec conscience*) or delusion without delusion (*délire sans délire*). These consisted of persistent thoughts, voices or visions recognized as not real.'[97] Guislain was one of the earliest alienists to classify delusions (and the patients experiencing them) according to *content*: the 'persecuted' (often seen in the deaf), the 'inspired' (erotic, religious, ambitious and hypochondriacal), the 'metamorphic' (who believed to be something they were not), and the 'hallucinated'.[98] During the second half of the century, the content of the delusion was to become the most important classificatory criterion.

JEAN PIERRE FALRET In his 1839 work on delusions, Falret[99] criticized Esquirol and insisted on the need to consider 'lack of insight' as a central criterion. Falret was fully aware of the semantic limitations of the French term *délire*[100] and held original views on the limitations of descriptive psychopathology which, he believed, had gone through three (bad) stages. During the earliest or 'novelistic' period, physicians had focused on the most bizarre and salient behavioural disorders. This meant that only disorders of functions considered as characteristically human (such as thinking) had attracted attention (hence why earlier definitions of insanity had been 'intellectualistic'). The second or 'narrative' period reflected efforts to describe, more or less empirically, whatever symptoms the patient produced. This attitude was naive, for description is 'never theory-free' (pace Jaspers). The third or 'psychological period' was characterized by the belief that psychiatric symptoms are describable in terms of normal psychology; sponsors of this approach, however, often had to 'force' symptoms into the available psychological categories thereby missing their real meaning. Falret sponsored a *fourth approach* based on the contextual description of symptoms; to do this the alienist needed to create special psychopathological categories.[101]

Falret first explored the *extension* of the term: '*délire* includes in its generality all disorders of the intellectual functions whatever their cause, origin and duration; this is why it cannot be used both to name a symptom (common to many diseases) and specific diseases such as *phrénésie*, encephalitis, meningitis, etc.'[102] Next, he criticized Esquirol: 'his definition, although descriptive, does not seem to us to include the essential attributes [of delirium]. It seems to us that a man who is preoccupied, distracted by false judgments, with a weak and capricious will, meets

all of Esquirol's criteria but is not yet in *délire*. What is missing in Esquirol's definition is a 'capital criterion', namely, the absence of awareness that he is wrong,
awareness that he can regain only if the delusion is interrupted.'[103]

Falret supported the 'ancient' view that there were three degrees of *délire*: mild,
easily giving way to reasoning, moderate, but susceptible to interruption by a
strong emotion, and the severe or 'tenacious' form.[104] It was also possible to tell
when the subject might develop *délire*: 'It is only the clever gardener, as Galen has
said, who can tell what plant a seedling will become as soon as it breaks the ground,
the same with the experienced alienist . . . this view of Galen also applies to *délire*.
If there is a great deal of agitation and violence, anyone can diagnose phrenetic or
manic *délire*, but it is far more difficult if all that there is is a minor change in
intellectual functions.'[105]

In regard to the mental function involved in *délire*, Falret wrote: 'psychologists
are busy trying to determine which mental faculty is involved in *délire*. In this
respect, the most respected opinion is that of Esquirol who claims that it is attention.' Falret felt that this might not always be right: 'nevertheless, it seems to me
that trying to isolate faculties in this way is highly arbitrary, and that one cannot
reduce the failure of all mental functions to that of one. Brain physiology, which is
not metaphysical, escapes these subtleties . . . it is not one but all intellectual faculties that are involved.'[106]

Délire was shaped by four factors: (*a*) the state of the brain, (*b*) the intellectual
and moral character of the patient, (*c*) circumstances surrounding the occasion
when *délire* had started, and (*d*) ongoing sensations (both internal and external).[107]
His choice of factors was consistent with his theoretical view that context was
always important. In this respect, he wrote: 'an attentive analysis of the characteristics of *délire* may reveal both its organic causes and circumstances of onset . . .
délire may reflect the most intimate preoccupations and emotions of the individual.'
Indeed, 'the features of *délire* may help to recognize what parts of the subject's
mental organization are suffering the most. Practitioners have given attention to
the relationships between *délire* and the character of the subject, and his intellectual
and moral make up . . . these same features may also give an idea of what organs
are involved, and what the morbid agent (*agent morbifique*) may be.'[108]

Against his initial intentions, Falret drifted in this work from treating *délire* as a
symptom (i.e. delusion) to seeing it as a disease (i.e. delirium). This is an important
indication of how close the two concepts were in the mind of nineteenth century
alienists, and how much the shaping of the modern concept of psychoses depended,
as has repeatedly been stated in this book, upon the phenomenology of delirium.

JULES GABRIEL FRANÇOIS BAILLARGER AND *DELUSIONAL PERCEPTION* On the
occasion of differentiating false judgments of normal sensations from illusions
proper, this great French alienist[109] offered (many years before Jaspers)[110] a clear
account of *delusional perception*. He believed that, in the former case, there was no

'illusion' for the *perception was normal*, i.e. patients only interpret 'in a particular manner' a sensation which was real, making a false judgment and developing a 'delusional idea on the occasion of a [normal] sensation'. In other words, he was here referring to 'false interpretations of sensations which were normal'. Baillarger reported the case of a patient who climbed a wall because he interpreted an (innocent) gesture of the administrator of the asylum as an order to do so. The gesture had actually been made, but a different interpretation was attached to it by the patient. He also reported a second patient who interpreted numbers written on a piece of material as 'meaning something special', and words in a letter as meaning that 'the patient had to be given special treatment'.[111] Ten years before the first edition of Jaspers' *General Psychopathology'*, Jules Séglas also emphasized the distinction between delusional perception and delusional idea; Jaspers did not quote him.[112]

ERNEST CHARLES LASÈGUE In 1852, Lasègue[113] introduced the view that paranoid delusions (*délire de persécutions*) constituted a separate disorder. He classified delusions into general and partial and believed that further subdivisions were unwarranted: 'delusions do not have either the homogeneity suggested by textbooks nor the variety hinted at by dramatists.'[114] Typical persecutory delusions were, however, a stable and 'new form'. Auditory hallucinations might be present but were neither cause or effect of the delusions. Indeed, the latter were primary phenomena: 'Persecutory delusions are not the consequence of any particular form of character; they appear in subjects with different mood, intelligence and social class; they are not seen in people younger than 28 and are more common in the female.'[115] Two years before his death, Lasègue proposed that alcoholic delirium (*délire alcoolique*) was a form of dreaming.[116] In their classical work, Taty and Toy[117] acknowledged Lasègue as the creator of the concept of persecutory delusions which was to become one of the pillars of French nosography until the second half of twentieth century.[118]

JACQUES JOSEPH MOREAU (DE TOURS) Until the 1850s, it was generally believed that delusions were not seen in the 'sane' (i.e. that they were always 'pathological'). Moreau de Tours[119] undermined this belief by suggesting that there was a 'continuity' between normality and alienation. To make his argument work, Moreau described subjects suffering from 'intermediate' mental aberrations such as those temporarily intoxicated with hashish. Their assessment showed that délire and hallucinations had in common a *fait primordial*: 'Thus, guided by observation . . . I believe to have identified the primitive source of all basic forms of *délire* . . . this is the fact that generates all other facts . . . I have called it *primordial fact*.' (my italics)[120]

This analysis required that symptoms were 'psychologized': 'I have postulated that *délire* has a psychological nature, identical to dreams.'[121] But the same delusional convictions (*convictions délirantes*) 'so common in mental alienation [were also seen] in hachisch intoxication.'[122] Moreau reported that once, after taking a large dose of the drug, he had been able to experience in himself a 'primordial change' (a state of 'excited imagination').

Based on these observations, Moreau went on to write: 'Locke has somewhere said, in regard to madmen, that 'they do not appear to have lost the faculty of reasoning, but having joined together some ideas very wrongly, they mistake them for truths' [but] 'is there any need to show how insufficient this view is? . . . [Locke] does not say, for example, how the anomalous joining together of ideas has taken place nor does he explain how patients allow themselves to be carried away by the false ideas and are impervious to reasoning' . . . 'is it not a fact of common observation that *we all have wrong associations of ideas* but do not allow ourselves to be guided by them?' (my italics).[123]

In 1859, Moreau also wrote on the clinical presentation of *délire*. Because insanity is continuous with normality, intermediate states do exist: 'Nature does not recognize any differentiations, here as everywhere else, *non facit saltus*. Manifestations of subtle mental activity can be found anywhere along the continuum . . . human intelligence is found operating both in the sane and in the madman . . . the mental faculties are not affected in all to the same degree.'[124] According to the function involved, four groups of patients could be identified: general sensitivity (the hallucinated), imagination (the fantasists), intelligence (the deluded) and combinations thereof.[125] There was also an 'intermediate' group: 'there is a class of subjects who should not be confused either with the sane or the alienated . . . this class finds its origin in the laws of heredity.'[126]

Moreau's contribution is very important. He conceived of delusion as a psychological phenomenon similar to a dream which could follow the 'excited imagination' caused by hashish intoxication. There was a continuity between the sane and the madman for 'excited imagination' could be experienced by anyone.[127] Moreau believed that his research with hashish had allowed him to identify the 'primordial fact' that led to delusions and hallucinations.

LOUIS JEAN FRANÇOIS DELASIAUVE Delasiauve[128] dealt with delusions in the context of his classification of mental disorders. The latter, he divided into general and partial, and the partial into pseudo-monomanias, partial insanities, and *délires*. His concept of *délire* fell between symptom and syndrome and included three forms: 1. isolated, fixed and systematized, constituting the central feature of the monomanias, 2. perceptual (*délire perceptif*) including hallucinations and illusions, and 3. moral, affective and instinctive.[129] Monomanic delusions were typical of the genre: 'False convictions, taking their power from mental impressions, keep themselves hidden in the mind before they dare to manifest themselves. Once they do come out, however, their action is tyrannical, they are impervious to objection and surround themselves of childish defences . . . incurability is the rule, cure the exception . . .

the main types originate from: (*a*) chimeric or ill-judged perceptions, (*b*) extravagant conceptions, often emerging from affective or moral experiences, and (*c*) other instincts'.[130]

The other forms of *délire* proposed by Delasiauve are difficult to fathom and illustrate the complexity of this notion in French psychiatry; for what is one to make of *délire instinctif*? Delasiauve explained: 'this is no longer about false beliefs. Intellectual functions are normal. The patient is under the control of his depraved appetites, by impulses so powerful that they push him ineluctably to violence, homicide, suicide, stealing, arson, and sexual crimes.'[131] Is the concept of *délire* being used here in a metaphorical way? Not necessarily. It is likely that there is a halo of connotations around *délire* that makes it hard to understand, let alone translate into English.

German-speaking psychiatry

ERNST FREIHERR VON FEUCHTERSLEBEN To this great Austrian physician[132] 'delirium is the erroneous combination of manifold ideas often united with the patient's own inclinations, without his being aware of the error or being able to overcome it. This erroneous idea gives rise to foolish speeches and actions.'[133] He proposed that delirium could be subdivided according to polar dichotomies: fixed vs wandering, quiet vs excited, cheerful vs wild, and acute vs chronic. Acute was usually accompanied by fever; chronic was not, and hence it could be confused with insanity.[134] Feuchtersleben had clear views on this: 'It will readily appear, from the preceding observations that the oft-agitated question, whether delirium and insanity be identical or not, is a superfluous question. It has been most frequently answered thus: that acute delirium with fever is to be distinguished from chronic without fever, which latter is to be designated insanity. But the *duration* of a state can by no means determine its essence; a corporeal disease cannot, because it is of long duration, be called a mental disease, and vice versa; nor can the presence or absence of fever, which is possible in every condition, decide the matter. . . Delirium therefore is not identical with insanity in its more *extended* signification' (my italics).[135] Delirium was thus a transitional state between physical disease and mental illness.

'Fixed delusions', Feuchtersleben described as secondary to the 'phantasms of coenæsthesis',[136] i.e. as pathological interpretations of somatic sensations, hallucinations, emotions, etc. They 'begin with a caprice, and represent a sensation or an impulse, which has absorbed the entire personality of the man; it is characterized by the predominance of one idea, or of a series of ideas constantly recurring.'[137] He dismissed the content of the delusion as unimportant: 'Whether this idea or series of ideas be sorrowful or joyous, is not essential . . . it is equally unessential what idea governs the patient, whether it concern body or mind; whether it be religious, political or scientific, etc. the disease consists in this: that some one idea is able to govern him, and therefore we can no more establish a genuine scientific division here, according to the object, than in the case of the impulses.'[138]

Feuchtersleben indicated that the content of the delusion may refer to the past, present or future and perceptively suggested that: 'most frequently to the future, where the reality of the present and the remembrance of the past do not put in their protest.'[139] Next, he classified delusions according to whether they are referred to the body or personality, or whether they are delusions of ambition, religion, love, or suicide.[140] In regards to causes he wrote: 'Pathological anatomy teaches us neither more nor less respecting fixed delusion than it does respecting folly. Sometimes the same abnormal conditions are met with, and sometimes none at all.'[141]

WILHELM GRIESINGER Griesinger[142] did not have a large clinical experience in psychiatry but showed an uncanny capacity to perceive connections, and re-interpret published cases in terms of the philosophical psychology he borrowed from Herbart. His textbook was one of the first to include a section on the 'elementary disorders of mental disease' (*Elementarstörungen der psychischen Krankheiten*).

He dealt with 'false contents of thought: delusional ideas' (*Falscher Inhalt der Gedanken: Wahnideen*) in the section on 'anomalies of thought'.[143] Griesinger reminded his readers that insanity was not necessarily accompanied by delusions (as an example, he mentions *Gemüthswahnsinn*, or emotional insanity). A supporter of the 'unitary psychosis' concept (melancholia led to mania and this to dementia),[144] he believed that all delusions had a 'secondary' origin: 'experience teaches us that, in the great majority of cases, the mental derangement does not cease here, that special insane ideas are developed . . . the mental affection which at the beginning was only an insanity of the feelings and emotions becomes also an insanity of the intellect' (*Irresein der Intelligenz*).[145] Delusions, therefore, are always 'secondary: 'the false ideas and conclusions, which are attempts at explanation and vindications of the actual disposition in its effects are spontaneously developed in the diseased mind according to the law of causality.'[146] For a moment, Griesinger pondered over the generalizability of this claim: 'All false ideas, however, are not to be considered as thus explicable; many originate with the fortuitous abruptness of hallucinations, or of those peculiar thoughts which spontaneously may intrude into the normal mind. They often originate from sensory disturbances, from dreams or from external stimuli; their persistence, depending on the mood of the patient or if the representation (*Vorstellungen*) can be tied up to some ongoing mental fact. We will find, however, that many such ideas are related to hallucinations, which are not that obvious.'[147]

Then diagnostic criteria are listed: 'the insane ideas of patients are distinguished from the erroneous views of the normal not only by the circumstances of their relation to the diseased subject himself, but also by numerous other characteristics: they are always part of a general disturbance of mental processes (e.g. emotions), they are opposed to views formerly held by the patient, he cannot get rid of them, they resist correction by the testimony of the senses and the understanding, they depend upon a disturbance of the brain which is also expressed in other symptoms (sleep disorders, hallucinations).'

Griesinger's views are extremely important. He considered delusions as 'symptoms', offered ten criteria to differentiate them from the erroneous beliefs of the normal, and proposed that all delusions were secondary to other morbid phenomena (e.g. pathological affect or hallucinations).[148]

English-speaking psychiatry

JOHN HASLAM Haslam's[149] views on insanity and delusions betray a great deal of clinical experience. But he also had linguistic interests, for example, in the Northern languages. On the etymology and implications of the diagnosis of *madness* he wrote: 'the importance of investigating *the original meaning of words* must be evident when it is considered that the law of this country impowers persons of the medical profession to confine and discipline those to whom the term mad or lunatic can fairly be applied. Instead of endeavouring to discover an *infallible definition of madness,* which I believe will be found impossible, as it is an attempt to comprise, in a few words, the wide range and mutable character of this Proteus disorder: much more advantage would be obtained if the circumstances could be precisely defined under which it is justifiable to deprive a human being of his liberty . . .'[150]

His views on delusion show the influence of both John Locke and Dugald Stewart:[151] 'But as madness, by some, has been exclusively held to be a disease of the imagination, and by others, to be a defect of the judgment; considering these as separate and independent powers or faculties of the intellect; it is certainly worth the trouble to inquire, whether such states of mind did ever exist as original and *unconnected disorders.* With respect to imagination, there can be but little difficulty; yet this will so far *involve* the judgment and memory, that it will not be easy to institute a distinction. If a cobbler should suppose himself an emperor, this supposition, may be termed an elevated flight, or an extensive stretch of imagination, but it is likewise a great defect in his judgment, to deem himself that which he is not, and is certainly an equal lapse of his recollection, to forget what he really is' (my italics).[152] This analysis makes the novel point (in early nineteenth century psychiatry) that there is an interaction between mental faculties, and that delusions result only when all three mental functions are affected.

Haslam also offered an interesting analysis of the relationship between hallucinations and delusions: 'By perception I understand, with Mr Locke, the apprehension of sensations; and after a very diligent enquiry of patients who have recovered from the disease, and from an attentive observation of those labouring under it, I have not frequently found, that insane people perceive falsely the objects which have been presented to them'. 'It is well known, that manics'[153] often suppose they have seen and heard those things, which really did not exist at the time; but even this I should not explain by any disability, or error of the perception; since it is by no means the province of the perception to represent unreal existences of the mind. It must therefore be sought *elsewhere*; most probably in the *senses*.'[154] In the early nineteenth century, 'senses' referred to 'reason' rather than to the windows of perception.[155] Haslam was here suggesting, as early as 1809, that hallucinations could, in fact, be *perceptual or sensory* delusions.

JAMES COWLES PRICHARD Prichard's[156] *Treatise* is a patchwork of cases and ideas often borrowed from others. Even his concept of 'moral insanity' (for which he is much quoted) is a combination of the French concept of *emotional monomanie* and some interesting observations of depressive cases: it has little to do with the current concept of 'psychopathy'.[157] The same is the case in respect to his views on delusion which were taken from French sources. This creates an interesting ambiguity in his book for he often conflates delirium, madness and delusion.

Prichard believed that actual disorders of sensation and perception (hallucinations and illusions) were not, in fact, common in insanity (on this he followed Haslam who, as we have seen, put forward the view that some hallucinations were in fact delusional in origin): 'That insanity does not consist in disease of the sensitive or perceptive powers appears the more clearly when we compare the state of the lunatic with that of individuals who have really laboured under affections of the organs of sense, giving rise to false impression on the sensorium.'[158] Then he asked: 'But in what disturbance of the understanding itself does insanity consist? What particular intellectual process is that which undergoes the peculiar modification characteristic of madness? And what precisely is this modification?'

To answer these questions, Prichard abandoned British empiricism for the views of Guislain (and through him) those of Pierre Laromiguière.[159] This is perhaps his best contribution to the British concept of delusion, as the great French philosopher, more than any other during his period, sponsored *an active, constructivist view* of the intellectual functions. Laromiguière's influence on Prichard shows clearly: 'Perhaps we may observe in general, that the power of judging and of reasoning [two of the three active functions in Laromiguière's philosophy] does not appear to be so much impaired in madness as *the disposition to exercise it* on certain subjects' (my italics).[160] And in respect to the effect of this view on delusions: 'There is often a manifest unwillingness to admit any evidence which appears contradictory to the false notion impressed upon the belief, while great ingenuity is even displayed in the attempt to find arguments which may seem to render it more reasonable.'[161]

Prichard's adoption of the Continental notion of partial insanity also drew his attention to the concept of 'insight' and its failures, indeed, he was one of the first British alienists to do so: 'It has been well observed by M. Georget, that insane persons uniformly entertain a full conviction of their perfect sanity ... in a word they believe themselves in perfect health ... yet, as the same author observes, there are some patients who are well aware of the disorder of their thoughts or of their affections, and who are deeply afflicted at not having sufficient strength of will to repress it.'[162] In this regard, Prichard noticed that there was 'a form of mental derangement in which the intellectual faculties appear to have sustained little or no injury, while the disorder is manifested principally or alone, in the state of the feelings, temper or habits.'[163] He was referring here to affective and volitional insanity, French notions referring to insanity unaccompanied by delusions.

JOHN BUCKNILL AND DANIEL HACK TUKE In 1858, these authors wrote: 'The word delusion is generally used by English writers, to include all the various *errors* to which reference has been made, whenever those errors are not corrected by the understanding' (my italics).[164] Bucknill and Tuke considered it advantageous to distinguish delusions from hallucinations and illusions, and defined the former as: 'a person may (*independently* of false inductions) have certain false notions and ideas, which have no immediate reference to the senses . . . as for example, when he believes himself or other person to be a king or a prophet; or that there is a conspiracy against his life; or that he has lost his soul. Or as another example, he may believe himself to be a tea-pot, without seeing or otherwise perceiving any change in his form. In all examples under this last head, a man is *necessarily* insane. He cannot have a false belief (not simply a false induction), but the result of disease, and unconnected with the senses, without the mind itself being unsound. When there is no pre-morbid perception, but only a false conception, the French employ the expressions, *conceptions fausses*, *conceptions délirantes*, and *convictions délirantes*.'[165] That their analysis was influenced by French ideas is not surprising, as during this period Continental influence was marked on British psychiatry. This is confirmed by Blount who in 1856 was able to write: 'we have been as much pleased with the general clearness in the use of these terms in all the French works we have studied, as we have been disappointed in our own authors.'[166]

The second half of the nineteenth century

French-speaking psychiatry

AXENFELD In keeping with the wide French notion of *délire*, Axenfeld distinguished between *délire de paroles* and *délire de action*, which he described in association with hysteria.[167] Attacks of *délire* could occur as part of an attack of grand hysteria or as a *substitute* for convulsions:[168] '*délire* or hysterical insanity[169] breaks out often without a cause or as a result of emotional strain, overwork or troubles with menstruation or pregnancy, accidents, severe physical disease, etc.'[170] By *délire de paroles* Axenfeld meant a form of 'incoherent overtalkativeness' that followed a convulsion, often lasting for hours and which was replaced by a *délire de action*, i.e. by exaggerated and aimless movements, a sort of 'ambulatory insanity' (*folie ambulatoire*) during which the 'patient ran about, climbed walls, jumped from roof to roof, absconded, hid behind corners, etc.' This *délire* was 'different from ordinary excitement in epileptics who are confused and have no idea of what they are doing.'[171]

Hysterical subjects had insight (*conscience du délire*) and their behaviour was reminiscent of alcoholic delirium in that it was accompanied by hallucinations (whose content reflected their ongoing preoccupations). Following Lasègue's view that the delirium of alcoholics was a dream, Axenfeld suggested that the same applied to 'hysterical delirium': 'it is observed, in fact, that in some cases hysterical delirium takes the form of a somnambulic state in that subjects are insensitive to external stimuli and show amnesia after the episode.'[172] Other clinical features of hysterical delirium included: exaltation of intelligence, flight of ideas, fixed ideas, automatisms, and erotic behaviour. Axenfeld's idiosyncratic use of *délire* not only reflects the fact that he was a general physician rather than an alienist but also that the concept itself remained blurred to the end of the century.

BENJAMIN BALL AND ANTOINE RITTI The crucial issue for these great alienists was to 'delimit *délire* from the normal state.'[173] *Délire* they loosely defined as: 'all morbid disorders of the psychological state, whether affecting the intellectual or emotional spheres, and the acts of will.'[174] Influenced by the emerging concept of unconscious cerebration,[175] Ball and Ritti wrote: 'All observers are now in agreement with Carpenter, Laycock, Onimus, Luys, etc. that there exist a number of manifestations of cerebral activity – frequently very complex – that constitute what has been called unconscious cerebration (*cérébration inconscient*) which differs from conscious and voluntary cerebral function in that it occurs automatically. This automatism of some cognitive acts is kept going by habit and transmitted by heredity. Cerebral automatism is of great help to conscious work; but it must not be allowed to get the upper hand as its preponderance would cause the anarchy that is *délire*.'[176] In attributing *délire* to cerebral automatism, these authors also acknowledged the influence of Baillarger.[177]

Then, Ball and Ritti re-affirm the wide French view: 'Which are the psychological functions affected in delusion? We know that psychological life includes four orders of functions: sensation, thinking, emotion, and action. Each of these can be impaired, so that there can be a sensory delusion (*délire sensoriel*), an intellectual delusion (*délire de la pensée*), an emotional delusion (*délire de sentiments*) and a delusion of acts (*délire des actes ou délire impulsif*).'[178] In the first group, Ball and Ritti included hallucinations; in the second, typical delusions (the *primordial Deliren* of the Germans) and obsessions; in the third, anhedonia-like experiences, and also made-emotions; and in the fourth, impulsions.[179] Their four criteria for *délire* were: spontaneity, bizarreness, conviction, and personalized meaning of the idea.[180]

Délire was subdivided into non-vesanic (delirium) and vesanic; the later corresponding to insanity: 'we considered as vesanic those patients with delusions who on post-mortem are found to have no lesions in the brain.'[181] Vesanic delusions can be general or partial, the former referring to generalized episodes of madness, the latter to hallucinations and delusions proper.

Lastly, Ball and Ritti localized delusions on the cortex: 'the cells of the cortical mantle, we are told, are the organ of intelligence; it is, therefore, right that to their disorder, whether anatomical or physiological, the production of delusions should be attributed.'[182] This view departs from Carpenter's mechanism of 'unconscious cerebration' which concerned subcortical structures.[183]

JULES COTARD Cotard[184] wrote two original papers on 'delusion'. *De l'origin psychosensorielle ou psychomotrice du délire* was read before the *Société Médico-Psychologique* in 1887; and *De l'origin psychomotrice du délire* was read on his behalf before the 1889 Paris Congress of Alienists, thirteen days before his untimely death.

In the 1887 paper, Cotard puts forward the view that the classification of delusions according to theme or level of systematization is insufficient, and that the criterion should be the physical state of the subject concerned.[185] Building on the voluntaristic psychology of Maine de Biran, he suggested that delusions were a cognitive expression of *motor function*. Thus, states in which motor behaviour was increased (e.g. mania) influenced the colour and content of delusions (i.e. made them grandiose), whilst nihilistic delusions were generated by motor retardation as seen in depressed patients.[186]

Cotard based these ideas on the view, popular at the time, that motor and sensory aphasia resulted from a loss of motor and sensory 'images' of words, respectively. He believed that images were in fact present in *all motor and sensory activities*, and hence the loss of 'mental vision' (which he thought was characteristic of psychotic melancholia) resulted in a loss of images: 'it can be concluded that the impossibility of invoking images, the loss of mental vision, both frequent symptoms in melancholia, might be explained by a psychical paralysis as well as by an anaesthesia of the sentiments.'[187] The important point in Cotard's speculation, is his emphasis on the relationship between motor activity, thinking, and mental content; observations which in the 1920s (in the wake of the epidemics of encephalitis lethargica)[188] were to develop in the French notion of 'bradyphrenia'.

British psychiatry

HUGHLINGS JACKSON'S CONCEPT OF DELUSION The only original view on delusion to appear in Britain during the second half of the nineteenth century was put forward by a neurologist, Hughlings Jackson,[189] as an offshoot of his model for symptom generation. The latter was built on four conceptual pillars: (*a*) evolution (and its counterpart, dissolution), (*b*) localization of higher mental functions on the cortex, (*c*) the doctrine of 'concomitance' (a crude form of dualism), and (*d*) the assumption that mental and brain functions were organized in a hierarchical manner.[190] Jackson had tried his model in stroke and epilepsy where *negative* symptoms (caused by the abolition of a function) and *positive* symptoms (caused by the adaptative release of inhibited functions) can be easily demonstrated.

Jackson considered the concept of 'mental disorder' as 'nonsense' and hence believed that mental symptoms such as obsessions, dementia and delusions should be explained by the same model:[191] 'illusions, delusions and extravagant conduct, and abnormal emotional states in an insane person signify *evolution* not *dissolution*; they signify evolution going on in what remains intact of the mutilated highest centres – in what disease, affecting so much dissolution, has spared.'[192] or 'disease only causes the (physical condition for the) negative element of the mental condition; the positive mental element, say a *delusion*, obviously an elaborate delusion, however absurd it might be, *signifies activities of healthy nervous arrangements*, signifies evolution going on in what remains intact of the highest cerebral centres.' (my italics)[193]

Jackson proposed a specific explanation for delusions. In this regard the issue was: what function had to be abolished and which 'released' for the delusion to appear? He suggested that: 'certain very absurd and persistent delusions are owing to fixation of grotesque fancies of dreams in cases where a morbid change in the brain happens suddenly, or when one increases suddenly, during sleep.'[194] This explanation was perhaps plausible for organic delirium in cerebral vascular accidents or epilepsy, but was it valid for ordinary delusions? Jackson never said. In regards to the function that is abolished he wrote: 'Suppose a patient imagines, to take one delusion as a sample of his mental condition, that his nurse is his wife. It is not enough to dwell only on the positive element, that he supposes the person attending on him is his wife, for this delusion of necessity implies the coexisting negative element that he does not know her to be his nurse (or some woman not his wife). His 'not-knowing' is a sample of the result of disease (dissolution of A); his 'wrong- knowing' is a sample of the outcome of what is left intact of his highest cerebral centres.'[195]

Jackson's model is interesting for he proposed that delusions were not themselves a manifestation of diseased brain tissue but the expression of healthy tissue released by the abolition of function in some higher centre. This view differed markedly from any which was (and is) being currently entertained. Jackson was more influential abroad than in his own country.[196] His views found fertile ground in France, particularly in the work of Ribot[197] and Janet,[198] and survived until after the Second World War in the work of Henri Ey.[199]

The twentieth century

French-speaking psychiatry

DÉLIRE AND ITS TYPES By the early twentieth century, four sources for delusion were recognized in French psychiatry: hallucinations (*délire hallucinatoire*), intuition (*intuition délirante*), interpretation (*interpretation délirante or délire d'intérpretation*), and fabulation or imagination (*délire d'imagination*).[200] The first has been dealt with in the chapter on hallucinations, the other three will be briefly mentioned here.

In 1892, Magnan and Sérieux developed the notion of 'chronic delusional state with systematic evolution' (*Le Délire Chronique á Èvolution Systématique*).[201] It comprised four stages: incubation (delusional mood), crystallization of the persecutory delusions, appearance of grandiose delusions and dementia (mental defect). A subtype, including bizarre and hebephrenic behaviour, was masterfully described by Auguste Marie the same year.[202] However, clinical vignettes included in the book by Magnan and Sérieux show that the new diagnostic category *did cut across* what currently would be called schizophrenia, psychotic depression and delusional disorders. As Pichot has rightly commented: 'it was a misleading construct defining a disorder found more readily in *theory* than practice.'[203] This work, however, gave the authors the opportunity to offer a developmental account of paranoid delusions and emphasize the importance of delusional mood.

Other French alienists continued analysing delusions in isolation. The most representative book from this period is that by Vaschide and Vurpas, published in 1903[204] where the authors dealt with the history and definitions of *délire* and its relationship to dreaming, and mapped its ever narrowing evolution from wide category to specific *trouble du raisonnement*. They also studied its nosological role in regard to *délire chronique*, paranoia, and mental confusion.

Paul Sérieux's interest in delusional states continued well into the new century, and in 1909 led to the publication (with Joseph Capgras) of an important volume on the 'delusion of interpretation' where the authors move away from Magnan's over-encompassing ideas: 'we shall detach from it a condition we want to call *délire d'intepretation*'. Whilst the psychoses leading to dementia include chronic hallucinations, our cases have exclusively delusions.'[205] They were, therefore, characterized by: (*a*) multiple and organized delusions, (*b*) absence of hallucinations, (*c*) normal intellect, (*d*) chronic course, and (*e*) incurability without terminal defect.'[206] This is likely to be an early description of delusional disorders.

However, the best study on *intuitions délirantes*, had to wait until the ideas of Bergson and Levy-Brühl percolated through in 1931. This book, by Targowla and Dublineau, included 60 case reports and explores the role of 'intuition', which, the authors concluded, was a *form of automatism*; delusions were generated by this mechanism and hence were unrelated to perceptions.[207] Delusion was thus: 'a self-evident judgement that, completely formed, suddenly and spontaneously appears in consciousness, has no sensory origin and is beyond the control of the will.'[208]

In 1905 Dupré coined the term *mythomanie* to refer to severe confabulatory delusions, which he subdivided into mythomania of vanity, and malignant and perverse mythomania; he later also described a 'wandering mythomania' shown by young subjects who, in addition to their confabulations, exhibited *Wanderleben*.[209]

PHILIPPE CHASLIN Chaslin published his great book on 'semiology' in 1912, that is, one year before Jaspers'. These two works can hardly be more dissimilar: Jaspers was only 28 when he wrote his work (bronchiectasis limited his physical activities, and he spent most of his time reading) and the book is a combination of philosophical discourse[210] and borrowed clinical experience. Chaslin, on the other hand, wrote his volume after an entire life of clinical work, which he spent actually living amongst his charges; indeed, the sample of patients reported covers a span of more than 20 years.[211]

Chaslin was interested in the suitability of the psychopathological language to capture information: 'I believe that the imprecision of terms is due to the imprecision of our ideas. But I also think that the inexactitude of the language may cause further inexactitude in our ideas.'[212] And referring to Germanisms and Anglicisms invading the language of 'mental pathology' in France he wrote: 'if only they helped to combat factual imprecisions, but the opposite is the case; it is often imagined that progress has been made simply because fancy names have been given to old things.'[213]

Chaslin wrote a number of papers on *délire*. In the most important of these, published in 1890[214], he explored the question of why persecutory delusions are more often accompanied by auditory hallucinations, whilst visual hallucinations are more commonly seen with religious delusions. To account for these associations, Chaslin suggested a neurophysiological hypothesis based on Tamburini's theory of hallucinations:[215] 'Delusion, like hallucination, is a physiological phenomenon of pathological origin; this genesis prevents the idea from corresponding to the reality of things . . . . I shall show that at the beginning of the disease the auditory hallucination and the delusion are the same phenomenon only that of different intensity' 'the content of the predominant hallucinations is determined by the mental content of the delusion . . . however abstract an idea might be it always contains an obscure image which in certain conditions may become distinct.'[216] To Chaslin, delusions and hallucinations were two sides of the same psychological and neurophysiological coin. These views were influenced by Cotard's ideas on the genesis of delusions.

In his 1912 book,[217] and in marked contrast to earlier theoretical discussions, Chaslin treated delusions (*idées délirantes*) descriptively:[218] 'delusions may present isolated or combined with hallucinations. Clusters of delusions may appear in the same patient, and these I call delusional states (*délire*). Delusions may be disconnected or form a system, i.e. as incoherent and systematized delusional states, respectively.'[219] The former were seen in subjects with low intelligence or dementia although a form of incoherence (*discordance générale, désharmonie entre les différents signes de l'affection*) was seen in conditions such as dementia praecox.[220] Primary and secondary paranoia were the best examples of systematized delusional states, in which there was a relative preservation of intellectual functions. Secondary paranoia was the remnant of a severe psychotic states, and could signify a transition to dementia.[221] But there were other types of delusion: persecutory, grandiose, hypochondriacal, nihilistic, auto-accusatory, mystical, religious and of possession.

Interestingly, Chaslin also wrote in 1912: 'delusional ideas seem to have their source in the *emotions of the patient* of which they are symbolic representations; but the difference between primary and secondary delusions may simply be one of intensity and presentation. One could illustrate the origin of delusions by recollecting the mechanisms of dreaming. Propensities, desires, and feelings from the waking state reappear in dreams in symbolic scenes . . . Freud has shown this to be the case.'[222] Chaslin explored the question of delusional contagion and concluded that it was rare, and that it occurred in people living closely together, particularly when one member was weaker than the other.[223]

German-speaking psychiatry

JASPERS Historical evidence included in this chapter shows that all aspects of delusion that have been attributed to Jaspers had already been fully discussed during the nineteenth century.[224] His views, however, were presented as new by the group of German émigrés who arrived in Britain during the 1930s.[225]

Jaspers's first writing on delusion (of jealousy) appeared in 1910,[226] and discussed the question of whether it was a 'development' of personality or a disease. It also reports eight cases and includes some nosological considerations; only German references are quoted. Soon after, in a paper on disorders of perception[227] and another on pseudohallucinations,[228] Jaspers returns to the issue of delusional belief and insight. Lastly, in a superb short paper on the 'feelings of presence', which Jaspers called 'vivid cognitions' (*Leibhaftige Bewusstheiten*), he explored the difference between intuitive and cognitive claims.[229] It is, however, in *General Psychopathology*[230] where Jaspers offers the longest account of delusions. Much has been written on this, however, and it would be unnecessary to rehearse his views again.[231]

What Jaspers[232] said sounded new to those who had little knowledge of the nineteenth century. In fact, the only new view in his model (new in that it is not present in nineteenth century psychiatric writings) is that of 'comprehensibility' which Jaspers borrowed from Wilhelm Dilthey.[233] It is clear, however, that the assessment of comprehensibility depends on the state of progress of psychological theory: delusions incomprehensible today may not be so tomorrow. Between Jaspers and Schneider, as Gerhardt Schmidt[234] showed in his classical review, no drastic change took place in the concept of delusion. The accumulation of clinical reports, however, led some credence to Kretschmer's view that personality factors may play a role in the generation and persistence of delusions.

British psychiatry

BERNARD HART AND THE PSYCHODYNAMIC TRADITION The other important influence on British views on delusion before the arrival of the German émigrés in the 1930s[235] was Freud and his school. This is well illustrated in the work of Bernard Hart[236] who explained delusion in terms of 'dissociation', a mechanism which he defined as 'a division of the mind into independent fragments, which are not coordinated together to attain some common end.'[237] 'The conception of dissociation enables us, again, to represent more clearly to ourselves the mental state of the patient who possesses a delusion. A delusion, it will be remembered, is a false belief which is impervious to the most complete logical demonstration of its impossibility, and unshaken by the presence of incompatible or obvious contradictory facts ... This tissue of contradictions seems at first sight inexplicable and incomprehensible, but the key to the riddle is clear as soon as we realisze that the patient's mind is in a state of dissociation.'[238]

The 1950 World Congress

Since the First World War, little that was new had been said on delusions in either Germany[239] or France.[240] This was the reason why it was decided to make delusions the theme of the First World Congress of Psychiatry held in Paris in 1950.[241] Its roll call included great men like Mayer-Gross, Guiraud, Morselli, Rümke, Delgado, Ey, Gruhle, Minkowski, Stransky, and Baruk.

Grühle re-asserted a definition that, since Hagen, had predominated in German psychiatry:[242] 'delusion is an interpretation without reason, an intuition without cause, a mental attitude without basis. It represents neither sublimated desires nor repressed wishes but is a sign of cerebral dysfunction. It is not secondary to any other phenomenon and has no relationship to the patient's constitution.'[243]

The Paris meeting did not generate new ideas but rehearsed most of the old ones.[244] For example, Honorio Delgado (from Perú) failed in his bid to make the English term 'delusion' be accepted as the international currency. Based on the work of Monakow and Mourgue, Guiraud offered a 'biological model' according to which delusions resulted from a failure of 'primordial psychological activity (*atteinte de l'activité psychique primordial*') distorted and masked by human cognitive and affective superstructures.'[245] The primordial activity included the feelings of existence, nutrition, reproduction, vigilance and growth. The self controlled such feelings or *pulsions* and satisfied them according to the rules of reality and logic. Focal or diffuse pathological changes in the brain caused selective or global failures (*une anomalie partielle ou globale du dynamisme psychique primordial*) which, in turn, might lead to a collapse in the logical organization of the self.[246]

Mayer-Gross stated that the choice of delusions as theme for the Congress was 'appropriate' for at the time there was a 'relatively low ebb of interest in the psychopathology of delusions.'[247] He noticed that the conventional definitions were unhelpful in practice, and suggested two ways of surmounting this difficulty: 'one can call a delusion pathological or, as Bumke put it, an error of morbid origin; or one can insist that delusions do not differ from other human beliefs in principle, that no line of demarcation exists. As Bleuler, whose views have so widely influenced psychopathological thinking all over the world, has pointed out, delusional ideas correspond to and are directed by the patient's affects and emotions.'[248]

E. Morselli[249] attempted a review of the neurobiological bases of some delusional states but did not go beyond listing toxic and metabolic states. H.C. Rümke undertook an analysis of the symptom delusion which he defined from the phenomenological point of view as an 'artificial abstraction.'[250] His contribution was, perhaps, the most important in that Rümke showed the uselessness of defining delusions as 'beliefs' and also the weakness of the conventional definitional criteria.

Summary

This long historical journey suggests that a definition of delusion had already crystallized by the end of the nineteenth century according to which it was fundamentally a speech act (although it may be, occasionally, expressed in non-linguistic behaviour) which was taken by the interlocutor to express a (pathological) belief about self or world. Such belief was characterized by unshakeability, insightlessness, imperviousness to reason, bizarreness of content and cultural dislocation. Little was said about the fact that evidential confrontation might, in fact, erode conviction.

The 'received view' that delusions are 'pathological' beliefs feels intuitively right. Delusions sound like any other declarative speech act, and it is plausible to assume that they must also convey information. Since the 'received view' was formed during the nineteenth century, it is legitimate to assume that it is based on views belonging to this period. If so, the current view of delusion encompasses an obsolete theory of language and the epistemology of introspection sponsored by classical psychology. Progress has occurred in all these areas and the notion of delusions needs updating even if such work might precipitate its disintegration. Such updating is beyond the scope of this chapter; what is not is the history of how such a view developed in the first place.

History of delusion as a belief

The view that delusions are 'wrong beliefs', was first formulated during the nineteenth century. So, it is dependent upon contemporary definitions of belief. Since the 1850s, the predominant British view was that of Alexander Bain who defined 'beliefs' as mental states which included 'some cognizance of the order of nature', but most importantly, included a volitional (willed) component. He suggested that the essence of belief was, in fact, the tendency by the believer to act out his belief.[251] This volitional element was incorporated by Bucknill and Tuke[252] into their own definition of delusion. In his later years, Bain did away with the volitional component.[253] The zenith of the intellectualist view of belief can be found in the work of H.H. Price.[254]

Some preliminary conceptual work is, however, required. The claim that a delusion is a 'wrong' belief, can be interpreted from the point of view of its *form* and *content*. In the first case it is assumed that delusions are misshapen structures, i.e. do not conform to conceptual blueprints; in the second case it is assumed that 'wrongness' concerns 'content' which is contrary to reality. The 'form' hypothesis is tested by using a model of normal belief; the 'content' interpretation is tested by demonstrating that contents are false. Confronted with this choice, Jaspers[255] opted for the latter: he was convinced that delusions were 'structurally sound' beliefs whose 'content' was discrepant with reality. This discrepancy was due to their pathological (morbid) origin. By re-asserting this nineteenth century view, he effectively led the descriptive psychopathology of delusions down a blind alley. It is clear from perusing current literature that researchers persist in viewing delusions as real 'ideas', as cognitive morsels of information about the world or self, upheld for 'morbid' reasons, and unsupported by evidence.

A conceptual analysis

The hypothesis must now be tested that, from the structural point of view, delusions are, in fact, beliefs. Price[256] distinguished four criteria. To believe that p is: (*a*) entertaining p, together with one or more alternative propositions q and r; (*b*) knowing a fact or set of facts F, which is relevant to p, q or r; (*c*) knowing that F makes p more likely than q or r, i.e. having more evidence for p than for q or r; and (*d*) assenting to p; which in turn includes a. the preferring of p to q and r and b. the feeling a certain degree of confidence with regard to p.

No current definition of delusion meets all of Price's criteria. First of all, clinical observation shows that it is rarely the case that the entertaining of delusion p is accompanied by the simultaneous entertaining of rival propositions q or r. Secondly, the set of facts F supporting the delusions is regularly absent, particularly so in the so-called primary delusions. Thirdly, no corresponding allocation of evidence is made by the patient in respect of p, q or r. In fact, assenting that p, is the only criterion that is regularly met. But even then, clinical observation shows that the nature of the *assenting* in the insane believer is different from that in the sane believer.

This difference, known since the nineteenth century, relates to what may be called a 'reality coefficient': i.e. a normal subject believing that p, does so within certain probability constraints which are determined by evidential strength, personality, emotional investment, etc. None of these factors is individually allowed to push the probability value to 1 (i.e. total certainty). Therefore, evidential strength is always assessed in terms of 'reasonable doubt' (i.e. a sort of 'pinch of salt' criterion), and emotional investment is normally kept at bay so that it does not unduly affect the probability values. Clinical observation shows that this probabilistic attitude may be impaired in the psychotic subject. However bizarre the content of speech acts might be, clinicians would not be happy to call them 'delusions', if at the same time they were upheld with certain coyness, and were accompanied by a correct probabilistic assessment of their reality.

The view that delusions are 'abnormal belief systems' has naturally led to the suggestion that probabilistic models (such as Bayesian inference)[257] may be used to explain the manner of their origin or persistence. Hemsley and Garety[258] have based their analysis on a probabilistic account of normal belief put forward by Fischhoff and Beyth-Marom[259] who also suggest that inferential failures may originate at each stage of the Bayesian procedure. The application of this model to delusions is not very helpful. Apart from the general point that an assumption of rationality (i.e. of the mind as statistician)[260] is not warranted in the case of psychotic subjects, and of the specific point made above that delusions may not be beliefs at all (and hence not a form of probabilistic knowledge), two other difficulties beset this approach: one relates to the assessment of *a priori* probabilities (in the case of delusional beliefs), and the other to the determination of what counts as *a posteriori* evidence. In fact, Hemsley and Garety[261] show that failures at each stage of the inferential procedure lead to 'phenomenological' situations resembling delusional 'beliefs'. It is unclear, however, whether these constitute so far unrecognized 'types' of delusions, and whether they are signposts for different brain sites. Finally, there is some evidence that, after all, 'normal' subjects do not often observe Bayesian inferential rules either.[262] So, a major overlap between deluded and normal subjects is to be expected. Discrimination between these two groups is likely to require the inclusion of variables external to the Bayesian model.

By the end of the nineteenth century, the concept of delusion as a morbid belief had become well established. So, questions began to be asked concerning its genesis, mechanisms, and types. Organic and psychological mechanisms became popular. For example, the 'seizural' hypothesis developed after 1880 in the wake of Tamburini's work on hallucinations[263] and the chemico-modular view of Luys and the French school in which phosphates played an important role.[264] Yet another was the Jacksonian hypothesis according to which delusions were expressions of normal and adaptative brain mechanisms released by the destruction of higher centres.[265] Jackson even suggested that one of the factors involved in the production of delusions might be personality and past history.[266] Ribot, Janet, Freud, Mourgue, and Ey followed this lead.[267] By the end of the nineteenth century, Wernicke[268] and Chaslin[269] had distinguished between primary and secondary delusions, the latter being misinterpretations of primary morbid phenomena, such as hallucinations or mood disorders.

Thus, it can be concluded that delusions are, from the structural point of view, so unlike 'normal beliefs' (incidentally, a similar conclusion is reached if other operational definitions of belief are used) then, it must be asked, why persist in calling them beliefs at all? Indeed, no heuristic pay-off seems apparent. Properly described, delusions are empty speech acts that disguise themselves as beliefs. To use Austin's felicitous term they are but 'masqueraders'.[270] So, although delusions purport to be real statements, and hence convey information, they may turn out to be epistemologically *manqué*. Their so-called content, like that of hallucinations, contains little information about the world, in spite of their often bombastic claims. A content of sorts, of course they have, but this is aleatory and detached from any evidential basis. The only information that it might carry relates to addresses for neurobiological events. But, given the amount of psychosocial noise in which they envelop themselves, even in this respect they may turn out to be unhelpful.

Special aspects: 'The predelusional state'

In clinical practice, delusions are but the culmination of momentous clinical and neurobiological events. As De Clérambault wrote: 'by the time the delusion appears the psychosis is usually of long-standing. Delusion is but a construct (*Superstructure*)'.[271] The psychopathological events immediately *preceding the crystallization of the delusion* will be called in this chapter 'the pre-delusional state' (PDS) and include cognitions, moods, conations, and motor acts (and combinations thereof) often fleeting and opaque to description. Although most classical authors mention PDS, only a few have explored them in any detail. Therefore, it remains to be seen whether PDS is actually the obligatory first stage in the process of delusional-formation or a non-specific prodromus to any and all psychoses. It will also be suggested here that the PDS is an important clinical event in that it helps to *differentiate sub-types of delusions* and, more importantly, in that it provides information on *brain localization* and *treatment effects*.

As stated earlier in this chapter, up to the early nineteenth century, delusions were simply considered as 'signs' of madness and alienists bothered little about their content. By the 1850s, interest began to develop in their 'form', particularly in the work of Baillarger and Falret. However, themes and contents became important during the second half of the century and complex classifications of insanity emerged.[272] The psychodynamic movement rendered this interest into a fine art and psychiatrists started seeking hidden messages and symbols with increasing keenness; but the hermeneutic rules on which the success of this search depends have unfortunately proven elusive. Although excessive interest in the content of delusions is a reason for the neglect of PDS, the most important, however, is likely to have been a practical one: PDS is not always available to clinical observation as it is often over before the subject is brought to hospital.

This elusive nature was well known to nineteenth century alienists. More than 120 years ago, when referring to 'delusional mood' (*Wahnstimmung*), Hagen wrote: 'the disturbed affect may not be recognized, not only because patients are able to control themselves or because doctors do not always investigate this possibility closely enough, but also – as a third reason – because the severity of the delusion itself may tend to mask or distract from the disturbed affect'.[273] Whatever the reason, PDS do not feature in current glossaries and hence have become 'invisible' to diagnosis.

An important student of PDS in the 1840s was Moreau de Tours who proposed that delusions originated out of a *fait primordial*. This concept, not dissimilar to the concept of *dissolution* in Jackson, reflected a general law of nature that led to a dismantling or disintegration of the self. To Moreau all forms of insanity resulted from the same set of causes, and were similar to dreaming[274]. The *fait primordial* included 'intellectual excitement, sudden or gradual dissociation of ideas, weakening of the coordination between the intellectual powers'. All these psychological causes have in common a 'molecular' mechanism: 'there is weakening of the power to direct our thoughts at will, insidiously strange ideas take over in regards to a particular object of attention. These ideas, which the will has not called upon, have an unknown origin and become progressively more vivid. Soon they lead to bizarre associations . . .. These cause 'a state of vagueness, uncertainty, oscillation and confusion of ideas that often leads to incoherence. It is a veritable disintegration, a dissolution of the intellectual system'.[275] By putting forward the notion of *fait primordial*, Moreau combined the psychological hypotheses of the 1840s with brain mechanisms.[276]

Based on Krafft-Ebing's four mechanisms for the formation of delusions (*Wahnideen*),[277] B. Ball and A. Ritti explored the pathogenesis of 'sudden' delusional formation and suggested that such phenomena result from 'a spontaneous internal irritation' and are accompanied by vegetative symptoms.[278] This seizural model was becoming popular at the time owing to the work of Tamburini.[279] Another original contributor to the debate was Jules Cotard who suggested that states of emotional hypo- or hypersensitivity were propitious states for the development of hypochondriacal delusions.[280]

Jules Séglas, in turn, separates delusional ideas which are simple and transient (*idées délirantes simples et passagères*) from *délires* proper. The former are 'secondary to interpretations of other symptoms such as hallucinations, emotions, intellectual events, perceptions and memories',[281] Séglas also quoted Meynert's view that delusions pre-exist in all normal brains only inhibited by normal mental function. Mental illness, however, causes a break in normal associations which together with the development of abnormal images facilitate the release of delusions.

Angelo Hesnard's work spans the first half of twentieth century French psychiatry. A keen exponent of psychoanalysis, his work during the 1920s was, however, marked by an imaginative eclecticism which included a view on the formation of the psychoses. In 1924, Hesnard proposed four stages: loss of physiopathological balance (humoral, etc.), an endogenous and disorganised over-production of affective experiences, the formulation of justificatory cognitions (e.g. delusions), and the full expression of the psychosis. Each stage gave rise to its own symptoms. PDS corresponds to the stages 1 and 2 of Hesnard's during which obscure and ineffable bodily changes are experienced by the subject.[282]

De Clérambault is one of the most original thinkers in early twentieth century psychopathology. His concept of psychological automatism, which is at the basis of all the psychoses, includes organic and cognitive disorders, and can be considered as the mechanism that underlies PDS. Clinically, psychological automatism can express itself in a number of disordered conducts, thought disorder, etc. and includes at a later stage hallucinations.[283] Hence delusions were always secondary, interpretative phenomena. De Clérambault highlighted the role of *coenestho-pathies*,[284] which included all manner of interoceptive and propioceptive sensations and constituted the magma out of which hallucinations and delusions emerged. He also spoke of 'sensitive automatism', i.e. of the eruption into consciousness of primitive, ineffable, sensations which caused perplexity and increased the likelihood of delusional formation.[285] Mourgue[286] and Morsier[287] also took seriously the possibility that hallucinations may originate in the 'vegetative' system.

Inspired by the work of De Clérambault, Targowla and Dublineau published in 1931 a classical book entitled *L'intuition délirante* where they made use of a combination of organic factors and the mechanism of intuition to explain the generation of delusions. Both were the result of what they call *automatisme psychologique*. The authors considered the actual delusional content as less important for it is but a stereotyped epiphenomenon that is the same in individuals of varying education and social class. What matters is the form and as part of it the delusional conviction which should be considered as primary a phenomenon as anxiety.[288]

Before embarking in his psychoanalytical career, Jacques Lacan wrote a substantial work on paranoid states in which he dealt with the formation of delusions.[289] Inspired by Jaspers,[290] he sought to identify a 'process' – both neurobiological and psychological – which would facilitate the crystallization of psychosis. He suggested the existence of a 'morbid factor X' which caused the development of both delusions and hallucinations. Lacan also recognized three stages in the evolution of the psychotic process: acute, affective and of consolidation and the first two are coterminous with PDS.

The Spaniard Marco-Merenciano also proposed that the 'delusional mood in schizophrenia exhibits all the features of an ineffable "aura" that tends to last a great deal . . . it can pass on or change itself into a sort of twilight state . . . or merge into the disease itself'.[291] These views are forerunners of current views on the association between epilepsy and schizophrenia.

THE NATURE OF THE PRE-DELUSIONAL STATE Since the nineteenth century PDS has been conceptualized as a disorder of cognition, affect, consciousness or motility. In general, PDS has been studied in relation to 'primary' delusions which since Baillarger[292] have been defined as delusions which are not secondary to other mental symptoms. The primary / secondary distinction will be explored in this paper as it is proposed that PDS is to primary delusions what hallucinations or pathological moods are to secondary delusions. It will also be suggested, based on a model of symptom formation developed by the author,[293] that PDS constitutes a form of *primordial soup* or pathological matrix out of

which, and depending upon certain coding rules either delusions or hallucinations will be formed.

PDS AS A DISTURBANCE OF COGNITION   According to this view, the primary component of PDS is an inchoate *cognition* which contains the kernel of a question
which the patient will eventually respond to by creating the delusion. What matters
here is the cognitive act of perceiving the world or self as *strange*. Once this has
happened, a process is triggered which culminates in a declarative statement. A
good example of this model is found in the work of Magnan and Sérieux on 'chronic
delusional states' where four stages are recognized: incubation or 'inner restlessness', persecution, grandiosity and 'dementia'.[294] The incubation period may run
unnoticed or be characterized by sadness, sombreness, anxiety, and an acceptance
by the subject of gradual increasing misinterpretations. Even less specific clinical
features such as anorexia, insomnia and hypochondria may occur. This state of
over-alertness may in due course lead to ideas of reference and eventually to crystallized delusions. These, in turn, will become systematized when 'confirmatory'
experiences such as hallucinations enter the picture.

  Similar 'cascade' models have been recently resuscitated. For example, Maher
proposed that delusions can be understood as attempts at making sense of 'anomalous experiences'; i.e. the psychotic patient would be like a 'scientist' or 'normal
theorist' testing hypotheses about his cognitive contents.[295] This approach is redolent of the notion of the 'reasonable man' as explored by Gigerenzer *et al*: 'the
reasonable man of the classical probabilists [has been] revived in psychology, and
along with him, the normative view of probability theory as a mathematical codifi-
cation of rational belief and action in uncertain situations'.[296] However, this view
needs to assume that apart from PDS other cognitive modules are in order for the
conclusions reached must be 'the best in the circumstances'. It is, however, likely
that PDS constitutes an all-pervading dysfunction which would hamper the reaching of 'reasonable conclusions'. Furthermore, the bizarre and contradictory clinical
nature of some delusions, would make it unlikely that they are actually explanations for anything, or indeed that they are fulfilling an adaptive or teleological
function. The cognitive approach remains popular and has been developed further
in the work of Helmsley and Garety,[297] Bentall,[298] Kinderman,[299] and Roberts.[300]
The latter author deals with the 'pre-psychotic state' as a convergence point of
'predisposing and precipitating factors' and attempts to reconcile cognitive and psychodynamic mechanisms; no discussion of PDS as such is, however, attempted.[301]

PDS AS A DISTURBANCE OF AFFECT   This has been a popular approach and writers since Hagen, Specht, and Bleuler have emphasized the 'affective' component of
PDS. An abnormal affect may disrupt the processing of information and linearity of
logical thinking or provide the context or medium in which delusional formation
takes place. For example, and based on associationistic psychology, Bleuler sug-

gested that the 'transforming' power of affect severely disrupts associations and overcomes logic. Although individual predisposition and distrust are also mentioned, Bleuler gives a special role to the 'cathathymic' forces.[302] For Lange, in turn, a special affect and perplexity are the basic components of 'delusional mood' (*Wahnstimmung*); he adds: 'it is unclear, however, what the relationship is between delusional mood and delusions. It may well be that both events result from a *third anomaly* and hence no cause–effect relationship can be established between the two' (my italics).[303]

KURT SCHNEIDER   The link between delusional mood and delusion was also explored by Kurt Schneider who found that they were often incongruent. In relation to delusional mood he wrote: 'We stated that delusional perception does not derive from any particular emotional state, but this does not contradict the fact that delusional perception is often preceded by a delusional atmosphere brought on by the morbid process itself, an experience of oddness or sometimes, though more rarely, of exaltation, and often in these vague delusional moods, perceptions gain this sense of something 'significant' yet not defined. The delusional atmosphere is, however, very vague and can offer no content pointing to the delusional perception that ensues later, nor can we understand the specific content of the delusional perception in terms of it. The most we can say is that these perceptions are characteristically embedded in this atmosphere but are not derived from it. There is no need for the delusional atmosphere to jibe exactly with the emotional tone of the following delusional perception. The atmosphere may be alien and uncomfortable, the delusional perception may be pleasant and cheering. Sometimes, however, the abnormal interpretation of a perception does seem to spring more understandably from the motiveless, perhaps anxiety-ridden atmosphere. We would then take this as one of the common paranoid reactions of a psychotic, the morbid process being the prerequisite. In practice, delusional perception and paranoid reaction may sometimes be difficult to distinguish. This provides occasion for leaving the diagnosis open for schizophrenia or cyclothymia. We have given the term 'preparatory field' to this delusional atmosphere that sometimes precedes delusional perception'.[304]

KARL CONRAD   Others have emphasized the *ineffability* and affective nature of delusional mood. For example, Wetzel explored the 'end of the world' experience in schizophrenics which he considers to be a special affective state, a 'sinister foreboding'.[305] But it was Karl Conrad who developed this view in detail. For this great German psychiatrist the development of schizophrenia included (roughly) five stages: *trema* (pre-psychotic state), *apophany* and *anastrophé* (development of delusions), *apocalyptic* (presence of catatonia and other syndromes), *consolidation* and *residual or defect state*. PDS is included in the *trema* stage which Conrad considers as predominantly affective in nature; indeed 'The number of cases of schizophrenia starting with endogenous affective symptoms (*endogener Verstimmung*) is high . . . trema can take the character of an endogenous depression'. Conrad notices that it is never observed that the latter can start with schizophrenic symptoms.[306]

KARL JASPERS Considering *Wahnstimmung* Jaspers wrote: 'If we try to get some closer understanding of these primary experiences of delusion, we soon find we cannot really appreciate these quite alien modes of experience. They remain largely incomprehensible, unreal and beyond our understanding. Yet some attempts have been made. We find that there arise in the patient certain primary sensations, vital feelings, moods, awareness: "Something is going on; do tell me what on earth is going on", as one patient said to her husband . . . A living-room which formerly was felt as neutral or friendly now becomes dominated by some indefinable atmosphere . . . the use of the word "atmosphere" might suggest psychasthenic moods and feelings perhaps and be a source of confusion; but with this *delusional atmosphere* we always find an "objective something" there, even though quite vague, a something which lays the seed of objective validity and meaning'.[307]

Lastly, Oepen has suggested that the relationship between affect and delusion may be based on 'cognitive lateralization', i.e. on the fact that affective messages (right hemisphere) are complemented by the left hemisphere.[308]

CHARLES BLONDEL Blondel is arguably the most original (and less well known to English-speaking mental health workers) writer in this field. In a classical book entitled *La Conscience Morbide*,[309] Blondel develops a explanatory model for the origin of delusions based on the view that the pre-delusional state is an expression of a highly personalized form of *cénesthésie viscerale*. This notion, central to French psychiatry at the beginning of the twentieth century, refers to stable and personalized patterns of proprioceptive information providing the experiential background of human consciousness.[310] In the 'normal state', human beings partake in a collective form of consciousness (*conscience socialisée*) (including a public language inadequate for the description of their subjective events) and hence suppress their own *cénesthésie*. The onset of mental disorder is marked by an increase in *cénesthésie* which forces the attention of the individual who soon realizes that his experiences have no equivalent in the collective consciousness. The ensuing affective restlessness or *conscience morbide* (or predelusional state) is handled by the patient in either of two ways. He may continue experiencing it as a mysterious anxiety and restlessness or may attempt a description. To do the latter, he borrows from 'normal discourse' and delusions are formed with a content made out of 'recognizable' material (which leads the observer to try and understand it). The referential function of such content, however, is *manqué*, in that it has no real referent. To use a concept described above, delusions are veritable 'empty speech acts' for their 'content' is really a foreign body irrelevant to anything in the patient's state (the content is, of course, trivially connected to the collective language of the period). La *conscience morbide* or predelusional state, on the other hand, is informative of the patient's actual experiences (and their origin).

PDS AS A DISTURBANCE OF CONSCIOUSNESS By disorganizing both cognition and affect, disorders of consciousness offer a fertile ground for PDS to develop. Deficits in any of the dimensions of awareness may disrupt the way in which information about world, body, or self is captured, organized or retrieved.

Friedrich Mauz, for example, has emphasized the fact that PDS may be accompanied by a feeling of 'increased awareness and lucidity'. This author believed that this was due to an accompanying feeling of 'transformation of the self' or 'psychological annihilation'.[311] Mauz also believed that this 'awareness of subjective change' (i.e. Berze's *Bewusstheit der Verändertseins*) was the hallmark of the schizophrenic process for it was the 'apperception of a threat to the self, or a weakening of individuality or an experience of insufficiency or a loss of capacity to act'.[312] Such experiences generated feelings of restlessness, uncertainty, fear, confusion, and perplexity. Mauz goes as far as saying that the quality of the awareness may have a prognostic value, namely, the more 'lucid' the subject is in regards to his state, the worse the prognosis will be. Lafora also supported the view that this sensation of transformation may be an important source for the 'primary symptoms' of schizophrenia.[313]

MANUEL CABALEIRO GOAS To the Galician psychiatrist Cabaleiro Goas, an important element in the development of PDS also was a disturbance of awareness. He agreed with the view that affective experiences might, on occasions, predominate but they were always 'associated with *hypotonia*[314] of consciousness'.[315] The central issue, however, was that 'an alteration of consciousness is required for the development of delusions . . .' 'we believe that in delusional mood there is something more than a disorder of affect, namely, a hypotonia of consciousness . . .' and 'delusional mood reflects more a profound disorder of consciousness than the perception of something uncertain'.[316]

BARTOLOMÉ LLOPIS By far the most important writer in this area is B. Llopis[317] who applied to delusional mood his own theory of the de-structuration of consciousness which he had developed in his work on pellagra psychosis.[318] Llopis proposed that the psychoses often caused somatic sensations which were experienced by patients as anxiety or euphoria. These affective changes, are therefore primary sensations perceived *ab initio* as *as if* experiences. The psychoses, however, also bring about a *fundamental change* in the content, level and structure of consciousness, and therefore, sooner or later patients lose control upon the cognitive organization of their world and no longer can hang on to the *as if* qualification. The net result is that they begin to perceive their somatic sensations as caused by an external agency. In this sense, the affective sensations are for Llopis the basis for PDS and delusions proper.[319]

Llopis also proposed an interesting distinction between what he called 'active' (*delusión viva*) and 'inert' (*delusión inerte*) delusions. The former was kept alive by emotions (delusional mood), the latter was but the 'corpse', or 'mnemic footprint' of a delusion. Due to their 'associationistic' nature, inert delusions might occasionally become kindled by an emotional upheaval. Showing great penetration, Llopis also called into question the time-honoured distinction between primary and secondary delusion, which he saw as the ends of a continuum. For him all delusions were incomprehensible in that they emerged from somatic changes; their content was unimportant.

HENRY EY This prolific French writer also sponsored the view that the psychosis (and therefore PDS) were a reflection of a subtle disorder of consciousness. Based on the hierarchical model of Hughlings Jackson and classical French psychopathology, Ey proposed that all mental disorders resulted from changes either in the longitudinal (diachronic) or cross-sectional (synchronic) structure of consciousness.[320]

PDS, according to Ey, varied in frequency and duration and was characterised by manifestations resulting from the physical changes caused by the psychoses such as nervousness, insomnia, hypnagogic experiences, irritability, mood disorder, lack of psychological stability, restlessness, agitation, anorexia, amenorrhoea, vasomotor and digestive disorders, and even soft neurological signs. These symptoms occurred in the context of a disorder of consciousness that he described as 'a reorganization of the boundaries of reality'. It was in this fertile ground that delusions crystallized.

The delusional state proper was characterized by (*a*) passivity, i.e. the subject's consciousness comes under the control of the delusion, (*b*) the *pur vecu*, i.e. the private experience of alone inhabiting a delusional state, and (*c*) the fact that delusions are just one aspect of the deeper process of 'going mad' (just like dreams relate to sleeping).[321] The acute delusional state always emerges in the context of a disorder of consciousness but whether or not it will become systematized and chronic depends on whether it becomes linked to personality and *the being* of the subject. In this way delusional states become traits.

The above authors agree on the view that disorders of consciousness are essential to the development of PDS. They differ, however, on how to define consciousness and on the manner of its becoming disordered. For example, Lange proposed a sort of 'hypertrophy' of awareness as the antecedent to the intuition or apperception of the delusion. Llopis and Ey, on the other hand, conceived of such disorder as a dislocation of structure. In general, the view that the psychoses result from an alteration of consciousness is an important theme in Continental psychiatry (Ey, Llopis, etc.). That it is not altogether intelligible to English speaking psychiatrists may be due to the fact that definitions and clinical markers for 'disorder of consciousness' differ between classic European and English speaking psychopathology. Whilst in the latter disorientation, confusion, and attentional syndromes are the crucial criteria, in Continental psychiatry subtle markers such as dysphoria, irritability, minor loss of cognitive grasp, situational as opposed to temporal disorientation, hyperaesthetic states, are also important.

DPS AS A DISTURBANCE OF MOTILITY Authors such as Störring and MacCurdy emphasized behavioural, motility and volitional aspects of PDS. One such was the syndrome of perplexity in which the bewilderment of the patient in regards to the ineffability of his experience is transmitted to the observer both in speech, motor postures and stereotypes.

GUSTAV E. STÖRRING Störring defined perplexity as 'the painful awareness of an inability to master external or internal situations, this awareness is 'lived' by the subject as something unexplicable that deeply affects the self'.[322] This state of perplexity (Ratlosigkeit) will disappear when the subject happens upon a delusion that 'explains' his feelings. A core of 'primary' anxiety, generated by the disease itself and related to a thalamic dysfunction, is always found at the centre of the perplexity state. Störring also studied the postures and motor disorder characteristic of perplexity. The gesturing and wide-eyed faces of the perplexed patient he compares with the Darwinian description of states of surprise and stupefaction. The state of perplexity is common in schizophrenia and appears in response to the primary feelings of strangeness or acute anxiety engendered by this condition.

JOHN MACCURDY MacCurdy was a Canadian who after 1926 taught in Cambridge.[323] Before coming over to the UK he had worked with Augustus Hoch and John Kirby and helped to edit Hoch's book on stupor.[324] Following Kirby, MacCurdy described perplexity as a two-stage process: subjective stupefaction was followed by over-retardation and perplexity. He believed that perplexity was the source for the formation of delusions: 'most often from this general matrix there emerges one dominating type of delusion and from the reaction ceases to be perplexity and becomes depression, anxiety or involutional melancholia, stupor or mania. Perplexity in the sense of a consistent psychosis tends, therefore, to be a brief reaction – a few weeks or months; it is often merely a brief interlude or transitory state and is commonest of all during the onset of manic-depressive attacks. Relatives describe the perplexity syndrome with great frequency when they tell how the psychosis began'.[325]

In regards to the specific role of perplexity in the formation of delusions, MacCurdy states: 'naturally, before the sense of reality is wholly lost, a patient may suffer from this kind of thinking (trying to reconcile the irreconcilable) and be puzzled until such time as the effort to be logical is relaxed. Hence, we may find – and often do – the symptoms of perplexity appearing in the earlier stages of

dementia praecox'.[326] Thus, for MacCurdy, as for Störring, perplexity is an important marker of early schizophrenia.

SUMMARY OF HISTORY OF PDS   The first question is whether in all patients PDS
is a *similar* experience (corresponding to a brain signal emitted by the same locus)
or a *composite* of experiences (corresponding to signals from various brain sites).
As described in the literature and observed in clinical practice, the experience
appears as *primitive* 'undifferentiated' and 'ineffable' corresponding to what has
been called elsewhere the 'primordial soup'.[327] Being described as 'ineffable', of
course, does not necessarily mean that it cannot be *conceptualized*; all it may mean
is that, at the time, the experience is surrounded by a mood of 'mystery' that makes
the patient declare that it is 'beyond words'.

Since the nineteenth century (if not before) such experience seems to have
changed little, and clinicians have found it as difficult to conceptualize as their
patients. Understandably, explanations have gone from the cognitive to the
emotional and volitional and consciousness related. In this chapter I would like to
suggest, as a working hypothesis, that PDS is a *homogeneous* experience and that
ab initio it is the expression of distress in a specific brain module. This also means
that I believe that the study of crystallized delusions is no longer of value in regards
to understanding the process of delusions formation or location in the brain. PDS,
on the other hand, is the actual expression of the mechanism of delusion generation: a patient in *Wahnstimmung* is one in whom we can 'see' such process in
operation. I propose that, once the delusion has been formed, it is set asunder from
this process and is stored away together with other knowledge-related engrammes.
Consequently, its localization should give little information on the brain locus in
which it was formed.

Bringing together the strands of this argument, the following can be stated. As
discussed elsewhere,[328] the 'received view' considers delusions as sharing the same
structure and contextual network with normal beliefs and other knowledge-
carrying statements, and locates the only real difference in the truth value of their
'content'. More recent approaches using attributional theory also assume the normality of the *structure* of delusions and concentrate on the demonstration that
cognitive biases affect the content of the delusion. I have argued that such a view
is likely to be mistaken as delusions share no structural similarity with normal
beliefs and suggested that they are best described as 'empty speech acts'.[329]
Delusions are called 'empty' not because they have no content (they all do!) but
because they have been 'shelled out' of all information in regard to the brain
address where they were formed, and because they no longer can be integrated or
'inscribed' in the pragmatics of a discourse between doctor and patient.[330] The
content of delusions is inscribed in a *different* discourse and reflects cultural and
personal codes: a consequence of this claim is that *crystallized* delusions become an
interesting detritus, a 'foreign body' the explanation of which is not necessarily

linked to that of delusion formation. If what has been said is the case, then correlating formed delusions with neuroimages will be of little help. We suggest here that the only window of opportunity to locate the *process* of delusion formation (which is a putative direct expression of the disease) is provided by PDS.

So far, it has not been specified whether all delusions are preceded by PDS. This concerns the all important question of whether all delusions are structurally similar regardless of aetiology. As far as it is known, there is no clear empirical answer to whether the delusion of mania, depression, schizophrenia, paranoia or organic delirium are the same phenomenon; indeed there is no meta-theory that allows for this distinction to be made meaningfully. This concerns one aspect of what has been called the problem of symptom heterogeneity,[331] and according to which delusions belonging to different diseases may be *different* phenomena. This difference would reside in the structure (form) of the delusions and hence go beyond the nineteenth century distinction between 'primary and 'secondary'. If such a view is correct, it would be heuristically unwise to generalize the PDS concept to all delusional forms. At this stage it might be wise to limit the clinical conclusions drawn in this historical survey to schizophrenia as other mechanisms may be responsible for the pre-delusional cognitive and emotional disorganization seen in organic delirium, drug-induced states, mania or depression.

The content of delusions

There has also been much discussion on the contents of delusions. During the early twentieth century a number of insanities were created on the basis of differences in content.[332] From nihilistic and parasitical to persecutory, erotomanic, grandiose and hypochondriacal, delusions were catalogued according to content and the unwarranted assumption made that each signified a different disease. This continued well into the twentieth century, with states such as the ones described by Capgras, Fregoli, and others,[333] some of which, thankfully, have by now been forgotten.

Since the nineteenth century, observational findings have persistently reported that delusions are extremely heterogeneous. Some have since suggested 'dimensions' to capture such differences. Such dimensions would include features such as insight, onset, course, dissolution, conviction, imperviousness to external pressure, emotional and volitional accompaniments, and behavioural consequences, and would be distributed in a hypothetical geometrical space.[334] Covariance does not seem to be a feature of these dimensions, and pattern recognition techniques extract rather trivial supervariables. Likewise, the clusters obtained seem bereft of clinical or neurobiological meaning.

The dimensional model has been considered by some to challenge the all-or-none model of delusions. The latter is, however, a figment of the researcher's imagination, and few experienced clinicians have ever upheld such a narrow view of delusions. The rejection of the all-or-none model has led to the unwarranted claim that a 'continuum' might then exist between overvalued ideas, obsessions and delusions. This very same view caused much confusion amongst nineteenth century alienists and was abandoned after 1870.

Final summary

In western culture, the symptom delusion is intimately linked to the notion of insanity itself. Most of what is current in the description and understanding of this phenomenon originated during the nineteenth century. Before 1800, the diagnosis of both insanity and organic delirium depended on the presence of delusions, and delusions, illusions and hallucinations were not considered as separate phenomena.

Conceptual changes that contributed to the shaping of 'delusion' during the nineteenth century include: (*a*) The new notion of 'symptom' as an elementary marker of mental disorder (as dictated by the anatomo-clinical model of disease),[335] (*b*) the decline of British empiricism and associationism and the growth of Faculty Psychology, (*c*) the conceptual divorce between knowledge and belief, and (*d*) the growth of theories of constitution and personality that allowed for the interpretation of delusions as personal or biographical events.

Delusion thus became a morbid belief. The morbidity factor was studied at individual level in terms of organicity, psychology and constitution. The content of the delusion became more important than its form, and sub-types were identified and considered as different diseases. Content was also used to identify congruencies or incongruencies between the delusion and other personal events. The notion of 'comprehensibility' originally used by Dilthey as a conceptual instrument in historical research, was borrowed by Jaspers and applied to delusions. Incomprehensible delusions were taken to signify primary events relating to the diagnosis of schizophrenia.

Since the nineteenth century, various criteria have accumulated to ascertain the diagnosis of delusions: conviction, unshakeability, bizarreness, cultural dislocation, and lack of insight. These have never been fully successful in the task of separating delusions from over-valued ideas, superstitions, and other forms of tightly held 'belief'. Clinicians have also remained puzzled over the relationship between delusions and behaviour, i.e. why the control of delusions upon behaviour is intermittent (on the history of this, little has been said in this chapter).

Delusions are likely to be empty speech acts, whose informational content refers to neither world nor self. They are not the symbolic expression of anything. Its 'content' is a random fragment of information 'trapped' at the very moment the delusion becomes crystallized. The frequency of certain themes (which changes from time to time) is likely to result from the fact that informational fragments with high frequency value have also a higher probability of being 'trapped'.

The pre-delusional state, although likely to be far more informative, particularly from the neurobiological point of view has been neglected. Such neglect can be explained by the bewitching effect of 'formed' delusions, the fact that they are easily available for study, the evanescent nature of the pre-delusional experiences, the fact that they occur in the context of subtle disorders of cognition and hence their recollection may be compromised, and finally, that no adequate techniques have yet been developed for their capture.

ACKNOWLEDGEMENT To Professor F. Fuentenebro, from the Universidad Complutense of Madrid, for his great help with the writing of the section on the Pre-Delusional State.

NOTES

1 pp. 168–179, Vaschide and Vurpas, 1903; also p. 43 Garrabé, 1989.
2 pp. 565–582, Berner and Naske, 1973; Huber and Gross, 1977; Spitzer, 1989.
3 The entry was probably written by Arnulfe d'Aumont, a graduate from Montpellier and professor at a minor University in Valence (Coleman, 1974). He also wrote the entry on *Démence* (Astruc, 1950).
4 p. 785, Arnulphe d'Aumont, 1754.
5 Arnulphe d'Aumont, 1754.
6 For an account of eighteenth century neurophysiology, see Brazier, 1984.
7 He said: 'all animals are provided with the faculties of distinguishing, feeling and moving', Chiarugi, 1987.
8 pp. 10–18, Chiarugi, 1987.
9 Blakey, pp. 206–215, 1850.
10 Chapter 8, p. 140, Hobbes, 1968. For a good account of Hobbes's psychology see Peters, 1967.
11 Chapter 8, p. 140, Hobbes, 1968.
12 Chapter 8, p. 141, Hobbes, 1968.
13 The religious dichotomy *possessio–obsessio* was the origin of the nineteenth century distinction between delusion and obsession.
14 Chapter 8, p. 142, Hobbes, 1968.
15 For an excellent analysis of Hobbes' style of analysing by contrast see Johnston, 1986.
16 Footnote, p. 526, Vol. 1, Locke, 1959.
17 On this see the excellent work by Sánchez, 1987: see particularly pp. 140–158 where Sánchez suggests that Locke gained direct acquaintance with the mentally ill during his French trip, and that this might have stimulated his interest in madness. This would explain why, whilst little mention of madness is made in the 1671 drafts of the 'Essay', Locke's 1675–1679 journals include many relevant entries which, in the event, were to appear in the 'Essay'.
18 Book II, Chapter XI, 12, Locke, 1959.
19 Book II, Chapter XI, 13, Locke, 1959.
20 Chapter 8, p. 141, Hobbes, 1968.
21 Book II, Chapter XI, 13, Locke, 1959.

22 Book II, Chapter XI, 13, Locke, 1959.

23 p. 139, Aaron, 1965.

24 Book II, Chapter XI, 13, Locke, 1959.

25 Book II, Chapter XI, 13, Locke, 1959.

26 Book II, Chapter XXXIII, 3 & 4, Locke, 1959. The 'continuity' view helped Locke to cope with the difficulty posed by the symptoms of madness to his empirical epistemology (see p. 142, Sánchez, 1987).

27 Book II, Chapter XXXIII, 5, Locke, 1959.

28 see Hoeldtke, 1967; Oberg, 1976.

29 For a general account of eighteenth century neurophysiology, see Carlson and Simpson, 1969; Jackson, 1970; Brazier, 1984.

30 p. 245, Hartley, 1834.

31 pp. 251–252, Hartley, 1834.

32 It has been suggested that Hartley's vibrationist neurophysiology is related to Newton's mathematical physics (see Smith, 1987).

33 p. 252, Hartley, 1834.

34 On Battie, see pp. 51–56, Leigh, 1961.

35 This view is also discussed by Hobbes: 'Every great agitation or concussion of the brain (as it happened from a stroke, specially if the stroke be upon one eye) whereby the optic nerve suffereth any great violence, there appeareth before the eyes a certain light, with light is nothing without.' (From Hobbes, 1651; quoted in p. 150, Rand, 1912.).

36 pp. 5–6, Battie, 1758.

37 p. 44, Battie, 1758.

38 p. 45, Battie, 1758.

39 p. 45, Battie, 1758.

40 p. 14, 'Introduction' by Hunter and McAlpine, 1962.

41 William Cullen (1712–1790) was an influential medic whose teaching attracted many to Edinburgh; he sponsored a form of 'neuralpathology' (the view that all diseases were diseases of the nervous system). Not much has been written on Cullen's psychiatric views. He is quoted *ad nauseam* for having coined the term *neurosis*. (see Bowman, 1975).

42 On this view Cullen was following Locke.

43 p. 167, Cullen, 1827.

44 p. 167, Cullen, 1827. This was at the time the accepted view. For example, Pargeter stated: 'The definition of madness, by the consent of all writers, is *delirium* [i.e. delusion] *without* fever' p. vi, Pargeter, 1792.

45 Carpenter, Thomas Arnold . . ., 1989.

46 pp. xv–xvi, Arnold, second edition, 1806.

47 Ralph Cudworth (1617–1688) was the leader of the Cambridge Platonists, said to have influenced Newton. He was professor of Hebrew, Master of Clare and then of Christ's College. Cudworth rejected the dualism of extended and thinking substance and postulated the existence of a sort of spiritual, plastic power in the universe. At her Oates home, his married daughter (Lady Masham) offered shelter to John Locke during his final years (see Passmore, 1951).

48 Henry St John Bolingbroke (1678–1751) was an English man of letters,

friend of Pope's, whose main contribution was in political philosophy. Controversy still reigns as to the real value of his work. He frequently quoted Locke but not always followed his views.

49 p. xvii, Arnold, 1806.

50 pp. 72–74, Arnold, 1782.

51 p. 59, Leigh, 1961; p. 469, Hunter and McAlpine, 1963.

52 Thomas Reid (1710–1796) was one of the central philosophers of the so-called Scottish School of Common Sense (which also included Dugald Stewart, Thomas Brown and to certain extent, William Hamilton) one of whose tenets was a return to a form of Faculty Psychology. In this sense, it was nearer to Kant than to Locke, Berkeley and Hume whose views they strongly criticized (see Marcil-Lacoste, 1982).

53 Karl Philipp Moritz (1757–1793) was a colourful German writer who suffered from a bipolar affective disorder, and whose work included fiction, grammatical textbooks, and an analysis of what can be called the philosophy of emotions (p. 267, *Biographie Universelle Ancienne et Moderne*, 1843–1847).

54 Salomon Maimon (1752–1800) was a distinguished Jewish philosopher and critic of the Lockean and Kantian separation between sensibility and understanding. His view was that if they constituted two different realms of knowledge, information could not flow from the one to the other as it does in the act of knowing. Maimon 'followed Leibniz and Wolff in the conception of sense knowledge as flowing from the same source as intellectual knowledge. They differ from each other only in clearness and completeness. While through understanding we attain clear and distinct concepts, sense knowledge is confused' (Atlas, 1967).

It is of some interest, therefore, that Crichton central argument was that Arnold's distinction was 'founded on a gratuitous distinction between ideas and notions' i.e. between sense and intellectual knowledge (p. xix. Crichton, 1798).

55 On the influence of Unzer on Crichton, an anonymous reviewer wrote some 50 years later: 'some of Crichton's principal merits are due to unacknowledged plagiarisms from the latter [Unzer] admirable treatise' (*Journal of Psychological Medicine and Mental Pathology* 1854). Supporting this view, in a handwritten note attached to the copy of Crichton's 'Inquiry' in the Library of the Royal College of Psychiatrists of the UK, Daniel Hack Tuke attributed this comment to 'Dr Laycock' (note opposite to page iv).

56 Crichton wrote: 'I received from Germany, among a number of works which had been recommended to me by my esteemed and learned friends, Professor Blumenbach and Professor Arnemann, of the University of Goettingen, one which greatly interested me. It was entitled *Magazine of Psychological Experience*. This work consists of no less than eight volumes, and was first published in numbers under the direction of two learned psychologists, Charles Philip Moritz and Salomon Maimon. In this work, I found what I had not yet met with in any other publication, a number of well authenticated cases of insane aberrations of mind . . .'

p. v, Crichton, 1798, *op. cit.*). For an analysis of some of these cases, see Förstl *et al.*, 1991; and Förstl and Rattay-Förstl, 1992.

57 The chapter of the *Inquiry* where Crichton dealt with delirium was translated into French by Pinel, and published as a separate pamphlet. It is one of the few references quoted by Esquirol (see next chapter) in his classical 1814 paper on *délire*.

58 pp. 137-138, Crichton, 1798.

59 Which was the conventional way of referring to hallucinations and delusions by British empiricists.

60 p. 138, Crichton, 1798.

61 pp. 140–141, Crichton, 1798.

62 p. 143, Crichton, 1798.

63 p. 147, Crichton, 1798.

64 p. 148, Crichton, 1798.

65 p. 176, Crichton, 1798. In spite of the fact that on this Crichton follows Battie's ideas, he calls his work 'wild romance' and sides with Monroe in the bruising exchange the two medics had in the 1750s (p. 157, Crichton, 1798).

66 For recent work on Pinel, see Garrabé, 1994; and for the general background Weiner, 1993.

67 See pp. 73-80, Riese, 1969.

68 See Postel, 1981.

69 p. 102, Pinel, 1809.

70 pp. 129–130, Pinel, 1809.

71 pp. 155–156, Pinel, 1809. This paragraph is already present in the first edition of this book although in a different section: pp. 149–150, Pinel, 1800. Interestingly, in a review of this first edition, Pinel's departure from the intellectualistic view is not noticed: 'The fourth section includes a classification of mental alienation. Without paying attention to earlier ones by other nosologists for they were not based, like his, on the clinical observation of large number of patients, Pinel identifies five species, according to the mode in which the intellectual functions (*fonctions de l'entendement*) are impaired.' (Jouard, 1880).

The earliest Pinelian reference I have found to the view that madness (*manie*) is not always the result of an impairment of the intellectual functions (*facultés de l'entendement*) dates from 1794: 'The idea of madness should not always carry the impression that it implies a total impairment of the intellectual faculties; on the contrary, the disorder may be partial affecting only the perception of ideas, judgment, reasoning, imagination, memory or psychological sensibility (*sensibilité morale*).'; p. 237, Postel, 1981. A recent English rendition of this text has also missed this point for the translator chose to render *facultés de l'entendement* as 'mental faculties'; see p. 729 in Weiner, 1992.

72 Pinel did not think much of the symptomatic method for it led to 'an infinite variety' of disorders; p. 5, Pinel, 1809.

73 p. 96, Pinel, 1809.

74 Destutt de Tracy, 1817. Destutt de Tracy (1754–1836) was the leader of

the so-called *Idéologues*, a group of thinkers trying to develop the views of Locke and Condillac.

75 Landré-Beauvais (1772–1840), disciple of Pinel and professor of Medicine at La Salpêtrière, was the author of a famous and influential book in which the symptoms of mental disorder were integrated with those of general medicine. This work, which went through numerous editions, can be considered as the first written from the point of view of a 'semiology' of disease (Landré-Beauvais, 1813).

76 pp. xxiii–xxiv, Landré-Beauvais, 1813.

77 pp. 4–5, Landré-Beauvais, 1813.

78 This was a clear reference to Locke's view.

79 p. 281, Landré-Beauvais, 1813.

80 p. 251, Esquirol, 1814.

81 p. 251, Esquirol, 1814.

82 p. 254, Esquirol, 1814.

83 On the French notion of *délire* see Lantéri-Laura, 1991.

84 The chapter on 'delirium' from Crichton's 'Inquiry' (1798) was translated and published separately by Pinel in the first issue of the *Recueil Périodique de Littérature Médicale Ètrangère* published by the *Société de Médicine* de Paris. Esquirol did quote this work; p. 259, Esquirol, 1814.

85 p. 354, Falret, 1864.

86 p. 333, Ball and Ritti, 1881.

87 Esquirol, 1838.

88 p. 12, Esquirol, 1838.

89 p. 191, Esquirol, 1838.

90 p. 38, Ey, 1939.

91 E.J. Georget (1795–1828), described as one of the great promises of early nineteenth century French psychiatry, died young. He qualified from Tours and Paris, and received his psychiatric training at the Salpêtrière under Esquirol, in whose arms he died.

92 p. 19, Georget, 1835. This entry was published posthumously and the list of references attached to the article was compiled by M. Dezeimeris, one of the editors.

93 p. 257, Georget, 1820.

94 p. 21, Georget, 1835.

95 Joseph Guislain (1797–1860), a follower of Esquirol, was born in Ghent, Belgium. He was both a thinker and a hospital reformer. His views influenced Griesinger and Morel.

96 p. 276, Guislain, 1852.

97 p. 278, Guislain, 1852. Some of the clinical examples suggest that he might have been referring to obsessions.

98 pp. 281–306, Guislain, 1852.

99 Jean Pierre Falret (1794–1870) trained under Esquirol and wrote on hypochondria and suicide, on administrative psychiatry, and against the concept of monomania. He was the father of Jules Falret (1824–1902), another important alienist.

100 This 50-page pamphlet entitled *Du Délire* is very difficult to obtain;

however, the entire text was reprinted in a later work, pp. 321–424, Falret, 1864.

101 For an excellent analysis of Falret's approach, see Lantéri-Laura, 1984.

102 p. 351, Falret, 1864.

103 p. 354, Falret, 1864.

104 p. 357, Falret, 1864.

105 p. 359, Falret, 1864.

106 pp. 360-361, Falret, 1864.

107 p. 361, Falret, 1864.

108 p. 362, Falret, 1864.

109 On Baillarger, see Chapter 3, On Disorders of Perception, this book.

110 Jaspers did not quote him, however, in the *Allgemeine Psychopathologie*, although Baillarger's book was in the library of the Heidelberg Clinic at the time he was there.

111 p. 291, Sérieux and Capgras, 1909.

112 p. 231, Séglas, 1903.

113 Ernest Charles Lasègue (1816–1883) trained first as a philosopher but influenced by Claude Bernard and Morel (with whom he had shared digs as a student), he switched to medicine and trained as a psychiatrist under Jean Pierre Falret. He is better known for his work on delirium tremens and anorexia nervosa.

114 p. 132, Lasègue, 1852.

115 p. 133, Lasègue, 1852.

116 pp. 85–105, Lasègue, 1971.

117 p. 22, Taty and Toy, 1887. This work was awarded a commendation when submitted for the 1895 Aubanel Prize.

118 See Pichot, 1982; Pichot, 1967; Porot, 1989.

119 Jacques Joseph Moreau de Tours (1804–1884) trained under Esquirol; he became interested on the effects of drugs (hashish) on mental state after accompanying a patient to the Near East (*Du Hachisch et de l'Aliénation Mentale*, 1845). His other great work appeared 14 years later (*La Psychologie Morbide*, 1859).

120 p. 44, Moreau de Tours, 1845.

121 p. 44, Moreau de Tours, 1845.

122 p. 83, Moreau de Tours, 1845.

123 p. 86, Moreau de Tours, 1845.

124 pp. 213–215, Moreau de Tours, 1859.

125 p. 215, Moreau de Tours, 1859.

126 pp. 211–212, Moreau de Tours, 1859.

127 For a discussion on concepts of normality and pathology during this period, see Canguilhem, 1966.

128 Louis Jean Delasiauve (1804–1893) had a wide range of clinical interests which included idiocy, epilepsy, psychiatric complications of physical disease and classification. In 1861, he started the *Journal de Médicine Mentale* which only lasted about 10 years.

129 p. 14, Delasiauve, 1861.

130 p. 12, Delasiauve, 1861.

131 p. 13, Delasiauve, 1861.

132 Ernst Freiherr von Feuchtersleben (1806–1849) was an Austrian
     physician, influenced by German Romanticism, whose theoretical interest
     in mental disorder led him to write two major books: *On the Dietetics of
     the Soul*, 1852 and *The Principles of Medical Psychology*, 1847.

133 p. 211, Feuchtersleben, 1847.

134 pp. 211–212, Feuchtersleben, 1847.

135 p. 213, Feuchtersleben, 1847.

136 p. 276, Feuchtersleben, 1847.

137 p. 276, Feuchtersleben, 1847.

138 p. 277, Feuchtersleben, 1847.

139 p. 277, footnote 3, Feuchtersleben, 1847.

140 pp. 279–282, Feuchtersleben, 1847.

141 pp. 283, Feuchtersleben, 1847.

142 Wilhelm Griesinger (1817–1868) was born in Stuttgart, qualified from
     Tubingen and trained as a psychiatrist under Zeller in Winnethal. As a
     young man he was actively involved in politics, and later in the strife
     between academic and asylum psychiatrists. In 1842 he founded the
     Archiv für Physiologische Heilkunde, and in 1867 the *Archiv für Psychiatrie
     und Nervenkrankheiten*. He was an internist with neuropsychiatric
     interests.

143 p. 71, Griesinger, 1861.

144 Berrios and Beer, 1994.

145 p. 71, Griesinger, 1861.

146 p. 72, Griesinger, 1861.

147 p. 72, Griesinger, 1861.

148 pp. 72–73, Griesinger, 1861.

149 For a rather flattering portrayal of Haslam, see pp. 94–147, Leigh, 1961.

150 pp. 5–6, Haslam, 1809. Haslam seems to be moving here in a
     medico-legal direction. On this, see Eigen, 1991.

151 Dugald Stewart (1753–1828) was another important member of the
     Scottish school of Common Sense (see Biographical Introduction by James
     M'Cosh, 1866). His views on the philosophy of mind were influential on
     the phrenological movement and through it on localisation theory and
     what nowadays is grandly called 'the modular view of the mind' (see
     Fodor, 1983).

152 pp. 15–16, Haslam, 1809.

153 'Mania' is being used here in its pre-nineteenth century sense, i.e. as a
     wide clinical category defined by an increase in the volume of behaviour
     and which may include schizophrenia, organic states, agitated depression,
     bipolar disorders, etc. It had little to do with current manic illness (see
     Berrios, 1981).

154 pp. 28–30, Haslam, 1809.

155 The *OED* describes this particular meaning as: 'The mental faculties in
     their normal condition of sanity; one's 'reason' or 'wits' and offers as
     illustration a quotation from 1794: 'Sometimes he would be in such fits
     of violence, that we almost thought he had lost his senses' (Mrs. Radcliffe
     Myst. Udolpho xli).

156 See pp. 148–209, Leigh, 1961; and on Prichard's work on anthropology see Stocking, 1973.
157 See Berrios, 1993.
158 p. 116, Prichard, 1835 (Prichard dedicated the book to Esquirol).
159 Prichard states that Guislain preferred Laromiguière to Locke, Condillac, Leibniz, and Kant (p. 118, Prichard, 1835). Pierre Laromiguière moved away from Condillac on the crucial point of the activity of the mind during the cognitive act (which he vigorously proposed). The teacher of Cousin, Jouffroy and Esquirol, Laromiguière is one of the origins of the spiritualist tradition in French philosophy which was to be so influential on French psychiatry during the nineteenth century (see pp. 1–20 in Taine, 1901; also pp. 110–128, Damirón, 1828; pp. 1–51, Cousin, 1826).
160 p. 120, Prichard, 1835.
161 p. 120, Prichard, 1835.
162 pp. 121–122, Prichard, 1835.
163 p. 4, Prichard, 1835.
164 p. 127, Bucknill and Tuke, 1858.
165 pp. 128–129, Bucknill and Tuke, 1858.
166 p. 496, Blount, 1856.
167 pp. 978–984, Axenfeld, 1883.
168 p. 978, Axenfeld, 1883.
169 On the history of hysterical insanity see pp. 209–312, Maleval, 1981.
170 p. 978, Axenfeld, 1883.
171 p. 981, Axenfeld, 1883.
172 p. 983, Axenfeld, 1883.
173 p. 332, Ball and Ritti, 1881.
174 p. 334, Ball and Ritti, 1881.
175 On unconscious cerebration, see Davies, 1873; on Carpenter, see Hall, 1979; on Laycock, see Leff, 1991; on the general intellectual background, see Young, 1970.
176 p. 336, Ball and Ritti, 1881.
177 p. 348, Ball and Ritti, 1883. They were here referring to a paper by Baillarger, 1856.
178 p. 338, Ball and Ritti, 1881.
179 For a discussion on impulsions, see Chapter 6, on Obsessions and Compulsions, this book.
180 p. 349, Ball and Ritti, 1881.
181 p. 384, Ball and Ritti, 1881.
182 p. 337, Ball and Ritti, 1881.
183 Walshe, 1957.
184 Jules Cotard researched into partial brain atrophy and softening, classification of insanity, aboulia, and hypochondria. His son, Lucien, also an alienist, died age 32 of a heart condition (see Berrios and Luque, 1995). For a full biography see p. 305, this book.
185 p. 366, Cotard, 1891.
186 p. 372, Cotard, 1891.

187 p. 421, Cotard, 1891.
188 See Berrios on the history of Parkinson's disease, 1995.
189 For information on Jackson, see Berrios on 'Positive and negative signals', 1992.
190 On the concept of hierarchy, see: Whyte *et al.*, 1969.
191 Savage, 1917.
192 pp. 415-416, Jackson, Vol. 2, 1932.
193 p. 418, Jackson, Vol. 2, 1932.
194 p. 482, Jackson, Vol. 2, 1932.
195 p. 415, Jackson, Vol. 2, 1932.
196 MacPherson, 1889; Stengel, 1963; also Berrios, 1977.
197 See Delay, 1957.
198 Rouart, 1950.
199 Ey, 1975; Evans, 1972.
200 p. 178, Porot, 1975.
201 Magnan and Sérieux, 1892.
202 Marie, 1892.
203 p. 478, Pichot, 1982.
204 Vaschide and Vurpas, 1903.
205 p. 2, Sérieux and Capgras, 1909.
206 pp. 4–5, Sérieux and Capgras, 1909.
207 p. 274, Targowla and Dublineau, 1931.
208 p. 300, Targowla and Dublineau, 1931.
209 Dupré, 1925.
210 Chaslin noticed this immediately and in a fine review of the book expressed surprise that, although 'in Germany there was a marked development of experimental studies in psychology . . . Karl Jaspers had utilized little these procedures' (p. 621) and 'he quoted little the French, except Janet' (p. 622); Chaslin Ph. *Allegemeine Psychopathologie* by K. Jaspers, 1914.
211 Phillipe Chaslin (1857–1923) was a French alienist who dedicated his life to clinical psychiatry (mostly spent at La Salpêtrière) and to mathematics. His encyclopaedic knowledge allowed the safe passage of French descriptivism from the nineteenth to the twentieth century. His concept of *confusion mentale primitive* marked the final separation of organic delirium from *délire*. He also wrote on mental handicap, epilepsy and other neurological diseases, and introduced the concept of 'discordance' as a description of, and an explanation for, schizophrenia (see Daumezón, 1973; Noël, 1984).
212 p. 17, Chaslin, La 'psychiatrie' est-elle une langue bien faite?, 1914.
213 p. 18, Chaslin, 1914.
214 Chaslin, 1890.
215 p. 46, Chaslin, 1890. On Tamburini's hypothesis, see Tamburini, 1990.
216 pp. 49–50, Chaslin, 1890.
217 Chaslin, 1912. This great book, about 1000-pages long, is a mine of clinical information.
218 The chapter is 16 000-words long and includes 45 clinical vignettes. To

emphasize its clinical nature, and not to make it overlong, Chaslin took
the decision – difficult for a man with an incomparable historical
knowledge – not to reference the book at all: 'it seems to me that this
work should be useful to the non-specialist who is forced to work as an
alienist, and also to the philosopher; like trainees, they should be
confronted with the facts . . . if by any chance a trained alienist did me
the honour of reading this book I should like to explain that a work
whose only aim is to be a practical guide . . . does not need to include
historical or bibliographical information.' (*Préface*, Chaslin, 1912).

219 p. 176, Chaslin, 1912.
220 For an analysis of the notion of *discordance* in the work of Chaslin see:
     Lantéri-Laura and Gros, 1984 (and re-issued in an expanded version:
     Lantéri-Laura and Gros, 1992). In 1926, Bleuler politely stated that: 'had
     the term "discordant insanity" been available [before I coined
     schizophrenia] I may well have used it'.
221 pp. 177–178, Chaslin, 1912.
222 p. 178, Chaslin, 1912. This shows how aware Chaslin was of new ideas,
     particularly for around the time he wrote his book, Freud was not yet
     well known in France; for this, see Hesnard and Laforgue, 1925.
223 p. 179, Chaslin, 1912.
224 Karl Jaspers (1883–1969) was a German philosopher who worked as a
     psychiatrist up to the First World War. In his early thirties, he
     abandoned psychiatry to dedicate himself to writing books on philosophy,
     and also political issues and intellectual biography. His psychiatric output
     includes 10 articles all written before 1913, when the first edition of
     General Psychopathology (*Allgemeine Psychopathologie*) was published. This
     book went through seven editions, the last in 1959. After the third
     edition, Jaspers delegated its updating to Kurt Schneider. This is
     important to those attempting a conceptual analysis of the 1963 English
     translation (in fact, the seventh German edition).
225 This area needs urgent research. For a general view, see Berrios, British
     psychopathology since the early 20th century, 1991.
226 Jaspers, 1910.
227 Jaspers, 1912.
228 Jaspers, 1911.
229 Jaspers, 1913.
230 pp. 78–90 *Das Realitätsbewußtsein und die Wahnideen*, in Jaspers, 1948.
231 See Walker, 1991; Hoenig, 1968; Koehler, 1976; Fish, 1968; Spitzer,
     1988. As a general background and information on German views, see
     the superb Huber and Gross, 1977; and Blankenburg, 1991.
232 Jaspers, 1963.
233 Hodges, 1952; Martin-Santos, 1955; Walker, 1988.
234 Schmidt, 1940.
235 See Berrios, 'British psychopathology since the early 20th century', 1991.
236 For information on Bernard Hart, see Berrios, 'British psychopathology
     since the early 20th century', 1991.
237 p. 42, Hart, 1916.

238 pp. 55–56, Hart, 1916.
239 Schmidt, 1940.
240 Ey, 1950.
241 Morel, 1950; Ey *et al.*, 1952.
242 Schmidt, 1940.
243 Ey *et al.*, 1952.
244 Morel, 1950.
245 Guiraud, p. 37, Morel, 1950.
246 Guiraud, p. 40, Morel, 1950.
247 p. 59, Morel, 1950.
248 pp. 60–61, Bleuler, 1906.
249 Morel, 1950.
250 Rümke, p. 182, Morel, 1950.
251 Bain, 1859.
252 Bucknill and Tuke, 1858.
253 Quinton, 1967.
254 Price, 1931.
255 Jaspers, 1963.
256 Price, 1931.
257 Iversen, 1984.
258 Hemsley and Garety, 1986.
259 Fischhoff and Beyth-Marom, 1983.
260 Gigerenzer *et al.*, 1989.
261 Hemsley and Garety, 1986.
262 Nisbett *et al.*, 1983.
263 Berrios, 1990.
264 Luys, 1876.
265 Berrios, 'Positive and negative symptoms' and Jackson, 1985.
266 Jackson, 1894.
267 Berrios, 1992.
268 Wernicke, 1906.
269 Chaslin, 1912.
270 Austin, 1962.
271 p. 466, De Clérambault, 1942.
272 Sérieux and Capgras, 1909.
273 Hagen, 1861.
274 p. 44 and p. 247, Moreau de Tours, 1845.
275 p. 47, p. 63 and p. 266, Moreau de Tours, 1845, see also p. 98, this book.
276 pp. 40–47, Paulus, 1941.
277 pp. 75–78, Krafft-Ebing, 1893.
278 p. 343, p. 414, Ball and Ritti, 1881.
279 Berrios, On a theory of hallucinations, 1990.
280 Cotard, 1891.
281 p. 224, p. 226, Séglas, 1903.
282 pp. 157–164, Hesnard, 1924.
283 pp. 484–5, Vol. 2, De Clérambault, 1942.

284 Dupré, 1925.
285 p. 435, De Clérambault, 1942.
286 Mourgue, 1932.
287 Morsier, 1938.
288 pp. 255-273, pp. 300–303, Targowla and Dublineau, 1931.
289 p. 207, p. 209, Lacan, 1975.
290 pp. 144–146, Jaspers, 1963.
291 p. 80, Marco-Merenciano, 1942.
292 p. 291, Serieux and Capgras, 1909.
293 Berrios and Marková, 1995.
294 Magnan and Sérieux, 1892.
295 pp. 15–33, Oltmanns and Maher, 1988.
296 p. 226, Gigerenzer *et al.*, 1989.
297 Helmsley and Garety, 1986.
299 Bentall *et al.*, 1991.
299 Kinderman, 1994.
300 Roberts, 1992.
301 p. 299, Roberts, 1992.
302 pp. 178–179, Bleuler, 1969.
303 p. 280, Lange, 1942.
304 p. 109, Schneider, 1959.
305 Wetzel, 1922.
306 p. 39, Conrad, 1958.
307 p. 98, Jaspers, 1963.
308 pp. 51–52, Oepen *et al.*, 1988.
309 Blondel, 1914.
310 See Dupré, 1913, 1925.
311 p. 34, Mauz, 1931.
312 p. 34, Mauz, 1931.
313 p. 10, Lafora, 1931.
314 Berze's sense of 'primary insufficiency' (Berze, 1914).
315 pp. 967–974, Cabaleiro Goas, 1966.
316 p. 1007, Cabaleiro Goas, 1966.
317 Colodrón, 1991.
318 Llopis, 1946.
319 pp. 23–26, Llopis, 1969.
320 Ey, 'Structure des psychoses aiguës et déstructuration de la conscience', 1954.
321 p. 36, Ey, 1950.
322 p. 90, Störring, 1944.
323 Berrios, On British psychopathology since the early 20th century, 1991.
324 Hoch, 1921.
325 p. 422, MacCurdy, 1925.
326 p. 422, MacCurdy, 1925.
327 Berrios and Marková, 1995.
328 Berrios, On delusions as wrong beliefs, 1991.
329 Berrios, On delusions as wrong beliefs, 1991.

330 Fuentenebro, 1995.
331 Marková and Berrios, 1995.
332 Sérieux and Capgras, 1909.
333 Christodoulou, 1986.
334 Kendler *et al.*, 1983; Garety and Hemsley, 1987.
335 Berrios, On historical background to abnormal psychology, 1988.

CHAPTER 6

Obsessions and compulsions

The terms obsession and compulsion name interloping and iterative thoughts and actions of a type and severity that may fracture behaviour. The condition is accompanied by feelings of distress, and *declarations* of resistance. Insight is assumed to be present but it may be belied by bizarre checking behaviour. Since last century, major works of scholarship on this condition have appeared.[1] But obsession-like behaviours can be found mentioned in the literature of the ages, often under social or religious labels;[2] and the question of whether such phenomena are neurobiologically equivalent to what is now called *obsessive–compulsive disorder* is tantalising. The *medical* concepts built into this diagnosis were tooled in Europe during the second half of the nineteenth century. This chapter deals with the historical process whereby such concepts and behaviours were brought together and transformed into a disease.

Obsession before 1800

In the *Anatomy of Melancholy*, Robert Burton reported an individual 'who dared not go over a bridge, come near a pool, rock, steep hill, lie in a chamber where cross beams were, for fear he be tempted to hang, drown or precipitate himself. In a silent auditorium as at a sermon, he [was] afraid he shall speak aloud at unawares, something indecent, unfit to be said . . .'[3] Bishop Moore of Norwich referred to subjects overwhelmed by 'naughty and sometimes blasphemous thoughts' which 'start in their minds while they are exercised in the Worship of God'.[4] David Hartley described states of 'frequent recurrency of the same ideas' 'When a person applies himself to any particular study, so as to fix his attention deeply on the ideas and terms belonging to it, it is commonly observed, that he becomes narrow minded' 'the perpetual recurrency of particular ideas and terms makes the vibrations belonging thereto become more than ordinarily vivid, converts associations into strong ones.'[5] Medieval terms such as *obsessio*, *compulsio*, and *impulsio* seem to have referred to behaviours redolent of obsessions; and so have vernacular words such as *scruple*[6] which since the 1500s (if not earlier) named repetitive thoughts of religious nature. The term appears in the autobiography of Ignatius of Loyola (the founder of the Society of Jesus) suggesting a (probable) organic obsessional disorder.[7] Likewise, in 1660, Bishop Taylor (1660) wrote: 'scruple is a great trouble of minde proceeding from a little motive, and a great indisposition, by which the conscience though sufficiently determined by proper arguments, dares not proceed to action, or if it does, it cannot rest.'[8] Terms such as superstition have also been used for the same purpose. For example, James Boswell wrote of Dr Johnson: 'He had another particularity . . . it appeared to me some superstitious habit, which had contracted early . . . this was his anxious care to go out or in at a door or passage, by a certain number of steps from a certain point, or at least so that either his right or his left foot (I am not certain which) should constantly make the first actual movement when he came close to the door or passage.'[9]

The nineteenth century

Terminology

During the nineteenth century, psychiatric terminology formed out of three sources: classical vocabulary (e.g. mania, melancholia, paranoia); *sermo vulgaris* which furnished terms to which technical meanings were attached (e.g. hallucination, obsession, stupor); and neologisms (e.g. lypemania, monomania).

GERMAN TERMINOLOGY In European psychiatry, the earliest *technical* term to refer to obsessions is *Zwangsvorstellung*, a compound word coined by Krafft-Ebing in 1867 to refer to irresistible thoughts.[10] It reflected the author's views on the *origin* of the disorder: *Zwang* derives from the high German *dwang* via *Twanc* which is the middle high German for 'to compel, to oppress'.[11] The word *Vorstellung*, in turn, meant at the time 'presentation or representation' and had been introduced by Wolff a century earlier to refer to the Cartesian 'idea'.[12] This noble term, of great importance in German psychology and psychiatry, was made popular by J.F. Herbart.[13]

Taking Krafft Ebing's term one step further, Westphal equated 'presentation' with the straightforward notion of 'idea' (until then the terms *had not been* regarded as synonymous), and concluded that obsessional states resulted from a disorder of intellectual function.[14] This 'intellectualistic' interpretation remained influential in German psychiatry until the twentieth century.[15] 'Presentations' were subdivided into 'pure mental experiences' (i.e. obsessive ideas or ruminations) and precursors of actions (i.e. compulsions); in this way, Westphal also started the view that compulsions were secondary or parasitical upon obsessions.[16] This ambiguity is responsible for a translational divergence that once upon a time had clinical significance, namely that *Zwangsvorstellung* was rendered as 'obsession' in Great Britain but as 'compulsion' in the USA; indeed, the term 'obsessive–compulsive disorder' was suggested as a compromise![17] *Zwang* also provided the stem for *Zwangshandlung*, *Zwangsphenomenen*, *Zwangszustand* all used to refer to iterative states and actions of various kinds.[18]

Before Krafft Ebing, Griesinger had already introduced another term, *Sucht*,[19] meaning 'disease, passion' to refer to states behaviourally coterminous with those named by *Zwangvorstellung*, and coined *Grubelnsucht* to name a subtype of ruminative behaviour;[20] the term gained additional force from the fact that Grubeln was an old German word meaning 'racking one's brains'.[21]

In a lecture delivered before the Royal Medical Society of Budapest on November 1895, Donath[22] proposed *Anancasmus*[23] as an alternative name for the syndrome that Thomsen had called *idiopathic obsessional state* (*idiopathische Zwangsvorgänge*).[24] The new term caught on for it lent itself to adjectival use[25] as in 'anancastic personality'.[26]

FRENCH TERMINOLOGY Obsessions travelled under various terms in French psychiatry.[27] Early in the nineteenth century, it was considered as a form of insanity, and brought under categories such as *manie sans délire*, *monomanie intellectuel*, and *folie lucide*. All three categories emphasized pathological changes in the 'intellectual' faculty and this reinforced the view that obsessions might also be a disorder of thinking.[28]

By the second half of the century, the view that emotions might be primarily involved in the aetiology of obsessions was developed by Morel and reflected in the appearance of a new term, *délire emotif*.[29] The word *obsession* (a derivative of the old Latin *obsidere*) gained its *medical* meaning in 1866 in the work of Falret.[30] Until this period, it had been used in the Medieval 'transitive' sense of being 'besieged' by an external agent.[31] Littré's dictionary did yet not recognize the new meaning,[32] although around the time of its publication the great Luys used *obsessions pathologiques* to refer to 'anomalous and repetitive, subjective events without external source.'[33] Luys' usage was also an important departure for he made obsessions into *internal*, private affairs. This novel view was soon accepted in French psychiatry.[34]

BRITISH TERMINOLOGY Terminology in the English language followed a similar path and a common term was 'fixed idea'.[35] The word 'obsession' had been in use since the sixteenth century to describe the act of being besieged by the devil,[36] but came into medical usage in 1892; indeed, at this time, D.H. Tuke still preferred 'imperative idea',[37] although in his translation of Legrain's entry[38] for the *Dictionary of Psychological Medicine*, he anglicized the corresponding French word to 'obsession and impulse'. As late as 1896, Mickle tried to introduce 'mental besetment'.[39] But the term 'obsession' was eventually adopted by *The Lancet* and the *British Medical Journal* at the beginning of this century.[40] Thus, in his 1904 review, Shaw wrote as if the word 'obsession' had been in use for some time.[41]

The term obsession also appeared in American literature by 1902.[42] In 1906, The Nomenclature of Diseases drawn up by the Joint Committee of the Royal College of Physicians in London (which included George Savage and Percy Smith as the psychiatric members) recognized 'obsessive insanity'.[43]

The history of the concepts

French contribution

ESQUIROL (1772–1840) Esquirol effectively opened a new nosological slot for what was to be known as obsessional disorder when he renamed *Mademoiselle F.'s délire partiel* as a form of 'reasoning or instinctive monomania'.[44] This he defined as 'involuntary, irresistible, and instinctive activity' that 'chained [the patient] to actions that neither reason or emotion have originated, that conscience rejects, and will cannot suppress.'[45] Mademoiselle F.[46] described her thoughts as 'irresistible' but had 'insight' into the fact that they were not hers. Esquirol oscillated between explaining her complaint as a disorder of ideas or of the will; this indecision beset French psychiatry to the second half of the century when a third aetiological mechanism, deranged emotions, was added.[47]

The fact that Esquirol regarded obsessions as a form of monomania did not help the inchoate clinical category for the concept of monomania itself came under attack by the 1850s.[48] Its critics claimed that it: (*a*) did not respond to clinical observation and resulted from a mechanical application of Faculty Psychology,[49] (*b*) encompassed too many clinical states and had little or nothing to say about individual cases,[50] (*c*) was based on cross-sectional observation and had no conceptual machinery to deal with longitudinal changes,[51] and (*d*) created medico-legal difficulties.[52] The knell of monomania was sounded at the 1853–54 debate of the *Société Médico-Psychologique* in Paris.[53] Its disappearance set obsessions asunder.

MOREL (1809–1873) Efforts to define the complaint as a disorder of intellect had been unsuccessful for the latter could not explain the emotional accompaniment of obsessions. B.A. Morel was keen on aetiological classifications[54] and suggested that obsessions might result from a dysfunction of the ganglionar (autonomic) nervous system. *Délire emotif* was to be not 'an insanity but a neurosis, that is, a disease of the emotions:'[55] 'What I call *délire emotif* corresponds to a particular type of fixed idea and abnormal act whose existence, however, does not entail a [primary] involvement of intellectual faculties.'[56] In this regard, 'compulsions' also resulted from a 'heightened *affective* state'.

Délire emotif was a broad category and included patients with vasomotor and digestive symptomatology, phobias, dysphoria, unmotivated fears, fixed ideas, and impulsions whose common feature was absence of 'cognitive impairment or hallucinations'. Almost 40 years later, Janet followed similar clinical boundaries to outline his notion of psychasthenia.[57]

Three reasons explain the success of *délire emotif*: the reputation of Morel, it provided an alternative to the German view that obsessions (*Vorstellungen*) were a disorder of thinking,[58] and it was flexible enough to fit both somatic and subjective symptoms, including generalised and paroxysmal anxiety.[59] However, Luys disagreed with Morel's view that all vegetative functions were localized in the ganglionar system, and suggested instead that obsessions originated in the cortex; furthermore, since ideas, emotions and actions had separate cortical localization, 'bizarre ideas', 'involuntary' emotions and compulsive acts originated independently.[60]

The reclassification of obsessions as a form of 'neuroses' re-opened the possibility that they might be an expression of pathology in brain sites related to emotions and volition. However, at this time, the meaning of neurosis itself began to change and no longer demanded a *focalized* lesion;[61] this was, for example, the view of Axenfeld.[62]

DAGONET (1823–1902) AND *L'IMPULSION* In the same way that obsession had to be separated off from 'delusion',[63] compulsion required separation from *impulsion*, a category of behaviour that since early in the nineteenth century[64] had been used in French psychiatry to name all manner of paroxysmal, stereotyped, and (apparently) *involuntary* actions.[65] Impulsion was for Dagonet an irresistible and involuntary act, that imposed itself upon the mind just like hallucinations or fixed ideas.[66] His view had, however, religious and moralistic connotations. This was corrected by Magnan: 'Impulsion is a mode of cerebral activity that forces actions that occasionally the will cannot prevent.'[67] Bourdin criticized this definition and proposed a four-fold classification of impulsions: conscious, unconscious, pseudo- and mixed. Conscious impulsions were secondary to obsessions; unconscious ones followed fleeting ideas which left no memory after the act was committed (e.g. epileptic impulsions); pseudo-impulsions followed a delusion or a hallucination and were typical of insanity; lastly 'mixed impulsions' were combinations thereof and characterized hysterical insanity.[68] In the work of Bourdin impulsions lost their moral connotation and mysterious irresistibility, and became incorporated into the general field of mental disorder. Pitres and Régis completed this process: 'impulsions have no special aetiology and their cause merges with that of insanity . . . impulsivity is a return to elementary reflex action which betrays a form of inferiority, whether innate or acquired.'[69]

Dagon et also resuscitated the notion of 'impulsive insanity' (*folie impulsive*) which included phobias, homicidal and suicidal tendencies, manic behaviour, hypochondriacal preoccupations, and epileptic seizures.[70] After offering a clinical and taxonomic analysis of this putative disease, he concluded that any subject suffering from insanity might show *impulsions violentes, irresistibles* which effectively led to a 'failure of the will' and were either primary or followed delusions, emotions or hallucinations.[71] To complicate matters, Dagonet included under impulsive insanity a disorder redolent of obsessions in which: 'the more one tries to discard the idea, the more it becomes imposed upon the mind, the more one tries to get rid of the emotion or tendency, the stronger it becomes.'[72]

LEGRAND DU SAULLE (1830–1886) The natural history of the obsessive disorder
was consolidated in the work of Legrand du Saulle who in 1875 reported a series
of 27 cases (11 his own).[73] He was one of the first to recognize that patients admitted to hospital were not typical in that they also showed psychotic symptoms or
depression. He was also aware of the fact that obsessions had a fluctuating course,
insidious onset, and tendency to change. He re-named the condition *folie de doute
avec délire de toucher* and proposed that it was a variety of *folie avec conscience*
('insanity with insight'). It tended to have *early* onset, and was more frequent in
females, high social classes, and fastidious and rigid personalities.

There were three stages in its evolution. The first was characterized by 'involuntary, spontaneous and irresistible thoughts without illusions or hallucinations'
accompanied by 'feelings of doubt, of brooding' and occasionally 'mental representations and images' of the thoughts. These symptoms engendered fears and anxieties which eventually led to rituals. The second stage was marked by the 'unexpected
revelations' made to relatives and friends of symptoms kept in secret for years.
Depression, anxiety and agitation together with suicidal brooding were common
but the latter rarely led to actual self-harm. 'Animal phobias', somatic (e.g.
vasomotor) symptoms, rituals, fear of touching objects, abnormal cleanliness, hand
washing, and 'eccentric behaviour' complicated the picture. Insight was not lost
and symptoms fluctuated in severity. The third stage started when rituals and
obsessional paralysis appeared that severely impaired psychosocial competence. On
follow-up (which in some cases was as long as 20 years), Legrand du Saulle found
that some patients remained house-bound, maintaining only a semblance of
insight, and showing a typical 'double book-keeping' behaviour. They often harbour
a 'darker, psychotic attitude'; however, no evolution towards dementia was ever
detected.[74]

Legrand du Saulle accepted Morel's concept of *délire emotif*, i.e. that obsessions
were a disorder of emotions. His acute clinical eye, however, had identified sufficient
patients with 'psychotic' symptoms to justify the use of terms such as *folie* and
délire. Under *délire emotif*, he included animal phobias, agoraphobia, vasomotor
phenomena, panic disorder and complex partial seizures.

BALL (1834–1893) B. Ball offered eight operational criteria for obsessions: presence of insight, sudden onset (subjects may even remember the day the disease
started), paroxysmal (severity varies; winter being a period of calm) and fluctuating
course (frequent periods of remission); absence of cognitive impairment; *release* of
tension by the compulsion; frequent somatic and anxiety symptoms; and, family
history (although acquired obsessions were common).[75] Ball also recognized three
subtypes: minor (only obsessions), moderate (presence of anxiety and major
hesitations), and major (compulsions). The disease could be brought about by
fatigue, major life events, puberty, sexual problems, pregnancy, puerperium and
menopause. Ball believed that obsessions resulted from impaired brain circulation

and advised against the use of morphine. The predominance of particular symptoms led to recognizing colourful subtypes: 'metaphysicians', 'realists', 'scrupulous', 'timids', etc.[76]

MAGNAN (1835–1916) Magnan classified mental disorders into: 1. organic, 2. psychoses (proper), and 3. mental retardations; and the psychoses into mania, melancholia, chronic delusional state, intermittent psychoses, and psychoses of degeneration (*folie des dégénérés*). Obsessions belonged to the latter, together with phobias, agoraphobia, sexual perversions, and hypochondriacal states.[77] Magnan believed that obsessions and its variants *onomatomanie* (the counting obsession)[78] and *erythromanie* (*facilité extrême à rougir*, blushing)[79] resulted from cerebral pathology[80] which 'appeared only in subjects affected by degeneration and [hence] merited to be considered as the psychological stigmata of degeneration psychosis.'[81] P.L. Ladame, himself a great specialist in obsessions, summarized well Magnan's contribution: 'Since Morel, the majority of authors have regarded heredity as an important factor in obsessions. No one had, however, considered the symptoms themselves as a sign of pathological heredity. This is what Magnan has successfully achieved. For him, obsessions and impulsions are but episodic presentations of the psychosis of degeneration, i.e. are psychological stigmata.'[82]

The German contribution

GRIESINGER, WESTPHAL, THOMSEN AND TUCZEK Obsessions were conceived of differently by German authors who tended to emphasize its 'intellectual' aspects.[83] On 28th March 1868, at a meeting of the Berlin Medico-Psychological Society[84] W. Griesinger read a paper on 'a little known psychopathic state' which he believed to be similar to the 'so-called *maladie de doute* de Falret.'[85] He reported three cases: a middle aged woman, a 34 year-old Russian prince, and a 21 year-old lad all suffering from obsessional ruminations (*Grübelsucht*) and self-questioning, and proposed that these complaints resulted from an 'impairment of ideas'.

At the 5th March 1877 meeting of the same Society, Westphal read his paper on: *Über Zwangsvorstellungen* in which he completed the German view of the disease. He knew of du Saulle's and Falret's work, and took into account Griesinger's *Grübelsucht*. Obsessions differed from delusions in that they were *ego-dystonic* (insanity of doubt); compulsive (*délire de toucher*), and impulsive. They reflected a pathology of thinking and not of emotions.[86] This latter conclusion was not accepted by Sander and Jastrowitz who in the discussion that followed defended the opposite view.[87]

But the most cogent case against the 'intellectual' thesis was put forward by the Swiss Ludwig Wille[88] who sided with the French in suggesting an emotional origin for obsessions. Wille believed that the symptoms were changeable and fluctuating, and could on occasions turn into insanity,[89] particularly of the *melancholic* type. Based on the analysis of 16 cases, he proposed that obsessions constituted a transitional state between neuroses and psychoses, and that with the affective psychoses they formed a new group: the hereditary psychoses.[90] Following this lead, Thomsen[91] went on to classify obsessions into *secondary* (*deuteropathische Zwangsvorgänge*) conditions such as hysteria, phobias, and neurasthenia and a *primary* or *idiopathic* group which also included tics, coprolalia, migraine, and somatic sensations. In the same year (1895), Donath coined in his Budapest address the term *anacasmus* to refer to Thomsen's idiopathic group. What is more important, he made a determined effort to reduce its size. *Anacasmus* has since been used in ways other than his originator intended.[92]

At the very end of the century, in an equally seminal paper, Tuczek suggested that obsessions only developed on the fertile ground of a particular *personality* structure.[93] Then Löwenfeld reported that although 70% of 200 'anancastic' patients showed family history of mental illness, the latter was so dissimilar that obsessions 'do not seem to form a unitary condition.'[94] Lastly, in 1915 Kraepelin proposed *Zwangsneurose* to name a 'series of conditions' including the phobic states. The impulsive psychosis, however, was separated out.[95]

The British contribution

In regard to obsessions, British alienists limited themselves to commenting upon Continental views. After reviewing the latter, Ireland concluded in 1885 that: 'it does not seem to me that we are able to explain the persistence of such ideas by a reference to known facts in the physiology of the brain'.[96] Julius Mickle dedicated his Presidential address before the *Medico Psychological Association* to 'mental besetments' which he defined as the 'state in which the mind is affected by some compulsive thought, of a kind, or irrational and often progressive fear; alone, or conjoined with an impulse which is, or tends to become, irresistible. Also an abulic form [*sic*].'[97] Under besetments, Mickle included agoraphobia and other phobic states, tics, the jumping disease, Myriachit, and Latah.[98] Feeling unable to take sides in the aetiological dispute, he backed all three views at once: 'But I think that here the proper 'organizing idea' is that, broadly viewed, besetments invariably tend to, and usually are, a blending of anomalies of all three: thought; feeling; will'.[99] The term mental besetments never caught on. Few years later, Claye Shaw published a review sensibly entitled 'Obsessions' and reported a solitary case with contamination fears.[100]

TUKE AND JACKSON During the last decade of the nineteenth century, the most interesting British event concerning obsessions is the debate between H.Jackson, D.H.Tuke and others on the 'mechanism' of obsessions.[101] It started on 1st March 1894 with a paper on 'Imperative Ideas' read by the elderly Tuke before the Neurological Society in London where he quoted Jackson's general point that, from a theoretical perspective, minor departures from mental health were as important as the severe ones.[102] He regretted that imperative ideas tended to be reported only when complicated by depression or delusions and objected to the French *obsession* for it evoked demoniac associations! His own view was that imperative ideas included emotions or impulses and that, whatever their intensity, these never acquired a delusional quality. Obsessions were frequently accompanied by a family history of epilepsy. Tuke bemoaned the fact that a plea of 'imperative ideas' had little value in English law.[103]

Although no cortical lesions had yet been found, it was possible to understand the impulsiveness of obsessions in terms of 'Laycock's doctrine of the reflex or automatic function of the cerebral cortex.'[104] According to this doctrine, 'by what is termed the association of ideas, the morbid action of vesicular neurine[105] be brought within the current of his thought he becomes utterly powerless to resist it, as much so as the electro-biologized (hypnotized) to resist the suggestions presented to their minds. The formation of these *substrata* is due to fixity of the mind on one idea or class of ideas, at a time when, from morbid changes, induced in the vesicular neurine (as by undue mental labour, intense emotional excitement, want of repose, the development of a dormant disposition, and the like), it is unusually susceptible to the operation of the unconsciously constructing mind, so that the fixed idea becomes deeply writ, as it were, on the vesicular neurine, in the same way as acquired instincts, habits, etc.; and are, in fact, as difficult to remove.'[106]

Laycock's speculative views on the neurobiology of memory were no longer current in the neurophysiology of the 1890s, but Tuke sympathized with Jackson's efforts to resuscitate them. This was because they provided Tuke with a mechanism for the acquisition of imperative ideas which preserved his belief that the content of obsessions was aleatory. Based on Jackson's model, Tuke went on to suggest that obsessions were exaggerated forms of behaviour released by the weakening of mental power (i.e. they were *positive* symptoms resulting from a *negative* symptom): 'With regard to those cases in which there is a morbid dread of dirt, I do not know that we can say more, in many instances, than that there is an exaggeration of the scrupulous cleanliness which in a marked degree characterizes some persons who are in perfect health, but the origin of the imperative idea may occasionally be traced to some affection of the skin, which has necessitated the attention being drawn to it, and has at last induced a morbid state of mind, not of introspection but of 'extero-spection'. Should the general mental power be lowered, or a hereditary predisposition exist, this tendency to attend to the state of the skin becomes a passion.'[107]

In what turned out to be a valediction (he died of a brain haemorrhage five days after delivering it), Tuke explained how imperative ideas were acquired and remembered (as per Laycock's hypothesis) and why did they manifest themselves the way they did (as per Jackson's hierarchical model).

Jackson had not been present at the meeting and submitted a reply stating that he had seen cases with imperative ideas as described by Tuke, but paid little attention to them.[108] Rather harshly, he stated that the view expressed in his Leeds paper (quoted by Tuke),[109] *did not apply to imperative ideas*: 'without qualification'. His view was that: 'certain very absurd and persisting delusions are owing to fixation of grotesque fancies or dreams in cases where a morbid change in the brain happens suddenly, during sleep.'[110] In the case of imperative ideas 'certain obtrusive thoughts which otherwise might be transitory become fixed, become 'imperative ideas', consequent on some *very slight morbid change* in the brain occurring during sleep' (my italics).[111]

Thus, Jackson seemed to be suggesting that the difference between delusion and imperative idea concerned the *severity* of the morbid change: mild in the latter, marked in the former. The alienist must: 'account for the existence of these quasi-parasitical states in cases where the general mental power is but little lessened.'[112] In the rest of the paper Jackson repeats his views and those of Monro and Anstie. He agreed with Tuke that 'the scientific study of insanities may be best begun in general hospitals.'[113]

George Savage, Charles Mercier, and Milne Bramwell also submitted replies to Tuke's paper. Savage criticised the use of the term 'imperative' for the 'ideas are not always the spring of action'.[114] In typical fashion, Mercier stated that what 'impressed me most was Tuke's complete acceptance of a doctrine that I have long held and preached.'[115] Milne Bramwell summarized Continental ideas and reported eighteen cases, stating that 'in nearly all the condition appears to have had an *emotional* origin' (my italics)[116] and challenged Tuke's view that obsession was an 'automatic' phenomenon: 'Are these acts automatic? An automatic act is simply an habitual voluntary one performed inattentively or unconsciously; while the so-called automatic acts of the sufferer from imperative ideas are carried out in opposition to his volition and frequently associated with intense and painful consciousness. Possibly with justice they might be called *reflex*, seeing that they are a 'fatal, unchosen, response to stimulation' (my italics).[117] This criticism was off the mark because Tuke's 'automatism' referred not to the content of imperative ideas but the mechanism by means of which they are acquired.

The aftermath

In the event, the view that obsessions resulted from disturbances of emotions was to prevail. The reasons for this were less scientific than social as there was no methodology then (as, indeed, there is not now!) to demonstrate that, at such level of abstraction, the emotional hypothesis is superior to the cognitive or volitional one. Anxiety-based explanations became acceptable not only because great men espoused them, but because during the second half of the nineteenth century there was a revival of 'affectivity', emotions, and of interest in the autonomic nervous system.[118] Furthermore, there were rivalries between Germany and France with great writers in the latter country (e.g. Ribot) championing the emotions. There was also the *Zeitgeist* factor: in France, this was a period of heightened social anxiety,[119] and the complaints brought to doctors often fell outside traditional insanity concepts. This is the period when notions such as neurasthenia, psychasthenia, and *surmenage* (all related to energy and emotions) made their appearance. Lastly, the work of psychologists like Ribot and Janet took place in a period when philosophical fashion favoured the emotions.[120] It was, therefore, predictable that 'diseases' such as agoraphobia and obsessions were re-conceptualized in emotional terms. A good illustration of this trend is the work of Janet.

JANET (1859–1947) Janet's views on obsessions owe much to his predecessors, including Pitres and Régis. His work, as his co-worker Raymond[121] once said, is more '*theoretical* than clinical' (my italics).[122] Obsessions resulted from an *engourdissement* of the mind;[123] they were the experiential concomitant of a 'feeling of incompletion' resulting from a defect in the 'function of the real'. In *L'Automatisme Psychologique*[124] Janet defined obsession as an *idée fixe* which, together with hallucinations, constituted 'simple and rudimentary forms of mental activity.'[125]

This view, heavy with the assumptions of late nineteenth century energetist psychology, amounts to no more than a metaphorical re-description of what patients say of their inability to bring tasks to completion. 'Psychasthénie' was carved out from the already inflated category of neurasthenia;[126] indeed, psychasthenia was itself an over-inclusive category soon to became, as Dubois called it, the new 'giant of neuropathology'.[127] Psychasthenia had no clear-cut clinical boundaries[128] and relied for its meaning on theoretical mechanisms such as 'reduction' of psychological tension[129] and 'incompletion' (*inachèvement*).[130] Schwartz, one of the great biographers of Janet, was right in referring to psychasthenia as 'a cluster of symptoms artificially demarcated to which the predominance of a 'typical (causal) mechanism' conferred a particular aspect.'[131] Indeed, analysis of the 234 cases reported by Janet shows that psychasthenia included, in addition to obsessions, panic, phobic and tic disorder, hypochondriacal and confusional states, and epilepsy.[132]

Summary

During the nineteenth century, obsession was successively classified as insanity (monomania), neurosis (old definition), psychosis (new definition), and finally made a member of the new class of 'neuroses'. 'Obsession' was a splinter concept from the parent category 'fixed idea', and compulsion from 'impulsion'. It was successively explained as a disorder of volition, intellect and emotions; the first and third views being more popular in France, and the second in Germany. In the event, the 'emotional' hypothesis prevailed. The description of the disease was completed by Legrand du Saulle in 1875 and not by Janet as it is often claimed. Indeed, psychasthenia was a retrograde nosological step, wider than du Saulle's, and a return to

Thomsen's old category. Obsessions, agoraphobia and other anxiety disorders travelled together until the end of the century when Freud separated them
successfully.[133]

NOTES

1 Pujol and Savy, 1968; Monserrat-Esteve *et al.*, 1971; Beech, 1974;
   Nagera, 1976; Rachman and Hodgson, 1980.
2 Mora, 1969.
3 p. 253, Burton, 1883.
4 Quoted on p. 163, Mora, 1969.
5 p. 249, Hartley, 1834.
6 Meaning 'small, sharp or pointed stone' in Lewis and Short, 1879.
7 Quoted in pp. 25–26, Saurí, 1983.
8 p. 208, Vol 1, Taylor, 1660. The concept of scrupulosity has been in use
   until relatively recently; see Weisner and Riffel, 1961.
9 Boswell, 1791.
10 Krafft-Ebing, 1879.
11 The etymological origin of 'twanc' being the Sanskrit 'tvanzkti' ('he pulls
   together'), see pp. 260–261, Walshe, 1951.
12 Abbagnano, 1961.
13 Erdmann, 1886; pp. 21–25, Ribot, 1885.
14 Westphal, 1877.
15 Schneider, 1918.
16 To current psychiatrists (and particularly psychologists) this is the
   'natural' way of understanding a compulsion, i.e. as the acting out of a
   thought. Indeed, it provides theoretical basis for treatment (see Beech,
   1974; Rachman and Hodgson, 1980). But this is *not the only way to
   conceptualize a compulsion*. As the French showed later on, it can also be
   seen as a disorder of the will.
17 p. 324, Rado, 1959.
18 Bräutigam, 1973.
19 The term was the nineteenth century version of the old high German
   suht which was related to *siech* (sick), and a cognate of the Armenian
   hiucanim ('I am ill'); Walshe, 1951.
20 In the same paper, which he published the year before his death,
   Griesinger reported three cases, see: Griesinger, 1868.
21 Walshe, 1951.
22 Donath, 1897.
23 From the Greek term for 'necessity' or 'obligation', p. 214, Donath, 1897.
24 Thompsen, 1895.
25 Kahn, 1928; Skoog, 1959; Blankenburg, 1973; Videbech, 1975; p. 39,
   ICD-10, 1992.
26 Schneider explained: 'As adjectival forms to refer to personality cannot be
   formed with the German term *Zwang*, we have to use a non-German
   word. The one I have chosen comes from Donath. Ziehen has objected

that it is insufficiently known. The expression *anancastic*, however, is
perfectly understandable and certainly less equivocal than 'obsessive',
borrowed by Ziehen from the French', see Schneider, 1950.

27 The following are only some of them: *manie sans délire* (Pinel, 1809); *folie
raisonnante* (Ladame, 1890); *monomanie raisonnante* (Esquirol, 1838);
kleptomanie (Marc, 1840); *idées fixes* (p. 62, Parchappe, 1850–1851); *idée
irresistible* (Brierre de Boismont, 1853); *délire avec conscience, délire sans
délire* (Guislain, 1852); *idées restrictives or mobiles* (Renaudin, 1854);
pseudomonomanie (Delasiauve, 1861); *folie lucide* (Trélat, 1861); *folie or
monomanie avec conscience* (Ritti, 1879); *délire de toucher* (Legrand du
Saulle, 1875); *folie de doute avec délire de toucher.* (Ritti, 1878); *folie de
doute* (Marcé, 1862); *obsessions pathologiques* (Luys, 1883, 3: 20-61); *folie
des héréditaires dégénérés* (Magnan, 1886–1887); *crainte de souillure*
(Eeden, 1892); *onomatomanie* (Charcot and Magnan, 1885; Séglas, 1891);
maladie du doute (Falret, 1864).

28 The change over to the new category, *folie avec conscience* (insanity with
Insight) merits a short comment. This was discussed in a famous debate
in the *Société Médico-Psychologique* in Paris, 1875. It marked a surrender
of the 'lack of insight' criterion (central to the insanities) and allowed for
a number of disorders such as obsession, agoraphobia, panic disorder,
and the hypochondriacal and homicidal monomanias to be classified as
'insanities'.

Under the increasing pressure of the new Kraepelinian concept of
psychosis, the category *folie avec conscience* itself disintegrated by the end
of the century (Berrios and Hauser, 1988). This did not affect obsession
for by then it had been given an alternative clinical and aetiological
interpretation.

29 Morel, 1866.

30 Falret, 1866. The current author has been unable to find the word
obsession mentioned in this paper (which started the debate on *folie
raisonnante* at the *Société Médico-Psychologique*), and which includes a
clear description of obsession (see pp. 413–416); it is also in this
intervention that Falret claimed that 'his father had coined for this
mental disorder the term *maladie du doute.*' (p. 414).

31 see Littré, 1877; p. 198, Jastrow, in Baldwin, 1901; and *Oxford English
Dictionary* (2nd edn.).

32 p. 784, Littré, 1877.

33 Luys, 1883.

34 Ball, 1892; Falret, 1889; Eeden, 1892.

35 Berrios, 1977.

36 *Oxford English Dictionary* (2nd edn.).

37 See Tuke, 1892; and also Tuke, 1894.

38 Legrain, 1892.

39 Mickle, 1896.

40 Editorial, Mental Obsessions, 1901.

41 Shaw, 1904.

42 Diller, 1902.

43 Royal College of Physicians, 1906.

44 Esquirol, 1838.

45 p. 332, Esquirol, 1838.

46 Mademoiselle F. was a tall, happy-go-lucky 34 year-old female
    accountant whose illness started suddenly at age 18 when she began to
    fear that she might take in 'her pockets objects belonging to her aunt'.
    She worried lest she got the accounts wrong, and that on touching
    money something of value might get stuck to her fingers. She accepted
    that her worries were absurd but could not help it. She started
    handwashing and fearing that her clothes might touch anything; when
    this happened she would rub her hands as if to get rid of some invisible
    substance. The fear began to include food and she had to be fed by her
    servant, etc. etc. pp. 361–364, Esquirol, 1838.

47 Billod, 1847; Ribot, 1904.

48 Winslow, 1856.

49 Falret, 1864.

50 Kageyama, 1984.

51 Linas, 1871.

52 Saussure, 1946.

53 *Société Médico-Psychologique*, Debate on Monomanie, 1854.

54 Morel, 1860.

55 Morel, 1866.

56 Morel's use of the word *délire* was unconventional in that it allowed for
    the presence of insight.

57 Janet, 1919; Pitman, 1987.

58 Meyer, 1906.

59 Doyen, 1885.

60 Semelaigne, 1932.

61 For a detailed analysis of this see López Piñero, 1983.

62 Axenfeld defined neurosis as: 'morbid states frequently apyretic, in which
    there are changes in cognition, sensibility, or motility (or all combined)
    which have two important characteristics: that they can occur in the
    absence of an appreciable lesion, and that they themselves do not cause
    serious lesions', p. 14, Axenfeld, 1883.

63 'Fixed idea' was their common ancestor. During the nineteenth century
    this term referred mainly to persistent thoughts or overvalued ideas,
    whether or not seen in a pathological situation (e.g. p. 74, Griesinger,
    1861). It thus served as the parent term for delusions, obsessions,
    phobias, and post-oniric ideas. When, after the 1880s, some of these
    symptoms were redefined, 'fixed idea' was kept as a synonym for
    obsession (Buccola, 1880) and phobia (Ireland, 1895). On occasions, it
    was given a definition that remained ambiguously posed between the
    normal and the pathological (Valery, 1933).

64 For example, it is fully discussed in pp. 270–308, Hoffbauer, 1827.
    Hoffbauer made the point, which was to re-appear in Magnan at the end
    of the century, that 'impulsion as an act may be strong without being
    irresistible. A scale is needed . . .' (p. 307, Hoffbauer, 1827). Esquirol also

discussed the concept of impulsion in the context of *Monomanie Homicide* (see pp. 376–393, 1838). Griesinger was more cautious in his discussion of impulsion which he included under 'disorders of the will': 'Whether, and to what extent, certain impulses in the insane, particular those ending up in criminal acts, are irresistible, is unclear. Few insane behaviours can be said to be forced or purely automatic; even in mania and according to reports from subjects who have recovered, many of their wild desires could have been restrained.' p. 78, Griesinger, 1861.

65 In the French language, the concept of *impulsion* was imported from the science of mechanics see: Littré, 1877. The term's 'explanatory' force came from its allusion to vestigial behaviours, drives, cravings, and appetites. By the 1860s, *impulsion* was caught between two dichotomies: description v explanation and internal v reactive. From the historical viewpoint, the view that it was of 'inner' origin was the earliest to appear (Dagonet, 1870; Porot, 1975). Versions of 'impulsive or instinctive insanity' had already been described under *manie sans délire* (pp. 156–160, Pinel, 1809). Georget, in turn, described similar cases as having an *impetuosité de penchans*. (p. 49, Georget, 1820).

66 p. 17, Dagonet, 1870.

67 Magnan, 1886.

68 pp. 238–239 in Bourdin, 1896.

69 p. 208 in Pitres and Régis, 1902.

70 Baldwin, 1901; Dagonet, 1870.

71 p. 15 in Dagonet, 1870.

72 p. 20 in Dagonet, 1870.

73 Legrand du Saulle, 1875.

74 Legrand du Saulle's quaint usage of the terms 'neurosis' and *délire* to refer to obsession may cause confusion. His work was transitional between the old and new concept of insanity (see Berrios on the Historical aspects of the psychoses, 1987).

75 Ball, 1892.

76 See pp. 605–622 in Ball, 1890.

77 Magnan, 1886–1887.

78 Ballet, 1881.

79 Boucher, 1890.

80 p. 1109 in Magnan, 1886–1887.

81 p. 1109 in Magnan, 1886–1887.

82 p. 381 in Ladame, 1890.

83 For a complete history of obsession in German psychiatry, see Warda, 1905 and Schneider, 1918.

84 Griesinger died of appendicitis, at the young age of 51, on 26th October of the same year. He had been the founder of the Berlin Medico-Psychological Society and of the *Archiv für Psychiatrie* in whose first volume his paper and obituary appeared together (Westphal, 1868). On the history of the Berlin Society, see Schultze, 1968.

85 p. 627 in Griesinger, 1868.

86 Westphal, 1877.

87 *Berliner Medicinisch-psychologische Gesellschaft*, 1877.

88 Ludwig Wille (1834–1912) was a German-born alienist who became a major figure in Swiss psychiatry and contributed to topics as wide apart as non-restraint, confusional states, self-harm, and obsessional disorders. His work has been sadly neglected (for a good biographical account, see pp. 99–121, Haenel, 1982).

89 The question of whether obsessions could become delusions split both German and French psychiatrists (for a good study, see Masselon, 1913).

90 Wille, 1881.

91 Thompsen, 1895.

92 See, for example, Skoog, 1959.

93 Tuczek, 1899.

94 Lowenfeld, 1904.

95 pp. 1823–1901, Kraepelin, 1910–15.

96 p. 200, Ireland, 1885.

97 p. 692, Mickle, 1896. The Presidential address was read before the 55th Meeting of the Medico-Psychological Society in London.

98 For a good account of contemporary knowledge on tics and other movement disorders, and why they were considered as related to insanity, the neuroses, and obsession, see pp. 46–64, Meige and Feindel, 1902. The English translation by the young S.A. Kinnier Wilson only includes an abbreviated and distorted version of the chapter in question (Meige and Feindel, 1907).

99 p. 699, Mickle, 1896.

100 Shaw, 1904.

101 for an analysis of this debate, see Berrios, 1977.

102 p. 179, Tuke, 1894.

103 p. 191, Tuke, 1894.

104 p. 192, Tuke, 1894.

105 It is easy to read 'vesicular neurine' anachronistically, i.e. as a forunner of a neurotrasmitter. It is not. It must be remembered that during Laycock's time even the notion of neuron did not exist. The word 'vesicular neurine' or 'substance' referred to whatever was the material that constituted the central nervous system. As late as 1876, and in the most popular physiology textbook of the period, it was defined thus: 'the nervous system of Man, like that of all other animals, is composed of ganglionic centres and nerve trunks; the former being essentially composed of "vesicular substance" (p. 582 in Carpenter and Power, 1876). And 'neurin' was further defined as 'term for the matter of which nerves are composed, and which is enveloped in neurilemma' (p.761 in Mayne, 1860). On the general background of neurophysiology during this period see Clarke and Jacyna, 1987; and Black, 1981; and on Laycock and the role he played in English neurophysiology, see Leff, 1991.

106 This quotation was taken by Tuke from a paper delivered by Laycock at the York British Association meeting of 1844 (published as Laycock, 1845). At the time, Laycock was a physician to the York Dispensary.

107 p. 195, Tuke 1894.

108 Jackson, 1895.

109 He was referring here to Jackson, 1889.

110 p. 355, Jackson, 1889.

111 p. 318, Jackson, 1895.

112 p. 319, Jackson, 1895.

113 p. 221, Jackson, 1895.

114 Savage, 1895.

115 Mercier, 1895.

116 p. 348, Bramwell, 1894.

117 pp. 347–348, Bramwell, 1894.

118 Gardiner *et al.*, 1937; Berrios, On Psychopathology of Affectivity, 1985. The philosophical reaction against 'materialism' and 'intellectualism' was led by Albert Lemoine and Paul Janet (Pierre Janet's uncle), starting in 1867 with the publication of Lemoine's *Le Cerveau et la Pensée*. At the time, Janet was the standard-bearer of the 'emotions-first' tradition in French philosophical psychology which had in fact started at the beginning of the century with Maine de Biran (Dwelshauvers, 1920; Moore, 1970), and kept alive by Royer-Collard (whose brother was a psychiatrist), Cousin, and Jouffroy (Ravaisson, 1885). Feelings and emotions, Pierre Janet declared in his popular Paris lectures were the 'centre of psychological organization' (Prevost, 1973*b*).

119 Zeldin has suggested that anxiety increased 'in the sense that traditional supports of behaviour were weakened, that people were left facing a larger world and a vastly greater range of problems, with far less certainty as to how they should treat them, and often with sharper sensibilities' p. 823, Zeldin, 1977.

120 Ravaisson, 1885.

121 Raymond and Janet, 1908.

122 Raymond, 1911.

123 Baruk, 1967.

124 Janet, 1889.

125 Janet, 1919.

126 Chatel and Peel, 1971; Cobb, 1920.

127 Dubois, 1905.

128 Hesnard, 1971.

129 Sjövall, 1967.

130 Prevost, 1973*a*.

131 Schwartz, 1955.

132 Berrios *et al.*, 1995.

133 Freud, 1953*a*.

CHAPTER 7

Mental Retardation

Although the *idea* that human beings have mental capacities to 'read into' (*intus-legere*) the nature of things is old,[1] the concept of *intelligence* as a psychological function is new. In earlier days, intellectual powers were not clearly differentiated from other mental faculties such as perception, emotions and will, nor from other information gathering mechanisms such as intuition or conjecture. Understanding is considered by Plato as superior to belief and conjecture,[2] and by Aristotle as depending upon the capture of the 'form' of the object in question: 'Now, if thinking is akin to perceiving, it would be either being affected in some way by the object of thought or something else of this kind. It must then be unaffected but capable of receiving the form, and potentially such as it, although not identical with it; and as that which is capable of perceiving is to the objects of perception, so must be the intellect similar to its objects.'[3] 'And I speak of as intellect that by which the soul thinks and supposes.'[4] Galen suggested that the active intelligence operated by means of mechanisms such as distinction, combination, solution, demonstration, enumeration, and classification.[5] For Aquinas, intellect is the function of 'apprehending something'[6] and has two components: an intelligence for simple ideas and another for 'complex understanding.'[7]

This *general* conception of understanding or intelligence lasted well into the eighteenth century and can be found in Kant:[8] 'if the power of knowledge in general is to be called understanding (in the most general sense of the term), understanding must include: 1. the power of apprehending, 2. the power of abstracting, and 3. The power of reflecting.'[9] During the nineteenth century, such broad power was subdivided into intuitive, operative and comprehensive understanding.[10] Intuition was neglected by classical psychology,[11] and after the 1880s, operative and comprehensive understanding were blended to form the current notion of intelligence. During this period, views on the relationship between intelligence and the brain follow the vicissitudes of the localization debate. For example, phrenologists believed that the faculties of intelligence (and there was no agreement as to how many there were) were sited on the *frontal part* of the brain; others – like J.H. Jackson – believed that 'the entire brain was involved in all intellectual process.'[12]

During the final years of the nineteenth century qualitative concepts of intelligence were superseded by quantitative approaches and the first efforts to test intelligence were made.[13] This led to many operational definitions which by 1910 had caused enough confusion for the *British Journal of Psychology* to publish the results of a symposium on the relationship between intelligence and instinct which included speakers such as C.S. Myers, C.L. Morgan, W. Carr, G.F. Stout, and W. McDougall.[14] In 1921, another effort was made by the editors of the *Journal of Educational Psychology* 'what do you conceive intelligence to be, and by what means can it best be measured by group tests? And what are the most crucial 'next steps' in research?. Controversy ensued, and some (e.g. B. Ruml and S.L. Pressey) even refused to answer.[15] Equally inconclusive has been a more recent exercise.[16]

The concept of mental retardation

There has been more historical work on the *management* of mental retardation than on its *concept*. Historical accounts, whether by Séguin[17], Barr[18], Kanner,[19] Lewis,[20] or Scheerenberger,[21] remain *presentistic*[22] and *decontextualized*. And yet it is only an analysis of the context (particularly in relation to the history of psychopathology) that will illuminate the otherwise complex notion of mental retardation. Such work will also throw light on the history of concepts such as cognition, development, psychometry,[23] and indirectly on the history of child psychiatry,[24] the infantile psychoses,[25] and the vexed question of the definition of man as a rational being.[26] Most of this work remains to be done. This chapter will limit itself to mapping the process whereby the *concept* of mental retardation was constructed in European psychiatric thinking during the first half of the nineteenth century. Historical changes after the 1860s will be barely mentioned.

Matters historiographical

The biographical approach has been the most popular in the history of mental retardation, and the ghosts of Pereira, Itard, Esquirol, Belhomme, Guggenbühl, Séguin, Howe, and Morel haunt most secondary sources. This technique, however, only works when it avoids anachronistic interpretation: otherwise, as for example is the case with Séguin's own historical views,[27] it can be unfair to earlier figures because no attempt is made to understand their intellectual and social context.

Likewise, efforts must be made to distinguish between the history of: (*a*) the *words* used for naming phenomena (semantic history), (*b*) the *behaviours* in question (behavioural palæontology), and (*c*) the *concepts* created throughout the ages to *understand* such behaviours (conceptual history). Confusing these three levels of analysis has led to historical error such as, for example, the claim that it was Esquirol who first *distinguished* idiocy from dementia.[28]

The approach to be used in this chapter assumes the existence of a mild form of social constructionism, i.e. of personal and social codes that modulate an *independent* biological invariant.[29] History tells us (and neurobiology predicts) that behaviours considered as pertaining to 'mental retardation' have existed from the beginning of time, irrespective of the fact that their *medicalization* might only have started during the seventeenth century,[30] and their *psychiatrization* two centuries later. This is probably the reason why Esquirol – who was writing from the point of view of mental alienism – is credited with creating the notion of idiocy.

Retardation before the nineteenth century

There is little doubt that 'idiocy' and 'dementia' were differentiated, *de facto* if not *de jure*, since before the nineteenth century. For example, such distinctions were made in Medieval Courts[31] where idiocy is found already associated with qualifiers such as 'congenital' and 'irreversible'. As Walker has written: 'The distinction between low intelligence and mental illness in English law is at least as old as the thirteenth-century Statute of the King's Prerogative which dealt with the management of their property.'[32] By the seventeenth century, legal definitions even included tests (based on the assessment of everyday behaviour, such as handling money) to decide on the level of mental retardation of a particular individual.[33] From a *medical* viewpoint, these definitions were sharpened by Thomas Willis[34] and later by Vicenzo Chiarugi[35] both of whom distinguished between insanity, dementia, and mental retardation. There was also an awareness that the latter could be congenital and irreversible.[36]

Cullen

To understand recent changes in the meaning of mental retardation one must take up the story at the time of William Cullen in whose nosography Class II: *neuroses* had as Order IV the *Vesaniae*, defined as: 'lesions of the judging faculty without fever or coma'. This rubric included four *genera*: *Amentia, Melancholia, Mania* and *Oneirodynia*. *Amentia*, the category relevant to mental retardation, was defined as: 'imbecility of the judging faculty with inability to perceive or remember', and classified into three species: congenital, senile, and acquired – the latter two corresponding roughly to dementia.[37] Under *Amentia* Cullen brought together a number of clinical categories: *Amentia, Stupidity, Morosis* and *Fatuity* (Vogel), *Amentia* and *Amnesia* (Sauvages and Sagar), and *Morosis* and *Oblivio* (Linné).[38] *Amentia congenita* is particularly important to the subsequent history of mental retardation because it was specifically defined by Cullen 'as a condition present from birth and which included *Amentia morosis* and *Amentia microcephala*', both recognizable types of idiocy. Indeed, the Latin term *amentia* was translated into the vernacular by Cullen's students as *folly* or *idiotism*.[39]

The first half of the nineteenth century

French views

PINEL Apart from being the translator of one of the French versions of Cullen's *Nosology*,[40] Pinel composed a nosography himself. His Class IV, *Neuroses*, included neuroses affecting the senses, cerebral function, locomotion, voice, nutritive function, and generation.[41] *Idiotisme* appears as one of the categories classified under the *Névroses des fonctions cérébrales*, where it is defined as an '*abolition*, more or less absolute, of the functions of understanding and feeling' which may be acquired or congenital (*originaire*).[42] Pinel did not deviate from this definition which he linked to the views expressed by the '*auteur of synonymes français*' on a '*échelle de graduation de la raison*'.[43] Thus, in 1801, Pinel defined *ideotism* as 'total or partial obliteration of the intellectual powers and affections: universal torpor; detached half-articulated sounds or entire absence of speech from want of ideas; in some cases, transient and unmeaning gusts of passion.'[44] He continued upholding the view that idiocy may be acquired or congenital. The same was repeated in the second and last edition of the *Traité*.[45]

Thus, Pinel's conception of idiotism can be described as fully medical (for example, it was included in his nosography), psychiatric (it featured together with mania, melancholia and dementia), and based upon his notion of disorder of reason or of the intellectual faculty.[46] Like Cullen (he also considered idiotism as a synonym of amentia), Pinel proposed that this condition may be either acquired or congenital. However, for the first time, he used the word *démence*[47] to refer to Cullen's acquired amentias, and included a discussion of *cretins*[48] which shows awareness of the fact that a variety of cases fall under the category idiotism.

ESQUIROL This great French alienist had the advantage of writing in the context of the much reduced psychiatric nosological system created by Pinel, and in the wake of the French Revolution, whose progressivism required that the distinction between idiocy and dementia (which was, as we have seen, already present in Cullen) be emphasized. It is one of the myths in the history of psychiatry that it was Esquirol who first distinguished idiocy from dementia; the *locus classicus* being: 'The demented is like the person who is deprived from his property after he has been able to enjoy it; is a rich person who has become poor; the idiot has always been poor and miserable'.[49]

Esquirol changed his mind about the nature of idiocy and in his later writings he seems to have been influenced by Georget (see below), although he does not mention him by name. Thus, whilst in the 1814 and 1817 entries to the Panckoucke dictionary[50] Esquirol stated that mental retardation *was* a disease, he changed his mind by 1838: 'idiocy is *not a disease* but a state in which the intellectual faculties are never manifested or *developed* for lack of education' (my italics).[51]

Chronology suggests that the *developmental* view originated with Georget, but this cannot be firmly stated. Esquirol seems also to have left a door open to the possibility, in some cases, of mental retardation resulting from pure cultural influence: for example, he discusses this in relation to the *cagots*[52] a cultural minority said to have had a high rate of mentally retarded children.

Esquirol provided a *psychological account* of dementia and idiocy.[53] Influenced by Faculty Psychology, he considered idiocy as a *disorder of intellect*, and hence, as a problem with which alienists ought to be concerned. He *did not*, however, consider idiocy as a form of insanity (*folie*) for at the time the latter condition was narrowly defined in terms of *délire*.[54] It was, however, a form of mental illness (*maladie mentale*). This was not meant to reflect any therapeutic pessimism: indeed, imbued by the optimism of the French Revolution, he encouraged Itard in his quest to educate the boy of Aveyron.[55]

But those who followed Esquirol, particularly after the 1850s, when the doctrine of *degeneration* began to take hold,[56] did not share in his optimism. There is little doubt that it was this new fatalism (and the negative consequences it engendered) that precipitated the challenge to the view that idiocy was a form of mental illness. The challenge was born out of the altruism of educators (e.g. Séguin) and of their belief that a 'psychiatric' approach would lead to suffering and hardship amongst the mentally retarded.[57] Current arguments concerning the separation between idiocy and mental illness are, therefore, redolent of those rehearsed during the nineteenth century. The problem then, as now, was not just a semantic one but the substantive point of whether mental retardation was on a *continuum* with normality. If it was, many thought, then mental retardation *per se*, could not be considered as a form of mental illness (although the mentally retarded, like anyone else, *might develop* mental illness). But even during Esquirol's time things were not that easy, for the observation had already been made that in severe forms of idiocy there was a high frequency of psychiatric and neurological disease.[58]

GEORGET AND THE *DEVELOPMENTAL* HYPOTHESIS However, an important departure of the 'disease concept' took place in 1820 when Georget[59] defined idiocy as 'failure in the *development* of the intellectual faculties'. Aware of his own originality Georget went on to state: 'idiocy *should not be made into a type of insanity (délire)* for a failure to develop cannot be properly considered as a disease (*maladie*)' ... 'idiots must be classified as monsters (*monstres*)' (my italics).[60] The expression of such unorthodox view by a man barely aged 25 needs explanation, particularly for he was a disciple of Esquirol who considered idiocy and imbecility as forms of *aliénation mentale*, and who, in general, paid little attention to the developmental aspects of mental disorder.

Georget's views were influential. For example, F.G. Boisseau included them in his great *Nosographie Organique*: 'some have said that idiotism is always congenital. This is a mistake, for whilst it is true that in many cases it is present at birth, in many others it results from a suspension in the *development* of the brain' (my italics).[61]

ONÉSIME ÉDOUARD SÉGUIN By the middle of the century, French views on mental retardation were divided between the medical views of Esquirol and followers and new social ones put forward by O.E. Séguin (soon to emigrate to America). For a while the former predominated. Thus, the anonymous reviewer for Fabre's influential encyclopaedia[62] starts with Esquirol and Belhomme and quotes Séguin only in his medical and *physiological* vein. Guislain – another popular author of the period – re-affirmed in his *Leçons* the conventional distinction between idiots and imbeciles but argued that he saw no reason to make of this group a variety of mental illness.[63] The new views of Séguin, however, soon started to dominate the scene.[64]

A lawyer turned educator and then physician, Séguin was also interested in metrication and thermometry (on both which subjects he wrote with enthusiasm).[65] After siding with the 1848 *républicains de la veille*, he felt (groundlessly) insecure in the France of Louis Napoleón and in 1850 left for the USA.[66] The first account of his work with idiots appeared in 1838 in joint authorship with Esquirol (*Résumé de ce que nous avons fait pendant 14 mois*), and the second writing a year later (*Conseils à Monsieur O **** sur l'éducation de son enfant idiot*). Three other works followed before the publication of his great volume of 1846.[67] He claimed that he had found 'in his soul' the resources needed to develop a theory which was not only important for 'idiocy but for education.'[68] It is unlikely, however, that these ideas were original.[69] Likewise, his anti-medical stance,[70] made it difficult for him to pronounce on whether mental retardation was a form of mental illness.[71]

After Séguin's departure, the medical view took hold. In 1874, when A. Foville wrote his review[72] he had no difficulty in repeating the old concepts except that, influenced by B. Morel, he emphasized the degenerative taint.[73] The same can be said of E. Chambard who, in his own review confirmed the medical approach, and stated that both idiocy and imbecility should be discussed under the rubric of *mental dysgenesis*.[74] Thus, it is not surprising that when Ball published his great work on mental disorder he called these states morphological insanities (*folies morphologiques*).[75]

German views

HOFFBAUER During the first half of the nineteenth century, a good example of German thought on idiocy is to be found in the work of Hoffbauer,[76] who dealt with the issue of legal responsibility in the mentally retarded and the deaf and dumb. He divided feeblemindedness (*Verstandschwäche*) into two subtypes according to whether the 'level' (imbecility-*Blödsinn*) or 'extension' (stupidity-*Dummheit*) of the intellect was involved. Both subtypes, in turn, could be congenital or acquired; in other words, mental retardation proper or dementia.[77]

HEINROTH Heinroth[78] made idiocy (*anoia*) into a *Genus* of mental disorder (*Störungen des Seelenlebens*) and divided it into four sub-types. He characterized idiocy as a disorder in which: 'the senses, especially the higher senses, cannot comprehend or grasp, and the intellect cannot collect any ideas from the sensations. The spirit is quite empty and is merely vegetating. The animal feelings and instincts, such as hunger or the sexual instinct, are however, stronger, and the patient can easily be excited into anger, which may become rage.'[79] The distinction between the four subtypes of idiocy was made in terms of accompanying symptoms: *anoia simplex* was the pure form; *anoia melancholica*, was accompanied by agitation and partial insight into the condition; *anoia abyole*, by lethargy, inactivity and lack of responsiveness; and *anoia catholica* which was the more severe form.[80]

Heinroth quoted Hoffbauer with approval: 'Idiocy has been sub-divided into several grades for the purpose of forensic medicine. The description of these fine differences must be credited, in the first place, to Hoffbauer.'[81]

GRIESINGER It has been suggested that W. Griesinger sponsored a form of unitary psychosis[82] because he believed that melancholia, mania and dementia might successively develop in the same individual. These changes were but the expression of a march of 'organic events' starting with neurophysiological depression (*Depressionszustände*) and proceeding to excitation (*Exaltationszustände*) then to weakness (*Schwächezustände*).[83]

Idiocy fitted in well into Griesinger's clinical cascade and was made (together with chronic insanity (*partielle Verrücktheit*), confusion (*Verwirrtheit*) and stupor or terminal dementia (*apathische Blödsinn*) the central example of *psychischen Schwächezustände*. Whilst the other three states were *acquired*, and constituted what, nowadays, would be called defect states,[84] idiocy was congenital: 'By the term idiocy (*Idiotismus*), we understand conditions in which the state of mental weakness exists from birth or early infancy, and in which psychological development has been impeded or prevented.'[85] Griesinger postulated a strong organic and hereditary hypothesis for such states of mental weakness, considering all social explanations as 'shallow' (*flache Auffassung*).[86]

VON FEUCHTERSLEBEN Von Feuchtersleben wrote:[87] 'Idiocy proceeds, as a psychopathy,[88] proximately from *anaesthesia*, weakness of attention, *amnesia*, and want of images. It represents, in some measure, an approximation of the human character to that of animals, and is characterized by an incapacity of judging, or even, in its higher degree, of contemplating. The alteration is more prominent in the direction of thought than in that of feeling and will, though, in the higher degrees, both feeling and will are also wanting (*Abulia*, Heinroth) . . . the lowest degree, which

Hartmann calls stupidity, is characterised by an incapacity of comprehending, judging, and concluding, even in affairs of what is called common sense . . . the higher
degree, idiocy *sensu strictiori*, shows total incapacity for mental activity.'[89] Von
Feuchtersleben's definition of mental retardation involves all mental functions.

British views

PRICHARD James Cowles Prichard, the British alienist and anthropologist,[90] did
not consider idiotism or mental deficiency as a form of insanity, and treated these
states in a separate chapter.[91] Idiotism he defined as: 'a state in which the mental
faculties have been wanting from birth, or have not been manifested at the period
at which they are usually developed. Idiotism is an original defect, and is by this
circumstance, as well as by its phenomena, distinguished from that fatuity that
results from disease or from protracted age.'[92]

Prichard quoted Esquirol, Fodéré, and Georget, discussed cretinism at length,
and supported Esquirol's continuity view: 'there is no exact line of demarcation
between idiotism and a degree of weakness which is generally termed imbecility';[93]
but he went one step further in linking these states to normality: 'There are different
degrees and varieties of mental deficiency, which scarcely amount to what is termed
either idiotism, or, in general language, imbecility. Persons so affected are commonly said to be weak in character, stupid, or of mean capacity.'[94]

Bucknill and Tuke also criticized what they believed to be Esquirol's pessimism:
'it would no longer be right to speak of the faculties of the idiot being doomed to
remain stationary',[95] and found contradiction between what Esquirol listed in a
table showing a decrease in the size of the heads of idiots and his claim in the text
that there was no difference with 'other men'.[96]

The second half of the nineteenth century

Views on mental retardation during the second half of the nineteenth century are
characterized by a transformation of the categorical approach: for example, quantitative bridges begin to be established between normal children and the mildly
retarded. This required a theoretical shift. Thus, Netchine has suggested that whilst,
up to this period, mental retardation itself was graded into sub-categories, there
was no general quantitative dimension to include the various levels of normality.[97]
This was to occur only after the important work of Sollier (sadly neglected)[98] and
that of Binet and Simon (often quoted) who introduced the first workable concept
of intellectual coefficient. This is also the period when specific syndromes such as
mongolism,[99] cretinism,[100] etc. were fully described.

PAUL SOLLIER Sollier trained under Bourneville at *Bicêtre*, and was for a while in
charge of the Pathological Museum. His aim was to deal with the general psycho-

logical characteristics of idiocy rather than with specific or rare cases. He complained that in France writings on idiocy were 'poor'[101] as compared with those in
America or England. The first problem he encountered was that 'idiocy was not a
clinical entity ... that the idiot was an abnormal being but that its abnormality
varied in many dimensions ... [on the other hand] he was not in a separate category but merged with the milder forms of the disorder.'[102] He suggested that it
might be possible to 'measure their mental state by seeking to compare it to a
particular age in the normal child.'[103] Sollier found an important obstacle: 'for this
principle to apply it would be needed that the cause of idiocy *was the same in each
case* ... unfortunately this is not the case' (my italics).[104]

To collect data, Sollier made use of a modified version of a structured interview
schedule developed by Voisin[105] which included sections on instincts, feelings and
affections, perceptual functioning, psychomotor skills, intellect, and physiological
and psychological functions. In spite of discussing quantification, Sollier's book
includes no actual numerical data; indeed, it is not even clear how many cases
were studied. His principles as much as his conclusions, however, are modern in
outlook and break with categorical thinking, to the point that Binet and Simon did
not need to think anew a justification for their psychometric work.

BINET AND SIMON In their classical paper of 1905,[106] these authors simply
repeated Sollier's view that there was a 'need to establish a scientific (quantitative)
diagnosis of the states of lower intelligence'. One year before Binet's death he published his final manifesto on the nosology of *l'arriération*.[107] After complaining about
the way in which alienists had neglected the study of these conditions, Binet and
Simon attacked anatomo-pathological classifications (a là Bourneville)[108] and Sollier's suggestion that imbecility was not accompanied by brain pathology.[109] They
re-affirmed the value of quantitative groupings but criticised Régis and Kraepelin for
not providing adequate operational definitions. Lastly, Binet and Simon commented
negatively on suggestions by psychologists that only one mental function was primarily disordered in mental handicap and stated that, in fact, all functions were.[110]

In the meantime, alienists continued searching for the best way of classifying
mental retardation. Séglas suggested that: *l'affaiblissement intellectuel* be differentiated from *la débilité mentale* in that the former was wider and included dementia
and amnesia.[111] Chaslin believed that acquired *arriération mentale* was a form of
démence infantile differentiable from *la faiblesse intellectuelle* which presented in a
variety of subtypes.[112]

The debate on the definition of feeblemindedness continued during the 1920s,[113]
and the following decade Lewis added the notion of 'subcultural deficiency'.[114] Current views are well reflected in DSM IV which requires quantitative criteria, and
assessments of genetic status, physical disability, behavioural adaptation, and social
competence. This Chinese menu system has improved the reliability of the descrip-
tors but does not guarantee validity nor does it offer a theory to unify the various

strands involved in the clinical expression of mental retardation. What is worse, it does not offer a conceptual framework to tackle the question: is mental retardation a form of mental illness?

Summary

The view that mental retardation was a defect of *intellectual* function different from insanity or dementia became well established during the first half of the nineteenth century. It was also during this period that mental retardation became burdened with an important ambiguity, to wit, whether or not it was necessarily a form of mental illness. This was not only due to definitional confusions. In fact, encouraged by the logic of Faculty Psychology, and the categorical view of idiocy, nineteenth century alienists felt entitled to claim that most forms of mental retardation were diseases. But following protestations by educators and anti-medical men such as Séguin, a compromise developed during the second half of the century which suggested a human variation type of continuum between normality, imbecility and idiocy (leading to the claim that members of the latter two groups could not be considered as mentally ill). This hypothesis was heuristic in that it encouraged the development of a quantitative view which, first with Sollier, and then Binet and Simon, led to the creation of the abstract notion of intellectual coefficient. Since early in the nineteenth century, however, there had also been awareness of the possibility that the frequency of neurological and psychiatric pathology increased *pari passu* with the depth of the mental retardation. The tensions that this observation created within the continuum model were not solved during the nineteenth century, and might not have been alleviated even today.

NOTES

1 pp. 33-51, Peterson, 1925; pp. 23–32, Sternberg, 1990.
2 Republic VII, 533e; p. 765, Plato: *The Collected Dialogues*, 1961.
3 Book III.4. 429a13., p. 57 in Aristotle's *de Anima*, 1968.
4 Book III.4. 429a18., p. 57 Aristotle, 1968.
5 p. 142, Siegel, 1973.
6 p. 74, Monahan (undated).
7 pp. 62–63, Kenny, 1980.
8 In this regard, Abbagnano has perceptively remarked: 'The definition of understanding as a 'faculty of thinking' was a common place of the eighteenth century and Kant simply repeated it', p. 409, Abbagnano, 1961.
9 Para 6.138, p. 19, Kant, 1974.
10 p. 410, Abbagnano, 1961.
11 p. 726, Ferrater Mora, 1855.
12 p. 159, Hollander, 1931.

13 see pp. 35–135, Peterson, 1925; also Young, 1923; Cattell, 1890; and Sokal, 1982.

14 pp. 209, *British Journal of Psychology*, 1910.

15 Editors, *Journal of Educational Psychology*, 1921.

16 p. 52, Sternberg, 1990.

17 Séguin, 1846.

18 Barr, 1904.

19 Kanner, 1964.

20 Lewis, 1961.

21 Scheerenberger, 1983.

22 By 'presentistic' it is meant here a form of historiography that describes events chronologically and as relentlessly progressive, i.e. it makes the assumption that the more recent development is necessarily superior. It has also been called by Herbert Butterfield 'the Whig interpretation of history'.

23 On this, see the penetrating study: Netchine, 1973; see also Pichot, 1948; Lang, 1965; and Mahendra, 1985.

24 Walk, 1964; Gontard, 1988; Duché, 1990.

25 Gineste, 1983.

26 For example, Sir Frederic Bateman's evocative title: *The Idiot; his Place in Creation and his Claims on Society*, 1902; or the debate initiated by Georget that the mentally handicapped were a type of monster: Georget, 1820. On the concept of monster and its relationship to the definition of man, see Davaine, 1874. After the 1860s, the notion of monstrosity became entangled with degeneration theory: see Talbot, 1898. The same ideological background inspired the debate on a classification of idiots based upon the physiognomic features of the 'great Caucasian family' which led to the coining of mongolism see Down, 1866.

27 Séguin, 1846. The English translation of this rare book, carried out by Séguin and his son for the American market (Séguin, 1866), did not include a large and telling section entitled: *Définitions de l'Idiotie antérieures á mes travaux* (pp. 23–71), in which the French writer describes and criticizes earlier definitions and classifications.

28 For example, Scheerenberger, 1983, pp. 54–55.

29 For example, Clarke, 1975; Rushton,1988.

30 Lewis, 1961; Cranfield, 1961; James; 1991.

31 Clarke, 1975.

32 p. 36, Walker, 1968.

33 See the seventeenth century definition: 'He that shall be said to be a sot and idiot from his birth, is such a person who cannot count or number twenty, and tell who was his father or mother . . .' (quoted in Bucknill and Tuke, p. 94, 1858); also Neugebauer, 1989.

34 Cranfield, 1961.

35 pp. 230–234 in Chiarugi, 1987.

36 James, 1990.

37 Cullen, Vol. 1, pp. 316–317, 1827.

38 Cullen, 1803. Cullen's contemporaries were already aware of the fact

that his category Amentia resulted from lumping together a number of
previous disparate clinical states. For example, the great Italian nosologist
Chiarugi stated: 'in his nosology, Cullen combined them in the same way'
(Chiarugi, 1987).

39 See, for example, the popular Vademecum of the London Hospitals, 1803.

40 Cullen, 1785. This translation seems to have been a financial failure due,
apparently, to the fact that E. Bosquillon, the Royal lecturer, published
another the same year.

41 Pinel, 1818 (first edition, 1798).

42 pp. 132–133, Pinel, 1818.

43 p. 132, Pinel, 1818; it is not easy to identify the work Pinel refers to.
However, it is likely to be the *Dictionnaire Universal des Synonymes de la
Langue Française*, 1792.

44 Pinel, 1806 (first edition: (Year IX)).

45 Pinel, 1809.

46 Although influenced by Cabanis and the French ideologues, Pinel used a
common sense form of Faculty Psychology which he is likely to have
borrowed from Dugald Stewart. On Pinel's psychological influences, see
Riese, 1969; Staum, 1980; Postel, 1981; d'Istria, 1926.

47 see Berrios, Dementia during the seventeenth and eighteenth centuries,
1987.

48 pp. 188–190, Pinel, 1809.

49 p. 77, Esquirol, 1838.

50 Esquirol first dealt with the notions of *idiotism* and *imbécillité* in 1814, in
the context of *démence* where he quotes Pinel, 1809: 'dementia should
not be confused with imbecility or idiotism. The faculty of reasoning in
the imbecile is undeveloped and weak; the dement has lost his ... idiots
and cretins are not able to have sensations, memory or judgement and
show only few animal instincts; their external shape shows that they are
not organised to think' (p. 284). In the same entry, he stated that
imbécillité was a species of *aliénation mentale*. The entry on *Idiotisme*
appeared in the same dictionary in 1817, and was reprinted in an
expanded form in pp. 76–132, Esquirol, Vol. 2, 1838.

51 p. 284, Esquirol, 1838.

52 *Les cagots*, referred to by Michel as one of the accursed races (*races
maudites*), include groups of peoples who, since the Medieval period, were
ostracized into various areas of Northern Spain and Western France, and
forbidden to enter into social contact with the rest of the population (see
Lagneau, 1869). Whether through inbreeding or social isolation and lack
of education, it was claimed that mental retardation was highly prevalent
in this group. Esquirol claims that this improved once their ostracism
ended (pp. 370–372, 1838).

53 Esquirol, 1838.

54 The French term *délire* (like the German *Wahn*) names a complex
psychiatric phenomenon which is not totally rendered into English by the
word 'delusion'. This has caused much difficulty over the years.

55 Nothing else will be said in this chapter about the boy of Aveyron and its

relevance to the conceptual debate on idiocy and its treatment in early nineteenth century France. Particularly important works on this topic are: Malson, 1964; Lane, 1977; Sánchez, 1982; Swain, 1976.

56 The notion of degeneration was introduced into psychiatry by Morel in 1857. Literature on this topic is now very large; for three different historical approaches, see Genil-Perrin, 1913; Huertas, 1987; Pick, 1989.

57 pp. 69–71, Séguin, 1846.

58 For example, pp. 487–521, Marcé, 1862.

59 Georget, 1820.

60 On the concept of monster, see Davaine, 1874; Talbot, 1898.

61 p. 263, Vol. 8, Boisseau, 1830.

62 pp. 553–576, Fabre, 1849.

63 p. 343, Guislain, 1852.

64 Kraft, 1961.

65 Martin, 1981.

66 Pichot, 1948.

67 Séguin, 1846.

68 p. 2, Séguin, 1846.

69 for a good analysis of the Saint-Simonian and 'moral treatment' origins of his method, see Kraft, 1961.

70 He started his medical training only in 1843, and had to quit the Bicêtre Hospital after entering into conflict with its physicians. His writing on the education of the idiot were praised by the *Académie des Sciences* and ignored by the *Académie de Médicine*. This may partly explain his anti-medical stance (Martin, 1961). Likewise, Séguin was displeased about a certificate issued by Esquirol and Guersant: 'The undersigned have the pleasure of acknowledging that Mr. Séguin has started with success the training of a child almost mute and *seemingly* retarded . . .' The use of the word 'seemingly' irked Séguin who felt that this betrayed Esquirol's belief in the incurability of idiocy (p. 14, Séguin, 1846). In the same work, Séguin mounted a savage attack on Esquirol and his disinterest in idiocy (pp. 24–30, Séguin, 1846). This text was omitted from the American translation: Séguin, 1866.

71 For example, he wrote: 'I hereby formally accuse physicians . . . of having confused idiocy with other analogous chronic conditions, of confusing it with concomitant pathological states that are not part or consequence of idiocy, of not dedicating sufficient time to their study . . .'. Séguin goes on to say that physicians entertain too theoretical a view, that their definitions are negative, and that there is too much emphasis on the intellectual defect (pp. 69–71, Séguin, 1846).

72 Foville, Vol. 18, pp. 363–375, 1874.

73 p. 354, Foville, 1874.

74 p. 508, Chambard, 1888.

75 p. 934, Ball, 1890.

76 J.C. Hoffbauer (1766–1827) was a professor of Philosophy and Law at Halle University from which he had to retire early on account of deafness. He collaborated with the German alienist Reil.

77 pp. 42–85, Hoffbauer, 1827 (first German edition 1808). This curious
    translation included frequent critical notes from both translator – a
    disciple of Esquirol – and the great man himself who clearly missed the
    point of Hoffbauer's work. For example, they derided his efforts to carry
    out a psychological analysis – in terms of Faculty Psychology – of the
    subtypes of feeblemindedness (for example, pp. 43–44). Instead,
    Chambeyron and Esquirol wanted clinical and frequential analysis of the
    phenomena involved, tasks which were irrelevant to Hoffbauer's brief (he
    was mainly writing for lawyers). A useful historical point, however, is
    made in a table composed by Chambeyron and Esquirol comparing
    Hoffbauer's classification of mental disorder with the ongoing French one.
    They concluded that: 'imbecility, idiocy and dementia are confused by the
    Germans under the general heading of feeblemindedness which they
    divide into imbecility and stupor'. It was, perhaps, wrong of them to
    generalize to all 'Germans' alienists as others, such as Heinroth, had a
    different view.

78 Historical misreading has created the myth that Heinroth believed that
    'the ultimate cause of mental disturbance is sin' (see p. 141, Alexander
    and Selesnick, 1966). For a timely correction, see Cauwenbergh, 1991.

79 p. 195, Heinroth, 1975.

80 pp. 195–199, Heinroth, 1975.

81 p. 198, Heinroth, 1975.

82 pp. 13–17, Vliegen, 1980.

83 pp. 22–59, Griesinger, 1861.

84 He wrote: 'Under this section are included morbid states which, although
    different in detail, form a sort of natural group. With some exceptions to
    be mentioned later, they look like each other in that they do not
    constitute primary, but secondary (*consecutives*) forms of insanity, and
    that they are remnants of the [acute] types already considered when
    these are not cured.' pp. 322–323, Griesinger, 1861.

85 p. 352, Griesinger, 1861.

86 p. 356, Griesinger, 1861.

87 Feuchtersleben, 1845.

88 A clarification is indicated here: circa 1845, the term 'psychopathy'
    simply meant mental disorder and had nothing to do with the usage it
    was to acquire after 1890 (Berrios, European views on personality
    disorders: a conceptual history, 1993).

89 p. 301, Feuchtersleben, 1847.

90 For an excellent account of his life and work, see Stocking, 1973.

91 Prichard, 1835.

92 p. 318, Prichard, 1835.

93 p. 324, Prichard, 1835.

94 p. 326, Prichard, 1835.

95 p. 93, Bucknill and Tuke, 1858.

96 p. 100, Bucknill and Tuke, 1858.

97 pp. 100–107, Netchine, 1973.

98 Sollier, 1891.

99 Down, 1866.

100 Cretinism is said to have been described by Platter during the sixteenth century (see James, 1990). During the nineteenth century, J.J. Guggenbühl made a determined effort to identify the aetiology of the disorder and the thyroid aetiology was masterfully dealt with by Wagner-Jauregg (Whitrow, 1990).

101 p. III, Sollier, 1891.

102 pp. 2–3, Sollier, 1891.

103 p. 3, Sollier, 1891. This view is persistently attributed to Binet and Simon.

104 p. 3, Sollier, 1891.

105 Voisin, 1843.

106 Binet and Simon, 1905. Binet has received far more attention than Simon. For a general introduction, see Wolf, 1973.

107 Binet and Simon, 1910.

108 Désiré Magloire Bourneville (1840–1909), a protégée of Charcot's, spent most of his creative career at Bicêtre, where he became the leading French specialist in mental retardation.

109 p. 350, Binet and Simon, 1910.

110 p. 351, Binet and Simon, 1910.

111 p. 187, Séglas, 1903. The difference between mental enfeeblement and amentia (congenital imbecility and idiocy) had already been discussed in British psychiatry, see p. 267, Clouston, 1887.

112 p. 237, Chaslin, 1912.

113 Goddard, 1928.

114 p. 303, Lewis, 1933.

CHAPTER 8

Cognitive impairment

As mentioned in Chapter 7, idiocy and dementia – the two syndromic forms of intellectual failure – were differentiated before Esquirol, although this alienist made their separation official. The history of acquired cognitive impairment, called here dementia for short, will also throw light on the history of the concept of cognition.

The current concept of dementia was constructed during the nineteenth and early twentieth centuries. This process can be described as one of pruning down the heterogeneous clinical content of dementia. The process started before 1800 and culminated in the early 1900s in what I have called the 'cognitive paradigm', i.e. the view that dementia just consisted of an irreversible disorder of *intellectual* functions.[1] Historical analysis shows that this view resulted more from ideology than clinical observation. For decades, the cognitive paradigm has prevented the adequate mapping of the non-cognitive symptoms of dementia and hindered research.[2]

Dementia before the eighteenth century

Before 1700, terms such as amentia, imbecility, morosis, fatuitas, anoea, foolishness, stupidity, simplicity, carus, idiocy, dotage, and senility (but surprisingly not dementia) were used to name, in varying degree, states of cognitive and behavioural deterioration leading to psychosocial incompetence. The word *dementia*, which is almost as old as the oldest of those listed above (for example, it is already found in Lucretius) simply meant 'being out of one's mind.'[3] Thomas Willis[4] described 'stupidity or foolishness', as that condition which 'although it chiefly belongs to the rational soul, and signifies a defect of the intellect and judgment, yet it is not improperly reckoned among the *diseases of the head or brain*; for as much as this eclipse of the superior soul proceeds from the *imagination and the memory being hurt*, and the failing of these depends upon the faults of the animal spirits, and the brain itself' (my italics).[5] Willis suggested that stupidity might be genetic ('original', as when 'fools beget fools') or caused by ageing: 'Some at first crafty and ingenious, become by degrees dull, and at length foolish, by the mere declining of age, without any great errors in living'[6] or caused by 'strokes or bruising upon the head', 'drunkenness and surfeiting', 'violent and sudden passions', and 'cruel diseases of the head' such as epilepsy.

The eighteenth century

The word 'dementia' first came into vernacular English in Blancard's *Physical Dictionary*[7] as an equivalent of 'anoea' or 'extinction of the imagination and judgement.'[8] The earliest adjectival usage ('demented') has been dated 1644 by the *Oxford English Dictionary*. The OED also dates the earliest substantival usage to Davies's translation of Pinel's[9] *Treatise of Insanity*. Sobrino's[10] *Spanish–French Dictionary* offers the following definition: 'demencia = *démence, folie, extravagance, egarement, alienation d'esprit.*'[11] It would seem, therefore, that the Latin stem *demens* (without mind) was incorporated into the European vernaculars sometime between the seventeenth and eighteenth centuries, and that after the 1760s, it acquired a medical connotation.

Further evidence for this usage can be found in the corresponding entry of the *Encyclopédie*: 'Dementia is a disease consisting in a paralysis of the spirit characterized by abolition of the reasoning faculty. It differs from fatuitas, morosis, stultitia and stoliditas in that there is in these a weakening of understanding and memory; and from delirium in that this is but a temporary impairment in the exercise of the said functions. Some modern writers confuse dementia with mania, which is a delusional state accompanied by disturbed behaviour (*audace*); these symptoms are not present in subject with dementia who exhibit foolish behaviour and cannot understand what they are told, cannot remember anything, have no judgment, are sluggish, and retarded. Physiology teaches that the vividness of our understanding depends on the intensity of external stimuli: in pathological states such understanding may be excessive, distorted or abolished; dementia results in the third case; abolition may follow: 1. damage to the brain caused by excessive usage, congenital causes or old age, 2. failure of the spirit, 3. small volume of the brain, 4. violent blows to the head causing brain damage, 5. incurable diseases such as epilepsy, or exposure to venoms (Charles Bonnet reports of a girl who developed dementia after being bitten by a bat) or other substances such as opiates and mandragora. Dementia is difficult to cure as it is related to damage of brain fibres and nervous fluids; it becomes incurable in cases of congenital defect or old age [otherwise] treatment must follow the cause.'[12]

But the *Encyclopédie* also offered a legal definition: 'Those in a state of dementia are incapable of informed consent, cannot enter into contracts, sign wills, or be members of a jury. This is why they are declared incapable of managing their own affairs. Actions carried out before the declaration of incapacity are valid unless it is demonstrated that dementia pre-dated the action. Ascertainment of dementia is based on examination of handwriting, interviews by magistrates and doctors, and testimony from informants. Declarations made by notaries that the individual was of sane mind whilst signing a will are not always valid as they may be deceived by appearances, or the subject might have been in a lucid period. In regards to matrimonial rights, *démence* is not a sufficient cause for separation, unless it is accompanied by aggression (*furour*). It is, however, sufficient for a separation of property, so that the wife is no longer under the guardianship of her husband. Those suffering from dementia cannot be appointed to public positions or receive privileges. If they became demented after any has been granted, a coadjutor should be appointed.'

These entries summarize well the state of knowledge on dementia during the 1760s. The clinical definition distinguished dementia from *mania* (a term which, at the time, described any state of acute excitement be it schizophrenic, hypomanic, or organic) and from *delirium* (which more or less corresponds to current usage). Dementia was reversible and affected individuals of any age. Reference to many aetiologies suggests that a 'syndromal' view of dementia was entertained.

The legal meaning survived the French Revolution and was enshrined in Article 10 of the *Code Napoléon*: 'There is no crime if the accused was in a state of dementia at the time of the alleged act.'[13] By the middle of the seventeenth century, the English judge Hale distinguished between *dementia naturalis*, *accidentalis*, and *affectata*, according to whether the intellectual incompetence was congenital, or due to mental illness or 'toxic disorders'.[14] Here is the kernel of the nineteenth century view of dementia as a disorder of the intellectual functions leading to behavioural incapacity and the view that duration depended on cause.

Cullen and amentia

Cullen used *amentia* to describe behavioural states now called dementia. The great Edinburgh physician based his nosology on clinical observation and used the principles of 'neuralpathology', i.e. the view that all diseases were, in the last instance, diseases of the nervous system.[15] Cullen simplified earlier classifications and defined 'neuroses' as diseases without fever due to a putative non-localized disturbance of 'sense and motion' of the nervous system. These wide criteria allowed him to include many syndromes into the 'neuroses' (of which the 'vesanias', i.e. the insanities, were just one order). *Amentia*, one of the neuroses, Cullen defined as a loss of intellectual functions and memory which could be congenital, senile, and acquired; the latter resulting from infections, vascular disorders, sexual excesses, poisons, and trauma. Cullen distinguished mental retardation from senile dementia and from brain damage.[16] When Pinel translated Cullen's nosology into French, he used the term 'dementia' throughout for Cullen's amentia.

Pinel and the end of the eighteenth century

Pinel was, by ideology and temperament, the last great nosologist of the eighteenth century. In the *Nosographie*[17] he dealt with cognitive impairment under amentia and morosis, explaining it as a failure in the association of ideas leading to disordered activity, extravagant behaviour, superficial emotions, memory loss, difficulty in the perception of objects, obliteration of judgment, aimless activity, automatic existence, and forgetting of words or signs to convey ideas. He also referred to *démence senile*.[18] Pinel did not emphasize the difference between congenital and acquired dementia.

Dementia during the nineteenth century

Eighty years after Pinel, 'dementia' is found referring to irreversible states of cognitive impairment mostly affecting the elderly. 'Amentia' had also changed meaning and named a 'psychosis, with sudden onset following often acute physical illness or trauma.'[19] This section of the chapter explores these momentous changes.

French views on dementia

ESQUIROL It is not accurate to say that Esquirol's views on dementia were more advanced than Pinel's;[20] first of all, Esquirol's views radically changed between 1805 and 1838. Thus, in *Des passions*[21] he used the word (as in *démence accidental, démence melancolique*) simply to refer to loss of reason. In 1814, he began to distinguish[22] between acute, chronic and senile dementia, and 'composite dementias' like those following melancholia, mania, epilepsy, convulsions, scurvy and paralysis. Acute dementia was short lived, reversible, and followed fever, haemorrhage, and metastasis; chronic dementia was irreversible and followed masturbation, melancholia, mania, hypochondria, epilepsy, paralysis, and apoplexy; senile dementia resulted from ageing, and consisted in a loss of the faculties of the understanding.

Esquirol's[23] later thoughts on dementia were influenced by his controversy with Bayle[24] who entertained an anatomical ('organic') view of the insanities and scorned Pinel's quasi-psychological views.[25] Esquirol (together with Georget) supported Pinel's 'descriptivist' approach. His 1838 chapter on dementia includes new terms, clinical vignettes, and post-mortem descriptions. He reported 15 cases of dementia (seven males and eight females) with a mean age of 34 years (SD = 10.9); seven of these suffered from general paralysis of the insane and exhibited grandiosity, desinhibition, motor symptoms, dysarthria and terminal cognitive failure. There also was a 20 year-old girl with a typical catatonic syndrome (in modern terms), and a 40 year-old woman with pica, cognitive impairment, and space-occupying lesions in her left hemisphere and cerebellum.

This assortment of patients illustrates well Esquirol's views. For example, no case of senile dementia was included – and although this is likely to reflect an admission bias at the Charenton Hospital – it is more likely that *age was not for him a relevant criterion*. Indeed, in early nineteenth century classifications, 'senile dementia' only appears as an afterthought. The same holds true for the 'irreversibility' criterion which is only mentioned in cases of severe brain damage: as to the rest, some improvement was expected.

The great nosographies of Esquirol's time define dementia in a similar way. Thus, F.G. Boisseau refers to a *weakness of thinking* caused by overexertion, abuse, old age, disease of the brain, etc. which may lead to apathy and damage of the faculty of thinking.[26] Dementia for Boisseau is a clinical state where perception, attention, thinking, language etc. are compromised and is accompanied by self-neglect and social incompetence; 'intermissions', however do occur.[27] In 1830, Léon Rostan considered idiotism and dementia as 'diagnostic signs' of dysfunction in the faculty of intelligence and hence as an expression of '*pathology in the cerebral cortex*'.[28]

General paralysis of the insane

Bayle[29] described under the name *arachnitis chronique* the pathological changes underlying what later was to be called 'general paralysis of the insane'. Whether this 'new phenomenon' resulted from 'a mutation in the syphilitic virus (*sic*) towards the end of the eighteenth century' is unclear.[30] Equally dubious is the claim that its discovery reinforced the belief of alienists in the anatomo-clinical view of mental disease;[31] in fact, it took more than 30 years for general paralysis to gain acceptance as a 'separate' disease. Bayle's 'discovery' was more important in another way, namely, as a challenge to the 'cross-sectional' view of disease; in the words of Bercherie:[32] 'for the first time in the history of psychiatry there was a morbid entity which presented itself as a *sequential process* unfolding into successive clinical syndromes' (my italics).[33]

By the 1850s, no agreement had yet been reached as to what mental symptoms were 'typical' of *periencephalite chronique diffuse* (as general paralysis was known at the time) or what mechanisms were involved in their production. However, three clinical 'types' were recognized: manic-ambitious, melancholic-hypochondriac, and dementia. According to the 'unitary view', all three constituted *stages* of a single disease, and the order of their appearance depended on the manner in which the cerebral lesions progressed. Baillarger,[34] however, sponsored a 'dualist' view according to which: 'paralytic insanity and paralytic dementia were different conditions'.

This debate had less to do with the nature of the brain lesions than with how, in general, mental symptoms were generated by such lesions. For example, how could the 'typical' 'grandiose content of the paralytic delusions be explained? Since the same mental symptoms could be seen in all manner of conditions, Baillarger[35] believed that chronic periencephalitis could only account for the *motor signs* – mental symptoms 'therefore, must have a different origin.'[36] The very fact that 'some patients recovered' suggested that there was no clear link between lesion and mental symptom.

Although great syphilis specialists such is L.V. Lagneau had reported from the beginning of the century that hypochondria, mania, dementia and idiotism could be seen in the wake of a syphilitic infection,[37] the view that *general paralysis* was related to syphilis[38] was resisted, and the term 'pseudo-general paralysis' was coined to refer to cases such as Lagneau's.[39] On account of all this, there is little evidence that alienists considered general paralysis as a 'paradigm-disease', i.e. a model for all other mental diseases; indeed, it can even be said that the new 'disease' created more problems than it solved.[40]

GEORGET Georget's *De la Folie* offered a dynamic approach to the description and classification of mental disorders and was published when he was 25.[41] He also outlined the new concept of stupidity or stupor[42] which Esquirol still called 'acute dementia'. 'Because all mental disorders were related to changes in the brain', Georget believed that Esquirol was wrong in claiming that the cognitive impairment of dementia was a primary deficit of attention. There were 'two irreversible states' in psychiatry: idiocy and dementia, and Georget proposed that both were characterized by an abolition of thought; the first originating from a 'vice' in the organization of the brain, and the second from weakening, old age, or intercurrent diseases.[43]

Georget criticized 'great men' such as Pinel, Esquirol, Crichton, Perfect, Haslam, Chiarugi, and Rush for they had feared to contradict extant philosophical or religious beliefs, and because they had limited themselves to describe mental illness: 'without touching upon causes, and considering the disorders of function without referring to the organs that supported them . . . giving the impression that it was the symptoms that constituted the illness and not the corresponding organic lesion.'[44] This organicism *á outrance* led Georget to develop a narrow and modern-sounding concept of dementia as well as raising the issue of irreversibility.

CALMEIL Aware of the importance of clinical description, Calmeil wrote:[45] 'it is not easy to describe dementia, its varieties, and nuances; because its complications are numerous . . . it is difficult to choose its distinctive symptoms.'[46] Dementia followed chronic insanity and brain disease, and was partial or general. Calmeil was not sure that all dementias were associated with alterations in the brain. However, in regard to senile dementia, he remarked: 'there is a constant involvement of the senses, elderly people can be deaf, and show disorders of taste, smell and touch; external stimuli are therefore less clear to them, they have little memory of recent events, live in the past, and repeat the same tale; their affect gradually wanes away.'[47] Although a keen pathologist, Calmeil concluded that there was no sufficient information on the nature and range of anomalies found in the skull or brain to decide on what caused dementia.[48]

GUISLAIN According to Guislain,[49] in dementia: 'all intellectual functions show a reduction in energy, external stimuli cause only minor impression on the intellect, imagination is weak and uncreative, memory absent, and reasoning pathological . . . There are two varieties of dementia . . . one affecting the elderly (senile dementia of Cullen) the other younger people. Although conflated with dementia, idiocy must be considered as a separate group.'[50] Amongst the 'acquired' forms, Guislain included the 'vesanic dementias': 'there is nothing sadder than seeing a patient progress from mania or monomania to dementia.'

In his *Leçons*, Guislain[51] even offered an operational definition for 'cognitive failure': 'The patient has no memory, or at least is unable to retain anything, impressions evaporate from his mind. He may remember names of people but cannot say whether he has seen them before. He does not know what time or day of the week it is, cannot tell morning from evening, or say what 2 and 2 add to . . . he has lost the instinct of preservation, cannot avoid fire or water, and is unable to recognize dangers; has also lost spontaneity, is incontinent of urine and faeces, and does not ask for anything, he cannot even recognize his wife or children.'[52]

MARC C.C.H. Marc published his classical treatise on forensic psychiatry in 1840. He wrote: 'In legal language the word dementia is considered as tantamount to insanity;[53] in medical language, however, it names only one of the forms of insanity.' His legal 'criteria' included weakness of the understanding and of the will as well as loss of memory and judgment. In five clinical situations, he noticed, doctors had difficulty in diagnosing dementia: in the early stages (i.e. when the mental faculties are well preserved); when there was a sudden onset (i.e. no prodromal features were present); in the presence of 'lucid intervals'; when there were early hallucinations and delusions; and in malingering. Marc was aware of the need to integrate the medical and legal meanings, and knew of the difficulties that expert witnesses faced in court. Similar developments were occurring in Germany, as attested by the work of Hoffbauer (see below).

MOREL Criticizing older taxonomies, Morel[54] wrote that in the past the mentally ill: 'had been categorized only in terms of a [putative] impairment of their mental faculties.'[55] He endeavoured to develop a 'causal' taxonomy, i.e. one based on the distinction between causes which were *occasionelle* (e.g. social precipitants) and *determinante* (e.g. genetic factors and brain changes).[56] Six clinical groups emerged: hereditary, toxic, associated with the neuroses, idiopathic, sympathetic, and dementia.

Morel believed that: 'if we examine dementia (amentia, progressive weakening of the faculties) we must accept that it constitutes a *terminal* state. There will, of course, be exceptional insane individuals who, until the end, preserve their intellectual faculties; the majority, however, are subject to the law of decline. This results from a loss of vitality in the brain ... Comparison of brain weights in the various forms of insanity shows that the heavier weights are found in cases of recent onset. Chronic cases show more often a general impairment of intelligence (dementia). Loss in brain weight – a constant feature of dementia – is also present in ageing, and is an expression of decadence in the human species.' [There are] 'natural dementia and dementia resulting from a pathological state of the brain ... some forms of insanity are more prone to end up in dementia (idiopathic) than others ... it could be argued that because dementia is a terminal state it should not be classified as a sixth form of mental illness ... I must confess I sympathize with this view, and it is one of the reasons why I have not described the dementias in any detail ... on the other hand, from the legal and pathological viewpoints, dementia warrants separate treatment' (my italics).[57]

Morel's view of dementia as a terminal state is in keeping with his theory of 'degeneration';[58] and he believed that insanity always pre-dated dementia. In the event, however, he came to realize that this was not always the case, and explained the anomalies in terms of ageing or degeneration. One problem with the 'terminal state' hypothesis was that it led Morel to believe that there were no specific brain alterations in dementia. Morel also coined the term *démence précoce*[59] which has been considered by some as a precursor of the notion of schizophrenia.[60] Dealing with this issue is beyond the scope of this book which deals with the history of symptoms.[61]

German views

HEINROTH Viewing Heinroth as a spiritualist physician who believed that 'mental illness was sin' is inaccurate.[62] He proposed that dementia followed all mental disorders, whether resulting from functional exaltation or depression. Exaltation gave rise to 'mania' (in the old sense of acute, raging insanity) which if chronic would lead to a situation where 'the intellect will be thrown overboard.'[63] The 'patient might appear to be sane, except for his understanding and judgment.'[64] On the other hand, 'melancholia' (defined in its old sense of retarded insanity – and *not* of depression) was caused by a decline in mental functioning which, if prolonged, would lead to idiocy and apathy. Both states gave rise to reversible stupor and cognitive impairment.

HOFFBAUER Early in the nineteenth century, *Blödsinn* and *Dummheit* were more or less the equivalent German terms to the French *démence*, and the English *amentia* or *dementia*.[65] *Blödsinn* referred to chronic and mostly irreversible states, and

Dummheit to acute, reversible forms.[66] The chronic group was sub-divided by Hoffbauer into senile (incurable) and secondary dementias, the final or defect stage of various mental disorders, and only rarely curable. This latter group was equivalent to the French 'vesanic dementias'.[67]

FEUCHTERSLEBEN Hoffbauer's broad definition of dementia remained influential in German-speaking psychiatry until the 1840s, when Feuchtersleben expressed the view that the category was tantamount to 'insanity'.[68] The Austrian physician provides a good account of the medical conception of senile dementia before the development of the 'cognitive paradigm'.[69] He made senile dementia equivalent to a state of idiocy occurring in the elderly, and defined it as an 'incapacity of judging, or even, in its higher degree, of contemplating. The alteration is more prominent in the direction of thought than in that of feeling and will, though in the higher degrees, both feelings and will are also wanting.'[70] Consistent with his view, Feuchtersleben did not even mention senile dementia in the section of the book on the memory disorders, where all other mnesic deficits are treated in detail.[71]

GRIESINGER Griesinger had an irreverent attitude to old classifications and broke away from Hoffbauer's. His own view of dementia was based on his theory that psychiatric disorder may result from exaltation, depression, or weakening of psychological function. Although *brain disease was* at the basis of all mental disorders, their full understanding required the intervention of psychosocial factors. He thus sponsored a modified form of 'unitary' psychosis according to which mania, melancholia, and dementia constituted three successive stages of the same basic insanity.

There were at least five mental disorders in which there was a weakening of mental faculties: chronic mania, dementia, apathetic dementia, idiocy, and cretinism. Dementia was a state of 'mental weakness without delusions': 'the fundamental disorder consists in a general weakness of the mental faculties. Increasing incapacity for any profound emotion, loss of memory, and the power of reproduction of the ideas is chiefly affected in this manner – than more recent events, things that occur during the dementia, are almost immediately forgotten, while not infrequently former ideas connected with events which happened long ago are more easily reproduced; complete remissions never occur.'[72] However fresh this definition may sound, it must not be forgotten that Griesinger was characterizing by it a general, third stage of insanity or 'terminal stage', which occurred at any period of life and followed any and all mental disorders from mania to schizophrenia or organic disorder. Although he outlined a sub-type called 'apathetic dementia' (which included senile dementia), he did not define it fully.

KRAFFT-EBING As early as 1876, Krafft-Ebing had emphasized the importance of separating insanity from senile dementia.[73] An age cut-off for any type of dementia, however, he found difficult to specify although he believed that senile dementia (*Dementia senilis* or *Altersblösinn*) rarely occurred before 65. He also believed that heredity and external causes were less important to senile dementia than the natural changes of ageing which included poor cerebral nutrition, anaemia, atheroma, and degeneration of the cortical cells. From the clinical point of view, patients with dementia were distractible, vacant, repetitious, disorientated, showed loss of memory, could not identify people nor recognise familiar places. As dementia progressed, mania or melancholia might supervene with hallucinations, paranoid delusions and fear of being robbed. His interest in dementia grew, and in the third edition of the textbook Krafft-Ebing dedicated a full section to senile dementia.[74]

British views

Although the word 'dementia' was used in English law since at least the seventeenth century, *medical* usage starts much later. *Clinical* states of cognitive disorganization, whether affecting the young or the old were, of course, recognized but named differently. For example, Sir John Roberts of Bromley was described by William Salmon in 1694 as 'decayed in his intellectuals'[75] and D'Assingy noticed that, in some cases 'it is impossible to remedy a decay'd memory.'[76]

PRICHARD With lucidity, the Bristol alienist wrote of dementia that: 'it may be thought scarcely correct to term this a form of insanity, as it has been generally considered as a result or sequel of the disease. In some instances, however, mental derangement has nearly this character from the commencement or at least assumes it a very early period.'[77] He felt unhappy about adopting 'a French term', and suggested the word *incoherence* instead, which described 'more than a mere breakdown in association of ideas.' In fact, Prichard wanted a term to name a general deterioration of mental life. 'Senile dementia is entirely distinct from that species of moral insanity which appears occasionally . . . in aged persons. The latter is merely a loss of energy in some of the intellectual functions . . . It is in senile decay that the phenomena of incoherence in the first degree (i.e. forgetfulness) are most strongly marked.'[78]

BUCKNILL AND TUKE By the middle of the century, contradictions in the definition of dementia were still concealed by the deft use of classifications. In their manual, Bucknill and Tuke summarised the views of Pinel, Esquirol, Guislain, and Prichard: 'they described how patients with mania, melancholia, old age, etc. may develop dementia, and discussed the definitions and types. Memory loss must be a central symptom'[79] but dementia could be either: 'primary or consecutive . . . acute or chronic . . . simple or complicated . . . occasionally remittent but rarely intermittent.'[80] The acute form was rare, the chronic irreversible, and the senile 'another variety although when established it differed little in its symptoms from the chronic form.'[81]

HUGHLINGS JACKSON Hughlings Jackson put forward a model relevant to mental illness, yet in principle he did not believe that any illness could be 'mental'. The 'insanities', he believed, were the behavioural reflection of the dismantlement of cerebral structures (a process called 'dissolution'). The functional layers of the brain were hierarchically deposited by evolution and ranged from the most primitive, stable, and organized (at the bottom) to the human and unstable (at the top).[82] Disease affected the top layer and obliterated function, this caused the negative symptoms. The release of the lower (*healthy*) structures led to exaggerated function, i.e. the positive symptom.

On the effect of age, Jackson wrote: 'we rarely, if ever, meet with a dissolution from disease which is the exact reversal of evolution. Probably healthy senescence is the dissolution most nearly the exact reversal of evolution.'[83] Coma, the deepest form of dissolution, he called 'acute temporary *dementia*: let us say that the patient is, or is nearly, mentally dead' (my italics).[84] For Jackson, dementia was the only form of insanity *without* positive symptoms. Jackson's treatment of dementia, like other mental disorders, was theoretical and related little to clinical practice. Though criticized by the alienists of his time, his model became influential on French psychiatry well into the twentieth century.[85]

MAUDSLEY In *The Pathology of Mind*, Maudsley included a chapter on 'Conditions of mental weakness' and treated 'weakness' as either a constitutional defect (idiots, imbeciles, amentias) or a secondary phenomenon, i.e. dementia. The latter was divided into primary or acute which 'followed some violent strain or shock, physical or mental, which paralysed mental function for a time or for life.'[86] Secondary dementia followed 'most frequently, but not invariably, some form of mental derangement.' Five causes were identified: (*a*) attacks of mental disorder which, 'lapse by quick steps of degeneration into terminal dementia', (*b*) habitual alcoholic excess. (*c*) frequent fits of established epilepsy, (*d*) positive damage from physical injury of the brain, and (*e*) 'failure of nutrition and deterioration of structure from the degenerational changes that condition the brain decay of old age. The resulting mental decay is known as senile dementia or senile imbecility.'[87]

Maudsley realized that describing senile dementias as 'secondary' sounded strange, and offered a bizarre way out: 'although chronic, it is really primary. But old age is virtually the slow natural disease of which a man dies at last when he has no other disease; one need not scruple, therefore, to describe his dotage as secondary. Moreover, there is the unanswerable argument that it is secondary to the feverish disease of life.'[88]

CLOUSTON In 1887, the Scottish alienist Thomas Clouston classified mental disorders as states of mental depression (*psychalgia*, e.g. melancholia), mental exaltation (*psychlampsia*, e.g. mania), and mental enfeeblement (e.g. dementia, amentia, congenital imbecility, and idiocy). In regard to the latter, there were: 'two great physiological periods of mental enfeeblement, viz. in childhood and old age . . . if the brain development is arrested before birth or in childhood, we have congenital imbecility and idiocy – amentia. Dotage must be reckoned as natural at the end of life. *It is not actually the same* as senile dementia, but there is no scientific difference' (my italics).[89]

All five types of dementia were incurable and 'the medical profession outside of public institutions has little to do with its treatment or management.'[90] Secondary dementia (*vesanic* for the French) was the commonest variety and followed mania or melancholia; 'senile dementia' is one of the senile insanities. Clouston's views are typical of the period, in that senile dementia starts to be classified as a separate and primary group resulting from an exaggeration of physiological senility.

CRICHTON BROWN In 1874, Crichton Brown, director of the West Riding Asylum[91] delivered a lecture on dementia that influenced twentieth century researchers such as Shaw Bolton and Frederick Mott. He reported a case of agitated depression, another of senile mania, and a typical senile dementia. In his time, these three patients would have been ordinarily grouped as 'senile insanity', but Crichton Brown considered them as representing *different diseases*.

Senile dementia was a condition in which there was 'a failure of memory, especially as to recent events . . . Long past occurrences, the incidents of youth and boyhood, may readily be recollected.'[92] Critchton Brown believed this to be due not only to 'dullness in perception . . . but also to enfeeblement of the conservative powers themselves.' *Delusions and hallucinations were part of the condition*, although dementia may show much 'dilapidation' (my italics).[93] Emotions were blunted, and there were marked changes in personality and physical appearance. He differentiated senile from 'apoplectic' dementia and claimed that, although vascular changes might be present on occasions, 'senile dementia may occur without any vascular degeneration.'[94]

Overview of the nineteenth century

By the 1880s, clinical states such as stupor, the vesanic dementias, melancholic pseudodementia, and most of the cognitive defects relating to brain injury began to be separated off from the old category of dementia. What was left constituted a more or less homogeneous clinical group containing senile and arteriosclerotic dementias. Historical forces guiding this process included the development of morbid anatomy,[95] the psychological re-affirmation of the intellectual (cognitive) functions,[96] and the view that senility was an exaggerated and / or pathological form of ageing.[97] This encouraged the development of histological techniques and also the clinical definition and measurement of dementia.

The choice of cognitive failure as the hallmark of dementia was guided by clinical and ideological factors. The former, because institutionalized patients were often found to be cognitively incompetent; the latter because, cognition was still considered as the defining feature of the human species, and hence it was not difficult to define dementia as essentially a pathology of 'intellect'.[98]

However, in clinical practice cognition proved too broad a function to assess, and those interested in its measurement soon realised that memory was the only cognitive function whose psychometry was adequately developed.[99] Consequently, mnestic deficits became, *de facto*, if not *de jure*, the central feature of dementia. The ensuing cognitive paradigm has served the profession well but may need broadening, particularly in relation to the clinical evaluation of the states of early and advanced dementia.

The twentieth century

French views

THE SEPARATION OF THE VESANIC DEMENTIAS At the beginning of the twentieth century, the clinical and neuropathological analysis of dementia was being hampered by the fact that many researchers still classified the vesanic dementias as part of the condition. The vesanic dementias corresponded to what nowadays would be considered as the *defect state* of the functional psychoses, particularly dementia praecox (schizophrenia). In 1900, in a classical article entitled *La démence terminale dans les psychoses*, Gombault offered a full review of the problem and concluded that dementia should be considered as a final common pathway to a number of chronic psychoses and organic disorders.[100] Bessière also supported the syndromatic view: 'under the influence of the German school, the boundaries of dementia have been much enlarged and now include four groups: praecox, terminal, senile, and that following a number of brain diseases. Whatever the group to which they belong, patients show the same symptoms, namely a weakening of intelligence, attention, judgment and will. Frequently, delusions are added to the clinical picture'.[101] This view was, however opposed by E. Toulouse who together with A. Damaye published in 1905 a fundamental article entitled *La démence vésanique: est-elle une démence?* where they argued that vesanic dementias did not exist, i.e. they were not the same as organic dementias either from the neuropathological or clinical viewpoints; they concluded that such states were simply chronic confusions.[102] By means of an instrument that included questions on orientation and general knowledge, arithmetic, and memory tests, Toulouse and Damaye showed that vesanic dementias were less impaired than the organic ones.

The view that the vesanic dementias should not be considered as genuine dementias was confirmed by A. Marie whose book was the most important to appear before the First World War. This superb volume included chapters on the history, psychology, pathology, epidemiology, and classification of dementia, which it defined as: 'an irreversible psychopathological state characterized by the weakening or partial or total loss of intellectual, emotional and volitional faculties'.[103] Régis followed a similar line and described Kraepelin's *dementia praecox* as a *confusion mentale chronique*,[104] thereby describing the vesanic dementias separately from *la démence* or *infirmité psychiques d'involution* which he deals with in another section of the book.[105] By the time Laignel-Lavastine's had established itself as the most popular textbook, the separation between vesanic and organic dementia had long been completed.[106]

German views

KRAEPELIN Kraepelin's views on senile dementia changed at least twice. In the first edition of his lectures,[107] he dealt with *senile imbecility* as a 'disorder of old age' together with melancholia and persecutory states. Kraepelin illustrated the new category by reporting the case of a shoemaker who after having broken his neck developed agitated depression, hypochondriacal delusions, and 'a pronounced inability to retain new mental impressions' in spite of his 'good memory for ideas formed long ago'. Recognition of these cases was important, Kraepelin believed for 'senile imbecility is of its very nature incurable, for it depends on the destruction of several constituents of the cortex.' Though depression or excitement might occur at first, 'the end will always be a high degree of mental and emotional feebleness'.[108]

It is likely that Kraepelin was influenced here by J. Noetzli from Zürich. In 1894, this author had reported 70 cases of senile dementia (the post-mortem studies were carried out by Auguste Forel who was head of department). In addition to degenerative changes all patients had a degree of *arteriosclerosis* and there was a marked reduction in brain weight. Patients were then subdivided according to whether in addition to (diffuse) degenerative changes there showed (focal) vascular lesions. The author found that focal lesions (30 cases) were more often accompanied by manic and melancholic symptoms and a rapid course. Senile mania, melancholia, and dementia were described, and it was found that, as far as the number of focal lesions was concerned (and irrespective of symptoms) there was no difference between the frontal, temporal and occipital lobe.[109]

In the second edition of the textbook, the corresponding chapter was entitled 'Senile Dementia' and included three clinical illustrations.[110] Lastly, in the 1909 edition, Kraepelin dealt separately with *pre-senile* and senile dementia. In the section on the latter, he discussed the psychological changes of old age and concluded that 'in the most serious cases', these alterations themselves led to 'the disease pattern of dementia', i.e. he seemed to suggest a continuity view.[111] He also described what was to become the typical profile of senile dementia: memory and cognitive impairment and changes in personality and emotions, and suggested some 'characteristic' neuropathological changes. It was in this section of the book that he mentioned that Alzheimer had described a 'particular group of cases with extremely serious cell alterations', which he baptised as 'Alzheimer's disease' (see below).[112]

ZIEHEN Theodor Ziehen, one of the most original German alienists of this period, was as concerned about the nosological position of the vesanic dementias as he was about the richness of neuropathological findings reported in the various types of 'dementias', particularly those of old age. His own classification, which with minor changes lasted up to the Second World War, included nine types: arteriosclerotic, senile, apoplectic (focal), post-meningitic, toxic (post-alcoholic, lead intoxication, etc.), traumatic, secondary to functional psychoses (vesanic), epileptic, and hebephrenic or praecox.

Ziehen defined senile dementia as 'mental disease affecting old age characterized by a progressive weakening of intellectual faculties and caused by cortical involution (without the intervention of causes such as alcohol or syphilis).'[113] 'Involution' of grey matter affected neurones and fibres directly and blood vessels occasionally; he believed that dementias starting before the age of 60 reflected 'praecox senility' which was hereditary in nature. Generalized arteriosclerosis, often affecting the heart, could also accompany dementia, as could history of head trauma. Overwork was dismissed as irrelevant to premature senility.

Memory failure affecting recent events, was for Ziehen the hallmark of senile dementia and he put it down to a defect in the formation of associations; important symptoms were also general intellectual and affective deterioration and hallucinations and delusions. This led him to describe a 'simple' form of senile dementia (characterised by cognitive impairment alone) and a complex form (accompanied by psychotic and affective symptoms); the latter was occasionally confused with the stuporous form of melancholia.[114] From the neuropathological point of view, Ziehen enumerated 13 putative brain changes in dementia.

JASPERS AND THE QUANTITATIVE APPROACH Jaspers' first paper on dementia dealt with its psychometry. After quoting Kraepelin's definition of dementia, Jaspers commented: 'It would seem that any failure in performance, whatever the way it is assessed, is called dementia. The concept is, therefore, so wide that, like other over-encompassing notions, it is in danger of being empty of real content.' His own suggestion was that dementia should be diagnosed 'in any situation when there is an omission of any of the necessary constituents of cognition, and as a result a situation of false thinking can be identified.'[115]

To the last edition of *General Psychopathology*, Jaspers continued recommending the old psychometric tests of Ebbinghaus and Stern. Intelligent behaviour failed in a number of clinical states but in 'organic dementia': 'the organic process usually destroys in a far-reaching manner the pre-conditions (*Vorbedingungen*) of intelli-gence, such as memory, powers of organization, and sometimes the apparatus of speech, so that, for instance, in senile dementia, we get a clinical picture in which a person forgets his whole life, cannot speak properly any longer, and can make himself understood only with difficulty.'[116]

Jaspers remained loyal to the view that 'intelligent behaviour' constituted a uni-tary mental activity whose success depended on the integrity of its various compo-nents.[117] This old associationistic approach has regained popularity in the current neuropsychiatry of dementia.

The view that the diagnosis of dementia must also be based in a quantitative assessment is, however, very important. In addition to Jaspers who realized its importance as early as 1910, the work of Revault d'Allonnes must be also men-tioned. In 1912 he made a determined effort to develop an instrument to assess dementia based on the identification of negative and positive behaviours and per-formance under effort of perception, memory, attention and ideation.[118]

British views

GEORGE SAVAGE Savage divided dementia into two categories: 'In one there was a destruction more or less complete of the mind, which can never be recovered from, and in the other there is a functional arrest, which may pass off . . . at the one end of life there may be inability to develop intellectually . . . amentia; and at the other end destruction of mind may leave the whole intellectual fabric a ruin . . . dementia.'[119]

Earlier, he had proposed the concept of 'partial dementia': 'Young adults, who have given way to excesses, especially when several varieties of excess have been indulged in at the same time, become unable to perform the duties for which they have been educated and fully prepared.' This was illustrated by a decline in per-formance and symptoms in what sounds like a case of simple schizophrenia. The partial dementia category did not thrive. In the fourth edition of the *Nomenclature of Diseases of the Royal College of Physicians*, the dementias were classified under the 'degenerations' and considered as: primary and secondary. There were six varieties, including senile and organic. Savage was one of the advisers on mental diseases to the Committee preparing this edition.[120]

BOLTON Whilst at the turn of the century alienists tried to improve the classifi-cation of the dementias in terms of clinical analysis, at the Claybury Hospital, Joseph Shaw Bolton carried out systematic post-mortem studies hoping to develop a neuropathological classification. He divided his patients into four groups: insanity without dementia, insanity with dementia, dementia with insanity, and severe dementia. To avoid brain lysis, Bolton stored the corpses soon after death in a new cold chamber developed by Frederick Mott.

In 1903, and based on the study of cortical neurones, Bolton offered a classification which included amentia, mental confusion, and dementia, the latter being subdivided into the 'dementia of worn-out neurons ... dementia of degenerates who owing to stress have become insane and ... the dementia of degenerates which is associated with premature vascular degeneration.'[121] That not all patients fitted into his classification, Bolton explained by the fact that 'they die at all stages of their mental diseases.'[122]

This classification, like others based on one or two aetiological principles, did not last beyond the First World War. Around this time, the theory of degeneration, which since Morel had provided a framework for the taxonomy of mental disorder, started to fall out of fashion, and with it disappeared versions of the doctrine related to dementia such as the notion of 'abiotrophy' – sponsored by William Gowers in the 1880s.[123] By the 1930s, a popular classification was that propounded by Mac-Donald Critchley who gave up identifying common aetiological denominators and simply listed the main groups: arteriosclerotic, syphilitic, traumatic, due to space-occupying lesions, epileptic, following chronic neurological and psychotic diseases, toxic-infective, and 'essential' which included Alzheimer's and Pick's disease.[124] When in 1944 Mayer-Gross was asked to review this field for a special issue of the *Journal of Mental Science*, he limited himself to confirm Critchley's classification.[125]

The fragmentation of the dementia concept

By 1900, senile, arteriosclerotic, and vesanic forms of dementia were still being recognized.[126] Many other cases, however, found no place in this three-partite classification but those which had been known for a long time such as general paralysis of the insane, dementia praecox, and *melancholia attonita* caused little problem as they were kept in their own nosological niche. Others, however, caused difficulty such as the dementias related to alcoholism, epilepsy, brain damage, myxoedema, 'hysteria', and lead poisoning.

This mismatch was resolved in various ways: some syndromes were re-defined as *independent* conditions (e.g. Korsakoff's syndrome and myxoedema), others were *hidden* under a different name (e.g. dementia praecox became schizophrenia and melancholia attonita stupor); yet others were explained away as *pseudodementias* (e.g. hysteria). The individual history of some of these states is worth telling.

Démence précoce *'becomes' schizophrenia*
The 'received' view on the history of this condition is that: (*a*) Morel coined the term *démence précoce* to refer to a state of cognitive impairment occurring during adolescence or soon after,[127] (*b*) Kraepelin used its Latinized version to name a composite 'disease',[128] (*c*) Bleuler renamed the same behavioural composite 'schizophrenia',[129] and (*d*) Kurt Schneider suggested a set of 'empirical' criteria to capture its symptomatology.[130]

Earlier reports of cases redolent of 'schizophrenia' can be found in Haslam,[131] Pinel,[132] and others;[133] however, there has been some debate as to its rarity before 1800.[134] The absence of early reports, however, may have been due to the absence before 1800 of the adequate language of description or to the fact that the disease was described under names such as mania and melancholia.

But what did Morel describe? The term *démence précoce* was first used by this alienist in 1860 to name a condition causing severe cognitive impairment and psychosocial incompetence in young people. In fact, Morel was referring to the clinical state that Georget had called *stupidité*, i.e. a syndrome of non-responsiveness. In 1853 Morel reported the case of a young man who developed religious preoccupations, delusions and hallucinatory excitement, and then 'generalized muscular contractions'. He was stuporous for months, maintained awkward bodily positions, did not answer questions, and was doubly incontinent. He remained lacking in initiative and showed automatic behaviour.[135] It is tempting to re-diagnose this case as a catatonic schizophrenia.[136]

Catatonic behaviour (under the name of *melancholia attonita*) was well known before Kahlbaum wrote his book in 1874.[137] This little monograph was not, of course, an attempt to describe a new disease but to put order in the confused field of *melancholia attonita*. Only 10 of Kahlbaum's 26 cases would be re-diagnosable as catatonias; the rest are a collection of cases with depression, epilepsy, and subcortical syndromes secondary to attempted hanging.[138]

So, Kraepelin demonstrated considerable foresight when he combined catatonia with dementia paranoides, simplex,[139] and hebephrenia[140] into a new disease (dementia praecox) characterized by bad prognosis and common anatomo-pathology.[141] Dementia praecox itself became 'schizophrenia' in a book published by Bleuler in 1911;[142] the idea probably having originated from a collective intellectual effort at the Burghölzli Hospital in Zürich.[143] Bleuler's notion of schizophrenia was shaped by Kraepelin's views but also by a combination of associationism, psychodynamic theory and a tinge of nationalism. Bleuler justified his preference for the word schizophrenia (which he had used for the first time in 1908) by saying that dementia praecox had developed a fatalistic connotation and was often taken literally to mean dementia affecting the young.[144] But as is often the case, the change in name led to a change in metaphor, and 'splitting' (*Spaltung*), a concept that has only meaning within associationism, became the image of the hour.[145]

Kraepelin had been careful not to offer a speculative pathophysiology of dementia praecox, and contented himself with a clinical description, a natural history, and a prognosis.[146] However, during the early years of this century, the view that symptoms were symbols of processes occurring beyond awareness became popular, and not surprisingly, there is much of this in the views put forward by Jung and Bleuler. Even motor and cognitive symptoms became 'psychologized'; thus stereotypies and echo phenomena were no longer considered as disorders of the motor system but of the will.[147]

Bleuler's conception became popular (particularly in the USA) for it offered a compromise between the old neuropsychiatry and the new psychodynamic ideas: symptoms were, to certain extent, 'understandable' although they might still be caused by some unknown toxin.[148] This remained thus until the 1970s, when the neuropsychiatric reaction encouraged, once again, an organic interpretation.[149]

During the late 1930s, Kurt Schneider reported a ranked classification of diagnostic criteria which he described as 'empirical' (i.e. non-theoretical). After a period of neglect (for example, they were paid little attention in the 1950 World Congress of Psychiatry where the psychosis were discussed in detail),[150] Schneider's first rank symptoms were re-discovered and have since become the foundation for a 'neo-Kraepelinian' definition. It would seem, however, that Schneider's first rank symptoms only capture a proportion of the clinical cases that Kraepelin called dementia praecox.

Pseudodementia and vesanic dementia

The concept of 'pseudodementia' was created during the 1880s to deal with cases of 'dementia' that recovered. At the time, cases of 'pseudodementia' were called *démence melancolique*[151] or 'vesanic', i.e. dementia secondary to insanity.[152] Mairet[153] reported that melancholic patients with cognitive impairment showed temporal lobe lesions, that such brain site was related to 'feelings', and that nihilistic delusions only appeared when the cortex was involved. Mairet's cases (some of which would now be called 'Cotard's syndrome')[154] showed psychomotor retardation, refused food, and died in stupor.

Another important contributor to the understanding of cognitive impairment in the affective disorders was George Dumas[155] who suggested that it was 'mental fatigue that explained the psychological poverty and monotony of melancholic depressions' and that the problem was not 'an absence but a stagnation of ideas'; i.e. he was, therefore, the first to explain the disorder as a failure in performance.

The *word* pseudodementia originated in a different clinical tradition, and was first used by Carl Wernicke to refer to 'a chronic hysterical state mimicking mental weakness.'[156] The term was out of fashion until the 1950s, when it was re-discovered.[157] Current usage is ambiguous in that it may refer to three different clinical situations: a real (albeit reversible) cognitive impairment accompanying some psychoses, a parody of such impairment, and the cognitive deficit of delirium.[158]

The term 'vesanic dementia' began to be used after the 1840s to refer to the clinical states of cognitive disorganisation following insanity; its meaning changed *pari passu* with psychiatric theory. According to the unitary insanity view,[159] vesanic dementia was a terminal stage (the end point in the sequence mania– melancholia–); according to degeneration theory, it was the final expression of a corrupted pedigree; and according to post-1880s nosology, it was a final common pathway to all the insanities. Vesanic dementias were occasionally reversible, and occurred at any age; risk factors such as old age, lack of education, low social class, and bad nutrition were reported to accelerate its progression and impede recovery.[160] The nosological position of the vesanic dementias was debated until the First World War.

The consolidation of 'senile dementia'

Concepts of ageing before the nineteenth century

In history, ageing has been portrayed as resulting from either internal changes or the buffeting of environmental factors.[161] The latter, or 'wear and tear' hypothesis, was popular during the early nineteenth century and was inspired in the observation that natural objects are subject to the ravages of time. Surprisingly, this view has not always been accompanied by a tolerant attitude to deficits in the elderly: in fact, across time and cultures, ambivalent attitudes abound. The Hebrew tradition and its Christian offshoot encouraged reverence to old age, particularly to those in positions of power,[162] but it was rarely extended to women or men in humbler stations.[163] It is likely, therefore, that even in these cultures ageing was considered as undesirable.[164]

Another interesting ambiguity related to whether ageing actually involved the mind. Whilst it was a palpable fact that the human frame decayed, not everyone accepted that this necessarily affected the soul or mind. Descriptions of the psychological changes caused by ageing (e.g. Cicero's)[165] suggest an early awareness of mental involvement. However, later theological speculation on the immutability of the soul, led to the view that it escaped wear and tear, and that humans could only grow wiser. This is likely to have encouraged the development of gerontocracies;[166] from the point of view of the history of cognitive impairment, it would be useful to know how such societies coped with dementia affecting the elderly in power.[167]

Buffon and Erasmus Darwin contributed to a change in ideas on ageing. For example, Buffon wrote: 'All changes and dies in Nature. As soon as it reaches its point of perfection it begins to decay. At first, this is subtle and it takes years for one to realise that major changes have in fact taken place.'[168] He put this down to a process of 'ossification' similar to that affecting trees: 'this cause of death is common to animals and vegetables. Oaks die as their core becomes so hard that they can no longer feed. They trap humidity, and this eventually makes them rot away.'[169]

Erasmus Darwin suggested that ageing resulted from a breakdown of 'communication' between man and his environment;[170] this followed a decrease in irritability (a property of the nerve fibre) and a consequent attenuation of response to sensations: 'It seems our bodies by long habit cease to obey the stimulus of the aliment, which supports us; three causes may conspire to render our nerves less excitable: 1. if a stimulus be greater than natural, it produces too great an exertion of the stimulated organ, and in consequence exhausts the spirit of animation; and the moving organ ceases to act, even though the stimulus is continued; 2. if excitations weaker than natural be applied, so as not to excite the organ into action, they may be gradually increased, without exciting the organ into action, which will thus acquire a habit of disobedience to the stimulus; 3. when irritative motions continue to be produced in consequence of stimulus, but are not succeeded by sensation.'[171]

Concepts of ageing during the nineteenth century

In 1807, Sir John Sinclair published a major compendium on ageing and longevity including references to pre-nineteenth century sources.[172] Soon after, empirical work started, like Rostan's[173] who was one of the most original members of the Paris school. He published in 1819 his *Recherches sur le Ramollissement du Cerveau* where the view was propounded that vascular disorders were central to brain ageing.[174] Equally important was his anti-vitalistic position[175] expressed in the claim that all diseases were related to pathological changes in specific organs.[176]

During the 1850s, Reveillé-Parise saw his task as writing on 'the history of ageing, that is, mapping the imprint of time on the human body, whether on its organs or on its spiritual essence.'[177] In regard to ageing he wrote: 'the cause of ageing is a gradual increase in the work of decomposition . . . but how does it happen? What are the laws that control the degradation that affects the organization and mind of man?'[178] Reveillé-Parise dismissed the toxin's hypothesis put forward by the Italian Lévy, according to which accumulation of calcium phosphates caused petrification, i.e. 'an anticipation of the grave.'[179] This view, Reveillé-Parise stated, had no empirical foundation and was based on a generalization from the effect caused by localised calcification. Instead, he proposed that ageing resulted from a negative balance between composition and elimination that affected the cardiovascular, respiratory and reproductive organs.

In 1868, J.M. Charcot offered a course of 24 lectures on the diseases of the elderly.[180] In the first, dedicated to the 'general characters of senile pathology', he commented that books on geriatrics up to his time had 'a particularly literary or philosophical turn [and were] but ingenious paraphrases of the famous treatise *De Senectute*'.[181] He praised Rostan for his views on brain softening, and also Cruveilhier, Hourman and Dechambre, Durand-Fardel, and Prus. He criticized Canstatt and other German physicians for their 'imagination holds an immense place at the expense of impartial and positive observation.'[182] Charcot developed the principle that: 'changes of texture impressed on the organism by old age sometimes become so marked that the physiological and pathological states seem to merge into one another by insensible transitions and cannot be distinguished.'[183]

The concept of brain arteriosclerosis

Reports of arteriosclerotic changes in systemic arteries abound before the eighteenth century.[184] By 1769, J.B. Morgagni had produced clear-cut descriptions of similar changes affecting the brain vessels.[185] So, when in 1833 Lobstein described the histopathology of arteriosclerosis,[186] little did he imagine that, during the second half of the century, it would become the favoured mechanism of 'senility'.[187] Motor and sensory deficits, vertigo, delusions, hallucinations, and volitional, cognitive and affective disorder soon were also attributed to arteriosclerosis.[188] Parenchymal and/ or vascular disorders affected the brain in a diffused or focalised manner; vascular changes included acute ischaemia (on which clinical observation was adequate)[189] and chronic ischaemia (on which it was not), the category having been invented by extrapolating from the acute syndrome.[190]

Of course, not everybody accepted the role given to arteriosclerosis, at least in relation to conditions such as the involutional psychoses.[191] In general, however, the old notion of 'arteriosclerotic dementia' remained alive until the 1960s.[192] It is important to remember that throughout this period alienists already knew that a drop in blood supply could cause diffuse or focal lesions; the latter called 'multifocal arteriosclerotic dementia' and equivalent to our multi-infarct dementia.[193]

Reviewing the issue, Hughlings Jackson[194] wrote: 'softening . . . as a category for a rude clinical grouping is to be deprecated.'[195] None the less, he followed Durand-Fardel's view that stroke could cause immediate or delayed mental symptoms; and recognized that major cognitive failure may ensue. Since emotional symptoms were instances of early 'release' phenomena,[196] Jackson believed that anxiety, stress and irritability were harbingers of stroke.

The concept of arteriosclerotic dementia

At the beginning of the century, old age was considered as a risk factor in arteriosclerosis[197] and melancholia;[198] and by 1910 a trend was afoot to consider 'cerebral arteriosclerosis' as a major risk factor in senile dementia.[199] Arteriosclerosis could be generalized or cerebral, inherited or acquired, and followed syphilis, alcohol, nicotine, high blood pressure, and ageing. In the genetically predisposed, cerebral arteries were thinner and less elastic. Mental changes resulted from narrowing of arteries and/or reactive inflammation. The view that arteriosclerotic dementia resulted from a gradual strangulation of blood supply to the brain was formed during this period; consequently, emphasis was given to prodromal symptoms and strokes were but the culmination of the process.

Some opposed this view. For example, Marie[200] claimed that such explanation was tautological as alienists claimed both that: 'ageing was caused by arteriosclerosis and the latter was caused by ageing',[201] and Walton expressed doubts on the relevance of arteriosclerosis to involutional melancholia.[202] Pathologists also worried lest they could not exclude 'cerebral arteriosclerosis in any single case' of senile dementia.[203] Based on this, Olah concluded that there was no such a thing as 'arteriosclerotic psychoses'.[204] The 'chronic global ischaemia' hypothesis, however, won the day, and continued into the second half of the twentieth century. For some it became a general explanation; for example, North and Bostock reported a series of 568 general psychiatric cases in which around

40% suffered from 'arterial disease', which – according to the authors – was also responsible for schizophrenia![205]

But the old idea of 'apoplectic dementia' also continued and achieved its clearest enunciation in the work of Benjamin Ball.[206] Apoplexy resulted from bleeding, softening or tumour and might be 'followed by a notable decline in cognition, and by a state of dementia which was progressive and incurable . . . of the three forms, localised softening (*ramollissement en foyer*) caused the more severe states of cognitive impairment.'[207] Ball believed that prodromal lapses of cognition (such as episodes of somnolence and confusion with automatic behaviour, with no memory after the event) and sensory symptoms were both caused by atheromatous lesions. Visual hallucinations, occasionally of a pleasant nature, were also common. After strokes, cognitive impairment was frequent. Post-mortem studies showed in these cases, softening of the 'ideational' areas of cortex and white matter. Ball also identified a laterality effect:[208] 'right hemisphere strokes led more often to dementia and left hemisphere ones to perplexity, apathy, unresponsiveness, and a tendency to talk to oneself.'[209] Following Luys, he believed that some of these symptoms resulted from damage to corpus striatum, insular sulcus, and the temporal lobe.

During Ball's time attention shifted from white to red softening. Charcot,[210] for example, wrote on cerebral haemorrhage (the new name for red softening): 'having eliminated all these cases, we find ourselves in the presence of a homogeneous group corresponding to the commonest form of cerebral haemorrhage. This is, *par excellence*, sanguineous apoplexy . . . as it attacks a great number of old people, I might call it senile haemorrhage.'[211]

Presbyophrenia and confabulation

In Kahlbaum's work, *paraphrenia* was an insanity occurring during a period of biological change. *Presbyophrenia* was a form of *paraphrenia senilis* characterized by amnesia, disorientation, delusional misidentification, and confabulation.[212] The term re-appeared in the work of Wernicke, Fischer, and Kraepelin. Wernicke's classification of mental disorders was based on his theory on the tripartite relationship between consciousness and world, body, and self.[213] Impairment in relationships with the *world* led to presbyophrenia, delirium tremens, Korsakoff's psychosis, and hallucinoses. Amongst the features of presbyophrenia, Wernicke included confabulations, disorientation, hyperactivity, euphoria, and a fluctuating course; acute forms resolved without trace, chronic ones merged with senile dementia.[214]

In France, Rouby conceived presbyophrenia as a final common pathway for cases suffering from Korsakoff's psychosis, senile dementia, or acute confusion.[215] Truelle and Bessière suggested that it might result from a toxic state caused by liver or kidney failure.[216] Kraepelin lumped presbyophrenia together with the senile and pre-senile insanities, and believed that such patients were older than Korsakoff's ones, were free from polyneuritis and history of alcoholism, and showed hyperactivity and elevated mood.[217] Ziehen wrote that 'their marked memory impairment contrasts with the relative sparing of thinking'[218] and Oskar Fischer suggested that 'disseminated cerebral lesions' were the anatomical substratum of presbyophrenia.[219]

During the 1930s, two new hypotheses emerged. On phenomenological grounds, Bostroem concluded that presbyophrenia was related to *mania* and resulted from an interaction between cerebral arteriosclerosis and *cyclothymic* premorbid personality,[220] but Burger-Pritz and Jacob questioned the relevance of such cyclothymic features.[221] Lafora, in turn, proposed that disinhibition and presbyophrenic behaviour were caused by a combination of senile and arteriosclerotic changes.[222] Bessiére then suggested that presbyophrenia could be found in senile dementia, brain tumours, traumatic psychoses, and confusional states.[223] More recently, it has been suggested that presbyophrenia may be a sub-form of Alzheimer's disease characterised by a severe atrophy of locus coeruleus or disruption of aminergic pathways in frontal and subcortical structures.[224]

The concept of senile dementia

Anecdotal cases of senile dementia abound in fictional and historical literature,[225] but the concept of 'senile dementia', as currently understood, was formed during the latter part of the nineteenth century. Indeed, it could not have been otherwise, as the neurobiological and clinical language that made it possible only became available during this period.[226] But even after the nosological status of senile dementia had become clearer, there were those who, like Rauzier, felt able to state: 'it may appear either as a primary state or follow most of the mental disorders affecting the elderly'.[227]

Following Rogues de Fursac,[228] Adrien Pic – the author of one of the most influential geriatric manuals during this period – defined senile dementia as: 'a state of intellectual decline, whether or not accompanied by delusions, that results from brain lesions associated with ageing.'[229]

Enquiries into the brain changes accompanying dementia started during the 1830s and were based on descriptions of external appearance.[230] Marcé carried out the first important microscopic study and described cortical atrophy, enlarged ventricles, and 'softening',[231] and the vascular origin of softening was soon ascertained.[232] However, the distinction between vascular and parenchymal factors in the aetiology of dementia was not made until the 1880s. From then on, microscopic studies concentrated on cellular death, plaques and neurofibrils. But Alzheimer's disease has become the prototypical form of senile dementia; indeed, the study of its history might throw light on the formation of the concept of dementia.

Alzheimer's disease

The writings of Alzheimer, Fischer, Fuller, Lafora, Bonfiglio, Perusini, Ziveri, Kraepelin, and other protagonists are deceptively fresh, and this makes anachronistic reading inevitable. However, the psychiatry of the late nineteenth century is still a remote country: concepts such as dementia, neurone, neurofibril and plaque were then still in process of construction and meant different things to different people. A detailed discussion of these issues is beyond the scope of this chapter.[233]

In 1906, Alzheimer reported the case of a 51 year-old woman, with cognitive impairment, *hallucinations*, *delusions*, and focal symptoms, whose brain was found on post-mortem to show plaques, tangles, and *arteriosclerotic changes*.[234] The existence of neurofibrils had, however, been known for some time,[235] for example, that in senile dementia 'the destruction of the neuro-fibrillae appears to be more extensive than in the brain of a paralytic subject.'[236] Likewise, on June 1906 (i.e. five months *before* Alzheimer's report), Fuller had remarked on the presence of neurofibrillar bundles in senile dementia.[237]

A putative association of plaques with dementia was not a novelty either: this had been reported in 1887 by Beljahow[238] and by Redlich and Leri a few years later.[239] In Prague, Fischer[240] gave an important paper in June 1907 pointing out that *miliary necrosis* could be considered as a marker of senile dementia. Nor was the actual clinical syndrome as described by Alzheimer new: states of persistent cognitive impairment affecting the elderly, accompanied by delusions and hallucinations were well known.[241]

As a leading neuropathologist Alzheimer was aware of all this work; so, did he *mean* to describe a new disease? The likely answer is no; indeed his only intention seems to have been to draw attention to the fact that the syndrome could occur in younger people.[242] This is confirmed by commentaries from those who worked for him at the time: for example, Perusini[243] wrote that for Alzheimer 'these morbid forms do not represent anything but atypical form of senile dementia.'[244]

Kraepelin coined the term *Alzheimer's disease* in the 8th edition of his Handbook: 'the autopsy reveals, according to Alzheimer's description, changes that represent the most serious form of senile dementia . . . the *Drusen* were numerous and almost one-third of the cortical cells had died off. In their place instead we found peculiar deeply stained fibrillary bundles that were closely packed to one another, and seemed to be remnants of degenerated cell bodies . . . The clinical interpretation *of this Alzheimer's disease* is still confused. Whilst the anatomical findings suggest that we are dealing with a particularly serious form of senile dementia, the fact that this disease sometimes starts already around the age of 40 does not allow this supposition. In such cases we should at least assume a *senium praecox* if not perhaps a more or less age-independent unique disease process.'[245]

Alzheimer himself showed some surprise at Kraepelin's interpretation, and referred to his 'disease' as *Erkrankungen* (in the medical language of the 1900s a term softer than *Krankheit*, the term used by Kraepelin). Others also expressed doubts.[246] For example, Fuller, whose contribution to this field has been sadly neglected, asked 'why a special clinical designation – Alzheimer's disease – since, after all, they are but part of a general disorder?'[247] In Russia, Hakkébousch and Geier saw it as a variety of the involution psychosis.[248] Simchowicz considered it as only a severe form of senile dementia,[249] and Ziehen did not mention it in his major review of senile dementia.[250] In a meeting of the New York Neurological Society, Ramsay Hunt told Lambert, presenting a case of 'Alzheimer's disease', that 'he would like to understand clearly whether he made any distinction between the so-called Alzheimer's disease and senile dementia' other than . . . in degree and point of age.' Lambert agreed that, as far as he was concerned, the underlying pathological mechanisms were the same.[251]

Lugaro from Italy wrote: 'For a while it was believed that a certain agglutinative disorder of the neurofibril could be considered as the main 'marker' (*contrassegno*) of a pre-senile form [of senile dementia], which was 'hurriedly baptised' (*fretta battezzate*) as 'Alzheimer's disease';[252] he believed that this was but a variety of senile dementia. Simchowicz, who had worked with Alzheimer, wrote 'Alzheimer and Perusini did not know at the time that the plaques were typical of senile dementia [in general] and believed that they might have discovered a new disease.'[253] These views, by men living in Alzheimer's and Kraepelin's time, must be taken seriously.[254]

Pick's disease and the 'frontal lobe' dementias

Dementias believed to be related to frontal lobe pathology are in fashion, and their sponsors persistently invoke the name of Arnold Pick.[255] It is little known, however, that when the Prague neuropsychiatrist described the syndrome named after him, all he wanted was to draw attention to a form of localised (as opposed to diffuse) atrophy of the *temporal lobe*[256] associated with dysfunctions of language and praxis diagnosable during life. Pick further believed that lobar atrophies constituted a stage in the evolution of the senile dementias.

The story starts, as it should, before Pick. Gratiolet[257] was responsible for re-naming the 'anterior' lobes after the 'frontal' skull, but made no assumptions in regards to any function sited on the 'anterior extremity of the cerebral hemisphere.'[258] Phrenologists before him had, however, suggested a relationship between the reflective and perceptive functions (qualitatively defined) and the forehead.[259] Empirical correlations between the frontal lobes and language and personality began to be found only during the 1860s.[260] These findings ran parallel to Jackson's consideration of the cerebral cortex as the seat for personality and mind.[261] Meynert believed that 'the frontal lobes reach a high state of development in man' and defined mental illnesses as 'fore-brain' failures (by this he really meant 'prosencephalon' or human brain as a whole).[262]

In 1892, Pick reported the case of a 71 year-old man with focal senile atrophy and aphasia,[263] and in 1901 that of a woman of 59 with generalised cortical atrophy, affecting her left hemisphere.[264] In neither case did Pick inculpate the frontal lobes; indeed, these are only mentioned in a fourth case, that of a 60 year-old man with 'bilateral frontal atrophy'.[265] At the time no one thought that Pick had described or intended to describe a new disease, least of all Pick himself. For example, Barrett considered the two first cases of Pick's as atypical forms of Alzheimer's disease,[266] and Ziehen did not see anything special in them.[267]

Liepmann, Stransky, and Spielmeyer also described similar cases with aphasia and circumscribed cerebral atrophy;[268] and Urechia and Mihalescu suggested that the syndrome should be named 'Spielmeyer's disease'.[269] This term did not catch on, however, and in two classical papers Carl Schneider constructed a view of the disease (*Picksche Krankheit*) by suggesting that it evolved in three stages – the first with a disturbance of judgment and behaviour, the second with localised symptoms (e.g. speech), and the third with generalized dementia. He recognized rapid and slow forms, the former with an akinetic and aphasic subtypes and a malignant course, and the latter with a predominance of plaques (probably indistinguishable from Alzheimer's disease).[270]

Creutzfeldt–Jakob disease

The condition nowadays called Creutzfeldt–Jakob disease (CJD) was described during the 1920s by two students of Alzheimer's.[271] ICD-10 defines the disease as: 'a progressive dementia with extensive neurological signs, due to specific neuro-pathological changes (subacute spongiform encephalopathy) which are presumed to be caused by a transmissible agent. Onset is usually in middle or later life . . . there is usually a progressive spastic paralysis of the limbs, accompanied by extra-pyramidal signs with tremor, rigidity, and choreoathetoid movements. Other variants may include ataxia, visual failure, or muscle fibrillation and atrophy of the upper motor neurone type. The triad consists of rapidly progressive devastating dementia, pyramidal and extrapyramidal disease with myoclonus, and a character-istic triphasic electroencephalogram is thought to be highly suggestive of the disease.'

In 1920, Creutzfeldt reported the case of Berta E., a 23 year-old woman who had been admitted in 1913 to the Neurological Clinic of Breslau University; Alzh-eimer was at the time in Breslau but it is not known whether he ever saw this case.[272] After an admission for an anorexic episode at age 21, and another admission a year earlier for a skin condition, the patient was noticed to have spastic legs, tremor, and 'hysterical' behaviour. Just before the neurological admission, her gait disturbance returned and she became unkempt and showed nihilistic delusions. On admission, she was emaciated and showed generalized muscle fibrillations, hyp-ertonia, and a fever.[273] She was disorientated, deluded, perseverative, incoherent, emotionally labile, and oscillated between excitement and stupor. Epileptic attacks supervened and eventually she died in status epilepticus. No cause or precipitating factor could be elicited. Her post-mortem revealed a 'non-inflammatory focal disin-tegration of cortical tissue showing also neuronophagia, glial and some vascular proliferation, and a marked fall-out of grey cells everywhere.' Creutzfeldt considered multiple sclerosis as a possible diagnosis, but drew no conclusion as to the nature of the disorder.

In 1921, A. Jakob reported four cases of a disorder 'resembling' the acute form of multiple sclerosis, and which he denominated 'spastic pseudosclerosis'.[274] The first was a 51 year-old woman with stiff legs, dizziness, fatigue, and later depression, ataxia, rigidity, and confusion; death occurred after one year of illness; the fourth case was that of a 43 year-old man, who drank heavily, and after sustaining a hip fracture was unable to work again. He complained of stiff legs, headaches, and later developed evening delirium with paranoid features, heard voices, and had bouts of excitement. Admitted to a mental hospital with the diagnosis of catatonia, he was intermittently stuporous, grimaced, and when occasionally accessible, was disorientated, confused, and confabulative. He died during an episode of severe confusion. All cases showed on post-mortem great loss of ganglion-cells, glial proliferation, and fatty degeneration, with the part of the brain most affected being the anterior part of the striatum and the thalami. Jakob stated that: 'there have been few cases like these in the literature. The nearest is that of Creutzfeldt's.'[275] And on the predominant cortical involvement he commented: 'the more widespread distribution found in Creutzfeldt's case, in the presence of similar lesions and symptoms, should not be taken as an important difference.' Creutzfeldt disagreed with this statement.[276]

For a time, the 'spastic pseudosclerosis of Jakob' became lost in the group of the degenerative states of the basal ganglia. Interest in the disease was later re-awakened by Gajdusek[277] whose work on Kuru suggested, together with Headlow's[278] research on scrapie, that CJD might be caused by a transmissible agent. In the event, brain tissue from a British patient affected with CJD was sent to Gajdusek and Gibbs who successfully transmitted the disease to a chimpanzee.[279]

Dementia associated with brain damage

Early descriptions of dementia following trauma can be found both in Willis and Cullen. The separation between 'traumatic neurasthenia' and 'traumatic dementia', however, was only achieved at the beginning of the twentieth century.[280] The former condition referred to states of irritability, headache, and hysterical dissociation occurring in the context of minor trauma; the latter to *cognitive impairment* occurring after severe brain injury. It was believed that traumatic dementia was more likely in open injury or when the blow was directed to the top of the skull; pre-morbid personality and history of alcoholism and arteriosclerosis were additional factors. Small haemorrhages and tissue tearing were described as responsible for the memory damage. For example, Marie noted that when the 'lesion is localized in the frontal lobes, there is rapid mental decline.'[281] During the latter part of the nineteenth century, traumatic dementia was mainly discussed in the context of epileptic dementia as it was believed that falls and brain injury were one of the factors causing the cognitive impairment.[282]

Summary

The history of the word 'dementia' must not be confused with that of the concepts or behaviours involved. By the year 1800, two definitions of dementia were recognized, both having psychosocial incompetence as their central concept. In addition to cognitive impairment, the clinical definition included delusions and hallucinations. Irreversibility and old age were not at the time features of the condition. Dementia was considered to be a terminal state to all manner of mental, neurological and physical conditions.

A major change in the concept of dementia followed the adoption of the anatomo-clinical model by nineteenth century alienists. Questions were asked as to the neuropathology of dementia and findings pertaining to the latter led, in turn, to re-adjustments of clinical description. The history of dementia during the nineteenth century is, therefore, the history of its gradual attrition. Stuporous states (then called acute dementia), vesanic dementias, and localized memory impairments, were gradually reclassified, and by the First World War the 'cognitive paradigm', i.e. the view that the essential feature of dementia was intellectual impairment, had become established. From then on, efforts were made to explain other symptoms such as hallucinations, delusions, and mood and behavioural disorders as epiphenomena, and as unrelated to the central mechanism of dementia.

There was also a fluctuating acceptance of the parenchymal and vascular hypotheses, the latter leading to the description of arteriosclerotic dementia. The separation of the vesanic dementias and of the amnestic syndromes led to the realisation that age and ageing mechanisms were central, and by 1900 senile dementia became the prototype of the dementias; by 1920, Alzheimer's disease became their flagship. Since then, the cognitive paradigm has been an obstacle to research, but a re-expansion of the symptomatology of dementia is fortunately taking place.

NOTES

1 Berrios, on memory and the cognitive paradigm of dementia during the 19th century, 1990.
2 Berrios, Non-cognitive symptoms and the diagnosis of dementia, 1989.
3 Berrios, Historical aspects of the Psychoses, 1987. This has improved of late as researchers turn towards the psychopathology of dementia (see Katona and Levy, 1992).
4 Willis, 1684.
5 p. 209, Willis, 1684.
6 p. 211, Willis, 1684.
7 Blancard, 1726.

8 p. 21, Blancard, 1726.
9 Pinel, 1806.
10 Sobrino, 1791.
11 p. 300, Sobrino, 1791.
12 pp. 807–808, Diderot and d'Alembert, 1765.
13 *Code Napoléon*, 1808.
14 Walker, 1968.
15 Rath, 1959; for a wider discussion of Cullen's ideological background, see López Piñero, 1983; Bowman, 1975; Jackson, 1970.
16 Cullen, 1827.
17 Pinel, 1798.
18 Paragraph 114, Vol. 3, Pinel, 1818. This disproves Cohen's point that 'the term senile dementia was first used by Esquirol' (see Cohen, 1983).
19 Meynert, 1890.
20 Tomlinson and Corsellis, 1984.
21 Esquirol, 1805.
22 Esquirol, 1814.
23 Esquirol, 1838.
24 Bayle, 1822.
25 Bayle, 1826.
26 pp. 250–251, Vol. 8, Boisseau, 1830.
27 pp. 261–262, Vol. 8, Boisseau, 1830.
28 pp. 349–340, Vol. 1, Rostan, 1839.
29 Bayle, 1822.
30 p. 623, Bayle, 1822; Hare, 1959; for a superb account, see pp. 160–175, Quétel, 1990.
31 This view was put forward by Zilboorg, 1941.
32 Bercherie, 1980.
33 p. 25, Bercherie, 1980.
34 Baillarger, 1883.
35 Baillarger, 1883.
36 p. 389, Baillarger, 1883.
37 pp. 353–356, Vol. 2, Lagneau, 1834.
38 Put forward by Fournier, 1875.
39 Baillarger, 1889. For a detailed account the pseudo-general paralysis see, pp. 160–175, Quétel 1990.
40 For a discussion of this issue, see Berrios, 'Depressive pseudodementia' or 'Melancholic dementia': a 19th century view, 1985.
41 Georget, 1820.
42 Berrios, Stupor, 1981; Postel, 1972.
43 p. 37, Georget, 1820.
44 pp.vii–viii, Georget, 1820.
45 Calmeil, 1835.
46 p. 71, Calmeil, 1835.
47 p. 77, Calmeil, 1835.
48 pp. 82–83, Calmeil, 1835.
49 Guislain, 1852.

50 p. 10, Guislain, 1852.

51 Guislain, 1852.

52 p. 311, Guislain, 1852.

53 p. 261, Marc, 1840.

54 Morel, 1860.

55 p. 2, Morel, 1860.

56 p. 251, Morel, 1860.

57 pp. 837–38, Morel, 1860.

58 Pick, 1989.

59 Morel, 1860.

60 It has also been suggested that the view that Morel 'discovered' the disease might have started in France during the chauvinism that followed the Franco-Prussian War (p. 685, Morel, 1983).

61 For a history of psychiatric diseases and the debate on the origins of schizophrenia see Berrios and Porter, 1995.

62 Cauwenbergh, 1991.

63 p. 163, Heinroth, 1975.

64 p. 169, Heinroth, 1975.

65 Kant called a similar disorder *Unsinnigkeit*. Interestingly enough, during the nineteenth century this term was translated as *démence* by the French (p. 136, Kant, 1863). The modern English translation has been to *Amentia* (p. 74, Kant, 1974); and so has the Spanish translation (p. 118, Kant, 1935). Reil, on the other hand, defined Blödsinn as 'abnormal asthenia of the understanding' (p. 402, Reil, 1803).

66 Hoffbauer, 1827.

67 The French rendition of Hoffbauer's book was by A.M. Chambeyron who saw the need to append 'clarificatory' (more often critical) footnotes either by himself or by Esquirol and Itard. For example, regarding Hoffbauer's suggestion that there were many varieties of mental weakness, a footnote reads: 'all the distinctions established by the author between stupidity and imbecility are unintelligible to French readers. In fact, the differences expressed are just degrees of dementia.' (see p. 60, Hoffbauer, 1827).

68 Feuchtersleben, 1845. Agreeing with him, his English translators used 'folly' for *Blödsinn*. (see Feuchtersleben,1847).

69 The cognitive paradigm refers to the view that memory deficit is the central symptom of dementia; see Berrios, Memory and the cognitive paradigm of dementia during the nineteenth century, 1990.

70 p. 301, Feuchtersleben, 1847.

71 pp. 237–240, Feuchtersleben, 1847.

72 pp. 340—43, Griesinger, 1861.

73 Krafft-Ebing, 1876.

74 pp. 654–660, Krafft-Ebing, 1893.

75 p. 778, Salmon, 1694.

76 p. 19, D'Assigny, 1706.

77 p. 6, Prichard, 1835.

78 p. 93, Prichard, 1835.

79 p. 119, Bucknill and Tuke, 1858.

80 p. 11, Bucknill and Tuke, 1858.
81 p. 122, Bucknill and Tuke, 1858.
82 Berrios, Positive and negative signals, 1992.
83 p. 413, Jackson, 1932.
84 p. 412, Jackson, 1932.
85 For example, in the work of J. de Ajurriaguerra who suggested that, in dementia, there was an ordered dismantling of functional layers which could explain the sequence of syndromes observed in Alzheimer's disease, including the presence of hallucinations and delusions (see Constantinidis *et al.*, 1978). On Ajurriaguerra, see Aguirre and Guimón, 1992.
86 p. 345, Maudsley, 1895.
87 p. 347, Maudsley, 1895.
88 There is also a sad side to this affair. In the early 1890s, Mrs Maudsley is said to have developed senile dementia forcing her devoted husband to give up most of his commitments to look after her. Since her life is likely to have been a tranquil one, would Maudsley still have felt able to say that all dementias were, after all, secondary to the 'feverish disease of life'?
89 p. 267, Clouston, 1887.
90 p. 271, Clouston, 1887.
91 Todd and Ashworth, 1991.
92 p. 601, Browne, 1874.
93 p. 602, Browne, 1874.
94 p. 602, Browne, 1874.
95 Maulitz, 1987; Ackerknecht, 1967.
96 Berrios, The psychopathology of affectivity, 1985.
97 Berrios, In Copeland *et al.* (eds.), 1994.
98 Likewise, at the turn of the century there were concerns about a putative loss of intellectual power affecting the European races; it is not a coincidence that a preoccupation of the British Eugenics movement was the intellectual betterment of the race (for this, see Kevles, 1985. For wider aspects of this problem, see Morton, 1988).
99 Berrios, Memory and the cognitive paradigm, 1990.
100 p. 248, Gombault, 1900.
101 p. 206, Bessière, 1906.
102 pp. 453–454, Toulouse and Mignard, 1914.
103 p. 5, Marie, 1906.
104 p. 316, Régis, 1906.
105 pp. 451–457, Régis, 1906.
106 Laignel-Lavastine *et al.*, 1929.
107 Kraepelin, 1904.
108 pp. 223–224, Kraepelin, 1904.
109 Noetzli, 1896.
110 Kraepelin, 1906.
111 p. 593, Kraepelin, 1910–1915.
112 pp. 627–628, Kraepelin, 1910–1915.
113 p. 282, Ziehen, 1911.
114 p. 299, Ziehen, 1911.

115 Jaspers, 1910.

116 p. 184, Jaspers, 1948.

117 see Chapter 7: Mental Retardation, this book.

118 Revault d'Allonnes, 1912.

119 p. 20, Savage, 1886.

120 p. 39, *Royal College of Physicians*, 1906.

121 p. 550, Bolton, 1903.

122 p. 550, Bolton, 1903.

123 Gowers, 1902; Similar notion was that of *nécrobiose* put forward by Schultze and Virchow (p. 317, Dastre (no publication date)).

124 Critchley, 1938.

125 Mayer-Gross, 1944.

126 Berrios and Freeman, 1991.

127 Rieder, 1974; Hoenig, 1983.

128 Kraepelin, 1919.

129 Bleuler, 1911.

130 Schneider, 1959.

131 Carpenter, 1989.

132 Wender, 1963.

133 Typical descriptions of 'schizophrenia' can be found under classical categories such as mania and melancholia; these terms have, of course, little to do with their modern counterparts.

134 Ellard, 1987; Jeste *et al.* 1985; Klaf and Hamilton, 1961; Hare, 1988*a*; Hare, 1988*b*; Boyle, 1990.

135 pp. 279–281, Morel, 1853.

136 Baruk, 1967.

137 Kahlbaum, 1874.

138 For an analysis of Kahlbaum's cases, see Chapter 14, this book.

139 Diem, 1903; also Klosterkötter 1983.

140 Hecker, 1871; also Petho, 1972.

141 Berrios and Hauser, 1988.

142 Berrios, Introduction to Eugen Bleuler, 1987.

143 Berrios, Introduction to Eugen Bleuler, 1987. This is why Jung's monograph contains similar concepts (Jung, 1907).

144 Berrios, 1987.

145 Lantéri-Laura and Gros, 1984.

146 Berrios and Hauser, 1988.

147 Berrios, Historical aspects of the Psychoses, 1987.

148 Berrios, 1987.

149 Johnstone *et al.*, 1978.

150 For a Discussion of the 1950 Paris Congress, see Chapter 5, this book.

151 Berrios, On melancholic dementia, 1985.

152 Berrios, Historical Aspects of the 1987.

153 Mairet, 1883; Albert Mairet (1852–1935), Professor of Mental Illness in the University of Montpellier.

154 Cotard, 1882. For a full review, see Luque and Berrios, 1994.

155 Dumas, 1894; Georges Dumas (1866–1946); *Normalien*, disciple of Ribot, editor of a famous *Traité de Psychologie*.

156 Bulbena and Berrios, 1986.

157 e.g. Madden *et al.* 1952; Anderson *et al.*, 1959; Kiloh, 1961.

158 Bulbena and Berrios, 1986.

159 Berrios and Beer, 1994.

160 p. 597, Ball and Chambard, 1881.

161 Grmek, 1858; Grant, 1963.

162 Cicero, 1923.

163 Kastenbaum and Ross, 1975.

164 Legrand, 1911; Gruman, 1966.

165 Cicero, 1923.

166 Minois, 1987.

167 Huber and Gourin, 1987.

168 p. 106, Buffon, 1774.

169 p. 111, Buffon, 1774.

170 Darwin, 1794–1796.

171 p. 365, Darwin, 1794–1796.

172 Sinclair, 1807.

173 Rostan (1791–1866). On this great French physician, see Chereau, 1877.

174 Rostan, 1819 and 1823.

175 On Vitalism, see Wheeler, 1939.

176 Rostan, 1833.

177 p. v, Reveillé-Parise, 1853.

178 p. 13, Reveillé-Parise, 1853.

179 Levy, 1850.

180 Charcot, 1881.

181 p. 25, Charcot, 1881.

182 p. 26, Charcot, 1881.

183 p. 27, Charcot, 1881.

184 Long, 1933.

185 See Letter LX, pp. 443–456, Vol. III, Morgagni, 1769.

186 Lobstein, 1838.

187 Demange, 1886; Grmek, 1958.

188 Marie, 1906; Albrecht, 1906.

189 Schiller, 1970; Fields and Lamak, 1989.

190 Grmek, 1958.

191 Walton, 1912.

192 Weitbrecht, 1968.

193 Potain, 1873; Ball and Chambard, 1881; Spielmeyer, 1912.

194 Jackson, 1875.

195 p. 335, Jackson, 1875.

196 For an analysis of this concept see Berrios, Negative and positive signals, 1992.

197 Berrios, In Copeland *et al.* 1994.

198 Berrios, Affective disorders in old age, 1991.

199 Barrett, 1913.

200 Marie, 1906.

201 p. 358, Marie, 1906.

202 Walton, 1912.
203 p. 677, Southard, 1910.
204 Olah, 1910.
205 North and Bostock, 1925.
206 Ball and Chambard, 1881.
207 p. 581, Ball and Chambard, 1881.
208 p. 582, Ball and Chambard, 1881.
209 p. 583, Ball and Chambard, 1881.
210 Charcot, 1881.
211 p. 267, Charcot, 1881.
212 Kahlbaum, 1863.
213 Lanczik, 1988.
214 Berrios, On presbyophrenia, 1986.
215 Rouby, 1911.
216 Truelle & Bessiére, 1911.
217 Kraepelin, 1910–1915.
218 Ziehen, 1911.
219 Fischer, 1912.
220 Bostroem, 1933.
221 Burger-Prinz and Jacob, 1938.
222 Lafora, 1935.
223 Bessiére, 1948.
224 Berrios, On presbyophrenia, clinical aspects, 1985; Zervas *et al.*, 1993.
225 Torack, 1983; also Howells, 1991.
226 Berrios, On Alzheimer's disease: a conceptual history, 1990; Schwalbe,
     1909.
227 p. 615, Rauzier, 1909.
228 Rogues de Fursac, 1921.
229 pp. 364–365, Pic, 1912.
230 Wilks, 1865.
231 Marcé, 1863.
232 Parrot, 1873.
233 Berrios, On Alzheimer's disease, 1990.
234 Alzheimer, 1907.
235 DeFelipe and Jones, 1988; Barrett, 1913.
236 p. 846, Bianchi, 1906.
237 p. 450, Fuller, 1907.
238 Beljahow, 1889.
239 Simchowicz, 1924.
240 Fischer, 1907.
241 Marcé, 1863; Krafft-Ebing, 1876; Crichton-Browne, 1874; Marie, 1906.
242 Alzheimer, 1911.
243 Perusini, 1911.
244 p. 143, Perusini, 1911.
245 Kraepelin, 1910–1915.
246 Alzheimer, 1911.
247 p. 26, Fuller, 1912.

248 Hakkébousch and Geier, 1913.

249 Simchowicz, 1911.

250 Ziehen, 1911.

251 Lambert, 1916.

252 p. 378, Lugaro, 1916.

253 p. 221, Simchowicz, 1924.

254 For a detailed discussion of these issues, see Berrios, on Alzheimer's Disease, 1990.

255 Niery *et al.* 1988.

256 Pick, 1892.

257 Jean Pierre Gratiolet (1815–1865), one of the most original histopathologist of the nineteenth century; his early death deprived France of a champion of the anti-localizationistic view.

258 Gratiolet, 1854.

259 Anonymous, 1832, On the science of phrenology: Combe, 1873; Lantéri-Laura, 1970.

260 Broca, 1861; Henderson, 1986.

261 Jackson, 1894.

262 Meynert, 1885.

263 Pick, 1892.

264 Pick, 1901.

265 Pick, 1906.

266 Barrett, 1913.

267 Ziehen, 1911.

268 Mansvelt, 1954.

269 Caron, 1934.

270 Schneider, 1927; 1929.

271 Traub *et al.* 1977.

272 Creutzfeldt, 1920.

273 Creutzfeldt, 1920.

274 Jakob, 1921.

275 Jakob, 1921.

276 Richardson, 1977.

277 Gajdusek and Zigas, 1957.

278 Hadlow, 1959.

279 Gibbs *et al.* 1968.

280 Ziehen, 1911.

281 Marie, 1906.

282 Ball and Chambard, 1881.

CHAPTER 9

Memory and its disorders

The historical analysis of the memory disorders must borrow from areas as wide apart as the history of neuropsychiatry, philosophy and psychology. Indeed, the decision of whether clinical phenomena such as *déjà vu*, fugues, confabulations or 'delusions of memory' are mnestic disturbances cannot be determined by empirical research alone and requires preparatory conceptual analysis.[1] Historical research may also inform us whether models of memory analogous to current ones have already been proposed in the past,[2] and to what extent they have also been inspired on the mnestic vicissitudes of few famous patients. This chapter will only scan what remains an uncharted territory.

Pre-nineteenth century issues

From earlier times, man's ability to retain, retrieve, or lose information whether about himself or the world has been motive of wonder, fear and much speculation.[3] Since the Classical period two memory 'stages' or 'capacities' have been identified: conservation and retrieval. The analysis of conservation was governed by 'spatial' metaphors (pertaining to storage spaces and containers) and these were easily retranslated into the current 'somatic' or 'organic' accounts. Retrieval mechanisms, on the other hand, were analysed in the temporal dimension or as Aristotle put it, they are 'always accompanied by time';[4] the guiding metaphors in this case were 'searching' and 'finding' and the ensuing models alluded to functions such as cataloguing, dating, and recognizing information. Since the time of Aristotle, interest on memory has oscillated between these two perspectives. References to 'memory' can be found in early documents including the Old Testament, the Talmud, and Plato's work, but there is agreement that Aristotle set the framework in relation to which the philosophy of memory has been discussed ever since.[5]

ARISTOTLE In his great essay *On Memory and Recollection*, Aristotle separated conservation (*mneme*) from recollection (*anamnesis*): 'First we must comprehend what sort of things are objects of memory; for mistakes are frequent on this point. It is impossible to remember the future, which is object of conjecture or expectation; nor is there memory of the present, but only conception; for it is neither the future nor the past that we cognize by perception, but only the present. But memory is of the past; no one could claim to remember the present while it is present'[6] 'memory, then, is neither sensation nor judgment, but is a state or affection of one of these, when time has elapsed ... all memory, then implies a lapse of time ... hence only these living creatures which are conscious of time can be said to remember ...'[7]

Aristotle described two stages: 'Memory of the object of thought implies a mental picture. Hence, it would seem to belong incidentally to the thinking faculty, but essentially to the primary sense faculty. Hence memory (*mneme*) is found not only in man and beings which are capable of opinion and thought, but also in some other animals.'[8] Recollection, on the other hand, can only be a human activity for it requires awareness and logical thought: 'Recollecting (*anamnesis*) differs from remembering (*mneme*) not merely in the matter of time, but also because, while other animals share in memory, one may say that none of the known animals can recollect except man. This is because recollecting is, as it were, a kind of inference (*sylogismos*).'[9] Aristotle provided an account of 'recollection' by describing a charmingly introspective act involving a geometrical inference.[10]

Aristotle also touched upon another three characteristics of memory. The first, concerns the 'referential' capacity of the 'recollected' mental act: 'if there is in us something like an impression or picture, why should the perception of just this be memory of something else and not of itself? For when one exercises his memory this affection is what he considers and perceives. How, then, does he remember what is not present? This would imply that one can also see and hear what is not present. But surely in a sense this can and does occur. Just as the picture painted on the panel is at once a picture and a portrait, and though one and the same, is both, yet the essence of the two is not the same, and it is possible to think of it both as a picture and as a portrait, so in the same way we must regard the mental picture within us both as an object of contemplation in itself and as a mental picture of something else.'[11]

The second characteristic refers to the 'awareness of the act of recollection', i.e. how does man know that he is remembering and not just experiencing something for the first time. Aristotle says: 'sometimes we do not know, when such stimuli occur in our soul from an earlier sensation, and we are in doubt whether it is memory or not. But sometimes it happens that we reflect and remember that we have heard or seen this something before. Now, this occurs whenever we first think of it as itself, and then change and think of it as referring to something else.'[12] This dissociation between experience and those elements required to render it into a memory, is of some importance to understand, for example, nineteenth century explanations of *déjà vu* and confabulation for it used to be claimed that these symptoms were first-time experiences taken (mistakenly) to be memories due to the action of some 'memory-converting' factor.

It would not be altogether surprising that Aristotle's source for this view was some clinical case, indeed, he writes: 'The opposite also occurs, as happened to Antiphenon of Oreus, and other deranged people (*egistamenois*); for they spoke of their mental pictures (*fantasmata*) as if they had actually taken place, and as if they actually remembered them.'[13] It is unclear whether Aristotle referred here to hallucinations or delusions of memory, such as *déjà vu*; the drift of the text suggests that it might have been the latter.

The third characteristic relates to the mechanisms that facilitate recollection and includes an account of the laws of association.[14] For reasons of space, this point will not be developed further in this chapter.

ST. AUGUSTINE AND BERNARDO DE GORDON Augustine includes memory, together with *intellectus* and *voluntas*, as one of the faculties of the soul. *Memoria* served as a repository for information temporarily unused and for the 'archetypal' ideas that made man a carrier of the divine truth.[15] Augustine's Platonism is nowhere better illustrated than in his view that the two functions of memory are to preserve and revive the data of experience, and store a complete referential system of knowledge. Echoes of these ideas re-appeared in Descartes, Freud and Jung.

The Classical metaphors for memory are still present in the late Renaissance and early modern period. For example, in 1495, Bernardo de Gordon writing on the 'corruptions of memory' stated that they resulted from 'corruption of the posterior part of the brain . . . and forgetting sometimes occurs in madness.'[16] A century later, Father Thomas Wright, asked: '57). How we remember? 58). In what part of the braine resideth the formes fit for memory? 60). How we forget? 62). What helpeth and hindereth Memory, and by what manner? 63). Why doth memory faile in old men? and 68). How can possibly be conserved, without confusion, such an infinite number of formes in the Soule?'[17]

DESCARTES Descartes developed a model of 'recollecting' based on a mental process akin to 'facilitation': 'Thus, when the soul desires to recollect something, this desire causes the gland, by inclining successively to different sides, to thrust the spirits towards different parts of the brain until they come across that part where the traces left there by the object which we wish to recollect are found; for these traces are none other than the fact that the pores of the brain, by which the spirits have formerly followed their course because of the presence of this object, have by that means acquired a greater facility[18] than the others in being once more opened by the animal spirits which come towards them in the same way.'[19] As Arnaud noticed, the problem with Descartes' model is that in order to have a memory it is not enough that an idea be reproduced, it must also be *recognized*.

Descartes attempted to answer this objection thus: 'all vestiges left by former thoughts are not of a kind to permit of recollection by us, but only those which enable the mind to know that they have not always been in us, but were formerly freshly impressed on the mind. For the mind to be able to recognize this, I consider that the first time these impressions were made, the mind must have employed a pure conception.'[20] True memories, therefore, still depend on an active participation of the mind.

HOBBES AND LOCKE Hobbes explored memory in relation to imagination, a power of the mind in which he was particularly interested.[21] In *Human Nature* he explains that forgetting or memory decay is analogous to walking away from something and gradually losing detail: 'why may not we well think of remembrance to be nothing else but the missing of parts, which everyman expecteth should succeed after they have a conception of the whole? To see at a great distance of place, and to remember at a great distance of time, is to have like conceptions of the thing: for there wanteth distinction of parts in both; the one conception being weak by operation at distance, the other by decay.'[22] Hobbes attempted to distinguish memory from imagination: 'But you will say, by what sense shall we take notice of sense? I answer, by sense itself,[23] namely by the memory which for some time remains in us of things sensible, though they themselves pass away. For he that perceives that he hath perceived remembers.'[24] And then, perhaps more clearly, 'Fancy and memory differ only in this, that memory supposeth the time past, which fancy doth not. In memory, the phantasms we consider as if they were worn out with time; but in our fancy we consider them as they are: which distinction is not in the things themselves, but of the considerations of the sentient.'[25]

Like Descartes, John Locke had little to say on the mechanisms responsible for the deposition of memories. Returning to Aristotelian associationism, he suggested that there were in operation rudimentary mechanisms which could be described in modern terms as 'semantic processing' and 'time-tagging': 'this laying down of our ideas in the repository of memory signifies no more but this, that the mind has a power in many cases to revive perceptions which it once had, with this additional perception annexed to them, that it has had them before.'[26] Rather interestingly, Locke felt that emotions could help to fix ideas in the mind. During the eighteenth century, English physiologists such as David Hartley, gave this view a neurophysiological interpretation.[27]

Pre-nineteenth century literature on memory is large, and in addition to clinical reports and philosophical theorising it includes works on *Mnemonics* or the 'Art of memory', an approach to the practical aspects of this mental function which, as Hutton has said: 'in the not too distant past held pride of place in the councils of learning . . .'.[28] This genre has been superbly studied by the late Francis Yates and will not be mentioned further.[29]

Memory during the nineteenth century

The time before Ebbinghaus has been called by Tulving the 'dark ages' in the history of memory.[30] However, the nineteenth century was, in fact, a period rich in studies on memory,[31] particularly after the 1820s, when the impact of phrenology began to be felt. Memory was then explored in relation to faculties and powers. This approach, common both to Britain and the Continent, emphasized the *content* of memory and its laws of retention and association.

Parallel to the psychological debate, there also was during the nineteenth century *the development of views on memory based on clinical observation*. For example, alienists included under the category 'amnesia' and 'paramnesia' phenomena such as confabulation, *déjà vu*, and 'memory delusions' which were alien to the quantitative approach taken by Ebbinghaus. At the time, the clinical approach attracted less attention but 'prototypical' cases soon accumulated and their interpretation was crucial to the development of theoretical models; indeed, most of current terminology was created within this tradition.

ROYER-COLLARD, VIREY, AND LOUYER-VILLARMAY At the beginning of the nineteenth century, concept of memory differed in England, France, and Germany. French views, inspired by the Scottish philosophy of Common Sense, are well represented in the work of Athanasius Royer-Collard,[32] brother of the great French alienist.[33] According to this thinker: 'the objects of consciousness are the only objects of memory. Properly speaking, we never remember anything but the operations and diverse states of our minds.'[34] This 'active' model of the mind, further developed by Victor Cousin, was to become a central piece in Ribot's theory.

Virey also offered a definition of memory: 'the faculty that conserves in the spirit the impressions and images of objects obtained via sensations, and that recollects these impressions in the absence of the object.'[35] Sexual abuse and drunkenness, Virey identified as the commonest cause of amnesia.

Louyer-Villarmay was able to distinguish between dysmnesia and amnesia and subdivided each into idiopathic and symptomatic (the latter being secondary to a recognizable disease).[36] He also described the law of regression (later attributed to Ribot),[37] and forgetting of recent events and intact remote memory in the elderly.[38] Via Bouillaud, these views were to continue in French psychiatry until the end of the century.[39]

FEARNS, MILLS AND BAIN English views remained firmly associationistic. Early in the century, John Fearns wrote: 'if we remember a thing brought in by association, this affection is, notoriously, forced upon us; but, if we try to recollect a thing, we will to put ourselves in this and that mood, or posture of thought, until at length the thing strike us by the medium of association.'[40] Fearn believed (as Descartes had done earlier on) that an act of specific attention was needed for the memories to be properly laid down.[41] James Mills, in turn, wrote: 'In memory there are ideas, and those ideas both rise up singly, and are connected in trains by association.'[42]

Alexander Bain followed these views in his *The Senses and the Intellect*[43] but later on he wrote: 'Retention, Acquisition, or Memory, then, being the power of continuing in the mind impressions that are no longer stimulated by the original agent, and of recalling them at after-times by purely mental forces';[44] he explained the mechanism of retention as: 'for every act of memory, every exercise of bodily aptitude, every habit, recollection, train of ideas, there is a special grouping, or coordination, of sensations and movements, by virtue of specific growths in the cell junctions.'[45]

NOAH PORTER This great American psychologist took a more eclectic approach and defined memory as that function by means of which: 'the essential elements of an act of previous cognition are more or less perfectly re-known, both objective and subjective, with the relations essential to each. These elements are not all recalled with the same distinctness, and hence there are varieties of memory.'[46] He criticized associationism for not explaining the process of recognition (just as Arnauld had criticized Descartes): 'The psychologists of the associational school provide for only half of the process – that of representation. Recognition they attempt to explain, but unsuccessfully, by the chemistry of association, i.e. by the union or blending of a present with a past mental state. Representation and memory may, however, with propriety and advantage, be ideally considered apart.'[47] Another important aspect of Porter's work is that he realised the theoretical importance of studying memory deficits, and included many such clinical references in his analysis.

HOLLAND In opposition to Bain, Henry Holland was a clinician who speculated on his observations. He realized early that *a priori* conceptualization was crucial to the understanding of memory disorders. For example, when commenting on the changes in the classification of memory suggested by Dr Brown,[48] he wrote: 'the whole discussion is another proof of the dominion which methods and phrases exercise over these abstruse subjects.'[49] Like Porter, Holland was also keen to emphasize that the efficiency of memory depended on the integrity of the brain: 'We merely express what alone we know as probable, that material structure, the excitement and instrument of the mental functions . . . is more closely connected with the operations of memory, than with those of any other faculty.'[50] After the middle of the century, this mechanistic model was re-interpreted in terms of an evolutionary framework, first by Herbert Spencer, and then by Hering, Hughlings Jackson, and William James.

FEUCHTERSLEBEN In Austria, and like Hobbes 200 years earlier, Feuchtersleben also discussed memory in relation to imagination. He accepted the laws of association but pondered over memory as a 'mental power'.[51] He also believed that memory capacity was directly proportional to brain size, to the 'consistency' of its medullary substance, and to its vitality. Memory naturally decreased in old age.[52] In regard to memory traces, he took an anti-Locke approach: 'It is at once self-evident that the notion of a *tabula rasa*, which is by degrees written over, is not tenable',[53] and suggested a dynamic mechanism: 'there probably remains to us only the conception of vital tension in the cerebral substance, such as occurs in the nerves on the occasion of every external impression.' There were three types of disorder of memory: heightened (hypermnesia), weakened (dysmnesia) and perverted memory (such as 'phantasms of memory', Feuchtersleben's name for *déjà vu*).[54]

GRIESINGER Griesinger also was critical of association theory – not so much as a theory in itself for, after all, he was a disciple of Herbart – but in its application to clinical problems. His definition of memory was straightforward: 'in so far as through the so-called association of ideas no new representations (*Vorstellungen*) are originated, but only some are awakened and reproduced out of the store of earlier presentations, this process is called the memory. The more intimate proceedings of this process of reproduction are obscure, and quite incomprehensible.'[55]

He believed that 'in many mental diseases, particularly in dementia (*Blödsinnigen*), the impossibility of judging correctly, and of drawing conclusions, is due to a deficit in memory.'[56] But this led to the crucial observation (later developed by Bonhoeffer)[57] that the brain has the tendency to respond to insult in a generalized manner:[58] 'Even slight changes in the cerebral state, as for example, the effect of alcohol, can retard the reproduction of ideas' 'The examples of partial loss of memory (*ganz partiallem Gedächtnissverlust*), so frequently the result of wounds or diseases of the brain, in which the loss of the apparatus devoted to a particular class of ideas might be inferred, appear in reality to be more general in their effects than might be first supposed. Here there appears to exist a general diminution of the reproductive power whereby those which are least connected with the individuality (*Individualität*) are the ideas most liable to be forgotten (Gratiolet).'[59] Griesinger seems to be saying here that autobiographical memories are more enduring than the others.[60]

HERING During the 1870s, a wider and more abstract view came into play. It developed out of Ewald Hering's lecture on *Memory as a universal function of organized matter* delivered before the Imperial Academy of Science at Vienna.[61] Therein, Hering made two crucial points. One was that: 'memory is a function of brain substance whose results, it is true, fall as regards one part of them into the domain of consciousness, while another part escapes unperceived as purely material processes.'; the other that: 'we have ample evidence of the fact that characteristics of an organism may descend to offspring which the organism did not inherit, but which it acquired owing to the special circumstances under which it lived' 'organized beings, therefore, stand before us as products of the unconscious memory of organized matter.' These materialist claims concealed two important points: that brain sites were important to memory, and that a Lamarckian mechanism was in operation. The timing of Hering's proposal was also right as both evolution[62] and degeneration theory[63] were in need of a machinery to explain the transmission of genetic information. Hering's views influenced Ribot[64] and culminated in the work of Semon[65] and others interested in the notion of engram.[66]

Hering's view was not lost to contemporary alienists. If memory was a property of matter, then its study should be advanced by exploring subjects with memory deficits. But such study required measurement instruments and at the time it was not clear whether tests for 'normals' could be applied to patients.[67] However, Hering's view that there was a 'continuity' between the normal and the pathological,[68] legitimized that endeavour.

The testing of abnormal subjects, however, uncovered phenomena which did not seem to fit into the old one-storage model of memory. For example, paramnesias such as false recognition, *déjà vu*, confabulation, delusions of memory, and the specific amnesic syndromes (see below) were not explainable within the traditional one storage retrieval model, and this caused some theoretical consternation.

Dementia, however, seems to provide a good instance of 'memory failure' in the traditional sense of the term. Thus, Ribot used it to illustrate the law of dissolution: 'to discover this law it is essential that the progress of dementia should be studied from a psychological viewpoint.'[69] To do so, he saw dementia as a 'syndrome': 'physicians distinguish between different kinds of dementia according to causes, classing them as senile, paralytic, epileptic, etc. *These distinctions have no interest to us*. The progress of mental dissolution is, at bottom, the same' (my italics).[70] In England, Shaw stated: 'sometimes, the existence of dementia is only shown by loss of memory or loss of energy and there are no positive signs of acute disturbance.'[71]

Kimball Young has suggested that in psychology the need to quantify first became apparent in psychophysics, assessment of difference limens, and mental and physiological measurement.[72] To these should be added the measurement of insanity.[73] All these, however, depended upon the legitimacy of quantifying psychological phenomena in general.[74] The work of Weber and Fechner (perception), of Hering (audition), and Donders (reaction time)[75] had suggested that psychological phenomena were ready for mathematical treatment.

In 1885, Ebbinghaus wrote: 'in the realm of mental phenomena, experiment and measurement have hitherto been chiefly limited in application to sense perception and to the time relations of mental processes' 'we have tried to go a step further into the workings of the mind and to submit to an experimental and quantitative treatment the manifestations of memory.'[76] At the turn of the century, this view was to encourage the development of the psychometry of dementia.[77] Ebbingaus's views,[78] however, led him to criticize Dilthey's notion of understanding[79] and its role in psychological inquiry.

Matters clinical

At the beginning of the nineteenth century, the term *amnesia* was already current in medical language[80] as was the distinction between memory for remote events and current retention. The terms 'anterograde' and 'retrograde' however only came into currency during the second half of the century.[81] By the 1890s, disorders of memory were an important topic of research as shown by Ribot's work.

From the vantage point of the present, this oft-quoted book makes quaint reading. After dwelling on Hering's view of memory as a 'biological fact', Ribot defined 'diseases of memory as morbid psychical states' [which might be] 'limited to a single category of recollections' [i.e. partial] or affect 'the entire memory in all its forms' [i.e. general].[82] Whether general or partial, amnesia was temporary, periodical, progressive and congenital. Epilepsy caused a typical form of temporary amnesia. The phenomenon of 'double consciousness', as described by Azam,[83] was an example of periodic amnesia. Senile dementia and cerebral haemorrhage cause progressive forms of amnesia. Congenital amnesias were seen in idiots and cretins.

Whilst Ribot was a philosopher–psychologist with limited clinical experience,[84] Falret, was a great clinician and his 1865 work on *Amnesia*[85] shows this. 'Amnesia' was then a *descriptive* concept and carried almost no assumptions in regard to reversibility or aetiology. Falret did not distinguish between physical and psychological causes of amnesia or between general and partial forms. His work is rich in clinical material and provides the modern neuropsychiatrist with instances of 'new' syndromes such as transient global amnesia, acute intoxication with anticholinergics, and state-dependent learning.

The paramnesias

'Delusions of memory' are rarely reported in current clinical practice and have elicited little historical interest.[86] It was otherwise between 1880 and the First World War when they were frequently written about. The symptom was defined as the reporting of 'memories' of (mainly) autobiographical events[87] which had not taken place. The symptom was considered as a *disorder of memory*, and classified as a *paramnesia* or *dysmnesia*. During the early years of the present century, however, changes in the concept of memory (and in that of delusion) led to the view that the symptom was not related to memory but was a *delusion*.

When the young Kraepelin[88] published his articles on false reminiscences[89] the symptom was well known.[90] Indeed, it had already been suggested[91] that it might be behind *metempsychosis*, i.e. the belief in the transmigration of the soul and in reincarnation.[92] Terms such as 'phantasms of memory', 'pseudo-reminiscences', 'paramnesias', 'fallacies of memory', and eventually *déjà vu*, were coined for it.

Paramnesias were said to occur both in confusion and clear consciousness; in psychosis and in normal people; in dreaming and in wakefulness. They might be fleeting or persistent; and memorable and vivid or only recollected with the help of hypnosis. Finally, and this stretched the credulity of some, the experience (object of the false memory) might even have taken place *before* the subject's birth. This latter belief goes a long way to explain the interest that many psychic researchers had in the paramnesias.

Sully classified these recollections into: (*a*) false (i.e. the recollected event had not occurred), (*b*) distortions of real event, and (*c*) time errors in the placing of a real event. It is not difficult to see that this classification was modelled on the old tripartite division of perceptual disturbances into hallucinations, illusions and sensory distortions. Although Kraepelin followed Sander's views[93] closely, he suggested a new name – pseudoreminiscences – for the same phenomena. His work concentrated on the study of Sully's first group, i.e. false recollections (or true hallucinations of memory), which he divided into 'simple', 'evoked' or 'provoked', and 'identified' pseudo-reminiscences. The first group included spontaneous images which, as they appear for the first time in the subject's mind, are accompanied by a 'feeling' of recollection; the second referred to real perceptions which evoke in the individual the feeling of having been experienced before; and the third, to new experiences which evoke the experience of being exact copies of earlier ones. Types two and three are often difficult to differentiate. Kraepelin's classification was important for it attempted to match the 'simple' type of false recollections with delusions, the 'evoked' type with illusions and hallucinations, and the 'identifying' type with *déjà vu*. Kraepelin reported 18 cases, some of which he had borrowed from von Gudden and Forel.

THE *REVUE PHILOSOPHIQUE*[94] DEBATE A series of papers on paramnesia appeared in the 1890s. André Lalande (a philosopher) started with a conceptual (rather than clinical) analysis based on the views of Sully, Ribot, Kraepelin, and Burnham. He noticed that: (*a*) the feeling of false recognition was 'instantaneous' and 'complete' (i.e. the subject did not say that the situation was similar but that it was exactly the same), (*b*) the experience was accompanied by a feeling of anxiety or apprehension, and (*c*) the subject felt that he could predict what was to follow. The phenomenon was not necessarily 'pathological' for (regardless of education) it was experienced by about 30% of the population.[95] Lalande also commented upon available explanations, ruling out 'reincarnation' and opting for a version of the 'double representation' view.

Dugas followed with a criticism of Lalande's views, although 'he had no theory to oppose it with';[96] he also felt that the concept of false memory had to be distinguished from the 'impression of *déjà vu*'. Dugas agreed that the experience was not necessarily pathological as those who experienced it often were balanced and intelligent people. The tendency might, however, be 'hereditary' and the experience was more common amongst young people (between ages 20 and 30). Dugas differentiated false memories on the basis of whether they were or not accompanied by a feeling of premonition (*pressentiment*). The latter, he called simple or incomplete and explained as resulting from a 'double perception' separated by a short period of absence. To explain the intensity of the first perception he resorted to Leibniz's concept of 'apperception'.[97] Dugas rejected Lalande's view that telepathy might be involved when *déjà vu* was accompanied by special foreboding, and suggested that this was just a case of 'double personality'.[98]

The next to participate in the debate on *paramnésie* was Jacques Le Lorrain who felt that Lalande's diagnostic criteria required tightening, and reported that as soon as this was done the phenomena became rare.[99] Paul Lapie put forward a 'coincidence' theory according to which the imagination of man creates situations that become deposited as 'memories', and on occasions, they might coincide with real life perceptions.[100] Two more writers intervened in the debate: van Biervliet[101] supported the double representation view, and the Italian Vignoli[102] put forward a three fold explanation for *déjà vu* which included dream work, the speed of psychological processes, and disordered imagination.

The history of déjà vu

Of all paramnestic phenomena, *déjà vu* seems to have attracted the most clinical and literary interest.[103] Together with 'confabulations' it has survived to this day although not, perhaps, as a 'real' disorder of memory. Although pre-nineteenth century descriptions suggestive of *déjà vu* can be found,[104] the phenomenon only became classified as a memory problem after the 1840s. Sir Walter Scott called it 'sentiment of pre-existence', and Wigan defined it as: 'a sudden feeling, as if the scene we have just witnessed (although, from the very nature of things it could never have been seen before) had been present to our eyes on a former occasion, when the very same speakers, seated in the very same positions, uttered the same sentiments, in the same words – the postures, the expression of countenance, the gestures, the tone of voice, all seem to be *remembered*, and to be now attracting attention for the *second* time, *never* it is supposed to be the *third* time.'[105]

A year later, and independently from Wigan, the Austrian Feuchtersleben described the phenomenon of 'phantasms of memory': 'for instance, when a person feels as if a situation in which he actually finds himself had already existed at some former time.'[106]

Hughlings Jackson also wrote on the 'sensation of reminiscence', one of the earliest references being a short note in 1876 suggesting that such feelings, seen in epileptic patients with 'intellectual aura', are 'not uncommon in healthy people.'[107] At this stage, Jackson seems to have 'believed to be a perfectly accurate account' the view that the condition was one of 'double consciousness' (à la Wigan). In 1888, Jackson returned to 'sensations of reminiscence' and referred to a medical colleague who reported his own temporal lobe epilepsy under the pseudonym of *Quaerens*.[108] To illustrate his feeling of reminiscence, *Quaerens* quoted from *David Copperfield*: 'We have all some experience of a feeling which comes over us occasionally of what we are saying and doing having been said or done before, in a remote time – of our having been surrounded, dim ages ago, by the same faces, objects, and circumstances – of our knowing perfectly what will be said next, as if we suddenly remember it.' In 1899, Jackson repeated his view that 'double consciousness' or 'mental diplopia' was an accompaniment of 'dreamy states.'[109]

ARNAUD AND THE *SMP* DEBATE The earliest usage of *déjà vu* is unclear. In 1894, Dugas used the expression *impression de déjà vu*, indicating that the term *déjà vu* had already been used by Paul Verlaine (1844–1896) in his poem *Kaléidoscope*,[110] and by *Loti* (Julien Viaud, 1850–1923).[111]

A more technical usage was started on 24th of February 1896 when, at a meeting of the *Société Médico-Psychologique*, Arnaud proposed: 'I believe that it would be better to abandon the words false memory and paramnesia that have the double inconvenience of being vague and inexact as the phenomenon in question may not be associated with memory at all. So, to keep things clear and make no theoretical implications, I would suggest *illusion of déjà vu*.'[112] Arnaud chronicled the history of the concept in the work of Wigan, Maudsley, Sully, Jensen, Sander, Pick, Anjel, Forel, Kraepelin, Ribot, Lalande, Dugas and Sollier, and attacked the prevalent view that the phenomenon was 'common in the normal': 'It is likely that the frequency of the illusion of *déjà vu* has been exaggerated for it has been confused with analogous states such as obscure memories, vague and remote recollections, etc. The true *déjà vu* has two features: the intensity of the illusion borders in conviction, and there is the feeling of *identity* between the subjective experience and that assumed to be recollected.'[113] Arnaud distinguished mild and severe forms of the disorder, the latter being delusional and hence *pathological*.

He then reported the case of Louis, a 34 year-old Saint Cyr trained officer, with family history of psychiatric illness (mother was said to be 'nervous') who had experienced *déjà vu* since infancy. After catching malaria in Tonkin, he returned to France in 1891 when he was found to be suffering both from anterograde and retrograde amnesia. By January 1893, his *déjà vu* experiences were frequent, for example, he 'recognised' newspaper articles which 'he (believed) to have written himself.' At the marriage of his brother, he had the feeling that he had attended the same ceremony a year before. After failing to get married (through opposition of the bride's parents), he became aggressive, and developed ideas of persecution and fears that his headaches were being caused by drugs. When receiving hydrotherapy, he felt that he had visited the same establishment the year before. In July 1894, he was admitted to the Hospital at Vanves, whereupon he claimed that he had already been there before, recognizing places, staff, their words and gestures. On meeting Dr Arnaud he said: 'You know me doctor! You also welcomed me last year, at the same time, and in this same room. You asked the same questions, and I gave you the same answers.'[114] He said the same after meeting the great Jules Falret.[115] The symptoms continued, but at no time did he have hallucinations. His *déjà vu* became constant and intense, involving both personal experiences and objective events; he claimed, for example, that his current existence was a repetition of last year's, and that he could 'recognize' all public events between 1894 and 1895 (such as the election of Félix Faure, and the death of Pasteur). His memory remained 'weak', and with both retrograde and anterograde deficits.

Arnaud believed that *déjà vu* was a *current* experience projected on the past and disagreed with earlier theories such as the double brain, metempsychosis, telepathy, delayed perception, parallel hallucination, and successive perceptions of the same event separated by a moment of distraction. In the debate that followed, Pierre Janet claimed that *déjà vu* was a *perceptual* rather than a *memory* disorder, but Paul Garnier stated the contrary.

LEROY'S STUDY The final stage in the history of *déjà vu* during the late nineteenth century is the survey by Eugène Bernard Leroy.[116] This researcher believed that, because the phenomenon was subjective, marked inter-individual differences were bound to exist, and hence single case reports (à la Arnaud) were an inadequate method of study. He undertook a survey based on a 36 questions instrument circularized with the help of the *Revue de Hypnotisme* and the *Proceedings of the Medico-Legal Society of New York*. Although there were 67 replies, the report was based on only 49. To these another 38 cases from the literature were added. This method of data collecting was fashionable at the time.[117]

The instrument included complex questions, such as: 'Have you ever experienced the feeling of so-called 'false recognition' alluded by Dickens in the following passage . . .'? or question 15: 'If you have experienced this, were you under the influence of alcohol, opium, morphine, ether, chloroform (please specify the dose)?' or question 35: 'Do you suffer from attacks, obsessions, phobias, panics, absences, convulsive tics or other neurological disorders?' No wonder, therefore, that respondents were mainly recruited from the educated classes (e.g. college students, philosophers, priests, medical doctors, psychologists and writers) and included great men such as Paul Adam, Emile Zola, Paul Borget, Fernand Gregh, Jules Lemaitre, and E. Boirac. Bernard Leroy concluded that the phenomena were heterogeneous and that no one hypothesis could account for all its instances.

THE AFTERMATH Since this time (and until the recent work by Sno *et al.*), little that is new has been said on the mysterious nature of *déjà vu*. In 1931, Berndt-Larsson suggested, once again, that a normal and a pathological form of *déjà vu* should be distinguished. The former type, which was transient and caused little emotional upheaval, resulted from a disturbance of perception akin to illusion; the latter, persistent and leading to perplexity and cognitive disorganisation, was a veritable delusional disorder.[118] In this regard, *déjà vu* was considered as related to misidentification syndromes such as intermetamorphosis[119] or Frégoli[120] in that both seemed to entail delusional misrecognitions: the former of a situation, the latter of people. Likewise, the *jamais vu* phenomenon may be matched to Capgras'[121] in that both seem to result from a pathological change in the feeling of 'familiarity'.[122]

FUGUES AND OTHER TRANSIENT 'AMNESIAS' The wide definition of amnesia entertained during the first half of the nineteenth century included all manner of total, partial, permanent, and transitory states all of which were considered as 'organic' in a vague kind of way. After the 1860s, however, this was gradually called into question as 'functional' explanations, principally related to experimenting with suggestion and hypnosis, began to accumulate. One consequence was the view that 'fugue' and transient memory loss might not, after all, reflect a brain lesion; another, that it might be related to inhibition, fatigue, and asthenia. By the end of the century, and after the development of psychodynamic ideas, new mechanisms were added such as repression, dissociation, multiple personality, and impulsive and wandering behaviour.[123] After 1910, the growth of psychoanalysis ensured the survival of these views, and to this day fugues (including forms of amnesia that involve loss of autobiographical memory),[124] are referred to as 'hysterical'. By the 1940s, however, the view once again developed that transient amnesias, particularly those in old age, might be organic. By the early 1960s, American writers decided to call these states 'transient global amnesias' (TGA), and a two-tier approach became established according to which fugues were functional, and TGA was organic. However, evidence for such a distinction has never been overwhelming; indeed, it has recently been asked whether it is warranted by the facts, i.e. to what extent TGA is always 'organic'.[125]

Descriptions of behaviours similar to 'fugues' can be found at least since 1851, when Aubanel reported the case of a patient with neurosyphilis who used to escape in a bewildered state. In 1861, Winslow described cases in whom 'sudden, transient, and paroxysmal attacks of forgetfulness, particularly if associated with an inability to articulate clearly' . . . ought to be regarded as harbingers of 'fatal attacks of paralysis, softening, apoplexy and insanity'.[126] The term 'fugue' seems to have been first used by Lasègue in 1868 to refer to the symptoms of an alcoholic subject during a dreamy, hallucinatory state.[127] The first important monograph on the topic is that by Achilles Foville who described a series of 13 subjects, mainly suffering from 'lypemania'[128] with a tendency to wandering away from home.[129] Foville concluded that psychotic subjects (depressives with paranoid and megalomaniac features) were inclined to wandering behaviour. In 1881, Luys reported a 39 year-old man suffering from what nowadays would be called a transient global amnesia,[130] and in 1884 Motet another who showed similar behaviour after a fall.[131] These, and other cases reported before 1888, concerned patients who, in the wake of an organic disorder, and whilst confused, wandered off for short periods of time.

On 31st November 1888, Charcot presented in his Tuesday Lectures the case of a 37 year-old epileptic who also presented wandering behaviour. He classified this 'somnambulism' into primary, post-hypnotic, and hysterical,[132] thereby suggesting that not all 'automatisms' were epileptic (comitial). Voisin availed himself of this new concept, and a year later reported a case of hysterical automatism.[133] From this period on, a series of cases were reported whose diagnostic background was hysteria, multiple personality, other forms of neuroses, and psychoses.[134] Benon and Froissart, in their review of 1909 defined fugue as: 'a disorder of action, which tends to be of sudden onset and is temporary and unplanned, and takes the form of wanderings and escapes.'[135]

Behr *et al.* have suggested that the history of the concept of fugue ought to be separated into three stages: psychiatric (from the earliest descriptions to the 1910s), psychopathological (up to the Second World War) viewing fugues as disorders of psychomotility, and clinico-psychological (up to present period) which see fugues as a disorder with multifactorial aetiology.[136]

The central feature of the fugue state was a transient loss of autobiographical information, including personal identity; this was highlighted by Abeles and Schilder in a paper on 'motivated' amnesia.[137] These authors reported 28 cases exhibiting personal disorientation but who had intact ability to retain information; all had spontaneous recovery and 'behind the superficial conflicts which precipitated the amnesia deeper motives were found.'[138] In 1937, Gillespie published his review on memory disorders in which he included 'psychogenic amnesia': a 'failure to recall . . . inhibition of recall may result from the activity of the ego itself.'[139] Two years later, Stengel started his series on the fugue state (compulsive wandering or *porimania*).[140] In his second paper, he reported 25 cases out of which 10 were related to epilepsy, one was schizophrenic, and the 'remaining were manic-depressives, hysterics and psychopaths.'[141] He found that most patients had a disturbed childhood, and a tendency to periodic changes in mood, compulsive lying, and twilight states. Parfitt and Gall studied a sample of 30 patients and concluded that organic and hysterical factors were important, that 'personal' recall was more often affected than impersonal recall, that these patients 'do not forget but refuse to remember', and that the difference between hysterical amnesia and malingering was only one of degree.[142]

In his 1947 paper on fugue and escape from oneself, Lagache emphasized the meaning of wandering behaviour in children.[143] In 1956, a re-evaluation of the fugue state was published based on 37 new cases; a comparison with Stengel's cases showed that alcoholism, hysterical mechanisms and brain injury were the more prominent factors and that a disturbed childhood might not, after all, be important.[144] The same year, a French review explored the definitional vagaries of the concept pointing out that whilst narrow definitions might miss out some forms of wandering behaviour, wide ones lost discrimination. The author opted for a 'pathological' view which separated fugues (as impulsive wandering followed by transitory amnesia) from behaviours found in travellers, vagabonds and tramps[145] whose mental state ranged from normality to psychosis, and in whom amnesia and secondary gain were conspicuous by their absence.[146] Little new has since been said on this topic.[147]

The current terms transient global amnesia[148] and *les ictus amnésique*[149] describe a clinical phenomenon which has been known, under different names, at least since the middle of the nineteenth century. Originally conflated with fugues and partial amnesias, the syndrome now includes cases which are not positively diagnosed as fugues and other so-called psychogenic losses of memory, which occur, in general, in a younger age bracket.[150]

Summary

This chapter has explored views on memory in both pre- and post-nineteenth century writers, and showed that its 'psychologization' was assisted by the combined contribution of associationism and Faculty Psychology. Then it showed how two parallel strands of thinking on memory developed during the nineteenth century – psychological and clinical – and each generated its own models and problems. It has suggested that, to a certain extent, these two strands have survived to the present day. The history of some memory disorders relevant to psychiatry, such as the delusions of memory and *déjà vu*, have also been explored in some detail.

NOTES

1   Edgell, 1924.
2   Burnham, 1888-89; see also Levin *et al.*, 1983.
3   For a superb discussion of memory before the fifth century BC see Simondon, 1982.
4   442b, 5, Aristotle, VIII, *Parva Naturalia*, 1986.
5   Sorabji, 1972.
6   449b, 10, Aristotle, 1986.
7   449b, 25, Aristotle, 1986.
8   450a, 10–15, Aristotle, 1986.
9   453a 5–10, Aristotle, 1986.
10 452b 5–30, Aristotle, 1986.
11 450b 10–25, Aristotle, 1986.
12 451a 5, Aristotle, 1986.
13 451a 10, Aristotle, 1986.
14 For a good discussion of this, see pp. 38–46, Sorabji, 1972.
15 x.xvii, Augustine: *Confessions and Enchiridion*, 1955.
16 Chapter xiii, p. jiij, Gordon, 1495.
17 p. 304, Wright, 1604.
18 *Ont acquis par cela une plus grande facilité que les autres*, p. 206, Descartes, 1919.
19 Article XLII, *The Passions of the Soul*, Descartes, 1967.
20 Letter to Arnauld, quoted in p. 152, Janet and Séailles, 1902.
21 This may be the reason why both Young, 1961 and Herrmann and Chaffin, 1988 miss Hobbes out altogether.
22 Hobbes, 1839–1845.
23 In regard to Hobbes's use of 'sense', Edgell explains: 'We thus have an epistemology which is subjective in that it regards the qualities predicated of both the inner and the outer world as depending on a sentient subject.

The knowledge yielded both by memory and by sense is knowledge of appearance as contrasted with reality. Sense and memory are on the same footing; their difference in value for knowledge is one of degree rather than kind' p. 54, Edgell, 1924.

24 p. 389, Hobbes, 1839–1845. Peters noticed a weakness in this view: 'Presumably, [Hobbes] meant that when we remember as opposed to perceive or imagine something, we have a fading image together with the conviction that we have had this picture before. But how then could a case of memory be distinguished from a case of perceiving for a second time?' p. 106, Peters, 1967.

25 Chapter 25, para 9, *De Corpore*, Hobbes, 1839–1845.

26 Book II, Chapter X, para 2, Locke, 1959.

27 For an account of physiological views on memory during the eighteenth century, see pp. 4–6, Gomulicki, 1953.

28 p. 371, Hutton, 1987.

29 Yates, 1966.

30 Toulving, 1983.

31 Murray, 1976.

32 A. Royer-Collard (1763–1845) was a follower of Maine de Biran, and of the Scottish Philosophy of Common Sense, and hence much opposed to the 'sensationalism' of Condillac.

33 On the interaction between the Royer-Collard brothers, see Swain, 1978.

34 p. 158, quoted in Janet and Séailles, 1902.

35 p. 278, Virey, 1819.

36 p. 303, Louyer-Villermay, 1819.

37 p. 321, Louyer-Villermay, 1819.

38 p. 307, Louyer-Villermay, 1819.

39 Bouillaud, 1829.

40 p. 277, Fearn, 1812.

41 p. 274, Fearn, 1812.

42 p. 328, Mill, 1829.

43 pp. 551-557, Bain, 1864.

44 p. 89, Bain, 1874.

45 p. 91, Bain, 1874.

46 p. 300, Porter, 1868.

47 Porter was here expressing his bias in favour of a functionalist and active view of the mind; both his interest on the 'philosophy of movement' and his criticism of associationism he learned from Trandelenburg in Germany (1802–1872): 'The fundamental defect, the *protos pseudos*, of the associational school, consists in this, that it does not distinguish between those activities of the soul by which, so to speak, objects are prepared for and presented to the soul for its varied activities, preeminently that of knowledge, and the activity which the soul performs with respect to them when so prepared and presented.' p. 57, Porter, 1868.

48 Holland was referring here to a book he knew well: Brown, 1828. In Lecture XLI, Brown proposed that 'certain supposed faculties', such as memory and conception, should be 'reduced' to 'simple suggestion', pp. 260–267, Brown, 1828.

49 p. 149, Holland, 1852.

50 p. 153, Holland, 1852.

51 p. 120, 'It would be well if, instead of speaking of the "powers of the mind" (which causes misunderstanding) we adhered to the designation of the several "operations of the mind" which most psychologists recommend' in Feuchtersleben, 1847.

52 p. 121, Feuchtersleben, 1847.

53 p. 121, Feuchtersleben, 1847.

54 p. 238, Feuchtersleben, 1847.

55 p. 31, Griesinger, 1861.

56 p. 31, Griesinger, 1861.

57 For further information on Bonhoeffer and his ideas see Chapter 10, this book.

58 Griesinger was here drawing a conclusion less from clinical observation than from his doubtful attitude towards brain localization: 'our knowledge of symptoms is not advanced enough to enable us to state with certainty whether, in a given case of insanity, anatomical changes exist and where they are', in p. 445, Griesinger, 1861.

59 pp. 31–32, Griesinger, 1861.

60 The meaning of the term 'individuality' is not clear here; Griesinger did not reference Gratiolet's name (1815–1865), but might have been referring to the anti-localizationist views of the French savant as expressed, for example, in his communication to the *Bulletin de La Société de Anthropologie*, 1861.

61 The lecture had European resonance: Hering, 1870 (available in English: Hering, 1913).

62 Mayr, 1982.

63 Saury, 1886.

64 Gasser, 1988.

65 Schachter *et al.*, 1978; and the superb Schatzmann, 1968.

66 Gomulicki, 1953.

67 Bondy, 1974.

68 On these two famous concepts in nineteenth century thinking, see Canguilhem, 1966.

69 p. 117, Ribot, 1882.

70 p. 117, Ribot, 1882.

71 p. 348, Shaw, 1892.

72 Young, 1923.

73 Walitzky, 1889.

74 On this issue, see Zupan, 1976.

75 Boring, 1942; 1950; 1961; Cattell, 1890.

76 p. xiii, Ebbinghaus, 1964.

77 See, for example, Jaspers, 1910.

78 Caparrós, 1986; Sahakow, 1930; Postman, 1968.

79 Dilthey, 1976.

80 The changes in the meaning of amnesia can be traced in successive dictionary entries: e.g. Louyer-Villermay, 1819; Andral, 1829; Fabre, 1840; Bernutz, 1865; Falret, 1865; also Rouillard, 1888.

81 p. 640, Régis, 1906; p. 827, Claude, 1922; p. 52, Galtier-Boissière, 1929;
    the word *rétroactive* is already found in 1865 to refer to loss of information
    acquired before the brain insult, (p. 739, Falret, 1865). The earliest usage
    of the word 'anterograde' I have found is p. 457, Arnaud, 1896.
82 p. 70, Ribot, 1882; Ribot pre-published a draft in his own journal: Ribot,
    1880.
83 On Eugène Azam and the case Félida, see Bourgeois and Geraud, 1990;
    the best account is by the author himself: Azam, 1876.
84 See Bertolini, 1991.
85 Falret, 1865.
86 For example, Buchanan, 1991.
87 For a useful study linking historical and current views on autobiographical
    memory see Ross, 1991. For a technical approach, see Conway *et al.*,
    1992.
88 Kraepelin was barely 30 at the time, and in the process of moving from
    Dresden to Dorpat, to take up his first chair.
89 Kraepelin, 1886–1887.
90 See Sully, 1894.
91 Amongst those suggesting the reincarnation idea were Bastian and
    Emminghaus, and probably St Augustine (Burnham, 1888).
92 Bonin, 1976.
93 Sander, 1874. In this paper, Sander – then working at Berlin – reviewed a
    number of phenomena including that of 'the doubles' (on the letter, see
    Dening and Berrios, 1994).
94 On the journal itself, its ideology, and the more specific issue of debates on
    memory, see the great work by Bertolini, 1991.
95 pp. 490–491, Lalande, 1893.
96 Dugas, 1894.
97 The concept of 'apperception' was a popular one at the time Dugas wrote
    his paper. It was defined as that part of attention that involved interaction
    between the presentation of the object attended to, the total preceding
    conscious content, and the preformed mental dispositions. The notion was
    originally introduced by Leibniz, taken up by Kant, and developed by
    Herbart. For details, see Lange, 1900.
98 The notion of *dédoublement de la personnalité* was also a popular one in late
    nineteenth century France. Then, as now, it helped to explain clinical
    phenomena in which the observer identified contradictory forms of
    behaviour.
99 Le Lorrain, 1894.
100 Lapie, 1894.
101 Biervliet, 1894.
102 Soury, 1894.
103 Sno and Lindszen, 1990; Sno *et al.*, 1992; Sno and Draaisma, 1993.
104 For example, references included in Hunter and McAlpine, 1963.
105 p. 84, Wigan, 1844.
106 p. 237, Feuchtersleben, 1847.
107 p. 274, Jackson, 1932.

108 pp. 388–389, Jackson, 1932. In regard to the identity of this patient, who probably was Myers's younger brother, see Taylor *et al.*, 1980.

109 pp. 467–468, Jackson, 1932.

110 Dugas, 1894.

111 Loti seems to have had a sensation of recognition on seeing the sea for the first time. He described this in a semi-autobiographical piece, *Roman d'un Enfant* (1890).

112 p. 455, Arnaud, 1896.

113 p. 456, Arnaud, 1896.

114 p. 458, Arnaud, 1896.

115 The Vanves clinic had been founded by Jean Pierre Falret (1794–1870) and Felix Voisin in 1822. At the time of the interview with the patient Louis, Jules Falret was 72 (he died in 1902).

116 Bernard-Leroy, 1898.

117 For similar surveys, see Chapter 3, this book.

118 Bernt-Larsson, 1931.

119 Bick, 1986.

120 On Frégoli syndrome, see Christodoulou, 1976; Pauw, 1987; for a critical analysis, see Marková and Berrios, 1994.

121 Derombies, 1935.

122 On the neurology of 'familiarity', see Critchley, 1989.

123 On the role of theories of memory in the origin of psychoanalysis, see Walser, 1974.

124 See Ross, 1991.

125 For the recent history of TGA, see the excellent work by Hodges, 1991.

126 p. 372, Winslow, 1861.

127 Lasègue, 1868.

128 Lypemania was the old term for depression, created by Esquirol 50 years earlier, and never fully accepted either in France or outwith it.

129 Foville, 1875. A related syndrome seems to concern the myth of the 'wandering Jew' (Meige, 1893).

130 Luys, 1881.

131 Motet, 1886.

132 Charcot, 1987.

133 Voisin, 1889.

134 For a full review, see Benon and Froissart, 1909.

135 p. 326, Benon and Froissart, 1909; see also presentation to the *Société Médico-Psychologique* a year before by the same authors (Benon and Froissart, 1908).

136 Behr *et al.*, 1985.

137 Abeles and Schilder, 1935.

138 p. 609, Abeles and Schilder, 1935.

139 p. 763, Gillespie, 1937.

140 His first paper in English was Stengel, 1938.

141 p. 597, Stengel, 1941.

142 Parfitt and Gall, 1944.

143 Lagache, 1979.

144 Berrington *et al.*, 1956.
145 On the historical and clinical aspects of the vagabond syndrome, see Mouren *et al.*, 1978.
146 Bergeron, 1956.
147 Akhtar and Brenner, 1979; Riether and Stoudmire, 1988; Pratt, 1977.
148 Hodges and Ward, 1989.
149 Benon, 1909; see also intriguing paper by Dromard, 1911.
150 Markowitsch, 1990.

CHAPTER 10

Consciousness and its disorders

The diaphanous nature of consciousness (as experienced by its owner) is more than matched by its opaqueness to analysis and description.[1] And yet a descriptive psychopathology which did not include this concept would be difficult to imagine. Thus, during the nineteenth century, many 'mental symptoms' were defined in terms of introspective data from consciousness (e.g. hallucinations, depersonalization, *déjà vu*, etc.). The subjectivity of the madman became a private theatre where phantasms played dramas to which the psychiatrist had no direct access. All he could do was get the privileged seer to describe the experiences and then believe that the patient was telling the truth. It goes without saying that such belief is based on the assumptions that consciousness exists and that the patient's descriptive capacity has been spared by the disease.

But in clinical practice things are more complicated than that. Sensations, images, feelings and impulses, often odd or never experienced before, must be recognized and put into words by a person who is simultaneously bemused, confused, upset, terrified or who may actually be participating in the inner drama. Therefore, what the psychiatrist may get is a prosaic, analogical, or bizarre paraphrase. Based on training and imagination, the interviewer will try to name and classify those descriptions that sound familiar. But what about the many which do not? In current practice, and due to the control of ready-made glossaries, it is likely that such descriptions will be quietly ignored. This is a pity for these unnamed experiences are also markers of disease. In the past, when alienists felt freer to describe madness, patients were listened to: that was the manner in which current symptoms were born.

In the early twentieth century, the need to describe subjective events was increased by the keenness on subjectivity brought along by the psychodynamic movement.[2] However, Freud has been criticized for not developing an adequate theory of consciousness.[3] Because all psychopathologies are dependent upon the contents of consciousness, it is difficult to imagine what the language of psychiatry would have been like had it come under the influence of the behaviourism of Watson, Skinner or Ryle.[4] This did not happen and psychiatrists have continued using nineteenth century notions. There are now clear signs that research into consciousness is moving again.[5]

The term 'consciousness' is a modern derivative of *con-scientia* and *sineidesis*, terms which meant 'sharing knowledge in common'. This etymological point is not altogether unimportant as it suggests that classical views of consciousness did not include reference to 'interiority' or 'self-reflection'.[6] The epistemological role of 'consciousness' was questioned by Aristotle: 'Since we can perceive (i.e. be aware) that we see and hear, it must be either by sight, or by some other sense. But then the same sense must perceive both sight and colour, the object of sight, or sight perceives itself. Again, if there is a *separate sense* perceiving sight, either the process will go on *ad infinitum*, or a sense must perceive itself' (my italics).[7] The problem of whether consciousness is a *separate* function that 'perceives' what is going on in all sense modalities, or is an *epiphenomenon* dogged this concept well into the nineteenth century.[8]

Plotinus widened the concept of consciousness by incorporating *sinaístesis*, i.e. the self-reflective function. Sir William Hamilton put it thus: 'The Greek Platonists and Aristotelians, in general, did not allow that the recognition that we know, that we feel, that we desire, etc., was the act of any special faculty, but the general attribute of intellect; and the power of reflecting, of turning back upon himself, was justly viewed as the distinctive quality of intelligence. It was, however, necessary to possess some single term expressive of this intellectual retortion . . . and the term *sinaístesis* was adopted.'[9]

With Christianity, the self-reflective function soon gained a moral dimension: 'This attitude of self-auscultation, which for Pagan philosophy was the privilege of the thinker, becomes in Christian philosophy the right of all individuals. Saint Augustine was the author of this conversion.'[10] These epistemological and moral meanings were to travel together until the seventeenth century when they became fully distinguished in the English language: *Consciousness* (as opposed to *Conscience*) was first used in an exclusive epistemological sense by Ralph Cudworth[11] and then by John Locke.[12] In German, *Bewußtsein* (as opposed to *Gewissen*) was first used by Christian Wolff in 1738.[13] Other languages, like French, Italian, and Spanish still have one term for both meanings.

The Cartesian contribution to the concept of consciousness is important for '*the cogito ergo sum* is the existential evidence of thinking as consciousness.'[14] Descartes wrote: 'By the word thought I understand all that of which we are conscious as operating in us. And that is why not alone understanding, willing, imagining, but also feeling, are here the same thing as thought.'[15] Consciousness thus ceases to be a fact amongst facts or a particular aspect of the soul to become *co-extensive* with the entire spiritual life of man. The certitude of consciousness becomes a solid ground from which man can call into question other certitudes.

On account of Descartes's ontological separation between mind and body, consciousness became imprisoned in 'mentalistic' discourse as a 'thinking substance'. This encouraged the creation of a subjective world well captured in metaphors such as 'inner theatre' and 'ghost in the machine', and its solipsist consequences prevented the development of meaningful links with the material side of man. More than 300 years later, the clinician still confronts this hiatus in the analysis of psychiatric symptoms (e.g. hallucinations,[16] depersonalization,[17] etc.)

The 'psychological' approach to consciousness, as hinted at in the work of Descartes and the British empiricist philosophers,[18] was developed during the nineteenth century together with the mechanism of introspection. Early in the century, James Mill was one of the last philosophers to argue against the 'independence' of consciousness: 'If we are in any way sentient, that is, have any of the feelings whatsoever of a living creature, the word conscious is applicable to the feeler, and consciousness to the feeling: that is, to say, the words are generic marks, under which all the names of the subordinate classes of the feelings of a sentient creature are included. When I smell a rose, I am conscious, when I remember, I am conscious, when I reason and when I believe, I am conscious, but believing and being conscious of belief are not two things, they are the same thing.'[19] Earlier, however, Thomas Reid stamped the seal of his authority on the psychological approach: 'Consciousness is a word used by philosophers to signify knowledge which we have of our present thoughts and purposes, and, in general, of all present operations of our minds. Whence we may observe that consciousness is only of things present . . . is it likewise to be observed, that consciousness is only of things in the mind, and not of external things'; and then opting for the independentist view: 'as that consciousness by which we have a knowledge of the operations of our minds, it is a *different power* from that by which we perceive external objects, and as these different powers have different names in our language . . .'[20]

William Hamilton complained about the difficulty in formulating a definition of consciousness.[21] Alexander Bain tried to explain why: the term, he said, was used to refer to a form of 'waking' and awareness,[22] to attending, observing, noticing, self-examination, indulging in emotions that 'have the self for object', as 'immediate knowledge of its operations', as belief and memory and also to passive, contemplative existence. He concluded that consciousness should be considered as tantamount to mental life (and opposite to mere vegetative functions) for anything that 'rendered mental life more intense was related to consciousness'.[23]

Bain's analysis can be contrasted with Adolphe Garnier's, written from a different perspective: 'Consciousness is the faculty by means of which the mind becomes aware of itself, if the mind was not aware of itself, then the notion of self would have no meaning for it refers to a cognition that grasps itself. It is consciousness that reveals to the mind the action of other faculties . . . If I had no consciousness of my own thinking, I could not use or understand language.'[24]

These two psychological views of consciousness were developed differently. The British view was 'physiologized' (starting with Bain) in the work of Laycock,[25] Carpenter,[26] and Bastian[27] and was of more relevance to neurology (for example, in the work of J.H. Jackson)[28] than to psychiatry. The French view, on the other hand, remained 'psychological' until the end of the century and gave rise to a rich descriptive psychopathology. Indeed, it was French alienists who started to ask whether there were primary disorders of the 'faculty' of consciousness and, if so, what role did they play in mental disorder.[29] Such question was asked in Britain only much later.[30]

Under the influence of Darwinian evolution, a further question was asked in regard to the psychological notion of consciousness, i.e. when did in the evolutionary chain consciousness appear. In *The Expression of Emotions in Man and Animals*, Darwin took an anthropomorphic perspective by stating that, in the lower species, bodily expressions resulted from the *experiencing* of an emotion;[31] however, in the *Descent of Man*, he wrote: 'It may be freely admitted that no animal is self-conscious, if by this term it is implied, that he reflects on such points, as whence he comes or whither he will go, or what is life and death, and so forth. But how can we feel sure that an old dog with an excellent memory and some power of imagination, as shown by his dreams, never reflects on his past pleasures or pains in the chase? And this would be a form of self-consciousness.'[32]

This was enough to open the gates. In 1888, to explain 'self-consciousness', Romanes proposed a form of emergentism: 'So in seeking to indicate the steps whereby self-consciousness has arisen from the lower stages of mental structure . . . When this advancing organization of faculties has proceeded to the extent of enabling the mind incipiently to predicate its own states, the mental organism may be said for the first time to be quickening into life of true self-consciousness.'[33] Lloyd Morgan moved further: 'Consciousness exists: of that there is no doubt. How did it come to exist? There seem three possible answers to this question: 1. it was specially created in man, or in some lower organisms from which man has evolved; 2. it has been directly evolved from energy; 3. it has been evolved, as I have suggested from infra-consciousness.'[34] Morgan argued against the first two options and settled for the third. 'Infra-consciousness was associated with all forms of energy which, to become consciousness, had to be helped by a mechanism called emergent evolution.'[35] A parallel development took place in France. Th. Ribot proposed a view of consciousness based on sustained attention, bodily movement and time, i.e. consciousness had meaning if it was sustained enough to straddle various periods in the life of the individual.[36] Also during this period, alienists such as Chaslin re-conceptualized confusion and delirium as primary disorders of consciousness. This allowed the nineteenth century notion of consciousness to survive in spite of the fact that in the wider field of psychology it came under attack and was eventually routed out; another casualty in this attack was the notion of introspection.

The fall of introspection

It was postulated during the nineteenth century that the capacity of the individual to examine the contents of his consciousness was based upon the existence of a special psychological mechanism called introspection.[37] The assumption of a form of introspectionism remains essential to the understanding of descriptive psychopathology. Introspectionism was based on the metaphor of the inner eye and hence shares in the epistemology of perception.

Confusion

The term confusion is still current in French[38] and British psychiatry[39] and in ICD-9.[40] *Verwirrtheit*, its German counterpart is, however, infrequently used in German-speaking psychiatry and is no longer differentiated from *Verworrenheit*.[41] The term has been dropped from DSM III-R[42] and it does not feature in PSE.[43]

In Roman times, *confusion* had a 'legal' meaning,[44] and during the medieval period it acquired a 'logical' one;[45] both usages were parasitical upon the Latin *confundere*. During the seventeenth century, an 'epistemological' dimension was added.[46] These quaint meanings were still present in the work of John S. Mill for whom the fallacy of confusion was an: 'indistinct, indefinite and fluctuating conception of what the evidence is'.[47] In 1813, the word *confusion* was introduced into medicine as the name for a disease of the eyes;[48] and in 1851, 'confusion of ideas' was used in a psychiatric context by Delasiauve.[49] From here on, the symptom seems to have been defined in terms of the theory of association,[50] the 'psychological' arm of British empiricism.[51]

Verwirrtheit, as well as *Verworren* and *Verwirren* were also used to described states of mental chaos and perplexity.[52] At the beginning of the nineteenth century, Heinroth, Ideler, and Spielman used these words as synonym of mental disorder,[53] but Griesinger connected them with dementia.[54] From then on, interest grew in Germany into the nosological meaning and independence of *Verwirrtheit*. Notable in this respect is the work of Fritsch suggesting the existence of symptomatic and idiopathic forms of 'confusion': the former seen in hysteria and epilepsy; the latter subdivided into its pseudo-aphasic and hallucinatory forms. Fritsch stated that the hallmarks of confusion were clouding of consciousness and impaired judgment.[55] Meynert became interested in *Verwirrtheit* as early as 1874, although at the beginning he thought that disorientation was *secondary* to the hallucinatory experiences.[56] Wille defined *Verwirrtheit* as 'an acute, functional disorder of the brain characterized by confusion, hallucinations, delusions, disorder of consciousness, and sometimes stupor'.[57]

Interestingly, the term 'confusion' does not feature in the dictionaries by Tuke[58] and Power and Sedwick;[59] although it was discussed in Baldwin's a few years later.[60] Thus, it would seem that, since the 1860s, 'confusion' has referred to a defect in the organization of ideas found in delirium, severe depression (for this see below), and other insanities. At the beginning, its presence did not entail organic aetiology but this was to change after the work of Chaslin.[61] The 'syndromatic' view, however, lived on.[62]

The terms confusion and *Verwirrtheit*[63] came into common medical use during the 1890s. The delay was due, at least in France, to Baillarger's insistence that confusion was just a form of melancholia. By the end of the century, however,

melancholia had been replaced by the narrower category 'depression'[64] which did
not include confusion as a symptom. Philippe Chaslin wrote his first paper on the
subject precisely during this period.[65] Only two years earlier, Conolly Norman had
published his paper on 'Acute confusional insanity' containing, in fact, most of the
clinical elements that were to be expanded by the French writer. Norman defined
confusional insanity as characterized by rapid onset, impairment of consciousness
and hallucinations.[66] Chaslin does not seem to have been aware of Norman's work
whose syndrome, nonetheless, survived in British psychiatry up to the present
century.[67]

The work of Chaslin

Chaslin's 1892[68] paper was an expanded version of a communication presented
earlier at the Blois Congress. Influenced by Wille, Chaslin made 'confusion' tantamount to delirium (i.e. used the word in a sense wider than that introduced by
Delasiauve). 'Confusion' became the anchor symptom to a panoply of others: hallucinations, stupor, delusions and physical symptoms. The syndrome was distinguished from mania, melancholia, *délire chronique* (schizophrenia) and even
febrile delirium. He speculated that confusion might be due to cerebral weakness.[69]
Chaslin's paper struck the right chord and a year later, at La Rochelle, a string of
supporting communications on confusion were presented. Séglas, in his *Salpêtriére*
lecture also acknowledged Chaslin's contribution and regretted the fact that Delasiauve's views had fallen into desuetude (due, he claimed, to the popularity of Baillarger's negative idea). Séglas agreed with the new meaning given to confusion (or
Verwirrtheit, Amentia or *Dysnoia*) for it referred 'not to a banal symptom
accompanying insanity but to a specific loss of voluntary control upon the intellectual faculties' (i.e. confusion was a manifestation of *mental automatisme*).[70]

Chaslin's great monograph on the subject appeared in 1895.[71] Not surprisingly,
he also linked *confusion mentale* to automatism.[72] The term gained international
circulation after Régis, together with a very young Hesnard, used it as title for their
contribution to the *Traité International de Psychopathologie*.[73] In this work, the
authors identified three stages in the evolution of the concept: a first period up to
1843 during which confusion, dementia and *stupidité*[74] were conflated; a second
period beginning in 1843 with Baillarger's paper[75] during which (melancholic)
stupor encompassed all the confusional states; and a third period starting in the
work of Delasiauve[76] and completed by Chaslin, Charpentier, Régis, Hannion,
Séglas and Marandon de Montyel, who had re-defined *confusion mentale* as a separate syndrome.

It was at this stage that Binet and Simon published their classic review of *confusion mentale*.[77] They had been criticized for not including this category in their
original work on mental disorders.[78] After stating that confusion was the new *caput
mortuum* of medicine, Binet and Simon identify two meanings: confusion as a symptom meant obscurity of comprehension or incoherence of purpose; confusion as a

disease included the condition first described by Chaslin and adumbrated by Delasiauve and others. The authors conclude that there was little reason to make a
disease out of what was simply a cluster of symptoms. Finally, Binet and Simon
consider it wrong, both from the psychological and clinical viewpoints, to conflate
confusion with dementia, for the mental state in these conditions is different: in
the former there is obscurity of thinking due to 'paralysis', in the latter 'abolition'
of the cognitive faculty.

In 1915, Chaslin[79] departed from his original view by conceding that confusion
was, after all: 1. a syndrome (not a *maladie*), 2. a *global* disorder of mental functions
(not only of intellect) and 3. always related to organic causes (by this time Bonhoeffer had already published his work on exogenous psychosis).[80] It was becoming
clear that a new debate was needed to clear the air. This took place in 1920,[81]
where, for the last time, an elderly Chaslin[82] rose to outline his ideas on confusion.
His intervention was motivated by a claim by Toulouse *et al.*[83] that confusion and
dementia were, after all, not clinically differentiable because both were disorders of
autoconduction.[84] These writers had also criticized, in a general way, the lack of
structure and sensitivity bedevilling psychiatric interviewing techniques at the time,
and proposed the use of standardized techniques and questionnaires.[85] Chaslin
reiterated that the crucial disturbance in confusion was a loosening of synthesis
affecting intellectual, affective and volitional functions, and stated (rightly) that
Toulouse's mechanism of *autoconduction* was just another name for the old notion
of synthesis. Chaslin concluded that the misunderstanding resulted not from real
clinical similarities between confusion and dementia but from the fashion of attributing prognostic value to the latter. He warned (with some prescience) that predictions of this nature were unwarranted unless longitudinal assessments were carried
out. One of the offshoots of the 1920 debate (and of Chaslin's defence) was that
the diagnostic criteria for delirium (for that is what it was about) were written in
stone, and linked up with clouding of consciousness.[86]

Confusion and stupor

The history of melancholic stupor is part of the history of confusion and must be
dealt with here, however briefly. During the nineteenth century, melancholic stupor
or *melancholia attonita* named a state of severe psychotic non-responsiveness
(whether depressive, schizophrenic or 'organic'). Subjects thus affected showed
confusion, posturing, psychomotor retardation, and delusions and hallucinations.
After the 1810s, the description and conceptualization of this clinical phenomenon
went through three stages, but only the first two are relevant to the history of
confusion.[87]

The earliest hypothesis (and period) concerning melancholic stupor was sensory
'numbness', i.e. the view that non-responsiveness was due to a temporal abolition
of perception. Pinel favoured this view and hence did not see the need to separate
stupor from idiocy.[88] Georget classified 'stupidity' as a separate genre of insanity

characterised by involvement of cognition and introduced a *post hoc* criterion: 'The mental content experienced by these patients is delusional in nature suggesting that stupidity should be separated from both idiotism and dementia.'[89]

The second period is characterized by the view that stupor resulted from an inhibition of higher mental functions rather than peripheral numbness. Thus, in his paper on *stupidité*, Ètoc-Demazy drew four conclusions: 1. 'stupidity' is not a genre of insanity but a complication of mania and monomania, 2. symptoms evolve in two stages: diminution of cognition and then suspension of relational functions, 3. none of the symptoms has predictive value in regard to outcome, and 4. *stupidité* and 'dementia' were different syndromes.[90] In order to apply some of these criteria, the alienist had to examine the mental state of his patient.

Thus, the 1840s witnessed the development of a view of stupor based on the analysis of subjective experience. For example, Baillarger believed that *stupides* were not devoid of mental experiences and that they were, in fact, suffering from 'melancholia'.[91] Baillarger concluded that: 1. patients diagnosed as 'stupid' often experience delusions and hallucinations, 2. delusions may be depressive in content including thoughts of self-harm, 3. illusions and hallucinations cause an internal, 'oniric' world of fantasy, and stupor is analogous to 'dreaming', and 4. 'stupidity' is an advanced state of melancholia.[92]

Baillarger's view did not go unchallenged, particularly because clinical counter-examples of non-melancholic stupors were easily found (such as, for example, cases to be later called catatonic stupor).[93] Sauze, however, supported Baillarger and offered narrow criteria for melancholic stupor.[94] Baillarger followed with a long paper making use of Sauze's cases.[95] His views predominated in France up to the 1860s when the issue was debated at the *Societé Médico-Psychologique*. It started with Legrand de Saulle reporting the case of Della F, a 32 year-old Italian patient who died in a stuporous state.[96] To deal with the issues raised by this case, Ritti suggested that stupor be classified into melancholic and symptomatic; the latter becoming a sort of rag-bag which included catatonic states.[97]

In Germany, Griesinger subdivided 'melancholic stupor' into a type characterized by rigidity, catalepsy, negativism, clouding, incontinence, fantastic hallucinatory and delusional experiences (recounted after recovery); and another consisting of 'a half-sleeping state without clear dreams or hallucinations' but marked abulia and melancholia.[98] In Scotland, Newington also distinguished anergic from delusional stupor, and intended these two categories to replace 'acute dementia' and 'melancholic stupor', respectively.[99] 'Melancholia with stupor' or 'melancholia attonita'[100] remained a source of controversy until Kahlbaum cut the Gordian knot by suggesting that stupor was, after all, the first stage of a new insanity (*vesania catatonica*).[101] At the turn of the century, Kraepelin brought catatonia under the umbrella of dementia praecox.[102] By this period, the view that stupor, confusion and *obtusion*)[103] might involve a change in consciousness began to be discussed. For example, Krafft-Ebing defined stupor as an 'elementary disorder of consciousness.'[104]

Disorientation

The symptom disorientation has an interesting conceptual structure. Like hallucination or delusion, it is meant to refer to an on-going mental state: but unlike these symptoms it relates to a failure in both 'knowing that' (verbal orientation) and 'knowing what' (behavioural orientation).[105] Indeed, since the time of Jackson, disorientation has been considered as a 'negative symptom', i.e. entailing a failure in a hypothetical orientation function.[106] Failure in orientation might thus result from a breakdown in: 1. perception; 2. updating of the internal map; 3. map-reading itself; 4. matching of retrieved script to incoming information; or 5. acting upon a detected mismatch. On occasions, the above system might be intact but, none the less, a temporary failure in orientation may occur resulting from updatings made according to a private, delusional reference system.

Considered as a general symptom rather than as a feature of delirium, disorientation had already been discussed by Meynert, Rieger and Sommer, and Grasset.[107] Wernicke proposed an abstract classification of *Ratlosigkeit* in terms of his three modes of consciousness (allo- auto- and somato-psychic). Alienists interested in a structured way of collecting information, such as Rieger and Sommer, suggested that the orientation questions be standardized.[108] By 1899, Finzi was able to write his classic paper on disorientation as a symptom,[109] and soon after testing techniques began to be developed. For example, Bouchard[110] tested time evaluation and orientation by asking subjects to 'produce' (by tapping or pacemaking) or to 'reproduce' time, i.e. to judge the duration of a given unit of official time.[111]

The English word 'orientation' derives from the French *orienter*[112] and was first used as a scientific term in astronomy.[113] Mott called 'imperfect orientation' one of the symptoms of cerebral arteriosclerosis.[114] By this time, disorientation had already been reported in association with acute brain syndromes,[115] transient memory disturbance[116] and reduction in mental function.[117] Janet used the term 'feeling of disorientation' to describe the loss of appreciation of spatial relationships[118] and König called disorientation the confusion observed in Parkinson's disease.[119] Jaspers recognized four types of disorientation: amnesic, delusional, apathetic and clouded.[120] Bleuler drew attention to the phenomenon of psychotic 'double orientation'[121] and Régis described a subgroup of patients suffering from dementia praecox who exhibited confusion and disorientation.[122] Jung proposed that, because dementia praecox patients paid preferential attention to their 'illusions', they might only give the impression of disorientation.[123] Likewise, Bleuler believed that in dementia praecox there was no 'primary' failure of temporal orientation,[124] and so did Kraepelin although he found that in the stuporous and severely agitated patient 'perception of the environment may be occasionally disordered.'[125]

It would seem, therefore, that these authors did not consider verbal descriptions alone as evidence for real time disorientation; later writers, however, such as Minkowski,[126] Schilder,[127] and Seeman[128] seem to have done. With Kurt Schneider[129] *clouding*[130] of consciousness became accepted in the German school as an 'axial' symptom of delirium, and temporo-spatial disorientation (as identified in the mental state examination) became its clinical counterpart. The perceptive observation by Chaslin that acute organic states may occur without clouding was also rescued by the German school when, in the 1950s, it recognized the *Durchgang* or transitional syndrome,[131] i.e. a reversible symptomatic (organic) psychosis without clouding of consciousness.

Since confusion and disorientation have been considered (at least since the late nineteenth century) as the hallmark of the so-called delirium syndrome, it is justified briefly to explore the history of this fascinating clinical phenomenon.

Delirium

Delirium (acute confusional state, exogenous psychosis) names a cluster of mental symptoms and behaviours, with fluctuating course and (often) incomplete presentation, occurring in the wake of acute brain disease.[132] Early this century, it was suggested that delirium might be a stereotyped,[133] (perhaps 'wired-in') brain response to a variety of insults. This could explain its transhistorical and transcultural stability (i.e. the fact that psychosocial noise seems not to distort its clinical presentation). This section will explore the way the current definition of this ancient mental disorder was shaped by the conceptual and empirical forces that operated during the nineteenth century. From typically being a state of excited *behaviour* accompanied by fever (*phrenitis*), delirium became a disorder of consciousness, attention, cognition, and orientation; the transitional concept of *confusion* playing a crucial role in this process.

During the same period *vesanic* and *non-vesanic*[134] forms of delirium were separated: the former becoming the current notion of delusion. Finally, it will be suggested that it was delirium, and not progressive paralysis of the insane,[135] that served as the clinical model for the current notion of psychosis.

Delirium before the nineteenth century

Reference to *phrenitis* and to an association between physical and mental disease can frequently be found in Ancient literature. For the Greeks *phrenitis*[136] was a disturbance of thought, mood, and action associated with physical disease. Jones wrote: 'The Hippocratic collection is rich in words meaning delirium: 1. those in which mental derangement is the dominant idea, and 2. those in which stress is laid upon delirious talk.'[137] As is well known, *phrenitis, mania, melancholia*, and *paranoia* were the core categories of Greek psychiatry.[138] Concepts similar to delirium can also be found in other cultures, for example, Hankoff has suggested that the Greek term *Kordiakos* was used in the Talmud to refer to temporary madness associated with wine drinking – probably a form of *delirium tremens*.[139]

Since Antiquity, absence of fever separated conventional madness (e.g. mania) from *phrenitis*. During the seventeenth century, Sydenham wrote: 'The patient falls into a brain fever, or into what is next door to it. He gets no sleep, he utters frequent exclamations, he uses incoherent language, he looks and talks wildly.'[140] Willis[141] and Cullen[142] fully agreed with this description. Indeed, the fever criterion remained central to Western medicine up to the early nineteenth century.[143]

With his usual historical sense, von Feuchtersleben asked: 'the question: are delirium and insanity identical? has been answered thus: that acute delirium with fever must be distinguished from the chronic variety which is called insanity', however, 'the presence or absence of fever, which is possible in every condition [cannot] decide the matter' ... 'Delirium is a symptom which indicates the transition of a purely somatic disease into a mental disorder'. In respect to the classification of delirium (here shifting its meaning to delusion) he wrote: 'it is fruitless, as has been frequently done, to consider differences in the object [of the delusion] as a ground for division [for] they do not express the essence of the disturbance.'[144]

Delirium and intellectual function

In Galen, delirium was co-extensive with *mentis alienatio*[145] and thus it remained until the eighteenth century. For example, Quincy defined delirium as: 'An incapacity in the organs of sensation to perform their function in due manner, so that the mind does not reflect upon and judge of external objects as usual; as is the case frequently in fevers, from too impetuous a hurry of the blood, which alters so far the secretion in the brain, as to disorder the whole nervous system.'[146] Dr Johnson defined delirious as 'light headed, raving and doting', 'people about him said he had been for some hours delirious, but when I saw him he had his understanding as well as ever I knew'. Quoting Arbuthnot, Johnson considered delirium tantamount to 'alienation of mind': 'Too great alacrity and promptness in answering, specially in persons naturally of another temper, is a sign of an approaching delirium. In a feverish delirium there is a small inflammation of the brain.'[147]

This (intellectualistic) view was challenged by Sutton who, when describing *delirium tremens* (or shaking delirium), played down the old view of *phrenitis*: 'As the disease advances, the faculties do not, generally speaking, show themselves in disorder by any extravagance of thought.' Sutton went on to suggest that *affective* and *motor disturbance* were, in fact, a central part of the new syndrome.[148] By the middle of the nineteenth century, the term delirium had accumulated a long list of medical synonyms.[149]

Délire, *delirium and delusion*

Up to the nineteenth century, the term delirium had a double meaning in most European countries.[150] For various historical reasons this fact seems to have been particularly troublesome to French psychiatry. For example, Pinel[151] used *délire* to refer both to specific errors of judgment (i.e. delusion) and to *phrenitis*.[152] Esquirol did likewise, and believed that *délire* was a primary disturbance of perception: 'A person is delirious when his ideas are not in keeping with his sensations, etc.' 'hallucinations are the most frequent cause of *délire'*.[153] Georget used the word to refer both to disorders of intellect and also to 'a disorder . . . resulting from general illness or illness of the brain', i.e. as *délire aigüe*. Georget composed a table showing the differential diagnosis between *délire aigüe* and *folie* and noticed the intermittent and reversible nature of the former.[154] In a posthumous article, he separated *délire aigüe* (or febrile) from *délire chronique ou sans fiévre* (tantamount to insanity proper).[155] By the 1860s, a differential usage had become established and *délire* mainly referred to *aberrant ideas* accompanying delirium. This shift from syndrome to symptom was consolidated by Lasègue[156] and Falret[157] and legitimized in Littré's dictionary.[158] In French psychiatry, this created the need for a term for organic delirium and the term 'confusion' was charged with this role. These linguistic ambiguities affected less British and German psychiatry where the early availability of the terms *delusion* and *Wahn* helped to separate the symptomatic from the syndromatic meaning (i.e. the organic syndrome was called *delirium* or *Verwirrtheit*, respectively).[159]

Delirium and insanity

The distinction between delirium and insanity remained an object of dispute up to the middle of the nineteenth century.[160] Brierre de Boismont, in a classical essay,[161] claimed that both shared the same 'moral' (psychological) aetiology and could not be told apart by post-mortem studies. He asked, 'is it the case that acute delirium is just an acute form of [ordinary] insanity'? He reported a sample of eleven patients in which the fever criterion had not worked. Brierre's views eventually crossed the Atlantic and the *American Journal of Insanity* presented them to American alienists twenty years later.[162] Griesinger also quoted Brierre in the second edition of his textbook.[163]

Indeed, the debate on whether acute delirium constituted a separate form of insanity went on until the end of the century.[164] For example, Calmeil[165] stated that delirium was caused by peri-encephalitis and that many insanities were only mild forms of the same lesion; if that was the case, he asked, is it not wrong to consider delirium insanity as totally different diseases? Worcester, however, felt that this 'continuity' view was no longer acceptable.[166]

The enduring nature of this debate is likely to be related to the popularity of the doctrine of unitary psychosis.[167] According to this view, clinical differences between all forms of insanity were explicable in terms of environmental and / or pathoplastic effects. Thus, if the insanities were on a continuum, i.e. expressions of one basic disease, why should delirium not be part of it? One reason why some alienists resisted this conclusion was clinical tradition; another that *there were* clinical differences, for example, in the type and distribution of symptoms and in outcome (there was a higher mortality in delirium).[168]

Only later in the century did involvement of consciousness become an *official criterion* to separate delirium and insanity. This does not mean that earlier descriptions of delirium did not, occasionally, include reference to confusion or other disorders of consciousness; indeed, they did: the issue here is that the same disturbances of consciousness were also attributed to ordinary insanity, and that no clinical stipulation yet existed that such disturbances were a hallmark of (organic) delirium. In fact, such stipulation only became possible after the psychoses had been redefined.[169] Thanks to degeneration theory,[170] the latter were now considered to be hereditary, i.e. capable of breeding through (which could not be said of delirium); likewise, insanities with chronic course were identified (i.e. *délire chronique*)[171] and shown to be different from delirium. Having found two external criteria to separate delirium from insanity, it only remained to compare their symptoms.

Delirium as a form of dreaming

The idea that hallucinations and delusions (particularly those seen in delirium) were dreams experienced during wakefulness was popular during the nineteenth century. This was well expressed by Griesinger: 'The acute febrile delirium, from which the insanities cannot be specifically distinguished, consists of active dreams during waking or half-waking.'[172] In his classical paper on *Alcoholic delirium is not a delirium but a dream*[173] Lasègue defined dreaming as a half-physiological, half-pathological state accompanied by visual hallucinations superior in sensory quality to those seen in insanity. He believed that alcoholic hallucinosis were gradually 'primed' by periods of disturbed sleep and dreaming.

But the most popular book on the subject during this period was written by a historian and politician.[174] In *Le Sommeil et les Rêves*, Alfred Maury reprinted some of his own published papers on the subject and discussed the physiology and psychology of sleep. The core of the book he dedicated to the view that hallucinations and delusions were related to dreaming.[175]

Onirisme, the name that the French gave to this putative mechanism, deserves a historical chapter of its own.[176] It was defined as a 'form of automatic mental activity constituted by visions and animated scenes similar to those experienced in dreams.'[177] Perhaps the best description of *délire onirique* is the one offered by Régis. This great alienist from Bordeaux remarked that although the tendency to compare delirium and dreams was ancient, earlier writers had only used the comparison analogically, and that only Lasègue had actually identified dreaming with alcoholic delirium from the *physiological* viewpoint. Séglas, Legrain, and Régis went on to extend the same explanation to febrile and toxic deliria. Régis described *délire onirique* as a state of somnambulism followed by amnesia and occasionally by fixed ideas, and recalled that it was in 1901 that he first presented his views: 'the typical form of toxic psychosis includes two elements: confusion and delusions . . . mental confusion is related to obtusion, disorientation, mental hebetude, and followed by

amnesia and occasionally dementia' . . . 'as far as delusions are concerned, these
are oniric in the strict sense of the term, i.e. born and developed during sleep, and
formed out of coincidental associations of ideas and fragments of hallucinatory
experiences related to old memories.'[178] Onirism and oniroid states played a descriptive and explanatory role in French psychiatry until the arrival of DSM III-R.[179]

Consciousness of illness and insight

Writing on the history of 'insight' (and its clinical derivative *insightlessness*) illustrates well the problem posed by ambiguous ideas. For which definition is to be
used as the guiding invariant?[180] A narrow, intellectualistic definition according to
which insight is just 'knowledge of being ill'? The equally narrow view implicit in
current empirical studies?[181] The wider idea that insight is a form of self knowledge?[182] Some form of psychoanalytical definition?[183] To be clear, the difficulty here
is not posed by the history of any one trend (tackled individually they are easy
enough) but by attempting to compose a 'valid' history, i.e. one that captures the
'theme' of insight, in its kaleidoscopic variety. The term 'theme', however, is a
portmanteau that needs unpacking.

Thus, soon enough the historian finds out that 'theme' may mean the history
of the *term* 'insight', of *behaviours* (whose experiential component seems highly
unstable), or of the *concepts* developed during the last 150 years to account for
such behaviours. Just as with empirical studies, the final choice will always be
'conceptual' or *a priori*. This is the case even if (as with 'empirical' studies) the
researcher chooses to deal with the reality of 'behaviour' (not to get entangled in
the web of concepts or ideas). For, unfortunately, 'insight' has less ontological stability than moles or murmurs, and what *makes* it a unitary behaviour or attitude
or set of thoughts or actions (putatively absent or disabled in some mentally ill
individuals) is a hidden concept already governing our perception of the *behaviour*.
Even if, as we all hope it to be, the basis of such behaviour has been fixed by
evolution (and has brain representation) it will remain 'attitudinal' in that its
expression is controlled by cultural instructions (e.g. the ongoing conceptions of
'mental illness'). In other words, 'behaviour' may prove to be less of an 'invariant'
than might be hoped. Should one then grasp the nettle and choose 'concepts' as the
invariant theme? This might not be very helpful either for concepts are particularly
vulnerable to cultural (and epistemological) change. Is the researcher then left with
the trivial option of writing on the history of a word? Even this will not be very
illuminating, for in regard to the word 'insight' and its linguistic equivalents, there
are major differences in usage between the French, German, Italian, British, etc.
psychiatric cultures.

Problems historical

Since, sometimes, problems become clearer when tackled at a lower level of abstraction, let us rephrase this against the context of the history of psychopathology. To

make things manageable, I shall concentrate on the history of insight in the psychosis rather than in dementia, obsessional disorder, or hysteria (where it poses serious definitional and psychometric problems). Until the early nineteenth century, the official view of insanity (offered by Hobbes and Locke)[184] was based on the presence of delusions, and the latter were defined as 'insightless' by definition. Within that particular discourse 'awareness of being deluded' had no meaning whatsoever and hence it is in principle understandable that the physicians of the period did not see it as a problem. Indeed, up to the end of the eighteenth century, the issue of 'awareness of illness' is raised more often by lawyers (challenging the notion of total insanity) than by physicians. Such challenges are a source for the concept of 'partial insanity' which, at the beginning of the nineteenth century, had two meanings: 'intermittent' (i.e. periods of madness interspersed with 'lucid' intervals),[185] and 'incomplete' (i.e. madness affecting one region of the psyche or monomania).[186]

In addition to partial insanity, there was at the beginning of the nineteenth century another development, also important to the history of insight. It was the challenge to Locke's intellectualistic (i.e. delusional) definition of madness.[187] Pinel, Prichard, and Esquirol (inter alia) proposed a definition of insanity in terms of Faculty Psychology, and this made possible the diagnosis of 'emotional' and 'volitional' insanities.[188] The latter were not definitionally linked to 'insightlessness', even if in practice patients with severe depression or mania or abulia might refuse to accept that they were 'ill'. To summarize, both the concept of 'partial' madness and of monomania allowed for the existence of an insanity which, to paraphrase Baillarger, 'was aware of itself'.

Changes in views on the causes of insanity opened up yet more space for the possibility of insight into mental illness. As an anonymous historian put it in 1840: 'all explanations of mental illness boil down to three options: they are localized in the brain . . . or in the soul . . . or in both.'[189] The former two options led to interesting implications: in general, the notions of monomania and partial insanity (and hence insight) were more readily accepted by supporters of the anatomo-clinical view of madness[190] than by those who believed that insanity was exclusively 'sited' in the mind or soul (l'âme) as it was difficult (in terms of the philosophical psychology of the period) to accept that the soul was 'divided up' and hence could become partially diseased. Such was the very argument that Jules Falret used before the Société Médico-Psychologique in 1866.[191]

The categorical changes listed above were made possible by a deeper shift in the notion of disease. Until the eighteenth century, 'total insanity' was but a reflection of what has been called the 'ontological definition of disease', i.e. being mad and losing one's reason was a sort of permanent (almost atemporal) state that affected the entire body/person. In a way, the problem at the time was to explain 'recovery'. On the other hand, the notion of partial insanity (which took foot after the momentous changes brought about by the ideas of Bichat)[192] assumed a 'modular' model of the mind[193] and more or less specific cerebral localization (both, at the time, sponsored by phrenology).[194] This allowed, as it has been seen, for the coexistence of sanity and insanity in the human mind.[195] Alienists during the 1830s were fully aware of the implications of the change and an important debate ensued on the legitimacy of such a mosaic-like model of the mind.[196] Others, like Maudsley, accepted this view but felt that in the insane all regions of the mind were affected: 'when an insane delusion exists in the mind, however circumscribed the range of its action may seem to be, the *rest of the mind is certainly not sound . . .* ' (my italics).[197]

Yet more conceptual space was provided to questions pertaining to 'insight' by the incorporation in psychiatry (during the nineteenth century) of noble concepts such as consciousness (awareness) and introspection,[198] and self[199] without which, it could be argued, the notion of 'insight' would be difficult to understand.[200] The acceptance of these concepts after the 1840s by the psychiatric brotherhood was facilitated (or accompanied) by determined efforts to incorporate *subjectivity* (i.e. descriptions of inner experiences) into the definition of insanity. Moreau de Tours[201] was important in articulating this need.[202] Encouraged by his work, alienists accepted the view that the way patients actually 'experienced' their illness was essential for diagnosis and classification. This belief paved the way for the development of a language of description (whose history this book is about!), of interviewing techniques, and of scientific questions as to the value and legitimacy of introspection.[203] As mentioned earlier, during the nineteenth century, the 'psychological' concept of consciousness was mainly understood as a form of *perception* (an inner eye). Not surprisingly, the force of this metaphor led to preferring the old English term *insight* to *inwit* (which could have been as useful but carried less 'visual' connotations).

The final facilitator for a development of a science of 'insight' was the arrival in psychiatry of the concepts of comprehension (*Verstehen*) (and later on of self-consciousness).[204] Important to the former were the ideas of Brentano,[205] Dilthey,[206] and eventually Freud, Husserl and Jaspers.[207] These grander concepts, however, were more ambitious than the mere 'looking into one's mind' (as suggested by introspection): they attempted to grasp the totality of one's mental and existential state (which includes regions of information which are not conscious or volition driven). Within this new conceptual frame, 'full insight' needs more than a mere definition as 'intellectual' knowledge of 'being ill': it demands to be based on deeper attitudinal processes involving emotions and volitions. The mechanisms that make such holistic insight possible will vary according to school of thought. In Brentano it concerned intentionality and particularly his mechanism of a 'third consciousness',[208] in Dilthey it pertained to the complex process of grasping the totality or *Verstehen*,[209] and in the psychoanalytical movement varied according to model of the mind.[210]

Insight: a convergence *manqué?*

I have now described three (no doubt there are more) conceptual spaces within which the history of insight could be explored. The question is, are they confluent and lead to a unitary phenomenon? Or are they parallel developments? Current empirical studies seem to assume the former, namely that there is such a thing as 'insightless behaviour' (as an ontologically given thing). What has been said so far suggests that the latter is the case, and that the so-called 'insightlessness' of schizophrenia (even if the latter is, as it is likely to be, fully organic) is, in fact, concept driven, i.e. reflects the way in which it is portrayed in contemporary culture. This generates a mild form of relativism (not fatal, in fact, to the neurobiological definition of schizophrenia), and that will be the perspective to be used in this section. The reason for this is that the process of 'symptom construction' (when *historically* studied) seems to result from the 'convergence' (at a point in time) of a term (insight, *Einsicht, conciencia de enfermedad*, etc.), a concept ('looking into', *Verstehen*, etc.) and some behaviours (which in the case of insight are probably partially dependent on the existence of deeper conceptual frames). The state of convergence may last only for a short period of time (as it happens when it dies with its proposer) or may become stable (a veritable 'word/concept/behaviour complex'). Some symptoms (e.g. depression, hallucination, etc.) have proven to be longer-lasting complexes. The convergence model also suggests that convergence can be very unstable. It is proposed here that this is the case with 'insightlessness', which can be said to belong to the category of convergence *manqué*.

The word

The history of the word is straightforward, and in this case less important. The OED provides various definitions, all governed by the same metaphor: 'internal sight, with the eyes of the mind, mental vision, perception, discernment' or 'the fact of penetrating with the eyes of the understanding into the inner character or hidden nature of things; a glimpse or view beneath the surface; the faculty or power of thus seeing'. The German term *Einsicht*, partially covers these meanings;[211] Italian, French, and Spanish paraphrase according to context. The earliest *clinical* usage of 'insightlessness' I have been able to find dates back to Kraff-Ebing: 'in chronic insanity, when delusions have become organized and defect has ensued, the patient is absolutely insightless to his disease'.[212]

The concepts

The history of the *concept* of insight, particularly in relation to the evolution of the notions of reason and consciousness in psychiatry, is more illuminating. Prosper Despine distinguished two meanings for the term 'lucidity': one concerned the state of recovery, the other the sparing of the intellectual faculty. The first, in turn, Despine divided up into two: improvement after the illness had lifted, and *lucidité pendant la folie même*. The latter included an inchoate form of the current concept of insight as 'awareness of illness'. This state, according to Despine, arose when delusions were limited to 'specific topics' and there was absence of a *passion pathologique* affecting the mind.[213] Others disagreed. Perhaps the best known work defending the old fashioned view of delusion as an insightless phenomenon was *Les Folies Raissonantes*, in which Serieux and Capgras, already during the early twentieth century, described around 19 cases with circumscribed delusional disorder, none of whom had any insight into their condition. Indeed, when exploring the natural history of their delusions, the authors do not consider the question of insight.[214] German writers tended to support this view. A young Gustav Störring defined delusions as not susceptible to correction and as insightless, regardless of whether or not the function of judgment was affected.[215] Mendel agreed with this view; and when discussing the issue of patterns of improvement from the psychoses, he wrote: 'the dictum of Willis, that 'no one can be regarded as cured till he voluntarily confesses his insanity' cannot be accepted in this categorical form. There are sporadic cases which, in spite of a limited residual insanity, may undoubtedly be considered as cure'.[216]

In a classical paper on *Conscience et Alienation mentale*,[217] Henri Dagonet recommended that alienists accepted a new (psychological) definition of consciousness: 'to comprehend mental illness further it is indispensable to examine the mental symptoms *in themselves* . . . the first to study amongst the latter should be the disorders of consciousness' (my italics).[218] Defined by Littré as 'the intimate, immediate, and constant monitoring of the activities of the self', consciousness had as one of its functions the detection of change: 'consciousness captures all the phenomena of our internal life, and commits them to memory: this includes the feeling of totality of the person. Consciousness should thus sense any transformation in the latter caused by mental illness.'[219] 'In the different forms of mental illness, the disorders of consciousness will depend upon what other faculties are involved . . . only in exceptional cases can cerebral automatism occur in clear consciousness'.[220] For example, in the case of hallucinated patients, some have no awareness of illness whilst others: 'preserve the sense of the strangeness of the hallucination and search for explanations.'[221] Dagonet explained such 'awareness of illness' on the basis of Luys's hypothesis that 'one cerebral hemisphere remained normal whilst the other was pathological'.[222] The notion of consciousness proposed by Littré and Parant was less popular in England. Maudsley, in his usual acerbic tone, wrote: 'it has been very difficult to persuade speculative psychologists who elaborate webs of philosophy out of their own consciousnesses that consciousness has nothing to do with the actual work of mental function; that it is the adjunct not the energy at work; not the agent in the process, but the light which lightens a small part of it . . . we may put consciousness aside then when we are considering the nature of the mechanism and the manner of its work . . .'[223]

Seven years earlier, Parant[224] had offered a full analysis of the problem. *La Raison dans La Folie* is an important book for it directly tackles the issue of legal responsibility in insanity. One approach to this problem Parant called *la conscience de soi dans la folie*. Awareness of illness in the context of insanity, he wrote, 'concerns the state in which the patient is aware of his experiences, acts, of all internal changes and of their consequences'. 'Thus understood, this awareness implies not only knowledge of illness but capacity to judge it by degrees'.[225]

Parant discussed 'awareness of illness' early in, during and after the mental illness. In the second group, and using combinations of awareness of quality of acts, of illness, and of emotional response to such knowledge, he recognized patients who may have awareness: (*a*) of the goodness or badness of their acts, but *not* of disease, (*b*) of being ill, but that the illness was *not* insanity, (*c*) of being insane, but not fully accepting it; (*d*) of being insane but unable to do something about it, and (*e*) like (*d*) but involved in serious acts.[226] In regard to group (*c*) Parant made the important point that 'the awareness of these patients is complex in that it probably results from conscious and unconscious factors'.[227]

The question of the role and state of consciousness in insanity continued troubling writers well into the twentieth century. For example, Claye Shaw inquired whether there was a disturbance of consciousness during the acute episode, and whether it could explain the lack of memory shown by psychotic patients of symptoms experienced during the attack. Indeed, he came close to explaining why there was no awareness of illness in delusion: 'there is evidence that both in dream states and in insanity the emotional side of the idea may be wanting, and this must have great effect on both memory and consciousness ... I have over and over again noticed that people with delusions of a very depressed type do not show the emotional tone which should co-exist with the delusions'.[228]

KRAEPELIN AND BLEULER The question of insight and its diagnostic and predictive value does not seem to have interested Kraepelin a great deal. He briefly touched upon it under 'judgement': 'what always surprises the observer anew is the quiet complacency with which the most nonsensical ideas can be uttered by them and the most incomprehensive actions carried out'.[229] But then he added: 'the patients often have a distinct feeling of the profound change which has taken place in them. They complain that they are 'dark in the head', not free, often in confusion, no longer clear, and that they have 'cloud thoughts'. But ultimately, 'understanding of the disease disappears fairly rapidly as the maladie progresses in an overwhelming majority of the cases even where in the beginning it was more or less clearly present'.[230] Bleuler was no different. The nearest he came to discussing awareness of illness was in the section on the nature of delusional ideas, but in the end he did not elaborate upon his views.

JASPERS Continuing in the tradition of Parant, Karl Jaspers wrote: 'Patients' *self-observation* is one of the most important sources of knowledge in regard to morbid psychic life; so is their *attentiveness* to their abnormal experience and the *elaboration* of their observations in the form of a psychological judgment so that they can communicate to us something of their inner life' (my italics).[231] Jaspers observed that in the early stage of their illness patients became perplexed; this was explained as an understandable reaction. As the illness progressed, patients tried to make sense of their experiences, for example by elaborating delusional systems. Jaspers then introduced personality as an explanatory concept and suggested that as it became involved in the illness, the patient's attitude changed; for example, patients appeared indifferent or passive to the most frightening delusions. As seen above, Shaw believed that this lack of reaction was due to lack of emotions.

Following Parant and earlier French psychiatrists, Jaspers also observed that transient insight may occur during acute psychoses, but that this soon disappeared. He believed that where insight persisted, the patient was more likely to be suffering from a personality disorder than a psychosis. In patients who recovered from the psychotic state, Jaspers made a distinction between psychoses such as mania and alcoholic hallucinosis where patients were able to look back on their experiences with 'complete' insight, and a psychosis such as schizophrenia where they did not show full insight. He described the latter patients as unable to talk freely about the contents of their experiences, becoming overtly affected when pressed to do so, and occasionally maintaining some features of their illnesses. In chronic psychotic states, he described patients who, from their verbal contents, often appeared to have full insight, yet in fact these verbal contents would turn out to be learnt phrases and meaningless to the patients themselves.

Jaspers's concept of insight was defined in terms of the patient's ability to judge what was happening to him during the development of psychosis, and the reasons why it was happening. So, he made a distinction between awareness of illness, that is experiences of feeling ill or changed, and insight proper, where a correct estimate could be made of the type and severity of the illness. These judgments, however, depended on the intelligence and education of the individual; indeed, because judgments of this nature are inherently a part of the personality make-up, in the case of patients with intelligence below a certain level (e.g. idiocy), it would be more appropriate to think of loss of personality rather than loss of awareness as the feature in their lack of knowledge of themselves.

Jaspers was aware of the difficulty involved in theorising about 'insight', and of the extent to which the outsider can hope to understand a patient's attitudes to his illness. In other words it was easier to assess objective knowledge, that is the ability of a patient to understand and apply medical knowledge to himself, than what he called the 'comprehending appropriation of it'. This latter function, Jaspers stated, is intrinsically linked to the patient's self, and cannot be divorced from knowledge of self-existence itself.

CONRAD Conrad carried out long-term observations on schizophrenic patients and described the development and progression of the psychotic state.[232] Although he did not use the term, his conceptualization of the awareness of change in the self and the environment due to mental illness is related to what Jaspers called 'insight'. Conrad named the early stage of the schizophrenic illness the 'trema'; during this stage patients found it difficult to express their feelings and experiences; some would talk about fear, tension, anxiety and anticipation, while others would describe feelings of guilt and helplessness. Conrad believed that the common theme was a feeling of oppression, an awareness that something was not right, and a sense of restriction of one's freedom. During the next stage of the illness, the 'apophany', patients attributed meaning to feelings and experiences; for example, when in the state of 'anastrophe', patients believed themselves to be the centre of the world.

Conrad described further stages during which destructive processes were followed by partial resolution as residual schizophrenic effects persisted, and postulated that schizophrenia was an illness affecting the higher mental functions which differentiate humans from animals. Thus, it affected the whole self-concept and, in particular, the ability of the individual to effect the normal transition from looking at oneself from *within* to looking at oneself from the *outside*, by the eyes of the world.

General summary

Until the 1850s, 'confusion' was considered as a type of melancholic stupor. It became a syndrome in its own right only towards the end of the century when the concept of melancholia was replaced by the narrower one of depression. The symptoms of delirium were considered by some as dreams breaking through into consciousness, and this model was reformulated during the second half of the century as being an instance of psychological automatism. On this, the influence of Jackson, via Ribot and Janet, is important. Difficulties in defining clouding of consciousness led to the acceptance of the clinical notion of disorientation. The final separation of the non-vesanic and vesanic forms of delirium encouraged the creation of the modern notion of psychoses. Indeed, the latter is modelled upon the symptom structure of delirium. At the beginning of the nineteenth century, delirium (*délire*) ambiguously named an acute organic disorder (*phrenitis*), and also the symptom 'delusion'. The two meanings were gradually separated on the basis of duration, reversibility, presence of fever, and confusion. This latter term was defined first in terms of the doctrine of association of ideas, and later as a disorder of consciousness.

In regards to the history of insightlessness, the following conclusions can be drawn: it is a symptom whose instability has resulted from an incomplete convergence between word, concept and behaviour. This makes life hard for the historian. Before 1850, there is very little on insightlessness in the clinical literature. This is likely to be due to the fact that questions concerning insight and awareness of illness were *meaningless* during a period in which insanity was specifically defined in terms of the presence of delusions. However, the development of concepts such as partial, emotional, and volitional insanity led, during the second half of the nineteenth century, to early questioning on the clinical value of evaluating the attitude of patients *vis-à-vis* their insanity. Equally important to the development of a concept of insight has been the availability of the (psychological) notions of consciousness, introspection and self. Whether the introduction of the notion of *Verstehen* has been equally useful remains to be seen. Current difficulties in mapping out the semantic structure of insight are due to the uncertain origins of the concept.

ACKNOWLEDGEMENT To Dr I.S. Marková from Cambridge for her great help with the writing of the section on insight.

NOTES

1 Wilkes, for example, has argued that the chances of consciousness ever becoming an *explanandum* are 'slim', p. 38, Wilkes, 1988.
2 In its relation to consciousness see Neumann, 1964; Gurwitsch, 1957; also the important chapter by Blanc, 1966; Valla, 1992 and Globus, 1975.
3 Globus, 1975.
4 Tolman, 1927; on the conceptual consequences of radical behaviourism, see pp. 49–89, Fodor, 1968, and chapters in Globus *et al.*, 1976; Burt's defence of consciousness against behaviourism remains fresh; Burt, 1962.
5 Ey, 1963; Lapassade, 1897; Vizioli and Bietti, 1966; Churchland *et al.*, 1988; Milner and Rugg, 1992. For a defence of the view that consciousness should be studied by means other than introspection, see Rosenthal, 1986. Of late, the field has started moving again although it remains to be seen whether these ideas will actually influence psychiatry (Baars, 1988; Dennett, 1993; Flanagan, 1992; Bock and Marsh, 1993; Rovonsuo and Kampinnen, 1994). For a pessimistic view on the accessibility of consciousness to philosophical or empirical study, see McGinn, 1991.
6 Abbagnano (1961) states in this regard: 'In truth, it does not seem to be the case that Greek philosophy recognized the privileged reality of mental interiority'. Hamilton (1859) is equally clear: 'In Greek there was no term for consciousness until the decline of philosophy . . . Plato and Aristotle, to say nothing of other philosophers, had no special term to express the knowledge which the mind affords of the operations of its faculties'
(p. 197).
7 425b, 10, 15, Aristotle, 1968.
8 Hamlyn has commented that the problem Aristotle poses is impossible to solve, p. 122, Notes. *Aristotle's De Anima*, 1968.
9 p. 199, Hamilton, 1859.
10 Abbagnano, 1961.
11 'Neither can life and cogitation, sense and consciousness ever result from magnitudes, figures, sites and motions' p. 93, Cudworth R. *The Intellectual System of the Universe*, London, 1837 (first edition, 1678).

12 'Consciousness is the perception of what passes in a man's own mind'.
    Book II, Chapter I, Para 19, Locke, 1959.
13 Jacobs, 1973.
14 Abbagnano, 1961.
15 Part I, Principle IX, p. 222, *The Philosophical Works of Descartes*, 1967.
16 A good example of this is a well-known lecture by Erwin Strauss where
    he spends a fair time dealing with Descartes's notion of consciousness:
    'More correctly, one should say, consciousness is alone with itself';
    p. 142, Strauss, 1958.
17 Cohen, 1984.
18 There is no space here for expanding upon the history of consciousness
    during the eighteenth century. For the contribution of the British
    Empiricists to the creation of *la conscience psychologique*, see Brunschvicg,
    1927.
19 p. 172, Mill, 1869.
20 pp. 222–223, Reid, 1854. In a footnote (p. 223), Hamilton commented:
    'Reid's degradation of Consciousness into a special faculty (in which he
    seems to have followed Hutcheson, in opposition to other philosophers),
    is, in every point of view, obnoxious to every possible objection.'
    Hamilton returned to this issue in his Lectures, see pp. 207–212 where
    he considers the view of consciousness as a 'special faculty' as a
    'degradation' of its higher role and 'untenable', Hamilton, 1859.
21 'Nothing has contributed more to spread obscurity over a very
    transparent matter, than the attempts of philosophers to define
    consciousness. Consciousness cannot be defined . . .' pp. 191–192,
    Hamilton, 1859.
22 According to the *OED* (second edition), the term awareness appeared in
    technical language only during the early nineteenth century and it is
    unlikely that its etymological history will contribute to an understanding
    of the phenomenon in question; hence it will be considered here as a
    synonym of consciousness.
23 pp. 599–610, Bain, 1859.
24 pp. 120–122, Garnier, 1852. Garnier was one of the French Roman
    Catholic spiritualist philosophers influenced by Thomas Reid.
25 Leff, 1991.
26 Davies, 1873.
27 Bastian, 1870.
28 Riese, 1954.
29 Dagonet, 1881.
30 Shaw, 1909.
31 Darwin, 1904.
32 p. 83, Darwin, 1883. Darwin follows on this a view which had been
    clearly expressed by Sir Charles Bell decades earlier: pp. 121–141, Bell,
    1844.
33 pp. 194–212, Romanes, 1888.
34 p. 335, Morgan, 1903.
35 On this concept, see MacKinnon, 1924. On 'supervenience,' the modern
    equivalent of emergence, see Kim, 1993.

36 pp. 74–75, Ribot, 1889. For a full discussion of Ribot's views on consciousness see: Evans, 1970.

37 The term had been in ordinary English at least since the seventeenth century (*OED*, 2nd edition). There is no space in this chapter to deal with introspection in any depth (for this see Boring, 1953; Danziger, 1980; Lyons, 1986).

38 pp. 35–38, Garrabé, 1989.

39 p. 83, Hamilton, 1974: 'unfortunately, this word is used in everyday speech to mean 'muddled', 'bewildered', or 'perplexed' and some English speaking psychiatrists use the word in this sense . . .'. This observation is correct, and the usage in question reflects (as it is explained below) the different conceptual pedigree of 'confusion' which during the nineteenth century was not conceptualized as a disorder of consciousness but of association of ideas!.

40 i.e. the *Ninth Revision of the International Classification of Diseases*, 1978. The term has disappeared from ICD-10.

41 Scharfetter, 1980.

42 American Psychiatric Association, DSM III, 1980.

43 Wing *et al.*, 1974.

44 Anonymous, Confusión, 1921.

45 Defined 'negatively', as an aberration of the logical doctrine of clarity and distinctness of thought (Abbagnano, 1961).

46 Eisler, 1904; Grimm and Grimm, 1956.

47 Mill, 1898.

48 Jourdan, 1813.

49 The terms *confusion de idées* and *obtusion* were used for the first time by Delasiauve in 1851 in the context of a famous analysis of the stuporous states associated with severe lypemania (depression). (Delasiauve, 1851).

50 Claparède, 1903; Warren, 1921.

51 Hoeldtke, 1967; Bricke, 1974; Billod, 1855.

52 Grimm and Grimm, 1956.

53 Wille, 1888.

54 p. 345, Griesinger (1861) calls Dementia *Die Verwirrtheit*.

55 Fritsch, 1879.

56 See, for example, his paper at the Vienna Medical Meeting in 1881 (Meynert, 1881). In 1890, Meynert proposed a separation of *Verwirrtheit* from the rest of the psychosis, suggesting as its central symptom the experience of bewilderment (*Ratlosigkeit*) (Meynert, 1890) (for an excellent study, Pappenheim, 1975; also Lévy-Friesacher, 1983).

57 Wille, 1888.

58 Tuke, 1892.

59 Power and Sedwick, 1892.

60 Therein confusion is defined both as a symptom ('a condition of embarrassment, distraction, or lack of clearness of thought and appropriateness of action') and as a disease (a variety of 'amentia', called also 'confusional amentia'. Another variety is stupidity or *amentia stupida*. A third variety is hallucinatory acute insanity . . .'). The subtypes were taken from Wille, 1888 (Morselli, 1901).

61 Chaslin, 1892; 1895.

62 Bleuler, 1911.

63 Zeh, 1960.

64 See Chapter 12, this book.

65 Chaslin, 1892.

66 Norman, 1890.

67 Bolton, 1906; Bruce, 1935.

68 On the life of this great mathematician and alienist, see Daumezón, 1973.

69 Chaslin, 1892.

70 Séglas, 1894.

71 Chaslin, 1895.

72 *Automatisme* names a psychological mechanism that since the 1880s has enjoyed much popularity in French psychiatry. It described the release of 'lower mental functions' from the control of higher ones resulting from weakening or dissolution. Ribot's interest in Spencer had led him to Hughlings Jackson, from whom he borrowed the central idea (Delay, 1953; Balan, 1989; Baruk, 1972. Janet followed Ribot's ideas (Janet, 1889). The hierarchical model of the mind implicit in Chaslin's definition of confusion was Jacksonian in origin.

73 Régis and Hesnard, 1911.

74 On the history of *stupidité*, see Berrios, 1981, Stupor: a conceptual history.

75 Baillarger, 1843.

76 Delasiauve, 1851.

77 Binet and Simon, 1911.

78 Binet and Simon, 1910.

79 Chaslin, 1915.

80 Karl Bonhoeffer started the view that delirium was a stereotyped response to any brain insult, and that symptoms did not reflect aetiology (Bonhoeffer, 1910; 1917; Bleuler *et al.*, 1966; Redlich, 1912. (On Bonhoeffer, see Neumarker, 1990; also Fleck, 1956.)

81 The debate is reported in the minutes of three meetings (29 March to 31 May) of the *Société Médico-Psychologique*, 1923.

82 Chaslin, 1920.

83 Toulouse *et al.*, 1920.

84 Auto-conduction was the name for a psychological mechanism that enjoyed transient popularity in France around the Great War. It meant something between 'self-deportment' and 'ego self-organization' and involved those voluntary and involuntary aspects of personality which are supposed to fulfil an adaptational function.

85 Toulouse *et al.* were not the first to suggest this approach. There had been already books and papers on the subject (Sommer, 1899; Binet and Simon, 1905; Jaspers, 1910).

86 Porot, 1975.

87 On these, see Berrios, On Stupor: a conceptual history, 1981; Berrios, On Melancholic Stupor, 1990. The history of melancholic stupor and that of confusion are also closely related to that of Catatonia.

88 Pinel, 1809.

89 Georget, 1820.

90 Étoc-Demazy, 1833.

91 During the 1840s, melancholia was still used in its old sense; hence, in addition to *psychotic depression* it included catatonic schizophrenias, what would now be called cycloid psychoses, and other functional and organic psychotic states (see Chapter 12, this book).

92 Baillarger, 1843; see also Camuset, 1897.

93 Delasiauve, 1851.

94 Sauze, 1853.

95 Baillarger, 1853.

96 The case was widely reported in the Parisian press, and the ensuing debate throws light on the uneasy relationship between press, alienists, and the public during the Second Empire. The central issue was whether Mr Della F. was a simulator. Although there is little doubt that he was suffering from catatonic stupor, at the time suspicions were aroused by the fact (common in this condition) that he occasionally talked to himself or showed defensive movements such as removing the bed cover from his face. The debate that followed, in which Morel, Moreau, Voisin, Linas, Berthier, and Foville intervened, shows how rigidly diagnostic criteria were adhered to: because it was assumed that stupor consisted of a total inhibition of psychological function, no movement or speech were allowed (societé-médico-psychologique, 1869).

97 Ritti, 1883.

98 Griesinger, 1861.

99 Newington, 1874.

100 Term introduced by Bellini during the seventeenth century (Berthier, 1869).

101 Kahlbaum, 1874; see also Mora, 1973 and Llopis, 1954.

102 See Chapter 8, this book.

103 Since the middle of the century (Delasiauve, 1851), *obtusion* had also been used to name the confusional state. However, the term was not fully synonymous with confusion in that it emphasized a different aspect of the mental state and derived from a different metaphor. Obtusion referred to blurring of consciousness and not to the incapacity to associate ideas.

104 Krafft-Ebing, 1893; Hoch, 1921.

105 Ryle, 1949.

106 Its role consisting in periodic updating of time and space information. Metzger, 1954.

107 See particularly the latter's great book: Grasset, 1901.

108 For example, Sommer asked: What is your name? Your job? Where are you? Where do you live? What year is it? What month? What date? What day? How long are you here? What town is this? etc. (Sommer, 1899).

109 Finzi, 1899.

110 Bouchard, 1926.

111 The relevance of this technique to time orientation has been since called into question (Benton *et al.*, 1964 and McFie, 1960).

112 Klein, 1967.

113 *Oxford English Dictionary* (second edition).

114 Mott, 1899.

115 Dupuytren, 1834; Sutton, 1813.

116 Falret, 1865; Winslow, 1861.

117 Bercherie, 1980.

118 Janet, 1919.

119 König, 1912.

120 Jaspers, 1963.

121 Bleuler, 1924.

122 Régis, 1906.

123 Jung, 1964.

124 Bleuler, 1950.

125 Kraepelin, 1919.

126 Minkowski, 1926; 1927.

127 Schilder, 1936.

128 Seeman, 1976.

129 Conrad, 1960; Schneider, 1948.

130 This symptom is a typical example of the ways in which the metaphor of perception has been applied to consciousness. The latter was said to have a focus and a periphery, and either could become disordered. Thus were born symptoms such as narrow, acute, oscillating, or clouded consciousness. The latter proved particularly difficult to define, and since the 1930s it was made tantamount to disorientation.

131 Wieck, 1961.

132 Lipowski, 1980.

133 Bonhoeffer, 1910.

134 Vesanic delirium was also called: cold, apyretic, or chronic; the non-vesanic hot, febrile or acute. The distinction was first made by Achilles Foville in 1869 (p. 357, Ball and Ritti, 1881).

135 General histories of psychiatry tend to claim that the modern concept of mental illness (by this it is usually meant the psychoses) is based on Bayle's 'discovery', i.e. that changes in the brain lead to changes in mental functioning. Whilst this may have confirmed the *causal* views implicit in the anatomo-clinical model of disease, it did not provide a clinical model, i.e. the view that the psychoses are characterized by hallucinations, delusions, behavioural disorder, insightlessness, and loss of cognitive grasp and reality testing. This originated from the analysis of delirium (Berrios, 1981; also Zilboorg, 1941; Leibbrand and Wettley, 1961; Acknerknecht, 1957).

136 Sakai, 1991.

137 Hippocrates, 1972.

138 Roccatagliata, 1973; Simon, 1978.

139 Hankoff, 1972.

140 1.4.42, p. 66, Sydenham, 1666.

141 1684, Willis, pp. 209–214.

142 Cullen, 1827.

143 Esquirol, 1814; Middleton, 1780; Sutton, 1813.

144 Feuchtersleben, 1845.

145 Siegel, 1973.

146 p. 103, Quincy, 1719.

147 Johnson, 1755.

148 Sutton, 1813.

149 Such as *Allophasis, Desipientia, Insipientia, Karabitus, Leros, Paracope, Paracrusis, Paranaea, Paraphora, Paraphrenesis,* and *Paraphrosyne* (Mayne, 1860).

150 Ball and Ritti, 1881.

151 Pinel, 1809.

152 This can be illustrated by the confusion caused by the translator of Pinel who rendered *délire* as delirium even when the context makes it clear that Pinel meant delusion (see Pinel, 1806).

153 Esquirol, 1814.

154 Georget, 1820.

155 Georget, 1835.

156 Lasègue, 1852.

157 p. 354, Falret, 1864.

158 Littré, 1877.

159 Such has been the linguistic confusion that in the first World Congress of Psychiatry (Paris, 1950) Honorio Delgado, a Peruvian psychiatrist, proposed that the word 'delusion' be universally used to mean what it does in English (p. 100, Discussion. Honorio Delgado. In Ey *et al.*, 1952).

160 Feuchtersleben, 1847.

161 Brierre de Boismont, 1845.

162 Leader, 1864.

163 Griesinger, 1861.

164 Ball and Ritti, 1881; p. 97, Gowers, 1893.

165 Calmeil, 1859.

166 Worcester, 1889.

167 For a full account of this doctrine, see Vliegen, 1980; Mundt and Saß, 1992; Berrios and Beer, 1994.

168 For example, of Brierre's eleven cases, seven died (Brierre de Boismont, 1845).

169 Sauri, 1972; Berrios, On historical aspects of the psychoses, 1987.

170 Degeneration theory is touched upon in other chapters of this book; see also Morel, 1857; Genil-Perrin, 1913.

171 Magnan, 1866–7; Magnan and Sérieux, 1911; Berrios and Hauser, 1988.

172 p. 115, in Griesinger, 1861.

173 Lasègue, 1881.

174 For a biographical account, see Paz, 1964; also Dowbiggin, 1990.

175 Maury, 1878.

176 A good start is the useful but incomplete essay by Ey, 1954.

177 p. 461, Porot, 1975.

178 1906, Régis, pp. 293–297.

179 See, for example, pp. 307–310, Ey *et al.*, 1974.

180 Lewis, 1934.

181 Marková and Berrios, 1995.

182 Marková and Berrios, 1992.

183 Richfield, 1954.

184 See Chapter 5, this book.

185 As late as 1875, Prosper Despine discussed in detail two senses of 'lucidité': 'in the work of the alienists, the word lucidity has been used in two ways; one is a synonym of reason and refers to the moment when the mental faculties become normal; ... the other has been defined by Trélat as the sparing of the intellect in cases where the other mental faculties are diseased' pp. 312–314, Despine, 1875. Ulysse Trélat (1795–1879) was a creative thinker whose busy political life prevented him from contributing further to psychiatry (see Morel, 1988). The work quoted by Despine was *La Folie Lucide*, a rather old-fashioned book, probably written much earlier, where Trélat studied a heterogeneous group of patients whose common denominator was that 'in spite of their illness, they responded exactly to the questions and did not seem insane to the superficial observer' although their behaviour betrayed their condition (p. XXX, Trélat, 1861). A few years earlier, in a very popular forensic work, Legrand defined the lucid interval as: 'an absolute albeit temporary suspension of the manifestations of insanity. It can be observed in about 25% of manics, less frequently in melancholia, rarely in monomania, never in dementia.' (pp. 109–110, Legrand, 1864).

186 On monomania, see Chapter 6, this book.

187 Well into the nineteenth century see Ernest Martini stating: *Le symptome propre et essentiel à la folie, celui qui commence et finit avec elle, est le délire* (p. 3, Martini, 1824).

188 See Chapter 5, this book.

189 p. 118, on Mental Alienation, in Fabre, 1840.

190 See Ackerknecht, 1967, López Piñero, 1983.

191 A typical example was Jules Falret who wrote: 'I firmly believe, both from a theoretical and practical point of view, that there is complete solidarity of the various faculties of the human mind both in the sane and the insane. In reasoning mania (*folie raisonnante*) clinical observation shows that, although the moral faculties are predominantly involved, there is also involvement of intellect'. 'The fundamental mistake in the work of alienists this century has been to import to the study of the mentally ill the divisions of the mind created by psychologists to study normal individuals' (pp. 384–385, Falret, 1866).

192 Xavier Bichat (1771–1802) developed a viable 'tissue theory' which forced changes in the very concept of the 'localization of disease' (see d'istria, 1926; Albury, 1977; Haigh, 1984).

193 On this admittedly anachronistic usage, see Fodor, 1983.

194 On the relevance of phrenology to the development of psychopathology, see Chapter 2, this book.

195 Kageyama, 1984.
196 société médico-psychologique, 1866.
197 p. 220, Maudsley, 1885.
198 For these three notions, see this Chapter, above.
199 For the notion of self, see Chapter 18, this book.
200 Unless a sort of 'dispositional', Rylean account is offered according to which to have insight is defined as 'the disposition to behave in a particular way' (pp. 116–198, Ryle, 1949).
201 Bollotte, 1973.
202 Moreau de Tours, 1845.
203 Lyons, 1986.
204 See Marková, 1988.
205 Brentano, 1973; Fancher, 1977.
206 Dilthey, 1976; Martin-Santos, 1955.
207 For background references, see Berrios, On Phenomenology and Jaspers, 1992.
208 'Experience shows that there exist in us not only a presentation and a judgment, but frequently a third kind of consciousness of the mental act, namely a feeling which refers to this act, pleasure or displeasure which we feel towards this act' (p. 143, Brentano, 1973).
209 Apel, 1987; McCarthy, 1972; Makkreel, 1975; López Moreno, 1990. *Verstehen* is not a transparent concept. Dilthey defined it in opposition to 'explanation' and hence it is supposed to be more mediate and to involve more mental functions than the mere intellectual grasping provided by explanations. 'Understanding presupposes experience and experience only becomes knowledge of life if understanding leads us from the narrowness and subjectivity of experience to the whole and the general' (pp. 187–188, Dilthey, 1976).
210 Richfield, 1954.
211 pp. 150–151, Pauleikhoff and Mester (in Müller, 1973).
212 *In den späteren Stadien des Irreseins, da wo systematische Wahn-ideen oder ein geistiger Zerfall eingetreten sind, ist der Kranke absolute einsichtslos für seinen krankhaften Zustand . . .'* p. 102, Krafft-Ebing, 1893.
213 pp. 312–314, Despine, 1875.
214 Sérieux and Capgras, 1909.
215 p. 210, Störring, 1907.
216 p. 147, Mendel, 1907.
217 Dagonet, 1881.
218 p. 369, Dagonet, 1881.
219 p. 370, Dagonet, 1881.
220 p. 389, Dagonet, 1881.
221 p. 393, Dagonet, 1881.
222 p. 20, Dagonet, part II, 1881.
223 p. 8, Maudsley, 1895.
224 Victor Parant was one of the great clinicians of the second half of the century. He also did important work in neuropsychiatry, particularly the mental symptoms of Parkinson's disease. See Chapter 17, this book.

225 p. 174, Parant, 1888.

226 p. 177–179, Parant, 1888. Echoes of Parant's classification can be found in twentieth century French psychiatry, in a recent tripartite classification of *la réaction consciente du malade á l'égard de son état morbide*' (pp. 85–88, Deshaeis, 1967).

227 p. 196, Parant, 1888.

228 pp. 406–407, Shaw, 1909.

229 p. 25, Kraepelin, 1919.

230 p. 26, Kraepelin, 1919.

231 p. 420, Jaspers, 1948.

232 Conrad, 1958.

PART III

Mood and emotions

CHAPTER 11

Anxiety and cognate disorders

Whilst the history of the neuroses[1] in general, and that of hysteria[2], hypochondria[3] and obsessive–compulsive disorder[4] in particular, have received historical attention, the evolution of what is nowadays known as 'generalized anxiety disorder', 'panic disorder', and 'phobia' has been neglected.[5] This may be due to their relative newness; or to the fact that the historical model used to account for the traditional *nervous disorders* is inappropriate for the *new neuroses*.[6]

This does not mean that the individual symptoms now included under the 'anxiety disorders' are themselves new. Indeed, they have been known since time immemorial;[7] the only difference being that, in the past, they were reported in different social and medical contexts. For example, during the eighteenth century such symptoms were considered to be specific diseases or, less frequently, included under the syndromic domain of other diseases. The *novelty* has been that, during the 1890s, these symptoms were rescued from their earlier niches and put together into what was then claimed were *independent* clinical conditions. The notion that these symptoms could all be the *manifestation* of a unitary construct called 'anxiety' is also new, at least is alien to pre-Freudian psychiatry. The historical and ideological factors that led to this state of affairs need disentangling.

By the 1860s, and before the final synthesis took place, such symptoms could be found in clinical realms as disparate as cardiovascular, inner ear, gastrointestinal, or neurological medicine. Basically, each symptom seems to have been taken *at face* value and treated as a real 'physical' complaint. This is one reason why they were mostly reported in *medical* (not psychiatric) journals. Likewise, their 'treatment' had little to do with 'psychiatric' practice; indeed, asylum alienists rarely dealt with such symptoms before the turn of the century.

Conventionally, the symptoms of 'anxiety' have been listed under two headings. Subjective ones (i.e. those felt as 'psychological' experiences) include fear, emotional worries, feelings of terror, depersonalization, etc, and also cognitive mental acts such as obsession-like thoughts concerning the safety of others, fear of dying, etc. Objective ones, also called somatic, (and sometimes anxiety equivalents) are referred to changes in a putative bodily system and include abdominal pain, nausea, vertigo, dizziness, palpitations, dry mouth, hot flushes, hyperventilation, breathlessness, headache, restless legs, and other bodily experiences sometimes indistinguishable from complaints caused by physical disease.

According to personality, culture, social class and other variables not yet identified, subjects may present these symptoms in different combinations. If some of these latter clusters are repetitive and stable enough, they may be called syndromes and even diseases. Sometimes, predominant somatic symptoms may mimic heart attacks or inner ear disorder; or subjective symptoms alone may present as phenocopies of physical diseases such as temporal lobe epilepsy. If the subjective symptoms are diffuse and more or less continuous they are called generalized anxiety disorder; if paroxysmal, panic attack. The latter are known to be mostly spontaneous but when triggered by a recognizable stimulus (whether heights, or going out, or spiders, etc.) they have been called 'phobias' and named after the stimulus. The current (fashionable) view that 'crises of anxiety' ('panic disorder') constitute a separate disease is very new. Since the 1900s, such attacks have been considered as part of the anxiety neurosis; before then they were associated with conditions such as neurasthenia and psychasthenia,[8] and even before considered to be cardiovascular[9] or inner ear disorders.[10]

A historical account of the origin of the modern concept of anxiety disorder and its allied clinical states should deal with questions such as: 1. Why were such symptoms and signs – often dissimilar in appearance – brought together under the same banner? 2. Was this the result of clinical observation or of theoretical and social pressure? 3. Were these states considered as exaggerations of 'normal' psychological phenomena, or as 'morbid' forms? 4. How relevant to their inception were late in neteenth century theories of emotion and developing views on the functions of the 'ganglionar' (autonomic) nervous system? It goes without saying that the history of anxiety can also be studied from a metaphysical, social, poetic and religious perspective. This chapter focuses only on its 'medical' aspects.

The word anxiety and cognates

The view suggested by Ey[11] that *anxiété* gained its *medical meaning* at the end of the nineteenth century needs rectification. Eighteenth century nosologists – including those whose mother tongue was French – already had made use of the Latin term to describe paroxysmal states of 'restlessness' and *inquietude*. For example, *anxietas* is used by Boissier de Sauvages, Linné, Vogel, and Sagar.[12] In addition, *panophobia*, *vertigo*, *palpitatio*, *suspirium*, and *oscitatio* (all redolent of anxiety and panic attacks) were used to refer to complaints that Continental nosologists considered as physical diseases. It is important to remark that no one of these clinical states was ever considered as belonging in the vesania category (i.e. with the mental disorders). The Scottish physicians McBride and Cullen were far more economical in their nosological classification, and the nearest Cullen got to describing a somatic symptom of anxiety was his *palpitatio melancholica*.[13]

Early in the nineteenth century, the French Landré-Beauvais[14] defined anxiety as: 'a certain malaise, restlessness, excessive agitation' and used the word *angoisse*; he suggested that such symptom may accompany 'acute' and 'chronic' diseases. There is little doubt that Landré attempted to conceptualize anxiety as a syndrome including both subjective and somatic components and which might accompany diverse diseases (see below). In 1858, Littré and Robin defined *angoisse* as 'feelings of closeness or pressure on the epigastric region, accompanied by a great difficulty in breathing and excessive sadness; it is the most advanced degree of anxiety'[15]; and *anxiété* as 'troubled and agitated state, with feelings of difficulty in breathing and pressure on the precordial region: inquietude, anxiety and anguish are three stages of the same phenomenon.'[16]

Lewis has analysed the way in which the etymology of anxiety, anguish, and angor influenced the clinical conceptualization of the anxiety states.[17] To this it must be added that, whilst the dichotomy 'anxiety-anguish' has little clinical meaning in Anglo-Saxon psychiatry (the term *anguish*, in fact, never gained a place in medical terminology), it found a comfortable niche in France, Germany, and Spain where the terms *Angoisse*, *Angst*, and *Angustia* (respectively) carry distinct meaning, and refer to the paroxysmal and more severe aspects of the disorder. Also playing on the etymology of the term anxiety, Sarbin constructed an argument to demonstrate that the symptom was but a metaphor.[18] Unfortunately, historical inaccuracy[19] and loose argument, mar his interesting ideas.[20]

'Anxiety'-related behaviours

Irrespective of the name these states travelled under (i.e. of the history of the words), or of how they were explained (the history of the concepts), *behaviours* recognizable as 'anxiety-related' are found described in the literature of the ages.[21] Altschule, for example, reminds us that writers such as Arnold, Locke, Battie, Mead, Smith, and Crichton described medical states of inquietude and uneasiness.[22] This chapter, however, will only deal with such behaviours, concepts or words as they feature in the clinical theatre of the nineteenth century and after.

By the early nineteenth century, anxiety symptoms began to be included under various medical categories rather than being considered independently (as had been customary the previous century); for example, Pinel included anxiety symptoms under 'epilepsy',[23] melancholia,[24] rabies (particularly of the 'spontaneous' variety),[25] and the 'motility' neuroses.[26] The same can be said of Georget in whose book some of these symptoms were discussed in the section on 'general and sympathetic symptoms'.[27] Likewise, Griesinger[28] – quoting Guislain[29] – reported that 9% of insanities start with acute 'fear'.

During this period, however, terms and meanings could not yet be easily exchanged between the languages of psychiatry of Germany, England and France. For example, where Guislain had written *craintes* and *frayeurs*,[30] Griesinger translated *Shrecken oder Angst*,[31] and Robertson and Rutherford (the English translators of Griesinger) 'shock or anxiety'.[32] This subtle drift of meaning from *frayeur* to *Angst* and anxiety reflects well the evolution of this symptom during the middle of the nineteenth century and after. For whilst Guislain was only referring to acute fear, Griesinger introduced *Angst*, a term which, after the publication of Kirkegaard's book in 1844,[33] had acquired a special meaning which went well beyond 'fear'. Apart from reflecting Kirkegaard's own morbid psychology,[34] the term brought into play the new epistemological and religious dimensions that Kirkegaard attached to his notion of 'anguish'.[35]

The term 'nervousness', used to encompassed most of the *subjective* aspects of the anxiety states, is another example. Thus, the anonymous reviewer[36] of Bouchut's book on *Nervosisme*[37] complained of its vagueness but remarked that there was no good alternative in the English language. It seems clear both from the points made by the reviewer, and from Bouchut's quotations, that the monograph was not only about hysteria or hypochondria (as it would have been expected during this period) but also about anxiety and its somatic accompaniments.[38]

'Anxiety' as a cause of mental disorder

Around this same time, and with his usual clinical acumen, Feuchtersleben wrote: 'Intense anxiety and grief lead us to expect organic affections of the heart and of the larger vessels, fretfulness, dejection, discontent and a disordered digestion.'[39] The Austrian writer was not discussing, however, diseases as such but the relationship of body and mind; hence his 'psychosomatic' remarks seem to have remained unnoticed. A few years earlier, Prichard had written along the same lines: 'Care and anxiety, distress, grief, and mental disturbances are by far the most productive causes of insanity', 'Anxiety and agitation of mind caused by political events have occasionally produced a very decided effect on the number of persons becoming deranged.'[40] Bucknill and Tuke echoed these words in their discussion of the effect of modern civilization on insanity: 'The very same person is possibly, also, the subject of ever-present anxiety and apprehension, in consequence of a precarious income.'[41] Amongst the unpublished manuscripts left by Alfred Wigan, there was a rambly piece on 'Anxiety' where the author describes the social difficulties caused by this experience.[42]

Thus, it seems clear that, by the mid-nineteenth century, the term anxiety was used in medical writings to describe a mental state that fell within the range of normal human experiences but was able to cause or lead to disease, including insanity.

MODELS AND EXPLANATIONS After the 1850s, the views that anxiety may be a cause of insanity but also a disease in its own right became increasingly conflated. Some have suggested that the work of Griesinger led to a period of rampant 'organicism' from which psychiatry was rescued by the work of Janet and Freud. This is inaccurate. It is true that the anatomoclinical model was influential, but it is also the case that its application to mental illness was governed by what here will be called (for lack of a better name) an 'open causal chain' mechanism; i.e. the belief that the brain lesions causing psychiatric symptoms were themselves caused by psychological trauma (anxiety being a prime candidate) and negative life events. In other words, psychological factors could start the causal chain leading to insanity. The analysis of the role played by anxiety during this period may illustrate this point. Thus, after the 1860s, *physiopathological* mechanisms were marshalled by alienists to explain how mental symptoms led to anatomical changes in the brain.[43]

By the early twentieth century, four views were available to account for the development of mental illness: 1. 'genetic', as expressed by degeneration theory,[44] 2. 'constitutional' as per Dupré[45] and Duprat,[46] 3. 'chaotic', according to which the breakdown in mental function resulted from total brain failure,[47] 4. 'hierarchical'[48] or 'ethological'[49] models, according to which mental symptoms resulted from the release of lower or atavic functions, and 5. functional accounts not dependent upon the anatomoclinical view.[50] Most of these views originated, in fact, during the nineteenth century, and alienists support combinations thereof.

Symptoms and syndromes

MOREL AND HIS *DÉLIRE EMOTIF* In 1866, Morel suggested that pathological changes (or a *neurosis* of) the ganglionic (autonomic) nervous system gave rise to symptoms which he called 'emotional delusions' (*délire emotif*). Analysis of his clinical reports shows that his view is an important departure from the traditional explanation of fears and anxieties. Morel's cases showed subjective (anxiety, phobias and obsessions)[51] and objective complaints, the latter referring to the skin, and the cardiovascular, gastrointestinal, and nervous systems. At least two of his patients showed classical 'panic attacks' and generalized anxiety disorder (although in retrospective diagnosis and on account of their age, they were probably secondary to a depressive illness).[52]

Morel combined recent knowledge on the 'ganglionar system' (started in the work of Bichat and Johnstone)[53] with Willis's metaphor of 'sympathy' of functions[54] to explain the particular clustering of symptoms which, until then, have been considered as unrelated. By making reference to the ganglionar system he also complied with the anatomo-clinical model of disease. He asked: What symptoms are directly due to pathological changes in the ganglionar system? His answer was that these included *both* subjective and objective complaints.

In 1860, Morel had proposed, in a separate work, to substitute symptomatic by aetiological classifications,[55] the idea being that dissimilar symptoms might prove to be related via the same anatomical locus. His 1866 paper provided alienists with the mechanism to bring together disparate symptoms on the grounds that they were all caused by a disturbance of the ganglionic system. But the paper also marks the point of origin of a group of 'neurotic' conditions (here called the 'new neuroses') which were to run parallel to the traditional ones (i.e. hysteria and hypochondriasis). It must be noted that, whilst these latter two conditions were beginning to lose their 'organicity' (via the notion of functional lesion and irritability),[56] the link with the ganglionar system kept the anxiety and obsessional[57] disorders linked to the 'organic' model for longer.

KRISHABER Morel's views found expression in Krishaber's 'cerebro-cardiac neurosis'. Maurice Krishaber (1836–1883) was a Hungarian ear–nose–throat specialist, trained and working in France, whose main area of research had, in fact, been the pathology of the larynx, and the physiology of singing.[58] In 1873, he published a classical monograph reporting 38 cases suffering from 'cerebro-cardiac neurosis'. After criticising the inadequacy of clinical categories such as nervousness, proteiform neuropathy, spasmodic state, etc. to describe his condition, he divided its symptoms into those affecting sensation, movement, circulation, and others. On clinical grounds, he differentiated the new disease from hysteria, hypochondria, chlorosis, cerebrovascular syndromes and toxic states. He also suggested that his illness was due to a pathological instability of the blood vessels and that its symptoms responded to caffeine. His patients showed remarkable homogeneity, with an even incidence (higher than 80%) of anxiety, light-headedness, vertigo, palpitations, tinnitus, tremor, gastrointestinal symptoms (nausea, indigestion and diarrhoea), intolerance to noise, photophobia and inability to concentrate.[59]

Krishaber died young but his views were influential. Instead of trying to encompass all the symptoms related to the ganglionar system, he chose those seemingly representing a 'lability' of the cardiovascular system. The new 'neurosis' provided internists with a God-sent explanation for the anxiety symptoms, and caffeine became for a while a popular form of treatment.[60]

VERTIGO AND ANXIETY The feeling of vertigo had been fully described in Classical times, but during the nineteenth century accounts began to be offered of its nosological associations.[61] For example, the work of Trastour on *vertigo nerveux*, and Axenfeld's discussion of subjects experiencing vertigo in social situations or after 'over-exertion' of the intellect.[62] In his award-winning study on vertigo in the insane, Millet reported cases where vertigo was part of a panic attack. The most illustrative of these being that of an ex-soldier who, on crossing la Place de la Bastille, would suddenly feel shaky, dizzy, with vertigo and experience an irresistible need to run; he would then become suicidal. Retrospective diagnosis of this case suggests an agoraphobic syndrome secondary to severe depression.[63] Weill also wrote on the *vertiges des névroses* characterised by 'anguish, palpitations, and headaches'[64] and which accompanied epilepsy, insanity, neurasthenia, and the 'cerebro-cardiac neuropathy' of Krishaber. These states are redolent of typical panic attacks.

In his full review, Leroux reported that vertigo was one of the central symptoms of agoraphobia (as described by Westphal in 1872 and Legrand du Saulle in 1877 – see below), and that it was similar to what Lasègue had called *vertige mental*.[65] Leroux also suggested that vertigo might accompany severe lypemania (i.e. depressive illness).[66] In this case the vertigo included: 'sensations of overwhelming precordial and epigastric anxiety, added to a feeling of impending fainting and collapse with weakness of the legs. There was also the sensation that the ground sunk, and that perceptions became misty. Anguish was the predominant component of the attack, and this translates itself in pallor, dyspnoea, cold sweating. The subject could not reason any more. He knew that there was no real danger but was incapable of controlling his worries. He might become paralysed or act in a discontrolled manner.'[67] A clearer description of panic attacks cannot be found. It is also likely that Haltenhof's cases of 'paralysing vertigo' were anxiety attacks.[68] Grasset also refers in his treatise to the vertigo of neurasthenia and hysteria.[69]

BENEDIKT, WESTPHAL, DU SAULLE, AND AGORAPHOBIA The 'organic' approach to the anxiety disorders also developed in other directions. For example, Benedikt[70] related panic attacks to pathological changes in the inner ear, and Westphal explained agoraphobia as vertigo of similar origin. Indeed, in his rueful autobiography, Benedikt[71] claimed that he had been the first to describe the condition of *Platzschwindel*, and that Westphal never acknowledged his idea.[72] Legrand du Saulle, however, with his usual clinical acumen was the first to realize that the feelings reported by these subjects were not, in fact, those of *objective vertigo* but only of *fear* that they might lose their balance. His description is classical: 'by the term *peur des espaces* I refer to a particular neuropathic state, characterized by a feeling of anguish and terror, without loss of consciousness, which occurs in an open space, and which is different from vertigo . . . This psychological disturbance has not been described in France, except by Perroud's writing on agoraphobia in 1873. This term, accepted by Cordes[73] and Westphal,[74] seems to me to be too narrow for it does not cover all the many symptoms of the cases described. Patients may fear spaces, but also streets and theatres, travelling by public transport, boats and bridges.'[75]

The nosological status of 'agoraphobia', however, was unclear at the time. Some alienists, like Ball and Gros, suggested that it was a form of psychosis.[76] Others, like Dagonet, regarded it as a hereditary, *sui generis*, mental disorder.[77] Hartenberg, in turn, suggested that agoraphobia was a learned behaviour in which anticipation played a major role.[78]

With hindsight, these difficulties were partially due to the fact that, up to this period, phobias and obsessions had not yet been clearly distinguished.[79] One of the first to attempt such separation was Ribot who, after criticizing the useless coining of 'pseudo-Greek' terms to name each specific phobia, distinguished between *pantophobia* (i.e. generalized anxiety states)[80] and specific phobias, and divided the latter into two groups: 'the first is connected with fear, and includes all manifestations implying in any degree whatsoever the fear of pain, from that of a fall or the prick of a needle to that of illness or death. The second is directly connected with disgust, and seems to me to include the forms which have sometimes been called *pseudophobia* (Gélineau). Such are the fears of contact, the horror of blood, and of innocuous animals, and many strange and causeless aversions.'[81] In the event, it was Freud who succeeded in separating phobia from obsession.

FREUD AND THE 'ANXIETY NEUROSIS' By the early 1890s, the concept of neurasthenia had become so large that it was threatening to engulf most of 'neurotic' states. Started by USA physicians, but taken over with some enthusiasm by their European counterparts (less so by alienists), neurasthenia included most if not all the symptoms of anxiety and panic disorder.[82] In 1894, Sigmund Freud published (in French) a classical paper entitled 'The justification for detaching from neurasthenia a particular syndrome: the anxiety neurosis' in which he marshalled clinical and theoretical reasons for the creation of the new disease. All symptoms were to revolve around the concept of 'morbid anxiety': 'general irritability, anxious expectation, anxiety attacks, and [somatic] 'equivalents' such as cardiovascular and respiratory symptoms, sweating, tremor, shuddering, ravenous hunger, diarrhoea, vertigo, congestion, parasthesiae, awakening in fright, obsessional symptoms, agoraphobia, and nausea.'[83] The symptoms could be found in various combinations and resulted from 'grave hereditary taint'[84] or from a 'deflection of somatic sexual excitation from the psychical field, and an abnormal use of it, due to this deflection.'[85]

A year later, Freud published another work on this subject[86] in reply to criticism levelled by Löwenfeld to his earlier paper. A full discussion of changes in Freud's sexual theory of the anxiety neurosis is beyond the scope of this book. Be that as it may, his actual suggestion that the anxiety states should constitute a separate condition received little challenge. This is surprising for, as he himself had stated in his original paper, he had 'adduced hardly any examples and quoted no statistics.'[87] In fact, it is likely that his suggestion was accepted less for his aetiological theory than for the fact that similar separatist views had been hinted at by Hecker, Krishaber, Ribot, and others. It should be kept in mind that, at this early stage in its history, anxiety neurosis was considered (by Freud included) *as a disease of the nervous system*: 'The nervous system reacts to an internal source of excitation with a neurosis, just as it reacts to an analogous external one with a corresponding affect.'[88] At the time Freud considered 'anxiety neurosis' as an example of 'actual neurosis', i.e. of acquired and reactive conditions unrelated to childhood events.[89]

Important alienists agreed with Freud's nosological views; for example, Hartenberg who only took issue against the 'sexual aetiology' and preferred the older mechanisms of Morel and Krishaber: 'anxiety neurosis originates in the sympathetic nervous system', 'the term anxiety neurosis is useful to differentiate from neurasthenia a distinct group of symptoms that may represent a 'primary disorder of the emotions' and which can provide an explanation for the development of phobias.'[90]

But there was also some disagreement. Pitres and Régis in their famous *Les Obsessions et les Impulsions* wrote: 'during recent years German authors have described what they call anxiety neurosis. According to Hecker,[91] this disorder would include all the symptoms of neurasthenia – the latter term being now reserved for simple spinal irritation. Freud, on the other hand, considers anxiety neurosis as an independent disorder characterized, in its pure form, by nervous overexcitement, chronic anxiety and anxious attention, attacks of acute and paroxysmal anxiety with dyspnoea, palpitations, profuse sweating.'[92] Pitres and Régis believed that: 'This is only a *syndrome* and hence may be found grafted, whether acutely or chronically, upon any neuropathic or psychopathic personality . . . It is associated with neurasthenia and melancholia but can also be seen in other neuroses and psychoses . . . *There is, therefore, no independent disorder called anxiety neuroses*'.[93] The same criticism was expressed at the Grenoble Congress of 1902, when Lalanne presented his oft-quoted historical account.[94] A young Capgras sided with the views of Pitres and Régis and reported two cases in their support.[95] Disagreements on the nature of the anxiety disorders gave rise to a plethora of treatment approaches; their study is also beyond the scope of this book.[96]

JANET'S VIEWS Janet was at the crossroads of three conceptual traditions, two French and a foreign one: positivism, as represented by Ribot, Taine, and Renan (who were his teachers); the spiritualist and introspective tradition of Maine de Biran, which had been transmitted to him by his uncle, the philosopher Paul Janet; and Jacksonism and the hierarchical approach to psychological functions.[97] The spiritualist view had also influenced Royer-Collard, Baillarger, Moreau de Tours, the so-called 'psychological alienists'.[98]

In Janet's model, 'feelings' were 'secondary' mental states and only served to guide the expression and termination of behaviour.[99] Their effectiveness depended on the level of energy (*force*) and integrative capacity (*tension*). Exaggerated energy or reduced integration led to a failure of feelings, and to the release of primitive behaviours. For Janet, anxiety and anguish were the main manifestations of such failures. Like Freud, he believed that both were accompanied by somatic symptoms. His interest was, however, in the description of the 'mental' or 'psychological' component of *l'angoisse* which he studied repeatedly[100] starting in 1903 with his work on *psychasthénie* (into which category he included all anxiety and panic symptoms).[101]

FERE AND 'MORBID EMOTIVITY' Féré published *La Pathologie des Emotions* in 1892. A disciple of Ribot and collaborator of Binet, he pursued an experimental approach in the study of emotions and their disorders. Of the 22 chapters of his book (covering all available knowledge on emotions), five are dedicated to 'morbid emotivity'. By this Féré meant emotivity 'characterized by reactions badly adapted to the interest of the individual or the species ... [it] presents itself in two forms: 1. diffuse and permanent morbid emotivity as a pathological character, and 2. systematic morbid emotivity induced by special conditions always the same for the same individual.'[102] Féré's examples of diffuse emotivity exactly correspond to current conceptions of generalized anxiety (what in his time was called pantophobia). Likewise, his examples of systematic morbid emotivity correspond to phobias (ranging from agoraphobia – which he mentions by name – to specific phobias). Féré believed morbid emotivity to be constitutional, and his view must be regarded as the origin of the idea of *constitution émotive* later on expanded by Dupré.[103]

BRISSAUD, *L'ANXIÉTÉ ET L'ANGOISSE* Éduard Brissaud was a neurologist with psychiatric interests.[104] His staunch organic position caused him to break away from Charcot on the issue of the psychogenesis of hysteria. He was equally firm in believing that anguish was not psychological in origin, and that its somatic symptoms resulted from brain stem lesions. Anxiety, on the other hand, was subjective and of cortical origin.[105]

Brissaud expressed this view repeatedly. In 1902, he was asked to comment at a meeting of the *Société de Neurologie* on a case of a docker who suffered from anguish without anxiety (*angoisse sans anxiété*), i.e. 'after more than a hundred attacks of severe chest pain, remained philosophical, lived from day to day, and had never developed either sadness (*tristesse*) or panic (*terreur*).'[106] Brissaud reaffirmed his 1890 views that there was a major difference between the two symptoms. Late in 1902, he repeated the performance at the 12th Congress of French Alienists and Neurologists at Grenoble when he confronted Lelanne,[107] and declared: 'Anguish (*l'angoisse*) is a brain stem phenomenon (*phénomène bulbaire*), anxiety is a cortical phenomenon (*phénomène cerebral*): anguish is a physical disorder that expresses itself in a sensation of constriction, of suffocation; anxiety is a psychological disorder that expresses itself in feelings of undefinable insecurity.'[108]

In 1938, Claude and Lévy-Valensi were still expressing agreement with his view![109] In 1945, in her classical work on *L'Angoisse*,[110] Boutonier[111] challenged it as a theory that 'had remained alive up to her time' because 'its clarity and simplicity were more apparent than real.'[112] She offered an integrated account instead.

HARTENBERG, TIMIDITE, AND SOCIAL PHOBIA Social phobia remains a confused construct whose meaning oscillates between avoidance personality disorder and specific social fears. The impression has recently been given that it was only recognized or defined in 1966.[113] This is reinforced by historical accounts showing a gap between the cases purportedly reported by Hippocrates or Burton and the present.[114] This is historically incorrect as there were two great books on 'Timidity' at the turn of the century.[115] The earliest (*Timidité*) by L. Dugas (known for his great contribution to the concepts of depersonalisation and *déjà vu*) is an introspec-

tive study, based on the classical psychology tradition. The second, by Paul Hartenberg (*Les Timides et la Timidité*) includes much clinical, theoretical and aetiological
discussion: indeed, the title of the book alludes to the possible mechanisms involved.

The author specialized in the field of fears and phobias, and in the same year
as his book on social phobias he published another major work on *La Névrose
D'Angoisse*.[116] A disciple of Ribot, to whom he paid warm tribute, Hartenberg
declared himself a positivist psychologist, interested in behaviour and not in the
soul. Like Ribot, he believed in the predominance of the 'affective life' and in the
James–Lange theory of emotions.

Hartenberg defined timidity as a combination of fear, shame, and embarrassment
felt in social situations and which affected psychosocial competence through attacks
(*accès*) of fear. From a clinical and experimental perspective, he studied subjective
and objective symptoms (including tremor, unsteadiness of gait, dizziness, blushing,
etc.). In Chapter 3 of his book he dealt with the timid personality and its tendency
to isolation, misogyny, pessimism, sadness, pride, irritability and suppressed anger.
Chapter 4 is dedicated to the origins, natural history, mechanisms and sub-types
of timidity. He distinguished between predisposing (inherited vulnerability), determinant (physical, social or psychological defect – real or imagined), and occasional
(learning situations) causes. Chapter 5 deals with situations in which timidity is
phobic and pathological, and Chapter 6 with treatments which include re-
assurance and self-administered behavioural therapies.[117]

FRANCIS HECKEL AND 'PAROXYSMAL ANXIETY ATTACKS' Heckel was a specialist in nutrition who managed to write one of the great works on *la nevrosse de
l'angoisse*, particularly on its *formes paroxystiques*, i.e. panic disorder. The book was
completed before the beginning of the Great War, but only published in 1917. In
12 chapters the author covers issues ranging from history to treatment. The first
three chapters are dedicated to *séméiologie* (i.e. clinical presentation) which Heckel
divided into paroxysmal and inter-paroxysmal. Then physical signs, mechanisms,
and causes are discussed. The paroxysmal states Heckel classified, according to
the predominance of a particular sign, into: cardiovascular, respiratory, digestive,
neurological, sensory, and endocrinological. Finally, the association of these states
is explored with generalized anxiety, obsessions, phobias, impulsions, and tics.[118]

Depersonalization

In 1898, Dugas defined depersonalization as 'A morbid state involving a loss of the
sense of personal identity and a feeling of the strangeness or unreality of one's own
words and actions; in extreme cases involving also an obsessive feeling of dissolution of the personality.'[119] Once again, although the term and concept were only
constructed during the 1890s, the behaviours to which they were meant to refer
had been known for a long time. For example, In 1847, Billod reported the case

of a woman in her 30s, with typical feelings of depersonalization: 'she tells me that she feels as someone who is neither alive or dead, who leaves in a dreamy state; and that things look as if they were wrapped up in clouds, and people as if they were shadows; their words seem to come from far away, from a different world.'[120] Similar experiences had been reported by Moreau de Tours as *erreurs sur le temps et l'espace* caused by hashish intoxication: 'I experience many times this illusion when walking along a boulevard, that people and things looked far away, as if seen through the wrong end of binoculars';[121] and also by Krishaber as a symptom of his so-called *névropathie cérébro-cardiaque*: 'the patient remains stupified, his head is empty, his mind is enveloped in vague, undefinable reverie . . . to recognize an object he must make the effort to remember its use; the simplest of thoughts cause him great effort'.[122]

Dugas is said to to have taken the word '*dépersonnalisation*' from the diary of Henri-Frédéric Amiel,[123] but somehow the term took a long time to make it into any of the great French dictionaries. In 1926 it is featured in Lalande's where it is claimed that it did not 'yet have any foreign equivalents'.[124] There is little doubt, however, that the behaviours and concept involved elicited great interest in France and, by the turn of the century, important literature began to accumulate. In *La Obsession at Psychasthenie*, Pierre Janet included a full section (and a series of cases) on *le sentiment de dépersonnalisation complète*. After summarizing the views of Dugas and Bernard-Leroy, Janet claimed priority for such ideas: 'In my lectures of 1897 and 98 on the sentiments intellectuels that accompany the exercise of the will and memory I had already attempted to show that the experiences of *déjà vu*, strangeness, and depersonalization are related to the feelings of loss of freedom and constraint that result from psychological automatism . . . that which characterizes the feeling of depersonalization is that the individual perceives himself as incomplete and unachieved (*incomplète, inachevée*)'.[125] Dugas' views need now to be expounded upon in some detail.[126] In a paper published in 1898 under the title *Un cas de dépersonnalisation*, he disclaimed any priority for noticing the behaviour in question first; indeed most of this work concerns the ideas of Taine, Ribot, Krishaber, and Pascal who according to Dugas had either dealt with the feelings of the self, or reported feelings of depersonalization. After reporting snippets of the case of M, the author suggests that the 'process' involved in depersonalization included apathy, dissolution of attention, release of automatic activity, and perception of the intellectual activity as if it were strange to the subject.[127] He concludes 'depersonalization is not illusory, or at least it is not an illusion without basis; it is a form of apathy . . . [which] is a loss of the sense of being a person'.[128] Nowhere in this paper is reference made to Amiel.

The same year, Bernard-Leroy[129] replied with a paper entitled '*Sur l'illusion de dépersonnalisation*'.[130] After pointing out that Dugas had already reported a case of depersonalization in a paper on *fausse memoire*,[131] Bernard-Leroy states that he has had personal experience with the disorder, and reminds the reader that in his survey on false recognition he had included five questions which specifically concerned the feelings of depersonalization; for example, Q32: Are your false recognitions accompanied by the impression that you are only a witness of the ineluctable and involuntary unfolding of your own actions, movements, thoughts and feelings, as if they belonged to some one else? and Q34: Have objects lost their natural aspect, do they look strange or surprising? 12 out of 65 replies, Bernard-Leroy claimed, were positive.[132] Their analysis suggested four types of depersonalization: (*a*) an analyzable feeling, as if reality is a dream; (*b*) a feeling of distance and remoteness, as if the subject is isolated from the world; (*c*) a feeling that only some actions or thoughts are actually strange and uncontrolled; and (*d*) the complete form of the feeling of depersonalization when all the above are felt at the same time. Lastly, he criticized Dugas for suggesting that one of the mechanisms of depersonalization might be the phenomenon of double personality: 'an impression of double personality is different from a double personality for in the latter the subject never experiences it directly ...'.[133] Without referring to Bernard-Leroy at all, Dugas dealt with the issue of *le dédoublement du moi* in 1910. He seemed to accept the point that there was no awareness of doubling, but then he insists: 'in fact, subjects are never properly *dédoublés*'.[134] Then in a book with Moutier he distinguished a 'positive and negative aspect' of the syndrome in that there was an illusion but there was also insight into the fact that the experience was illusory.[135] A year later, he returned to the topic to claim that 'a theory of depersonalization will not be established until a large number of subjects has been studied. It might then be possible to isolate the symptom as usually it is combined with other mental symptoms'.[136] He concluded that, whatever else depersonalization was, it was not a delusion but a specific disorder.[137]

Other writers then joined the debate. Chaslin made the important suggestion that the feeling of strangeness could be due to 'an alteration of the self of the patient'.[138] Régis viewed depersonalization as a disorder of the 'conscious personality'.[139] Following earlier definitions, a young Schilder wrote: 'The patient feels separate from his earlier being; he cannot recognize himself as a person. His actions seem automatic, and he behaves as if he were a witness of his own actions. The external world appears strange and new and unreal. The self feels different'.[140] In a paper read before the British Psychological Society, Mayer-Gross criticized Schilder: 'in this definition, I would rather call it a short description, two different symptoms are joined together under the heading of depersonalization ... on the one hand *changes of the self*, depersonalization in a narrow sense, and on the other *changes in the environment*, feelings of unreality, alienation of the outer world' (my italics).[141] He went on to say that, although there were theoretical grounds to combine both types of symptoms, in clinical practice they are not always found together. This view, that depersonalization and 'derealization'[142] are often dissociated proved to be an important one. Lastly, in 1931, Ehrenwald drew attention to the association between left-sided stroke and other neurological disorders, depersonalization experiences and anosognosia.[143]

Clinical descriptions and definitions do not tell the whole story about what was being debated in the literature on depersonalization. First of all, there is the nineteenth century principle on which descriptive psychopathology was based, namely that symptoms are always disturbances of a mental function. Hallucinations were a disturbance of perception, and obsessions might be of thought or the will. But what about depersonalization? The variety of complaints included in its definition suggested that many functions might be involved. Thus there seem to be a defect in emotions and feelings, in attention, in perception, in the sense of the real, etc. Since the time of Billod and Krishaber, this had caused much grief and many proposals had been made as to what was the primary disorder. However, the very utilization by Dugas of the word depersonalization suggests that by the turn of the century, as the notion of person and self was beginning to take shape in French psychology (it was a very old one in metaphysics and theology), it seemed possible that the clinical phenomenon in question was in fact a disorder of the self. That the notion also became attractive to German psychiatry suggests that the convergence point was indeed the notion of *Ich-Bewusstsein*[144] and *Persönlichkeitsbewusstsein*.[145] In his paper on the disorders of the self, Pick reported a case with depersonalization and derealization (objects were 'perceived as far off');[146] and Packard conceived of depersonalization as a disturbance in the mechanisms that underlie the notion of personal identity, namely the *Apperceptionsystem*.[147]

Since those creative days there has been little real progress: it remains unclear whether there is any point in separating depersonalization from derealization, whether the phenomenon is the same in schizophrenia, depression, obsessional disorder, epilepsy, panic attacks, etc., whether depersonalization is a disturbance of a unitary mental function called the 'self' or whether it simply is a vestigial behaviour which once upon a time had an adaptive function. However, discussion of these important issues brings the *history* of depersonalization uncomfortably close to the present.

Body dysmorphic disorder

Unrealistic fears of personal deformity or ugliness are likely to have been part of the self-consciousness of mankind, particularly since the time reflective surfaces became widely available. Whether in earlier times such behaviours were considered as deviant or pathological is unknown, although it is likely that they might have been frowned upon by long-suffering friends or relatives. Historical and transcultural literature suggests that since classical times,[148] humans have considered their 'body' and appearance as special objects of aesthetic[149] and symbolic inquiry.[150] Since self-reflective behaviour is also 'attitudinal' in nature, it is to be expected that the perception of one's own body is controlled as much by reality as by emotions, fashion, and the pragmatics of the situation.[151] In individuals with psychobiological vulnerability[152] or brain lesions,[153] this host of factors might offer a propitious setting for the development of deviant or pathological views about one's own body.[154]

Rather unsuitably, Stutte has suggested that such behaviour should be called the 'Thersites-complex'.[155] *Thersites* was 'the most ugly and the most impudent talker amongst the Greeks at Troy';[156] he was cross-eyed and limped, but there is little evidence that he ever worried over his all too real ugliness (unless his persistent verbal aggression and nastiness are to be considered as an emotional equivalent). The name 'Quasimodo Complex' has also been suggested: 'if anxiety, hostility, social withdrawal, and abnormal personality traits are produced by emotional reaction to physical deformity'.[157] Needless to say, the implication is a false one: all the features listed do exist but their clustering does not entail the existence of such a syndrome.

During the late nineteenth century, worries and complaints over one's deformity were named by Morselli[158] as 'dysmorphophobia'. In keeping with the psychopathology of the period, he conceptualized them as 'phobias', 'obsessions' and 'fixed ideas' (all three terms used in their pre-1895 sense). *Dysmorfia* is reported as having been the ugliest woman in Sparta.[159] The interesting point has been made by Philoppopoulos that the most appropriate transliteration of the term into English should be *dysmorfiophobia*.[160] Since then, both the boundaries of the *concept* and *behaviour* associated with 'dysmorphophobia' have repeatedly changed. The ensuing confusion has been blamed on the fact that the term itself is ambiguous for it includes the suffix 'phobia'.[161] This argument is spurious for terms are always arbitrary: what matters is the associated concept which, in this case, has changed since the last century and is likely to do so again. (If *terms* were important, then *melancholia* could not be used, as it is not the case that such patients suffer from black bile.) To deal with the so-called 'neurotic' end of the disorder, DSM III-R introduced the term *body dysmorphic disorder*, whilst classifying cases exhibiting 'delusional' intensity as *delusional (paranoid) disorder, somatic type*.[162] DSM IV has added the criterion of 'clinically significant distress or impairment' in psychosocial functioning.[163] ICD-10 includes both body dysmorphic disorder and non-delusional dysmorphophobia under *hypochondriacal disorder*; so-called delusional dysmorphophobia, on the other hand is classified under *other persistent delusional disorder*.[164]

Historical analysis shows how, from a set of ancient negative attitudes towards the self, Morselli separated off a *sub-type* which he mainly related to bodily deformity and explained in terms of the descriptive and nosological categories of his day. To say now that he 'got it wrong', for 'dysmorphophobia' includes over-valued ideas, delusions, obsessions and phobias is unhelpful because the term is meant to refer to 'symptoms',[165] and because there is little *empirical* evidence that the current classification is definitive or superior to the one reigning during the second half of the nineteenth century. Indeed, Morselli was aware of the fact that the meaning of phobia was changing. Renaming the entire set of deviant attitudes as 'body dysmorphic disorder' has not dispelled the conceptual ambiguities attached to dysmorphophobia.[166,167]

New syndromes, plastic surgery, psychoanalytical views on the pathological perception of the body,[168] and imported transcultural clinical phenomena have all added to the *caput mortuum*. Thus, to cope with the heterogeneity of complaints, and based on their content[169] and response to medication,[170] specific delusions have been considered as independent entities. Likewise, the appearance on the scene of the eating disorders has contributed a sizeable group of patients said to be suffering from 'body dysmorphic disorder' (indeed, some consider this to be the central symptom).[171] Secondly, the frequent failure of plastic surgeons to satisfy their customers after correcting real or illusory disfigurement has created a pool of subjects claimed to entertain 'abnormal attitudes' to their bodies, and it has been concluded that some of these may suffer from body dysmorphic disorder.[172] Lastly, the Chinese and Japanese cultures have long recognized *koro* and *Taijin-Kyofu*;[173] subjects affected by these syndromes express severe anxiety about the penis retracting into the abdomen or about selective social interactions, respectively. Originally considered as culture-bound, some of these states have now been described in the West.[174] It would seem therefore, that the term 'body dysmorphic disorder' has imposed only a superficial order and clarity upon the gamut of the dysmorphophobias. By analysing its history, this section means to replace this group of disorders back into their old context, namely, the wide category of 'pathological attitudes towards the self'.

Matters conceptual

One of the tasks of the historian is to determine whether the 'feelings and behaviours' brought together by Morselli under the term dysmorphophobia have been stable in time and space. Stability is, of course, a relative concept in that it depends upon the temporal perspective of the observer. Nonetheless, when present, it can be surmised to result from biological (evolutionary), psychological and social invariants (or combinations thereof). Candidacy for biological invariance (i.e. for brain representation) requires that the behaviour in question is functionally meaningful and (even better) neuropsychologically accessible. In the case in hand, the existence could be postulated of a brain programme, wired-in by evolution, and dedicated to the monitoring of the boundaries and integrity of the human body. Failure in any of its matching mechanisms or templates (containing updated images of the body) could then give rise to dysmorphophobia-like behaviour. Such a model would also have to account for the acute sense of dissatisfaction that accompanies dysmorphophobia.

The (wider) model to be used in this chapter is based on the assumption that, in addition to any monitoring of the integrity of their body, human beings entertain 'attitudes' about their appearance, including both descriptions and prescriptions. The former have become organized into what is now known as the 'biological human sciences' and correspond to what Kant called *Physiologie*, i.e. the science that studies the way in which *'nature made man'*. The latter, on the other hand, refer to what he called *Anthropologie*, i.e. what 'man has made of himself'.[175] This corpus of knowledge should include evaluative attitudes towards the body (violations of which might lead to some forms of dysmorphophobia). Such evaluative attitudes include cognitive, emotional and volitional components, and each age has favoured one upon the other. In regards to the behavioural phenomenon of 'disliking the self', the nineteenth century (like ours) tended to emphasize (as the work of Morselli and Ribot shows) the cognitive component.

Matters historical

PRE-NINETEENTH CENTURY ISSUES Since Classical times, writers have been concerned about those who thought little of themselves, whether of their mind or body. For example, in *Anatomy of Melancholy*, Burton dedicated space to arguments used in classical times to convince those who had physical handicaps (or had acquired disfigurements in battle) that their bodies mattered little: 'deformities or imperfections of our bodies be they innate or accidental torture many men: yet this may comfort to them, that those imperfections of the body do not a whit blemish the soul, or hinder the operations of it, but rather help and much increase it.'[176] It is doubtful, however, whether such advice has ever worked! In her *Psychologie du Corps*, Maisonneuve and Bruchon-Schweitzer refers to the belief that 'what is beautiful must be good' as one of the more nocive ones to be found in western culture.

THE NINETEENTH CENTURY The nineteenth century was not immune to similar concerns. Alienists, therefore, took seriously complaints about facial deformity, and depending upon their intensity, considered them as hypochondriacal or melancholic in origin (both were then defined as restricted delusional states).

Enrico Morselli When Morselli (1852–1929) began to work in this field he had already been out of Modena Clinical School for 12 years. After training under Canestrini, he learned phrenology at instigation of Gaddi, the great anthropologist, who believed that this discipline was 'the most scientific of all psychiatric specialisms'. Morselli completed his psychiatric training at the mental hospital of *Reggio Emilia* under Livi. He won a scholarship to the *Instituto di Studi Superiori* of Florence where he worked with the physiognomist Paolo Mantegazza. He joined Tourin University in 1880, where he was to deliver the lectures included in his *General Anthropology* and was also to write his famous book on suicide. In 1881, he founded the *Rivista di Filosofia Scientifica*, one of the acknowledged organs of Italian positivism. In Turin, he built up a rich private practice, probably his main source of dysmorphophobic patients (in general, these complaints were very rare in asylums for the insane).

In 1885, he published *Manuale di semejotica delle malattia mentali*, a popular textbook of descriptive psychopathology. In 1890, Morselli moved to Genoa by which time he had grown unhappy with neuropathological explanations as shown in the second volume of his *Semejotica*. Published in 1894, this book emphasizes the role of emotions in the generation of mental symptoms. But, during the early 1880s, when collecting his 'dysmorphophobic' patients, Morselli was still infatuated with the brain. There is little doubt that this interest had to do with his training in physical anthropology.

Morselli defined dysmorphophobia as *an idea ossesiva, desolante, della deformitá corporea* and classified it as a 'rudimentary paranoia' or 'abortive monomania'. This double classification makes sense in terms of the 1880s European debate on the clinical boundaries of these two clinical categories. The dysmorphophobic idea threatened the sense of 'personal integration' of the individual. According to whether it was a defence against a direct injury or a manifestation of a deeper psychological disturbance, the idea was primary or secondary, respectively.

The clinical phenomenon (but not the word) was widely discussed during the early part of the twentieth century. For example, fears of ugliness were studied as early as 1892 by H. Kaan in his book on neurasthenia and obsession.[177] In 1901, Hartenberg referred to similar worries in his book on timidity.[178] In 1907, Dupré explained such fears as resulting from a disturbance of proprioceptive information, and Janet called them 'feelings of shame of the body'.[179] In their useful review, Korkina and Morozov point out that early in the century, Korsakov, Betcherev, and Suchanov had already reported similar clinical phenomena in the Russian literature, and that in 1912 Osipov introduced the term dysmorphophobia in that country as the diagnosis for a 27 year-old woman who believed that 'she was too big', and that the 'lower part of her face was deformed'.[180]

The *term* 'dysmorphophobia' took some time to catch on in English and German. It probably first came into English in the translation of Tanzi's *Textbook of Mental Diseases* where, linked to Morselli's name, is mentioned in the section on obsessive ideas.[181] In 1915, it was legitimated by Kraepelin in his chapter on *Die Zwangsneurose (Dysmorphophobie)*.[182] Kraepelin, however, did not refer to Morselli, thus giving the impression that he had coined the word himself. Koupernik, for example, has fallen into this trap.[183] Kraepelin also discussed the same clinical phenomenon under a different rubric (*Ereuthophobie*). Many other terms have since been coined to deal with the same theme: shame of the body, psychosis of ugliness, hypochondria of beauty, madness of introspection, etc. It is unlikely that such new terms have advanced our knowledge of the disorder.

Summary

Terms and behaviours relating to anxiety were well known before the nineteenth century. After the 1810s, severe forms of anxiety were included with the insanities, but the view remained that anxiety was a form of 'social' stress and a potential *cause* of insanity. In 1866, Morel introduced the view that both subjective and somatic forms of anxiety (together with obsessional disorders) might result from a disorder of the autonomic nervous system.

For the next decades, somatic symptoms were repeatedly considered as separate diseases; for example, typical panic attacks were considered by Krishaber to result from cardiovascular pathology, and by Benedikt from inner ear disease. It was in this medical milieu that the concept of 'agoraphobia' was developed by Benedikt, Westphal, Cordes, and du Saulle. In 1980, Brissaud proposed that generalized anxiety and panic disorder (*angoisse*) were separate symptoms, the one generated in the cortex, the other in the brain stem. For a time, some believed that all the symptoms of anxiety were part of neurasthenia, the new 'disease' that during the 1880s threatened to engulf most of the neuroses.

In 1895, Freud proposed that 'anxiety neurosis' ought to be separated from neurasthenia and considered as a disease in its own right; and also that phobias and obsessions were different symptoms. In 1902, Hartenberg outlined both the concept of panic disorder (later to be confirmed by Heckel) and also that of social phobia. Soon after, the notion of 'emotive constitution', that had been suggested by Féré, was completed by Dupré.

However, the integrative power of the Freudian view tended to predominate, and all manner of symptoms were brought together under the construct 'anxiety' which by the 1920s was no longer a 'symptom' but had become a full explanation. The view that panic (*angoisse*) was a brain stem disorder managed to last in France up to the second World War, when Boutonier sounded its death knell. Lastly, the history of depersonalization and dysmorphophobia were also explored.

ACKNOWLEDGEMENTS Dr Chris Link, UK, greatly helped with the writing of the section on anxiety, Dr Simon Barnett, UK, with the section on depersonalization, and Dr Kan Chung-Sing from Hong Kong with the section on dysmorphophobia.

NOTES

1 Raymond, 1911; López Piñero, 1983; Rosenberg, 1989; Drinka, 1984; Cottereau, 1975; Oppenheim, 1991.
2 Veith, 1965; Owen, 1971; Trillat, 1986; Roccatagliata, 1990; Bannour, 1992.
3 Michéa, 1843; Gillespie, 1928; Kenyon, 1965; Meister, 1980; Place, 1986.
4 Berrios, On Obsessive–compulsive disorder, 1989.
5 The standard of historical scholarship in this field is mediocre: see, for example, Boulenger and Uhde, 1987; Zal, 1988; Errera, 1962; Kuch and Swinson, 1992; May, 1968; Saurí, 1979. The only exception is Ey, 1950.
6 By these are meant here conditions such as the anxiety disorders,

vascular neuroses, neurasthenia, obsessive–compulsive disorder and neurotic depression which were not included (in name at least) amongst the original 'nervous disorder' of Willis, and which were conceptualized as *neuroses* only during the late nineteenth century.

7 For example Burton collected many such symptoms in the *Anatomy of Melancholy*.

8 Before this period, they were described as cardiovascular disorders.

9 Krishaber, 1873.

10 Benedikt, 1870.

11 p. 386, Ey, 1950.

12 Cullen, 1803.

13 Cullen, 1803.

14 p. 327, Landré-Beauvais, 1813.

15 p. 77, Littré and Robin, 1858.

16 p. 93, Littré and Robin, 1858.

17 Lewis, 1967.

18 Sarbin, 1964; 1968.

19 For example, his claim that 'the word anxiety was hardly used in standard medical and psychological textbooks until the late 1930s. It was a result of Freud's writings about Angst, translated as anxiety' (Sarbin, 1964).

20 For a good discussion of the etymology involved, see López Ibor, 1950.

21 See Errera, 1962.

22 pp. 119–124, Altschule, 1976.

23 p. 80, Pinel, 1818.

24 p. 85, Pinel, 1818.

25 p. 156, Pinel, 1818.

26 p. 159, Pinel, 1818.

27 *Symptômes Généraux ou Sympathiques* in Georget, 1820.

28 Griesinger, 1861.

29 Guislain, 1852.

30 p. 45, Guislain, 1852.

31 p. 169, Griesinger, 1861.

32 p. 165, Griesinger, 1867.

33 Kirkegaard, 1959.

34 Jolivet, 1950.

35 McCarthy, 1981.

36 Anonymous, 1860. The reviewer was probably Forbes Winslow himself.

37 Bouchut, 1860.

38 Zeldin, in his otherwise inaccurate historical account of developments in French psychiatry during the middle of the nineteenth century, suggests that 'nervousness' was increasingly recognized as a complaint after the 1850s, and quotes Bouchut in this regard (p. 833, Zeldin, 1977).

39 p. 193, Feuchtersleben, 1847.

40 pp. 182–183 in Prichard, 1835.

41 p. 38, Bucknill and Tuke, 1858.

42 'Is there a human breast in which this awful word fails to produce an

echo? – from the youth who fears to be superseded in the affections of the object of his love, or the parent, etc. etc.' Wigan, 1849.

43 Feuchtersleben, 1847, this illustrates early attempts at using a 'vascular' model to account for the link between emotion and brain.

44 Genil-Perrin, 1913.

45 Dupré, 1919.

46 Duprat, 1899.

47 As in Luys, Meynert, Chaslin, Mairet and many others.

48 As in the work of Jackson and his followers in the Continent such as Ribot and Janet.

49 Houzeau, 1872; and also the work of Romanes, Spalding and Morgan in Britain.

50 Although both Janet and Freud paid lip service to anatomical explanations, they offered models according to which symptoms resulted from shifts in the level of a putative psychological energy. Both were influenced by Jackson.

51 Berrios, 1989.

52 Morel, 1866.

53 Clarke and Jacyna, 1987.

54 Clarke and Jacyna, 1987.

55 Morel, 1860.

56 López Piñero, 1983.

57 Berrios, 1989 (also Chapter 6, this book).

58 Dechambre, 1889. It is reported that Krishaber also tried to inoculate monkeys with serum from syphilitic patients. Apparently he died of a 'mysterious infection which also killed his family and his experimental animals' (p. 152; Dugas and Moutier, 1911).

59 Krishaber, 1873.

60 These observations are likely to have provided the background from which was to emerge the James–Lange theory of emotions. For an account of this theory, see pp. 295–299 and pp. 326–328 in Gardiner *et al.*, 1937.

61 It is a pity that the history of the concept of vertigo has been neglected as it is likely that under its wide umbrella typical cases of anxiety attack were included during the nineteenth century.

62 p. 268, Axenfeld, 1883.

63 p. 208, Millet, 1884.

64 p. 64, Weill, 1886.

65 Leroux, 1889 claimed that Lasègue had, *faute de mieux*, included under 'vertigo' the same clinical states that Westphal (1872) (see below) was to call agoraphobia (with *Schwindel* as the central symptom). Lasègue listed his operational criteria: (*a*) somatic symptoms often precede the eruption of acute anxiety; (*b*) the latter is out of proportion to the former; (*c*) the anxiety is overpowering; (*d*) it often has sudden onset and is unprecipitated; and, (*e*) once it started it must follow its course.

66 pp. 152–153, Leroux, 1889.

67 pp. 168–169, Leroux, 1889.

68 Haltenhof, 1887.
69 p. 203, Grasset, 1901.
70 Benedikt, 1870.
71 Benedikt, 1906.
72 There seems to have been an earlier and typical case: López Ibor, in his excellent historical review, quotes a 1832 paper by Brück in *Huffeland's Journal* reporting the case of a priest who complained of severe vertigo and anxiety as soon as he was outdoors. To feel better, he needed to take shelter under a roof (see p. 25, López Ibor, 1950).
73 Legrand was here referring to Cordes's paper published the same year as Wesphal's: Cordes, 1872.
74 A recent translation of this paper neglects to quote the French contribution and the important paper by Legrand (Knapp and Schumacher, 1988). Late in 1872, Westphal published a *Nachtrag* clearly addressed at dealing with any priority claims: Westphal, 1872.
75 pp. 405–406, Legrand du Saulle, 1876.
76 Gros, 1885.
77 pp. 424–426, Dagonet, 1894. A recent French paper on the history of agoraphobia misses the opportunity to study this important problem. For example, it claims that after Legrand du Saulle agoraphobia 'was forgotten at the beginning of the twentieth century and only retaken in the work of Marks'!! (p. 115, Boulenger and Uhde, 1987).
78 p. 692, Hartenberg, 1901a.
79 For a good account of this period, see p. 91, Leguil, 1979, where Westphal is quoted as saying that phobics and obsessives inhabit a borderland (*Grenzgebiet*) between neuroses and psychoses.
80 'This is a state in which the patient fears everything or nothing, where anxiety, instead of being riveted on one object, floats as in a dream . . .' (p. 213, Ribot, 1897). The best discussion of *panophobie* during this period is to be found in the book by Pitres and Régis. They also called it *émotivité diffuse* (see pp. 20–34, Pitres and Régis, 1902). Devaux and Logre protested that the term should be 'pantophobic and not panophobic, a word which in good etymology refers to worshipping of the god Pan' (see footnote, p. 35, Devaux and Logre, 1917).
81 p. 213, Ribot, 1897.
82 Fleury, 1901.
83 Freud, 1953a.
84 By accepting degeneration theory, Freud simply showed that he was a child of his time.
85 p. 97, Freud, 1953.
86 Freud, 1953.
87 p. 108, Freud, 1953.
88 p. 102, Freud, 1953.
89 pp. 10–12, Laplanche and Pontalis, 1973.
90 p. 699, Hartenberg, 1901a.
91 Here the authors are referring to E. Hecker whose 1893 paper is acknowledged by Freud: 'I believed that this conception of the symptoms

of the anxiety neurosis had originated with myself until an interesting paper by E. Hecker came into my hands, in which I found the same idea expounded with the most satisfying clearness and completeness. Although Hecker recognizes certain symptoms as equivalent or incomplete manifestations of an anxiety attack, he does not separate them from neurasthenia as I propose to do' (p. 77, Freud, 1953a). Freud had started thinking about this problem as early as 1983 (see p. 39, Laplanche and Pontalis, 1973). For an excellent treatment of this period, see Levin, 1978.

92 p. 250, Pitres and Régis, 1902.

93 p. 251, Pitres and Régis, 1902.

94 Lalanne, 1902.

95 Capgras, 1903.

96 Dubois, 1905; Dejerine and Gauckler, 1911; Thomas, 1913; Levy, 1917; and for a history and general summary the monumental: Janet, 1919.

97 Rouart, 1950.

98 López Piñero and Morales Meseguer, 1970.

99 Fouks et al., 1986. For a general analysis of recent work on Janet, see Brown, 1991.

100 These include Janet, 1898; 1909; 1926.

101 pp. 220–265, Janet, 1919.

102 p. 360, Féré, 1899.

103 Dupré, Préface. In Devaux and Logre, 1917.

104 Freeman, 1970.

105 p. 410, Brissaud, 1890.

106 Souques, 1902.

107 Lalanne, 1902.

108 Brissaud, 1902.

109 p. 24, Claude and Lévy-Valensi, 1938.

110 Boutonier, 1945.

111 Juliette Favez-Boutonier was a psychiatrist and psychologist with psychoanalytic interests (Personal Communication by Professor Pierre Pichot, London, September, 1991). Her 1938 doctoral thesis in Medicine was on La Notion d'Ambivalence. During the 1960s, and together with Didier Anzieu, Boutonier fought for the independence of clinical psychology from the academic control of philosophy and medicine. This was obtained after the student movement of 1968. She then became director of the Centre Psychopédagogique Claude-Bernard. She died in 1994. (pp. 255–256, Parot and Richelle, 1992).

112 p. 18, Boutonier, 1945.

113 Liebowitz et al., 1985.

114 p. 152, Marks, 1969.

115 Dugas, 1898; Hartenberg, 1901b.

116 Hartenberg, 1901a.

117 Hartenberg, 1901b.

118 Heckel, 1917.

119 Dugas, 1898.

120 Billod, 1847.

121 p. 69, Moreau de Tours, 1845.

122 p. 105, Krishaber, 1873.

123 p. 302, Hécaen and Ajuriaguerra, 1952. Taylor and Marsh (1980) wrongly claim that the word was coined by Dugas).

In fact, Dugas wrote: *Le mot dépersonnalisation avait été employé avant nous par Amiel* (p. 3, Dugas and Moutier, 1911). The actual quotation goes as follows: '*Tout m'est étrange; je puis être en dehors de mon corps et de mon individu; je suis dépersonnalisé, détaché, envolé*' (Amiel H.F.: *Journal Intime*, Vol. 2, pp. 300–301; quoted on p. 5, Dugas and Moutier, 1911). Henri-Frédéric Amiel (1821–81) was a professor of Aesthetics and Philosophy at Geneva University. Of Protestant ancestry, he became well known when after his death it was discovered that he had kept an intimate diary for years. It was a 'remarkable piece of introspective writing' (Harvey and Heseltine, 1959) where many abulic, depersonalization and derealization experiences are described.

124 p. 216, Lalande, 1976.

125 p. 325, Vol. 1, Janet, 1919.

126 L. Dugas was born in *Portici*, Italy in 1871. Trained under Ribot, he relentlessly pursued the view that emotional factors were more important than intellectual ones in psychiatry and education. In regard to the latter, he was fond of citing that of John Stuart Mill as a complete failure. During the second half of his life, he became increasingly interested in education and with L. Cellerie, in 1911 became editor of the influential *L'Anne Pedagogique*.

127 p. 505, Dugas, 1898.

128 p. 507, Dugas, 1898.

129 Eugene Bernard Leroy (1871–1932) was born the same year as Dugas. After training as a physician in the Hôpitaux de Paris, he graduated as a doctor in medicine in 1898. In addition to working in the psychology of memory he was very interested in the psychology of religion, language, dreams, hallucinations, etc. (see obituary by Janet, 1933).

130 Bernard-Leroy, 1898.

131 Dugas, 1894.

132 For an analysis of Bernard-Leroy's survey, see Chapter 9, this book and Bernard-Leroy, 1898.

133 p. 162, Bernard-Leroy, 1898.

134 p. 489, Dugas and Moutier, 1910.

135 p. 8, Dugas and Moutier, 1911.

136 pp. 43–44, Dugas, 1912.

137 p. 47, Dugas, 1912.

138 p. 186, Chaslin, 1912. For a history of the notion of self in psychiatry, see Chapter 18, this book. On the French notion of *conscience de soi*, see Follin and Azoulay, 1978. This notion, in turn, is an offshot of the nineteenth century concept of *le sens intime*, one of the noblest in French spiritualist psychology (pp. 87–124, Tiberghien, 1868).

139 Régis, 1914 quoted in Le Goc-Diaz, 1988.

140 p. 54, Schilder, 1914.

141 p. 104, Mayer-Gross, 1935.

142 He suggested in the same paper the adoption of the term derealization, 'created by Dr Mapother', p. 104, Mayer-Gross, 1935. Historians accept this to be the *fons et origo* of derealization (Follin and Azoulay, 1979; Weckowicz, 1970). However, I have been unable to locate the *printed* source where Mapother actually makes the suggestion nor have I found the noun derealization in use before 1935. The verb *derealize*, however, was used by William James in 1904: 'We have no transphenomenal absolute ready, to derealize the whole experienced world by, at a stroke' (in *OED*, second edition).

143 Ehrenwald, 1931.

144 Bergmann, 1896; a similar interest existed in England, see Marshall, 1901.

145 Schilder, 1914.

146 Pick, 1904.

147 Packard, 1906.

148 Laín-Entralgo, 1987.

149 Maisonneuve and Bruchon-Schweitzer, 1981.

150 Bruchon-Schweitzer, 1990.

151 Kogan, 1981.

152 López Ibor and López-Ibor, 1974.

153 Hécaen and Ajuriaguerra, 1952.

154 Cash and Pruzinsky, 1990.

155 Stutte, 1962–1963.

156 p. 1099, Smith, 1869.

157 p. 204, Masters and Greaves, 1987.

158 Morselli, 1891.

159 Herodotus, 1971.

160 Philippopoulos, 1979.

161 Munro and Stewart, 1991.

162 APA, DSM III-R.

163 APA, DSM IV.

164 ICD-10.

165 Thomas, 1984.

166 Vallat *et al.*, 1971.

167 Fava, 1992.

168 Vanini and Weiss, 1972.

169 Marková and Berrios, 1994.

170 Hollander *et al.*, 1989.

171 Buvat and Buvat-Herbaut, 1978.

172 Reich, 1982.

173 Yamashita, 1993.

174 Berrios and Morley, 1984.

175 p. 3, Kant, 1800.

176 p. 379, Burton, 1883.

177 Kaan, 1892.

178 Hartenberg, 1901*b*.
179 Janet, Les obsessions . . . 1919.
180 Korkina and Morozov, 1979.
181 p. 150, Tanzi, 1909.
182 pp 1823–1901, Kraepelin, 1915.
183 Koupernick, 1962.

CHAPTER 12

Affect and its disorders

For most of the nineteenth century, alienists had a preferential interest in the intellectual functions and their disorders;[1] consequently, the semiology[2] of 'affectivity' remained underdeveloped and contributed little to the emerging definitions of mental disease.[3] This attitude was a legacy from Classical times when 'passions' were considered as the dark and lesser aspect of man.[4] During the late eighteenth century there was a period when it seemed as if the passions might play an important role in the definition of man[5] but this soon passed.[6] Nineteenth century alienists were also limited in their capacity to deal with affective constructs by associationism and classical psychology.[7] Such views markedly contrast with the extolling of emotions that characterized the Romantic movement.[8]

This historical preference for the rational aspect of man is not, however, the only reason for the underdeveloped state of the semiology of affectivity. 'Feelings', 'emotions', 'moods', 'affects', and 'passions' are states whose experiential and behavioural components elude definition;[9] to this day, for example, there is no agreement as to what should count as a valid report for an emotion.[10] Secular efforts to capture these states in words only succeeded in creating a terminological palimpsest.[11] During the second half of the century, however, there was a growing interest in affectivity as illustrated by the work of Brentano,[12] the hypnotists,[13] and later on by that of Janet[14] and Freud.[15]

A general preference for an intellectualistic account of mental disorder has not yet abandoned Western psychiatry. For example, depression, one of the few conditions considered as a 'primary' disorder of affect by nineteenth century alienists, is currently undergoing subtle revision. Indeed, the theoretical claim that negative 'cognitions' cause depressed affect assumes that thinking has primacy over affect.[16]

Conceptual aspects

The elusive nature of feelings

Although clearly recognizable each time they flood some subject's consciousness, affect states are mostly diffuse and ill defined in the time dimension;[17] equally unclear is the role played by social triggers and overt behaviours.[18] These difficulties notwithstanding, feeling states are expected to be recognized and analysed out into sensations and mediating images.[19] Once upon a time, introspection was supposed to provide the sentient subject with a 'privileged' position. This nineteenth-century approach, however, came to grief when doubts were voiced concerning: 1. the existence of an 'inner space' where emotions actually inhabit,[20] 2. the 'usefulness' of introspection, 3. the ability of the subject to tease out mixed affective states into primary components, and 4. the wisdom of using emotion words as names.[21]

News from these debates has hardly reached descriptive psychopathology. In psychiatric practice, the mentally ill patient is expected to describe his emotional states in spite of the fact that often he is unable to behave as a rational observer, i.e. often enough delusions, agitations and distractions cloud his introspection and distort his reporting. His 'privileged' position may also be unhelpful if the mood disorder to be reported is a new experience.

To locate and interpret mood states, clinicians utilize parameters such as duration, intensity, quality, saliency, intentionality (object), pleasantness, diurnal variation, interference with psychosocial competence, behavioural control, etc. Rarely can those acutely ill rate their mood or affect according to these dimensions. In spite of all this, clinicians are surprisingly successful in the assessment of affect and mood. Thus, it is not unreasonable to assume that they use other clinical data as well. Past history, concurrent symptoms, personality, non-verbal behaviour and psychopathological 'credibility' may also play an important role. In fact, historical evidence shows that, since the nineteenth century, mood states have been assessed and classified by taking into consideration somatic, behavioural and metapsychological elements.[22] If so, such assessments should work particularly well when doctor and patient share the same signal system.[23] Both cultural and biological determinants play a role in the acquisition of such systems.[24]

The terminology

Mood, affect, feeling, sentiment, emotion, passion, agitation and propensity (*inter alia*) constitute a family of terms with a protean referent, and different etymology and historical origin. The view that they are members of a 'dramatic' language enshrining the wisdom of the ages is attractive but remains unproven.[25]

Sentiment, emotion and passion have been customarily distinguished from mood, affect and feeling in terms of criteria such as duration, polarity, intensity, insight, saliency, association with an inner or outer object, bodily sensations and motivational force. Sentiment, emotion and passion are defined as feeling states that are short-lived, intense, salient, and related to a recognizable object.[26] Emotion and passion (the latter of which is purported to be an intense version of the former) are assumed to be accompanied by bodily changes and hence to possess motivation properties.[27]

Mood and affect, on the other hand, are defined as longer lasting and objectless states capable of providing a sort of background feeling tone to the individual.[28] Upon this basic mood, emotions of congruent (synthymic) or incongruous (catathymic) value can be superimposed.[29] Affect is also said to be 'dispositional' in nature, i.e. being in 'affect A' means that if certain conditions are met the subject will behave in a particular way.[30] The tone and consistency of the experiences and behavioural forms ordinarily called mood and affect are probably controlled by neuroendocrinological variables, and subject to both genetic and environmental control. Attempts have also been made to redefine affect as a symbolic category, closely related to the action systems of the individual.[31]

'Feeling' is the widest and more abstract term of the entire family;[32] defined in a negative fashion, it refers to those aspects of human experience which are neither cognitive nor volitional. Sensations when elicited by an external stimulus have an informational and a non-informational consequence. The latter, i.e. the capacity to cause a modification in the subjective experience of the individual, constitutes the 'feeling'. There is disagreement on the extent of the contribution made to the formation and definition of a feeling by both the external stimulus and the sentient subject; there is also disagreement on the number of 'elementary' feelings, and on how these come together to form complex emotional states (e.g. see Condillac's allegory of the statue).[33] Be that as it may, these views and debates may be too abstract to be harnessed into everyday descriptive psychopathology.

Historical aspects

Passions and the nature of man

Passions have played an uncertain role in the development of the western view of man. Plato[34] and Aristotle[35] considered 'reason' as the defining human characteristic, the instrument of knowledge, and the guarantee of ethical freedom. The absence or obliteration of reason led to error and evil with the 'passions' being the main source of perturbation and chaos. This view, however, needed to be reconciled with the belief that passions constituted the animal part of man and, as such, his source of energy. This was resolved by accepting the existence of feelings but in a subordinate or 'reduced' capacity. It is not a coincidence that, since Classical times until the end of the eighteenth century, emotions were considered either as a residue from sensation or as a component of volition, but never as entities in their own right.[36] Even Faculty Psychology philosophers such as Reid only recognized 'intellectual' and 'active' powers in the human mind including the emotions in the latter.[37]

The first important revision of these views was due to Aquinas when he suggested that the psychological study of passions should start with the examination of everyday behaviour. He identified the biological (e.g. growth, reproduction) and relational functions (e.g. sensory perception, locomotion) which man shared with animals, and distinguished these from the cognitive and appetitive faculties exclusive to man. He also identified 11 appetitive functions and divided them broadly into two classes: concupiscible and irascible. The passions or appetitive functions were the expression of the 'powers' of the soul which was independent of the body.[38] Three consequences follow from his approach: affective macroconcepts can serve as primary units of analysis; feelings are related to inner representations or structures; and their definition does not necessarily include bodily concepts.

Descartes modified this view by defining passions as 'perceptions, feelings or emotions of the soul which related specially to it, and which are caused, maintained and fortified by some movement of the spirits.'[39] This definition still emphasized the special nature of affective macroconcepts, but challenged the view of emotions as disembodied phenomena; according to Descartes, bodily manifestation must be included in the definition of feeling.[40] His view of the soul as a substance separated from the body led, however, to a neglect of the somatic component of the feelings. Cartesian subjectivism encouraged the view of emotions as independent mental functions. This process culminated in Kant's work.[41]

During the eighteenth century, the negative view of the passions was called into question,[42] but not by everyone and to many it remained as the received doctrine.[43] During the early nineteenth century, both Romantic and Positivist medicine endeavoured to incorporate the passions into the concept of disease.[44] For example, Comte characterized madness as an *excés de subjectivité*.[45] On this Lewes wrote: '*Agir par affection, et sentire pour agir*, such is the motto of Comte's system, which indicates the predominance given to the emotive over the merely intellectual – in opposition to the old psychology which always sub-ordinated the emotions to the intellect.'[46]

During the nineteenth century the psychiatric role of emotion became clearer: it could either cause or result from mental disease. The causal role was the earlier[47] and led to the view that the manipulation of the emotions could have therapeutic value; this, called the 'moral treatment',[48] was well described by Esquirol as early as 1805: 'Previous discussions and the facts upon which they are based show the relationship between emotions and insanity; they indicate better than any definition what 'moral treatment' means. If it is essential to provoke violent shocks and excite this or that emotion to control the lunatic . . . it is no less important to be kind and affable to him.'[49]

Passions as causes of madness

In Greek culture, affective excitement culminating in irrationality was considered as a common mechanism of insanity.[50] This view remained unchanged throughout the Medieval period,[51] Renaissance,[52] and up to the nineteenth century.[53] The mechanisms whereby passions induced madness were rarely specified although they may have included pathological changes in 'imagination'[54] and constructs such as 'reaction'.[55] There is some evidence that the concept of 'imagination' may be a forerunner of the current notion of 'psychogenesis'.[56]

The naturalistic view of the passions started by Descartes began to show in the medical literature towards the end of the eighteenth century. Alexander Crichton summarized it thus: 'the passions are to be considered from a medical point of view as part of our constitution, which is to be examined with the eye of the natural historian, and the spirit and impartiality of the philosopher. It is no concern of this work whether passions be esteemed natural or unnatural, or moral or immoral affections. They are phenomena and produce constant effects on our corporeal frame; they produce beneficial and injurious effect on the faculties of the mind.'[57]

It is unclear why this novel view of the passions as a natural phenomenon did not encourage clinicians to develop a descriptive psychopathology of affectivity. It would seem that the main obstacle was still the received view of madness as a dislocation of the intellect. Nowhere is this clearer than in the opposition by early nineteenth century alienists to the existence of an 'affective monomania'.[58]

The received view of madness

The definition of madness inherited by the nineteenth century was intellectual-istic in nature. Irrationality and overt behavioural disturbance had since Greek times been the two central features of madness.[59] *Paranoia*, *phrensy*, *mania*, *melancholia* and *lethargy* were defined in these very terms.[60] Melancholia, for example, was defined as a mixture of irrationality and reduced behavioural output.[61] Sadness of spirit, although occasionally mentioned, was not a necessary or sufficient diagnostic feature. This view of melancholia remained unchanged until the Modern Period.[62]

The *Anatomy of Melancholy*[63] and other writings of the period illustrate this well.[64] Burton did mention sadness and sorrows as accompaniments of melancholia but also included obsessions, delusions, suicidal behaviour and hypochondriacal complaints. He considered the latter not as secondary complications but as primary symptoms of melancholia. In fact, he defined as melancholic any mental disturb-ance characterized by an exaggeration of function, irrespective of whether or not it involved the affective life.[65] Thus, the word melancholia acquired at least two mean-ings around this period: a popular usage related to sadness, suicide and nostalgia[66] and, the technical usage – successor to the old theoretical speculations – according to which melancholia was a form of delusional insanity.[67] Early nineteenth century psychiatrists commented upon these two meanings: 'The word melancholic, conse-crated in vulgar language as the name for ordinary sadness (*tristesse*) should be left to moralists and poets.'[68] The other disorders, namely phrensy, paranoia, lethargy, and mania were also defined in terms of intellectual disorder.[69]

Changes in the received view of madness

During the early nineteenth century, theoretical changes and the clinical demands of the new medicine caused a revision of the intellectualistic view of insanity. Four historical factors will be briefly discussed: 1. the establishment of affectivity as an autonomous mental function in psychology, 2. the transient predominance of feelings and emotions caused by the Romantic Movement, 3. the clinical limitations of the intellectualistic account of insanity, and 4. the development of the new medical science of signs and symptoms.

After 1800, Faculty Psychology became a psychological alternative to Associationism.[70] To this contributed the Scottish Philosophers[71] as well as Kant.[72] Faculty Psychology provided phrenology with its conceptual basis[73] and encouraged work on brain localization.[74] According to most versions of Faculty Psychology, the affective functions constituted a primary, autonomous and irreducible faculty of the mind. This encouraged the view that there might be primary disorders of affect,[75] and soon enough 'emotional' forms of insanity were proposed; in due course melancholia was re-defined along these lines. Esquirol, for example, attempted to emphasize the role of sadness in the development of melancholia (he coined the term 'lypemania') but, in the end, fell back on the partial insanity (monomania) concept.[76] Heinroth was far more direct: 'the presence of an *idée fixe* does not mean that the disease is an affectation of the intellect; the intellect is the mere servant of the sick disposition ... the *idée fixe* may not be present but melancholia remains what it is: depression of the disposition, withdrawal into oneself, detachment from the external world.'[77]

The glorification of the feelings is one of the central features of the Romantic Movement.[78] Such emphasis on subjective experiencing as a source of aesthetic knowledge encouraged the development of introspection and, later, of the psychological notion of consciousness.[79] This drive towards mentalism changed medical attitudes towards the definition of disease. Most important, it caused a redefinition of the traditional concepts of 'sign' and 'symptom'.[80] Alienists responded to these changes, and in due course disturbances of subjective experience were to be added to the symptomatology of madness.[81] In a general sense, writers such as Maine de Biran,[82] Royer-Collard,[83] and Moreau de Tours[84] made possible the incorporation of subjective information into the descriptive language of mental illness.[85] Complex inner experiences began to be painstakingly described and catalogued according to the analytical method of the philosophy of ideology.[86]

The intellectualistic view of madness, although in keeping with the empiricist epistemology of the period, was of limited clinical use. In the event, its main role was to facilitate the development of the concept of 'partial insanity'. This term had three meanings during the early nineteenth century: a mild form, involvement of one faculty, or monothematic delusions, the latter being called *délire exclusif*.[87] The concept of partial insanity was mostly popular in forensic psychiatry.[88] The clinical usefulness of the intellectualistic definition of insanity was challenged early in the nineteenth century by Pinel,[89] Prichard,[90] and Heinroth.[91]

The need to describe signs and symptoms was a requirement of the anatomoclinical view,[92] but the search for lesions to match signs and symptoms was unsuccessful in psychiatry.[93] Practical needs were also important; for example, the involvement of medical practitioners in the running of asylums for the insane occasioned the need to keep good clinical records. Finally, the observation of patient cohorts created the need to register symptoms independently[94] and to introduce 'time' as a dimension of mental illness.[95]

The semiology of affectivity

It remains to be explained why, in spite of all these favourable changes, affectivity failed to play a role in the new psychiatric semiology. One reason might have been that, during the last century, psychologists and philosophers of mind continued (overtly or covertly) reducing affective behaviour to cognition or volition.[96] Psychiatrists, in turn, found clinical mood disorders lacking in stability, and reliable behavioural indicators for their presence were unavailable.[97] Even writers who sponsored Faculty Psychology, like Benjamin Rush, shared this difficulty.[98] On this it has been written: 'Rush has little to say of the passions considered intrinsically. His treatment is mostly occasional, where the passions are associated with other faculties, operations and diseases.'[99] Pinel was equally parsimonious on the passions, in spite of his criticism of Locke's view.[100]

Yet another illustration is found in Esquirol whose thesis was entitled *The passions as causes, symptoms and means of treatment of mental illness*.[101] In this work he signally failed to develop a semiology of affectivity; more surprisingly, his very concept of lypemania, only emphasized the 'partial' nature of the delusional thoughts (i.e. *monomanie*).[102] Feuchtersleben, for all his psychological proclivities, defined melancholia in similar terms;[103] and even an idiosyncratic writer like Broussais[104] preferred the bodily aspects of the passions and subscribed to an intellectualistic view of insanity. Laycock[105] equally emphasized the physiological aspect of the 'emotions and passions,' and his list of affective macroconcepts is unconvincing. Bucknill and Tuke dedicated no separate section in their Manual to the disorders of affect.[106]

Griesinger, on the other hand (and in spite of having been accused of exaggerated organicism), was one of the first alienists to deal separately with the 'anomalies of sentiment'.[107] Falret attempted a similar approach, and included the 'derangement of the emotions' as a subsection of his 'general symptomatology of insanity'.[108] His treatment of the topic is, however, jejune which is not surprising in view of his belief that no faculty could become impaired in isolation, i.e. he supported what was then called the principle of solidarity of the mental faculties.[109] Morel wrote on 'symptoms originating in the affective functions' and endeavoured to define 'feelings, instincts, etc.'[110]

The lost opportunity

During the second half of the nineteenth century the chances of developing a descriptive psychopathology of affectivity were negatively affected by Darwinian evolutionism,[111] by the development of a peripheralist view of emotions[112] and by advances in brain localization studies.[113]

Darwin resuscitated the view that emotions were ancient and stereotyped behaviours shared by man and lower animals.[114] It is not surprising, therefore, that greater emphasis was put on the analysis of overt 'expression' than subjective experience: 'the main difficulty in elucidating emotions consists in the fact that the major part is due to historical antecedents registered in the susceptible organisms, but little to individual acquisitions. No experience of the individual can account for the strength or the direction of feeling. If any one should be found to doubt the cumulative and permanent effect of racial influences he has only to attempt to explain without such reference any of the more pronounced passions and affection. One need not be surprised therefore that so little progress has as yet been made in this department of psychology, *owing to the excessive reliance on the introspective method*, a method which leads no further than to description' (my italics).[115]

Ribot wrote along the same lines, castigating 'intellectualism' and siding with the 'physiological school', according to which 'all states of feeling (are connected) with biological conditions.'[116] Lloyd Morgan agreed: 'I think that comparative psychology may fairly assume that throughout the range of the sense experience, common to men and animals, their emotional states are of like nature with ours.'[117]

The so-called peripheralist theory reduced the analysis of emotions to incoming sensations. Ziehen for example, wrote: 'The older psychology regarded the emotions as the manifestation of a special independent faculty of the soul. Kant placed the feeling of pleasure and pain between the cognitive faculty and the appetitive (volitional) faculty; ultimately, the emotional tone of all ideas may be reduced to the emotional tone of sensations.'[118] Peripheralist views such as this, and the James–Lange hypothesis[119] did little for the semiology of affect.

Work on brain localization, for all its great importance to the development of neuropsychology, did not serve the emotions well, as it concentrated on speech, perception and movement.[120] Questions on the localization of the emotions were usually referred to the ganglionar nervous system.[121] Workers like Mairet, attempted to localize affectivity in the temporal lobe but their work fell on deaf ears.[122] The problem with referring to the ganglionar system was that this structure could be considered as either a generator or a simple instrument for the expression of emotions.[123]

In the event, it was not an experimental worker but a clinician, Bernard Hollander, who was to reassert the old view: if delusional insanity 'can only be explained by disease of one part causing derangement of some of the intellectual faculties . . . then diseases in another part may not disturb the intellect but derange the moral powers or propensities.'[124] This author collected about 50 cases of melancholia in which neuropathological studies seemed to show lesions in the angular and supramarginal gyri of the parietal lobe. Hollander made no mention of Mairet's seminal work.[125] The frontal lobes were also mentioned in relation to feelings;[126]

for example, Bianchi reported experimental work in monkeys showing changes in complex emotions after frontal lobe excisions; his methodology was later criticized by Lashley.[127] Localization studies did not encourage work on the phenomenology of affectivity.

Reactions against reductionism

The reductionistic approach entertained during this period was unhelpful to the development of a semiology of affectivity, and a reaction started in some quarters. For example, there was a determined attempt by Brentano[128] and later by Ward[129] to return to a phenomenology of affective macroconcepts; and Freud, in general, followed this view[130] although, as Green rightly said, 'he struggled with the problem of affect all his life.'[131] This probably stemmed from the fact that affect played too complex a role in Freud's system; not only was it a descriptive category (in the traditional nineteenth century sense), but also a mechanism and a source of energy. Surprisingly enough, these over-extended conceptions contributed little to the semiology of affect.[132]

Bleuler, on the other hand. wrote with some sensitivity on affect[133] but later on he reverted to a conventional view.[134] Bianchi included in his textbook a large section on the symptomatology of disordered affect, but his treatment is excessively physiological.[135] Régis restricted the role of the disorders of mood to that of precipitants of 'delusions and hallucinations'.[136] Even Jaspers dedicated just five pages to affect which are amongst the less inspired of his textbook.[137] Thus, lost somewhere between the evolutionary, the peripheralist, the psychodynamic, and the 'phenomenological' views, the clinical disorders of affect struggled for recognition.

Kraepelin's distinction between dementia praecox and manic-depressive insanity appears to be based on a distinction between thinking and affect, respectively.[138] Analysis of the eighth edition shows, however, that his defining criteria of manic-depressive insanity were: 1. uniform and good prognosis, 2. differential heredity,[139] and 3. presence of excitement or inhibition.[140] As far as this writer has been able to determine, nowhere did Kraepelin say that manic-depressive insanity was a *primary disorder* of affect.

Schneider included in his psychopathology a short Appendix on 'Abnormal feeling' and made much of their positive and negative polarity.[141] Even Minkowski, whose self-given brief was to develop a 'phenomenological psychopathology', produced a quasi-mechanistic characterization of mood disorders, according to which symptoms may result from weakness, inhibition, disjunction, dysrhythmia and immaturity of the affective faculty.[142] Perhaps Bash's analysis is the most serious and relevant to clinical practice to date.[143]

Summary

The aim of this section has been to explain why the semiology of affectivity is not as well developed as that of the intellectual functions. It has been suggested that this resulted from a long-term neglect and also from the obscurity of the subject matter itself. This led to an undue predominance of 'intellectualistic' symptoms such as delusions, hallucinations, obsessions, and memory deficit.

The history of depression and mania

The group of conditions nowadays called 'affective disorders' has resulted from the convergence of certain words (e.g. 'affective' and its cognates), concepts (theoretical notions accounting for 'mood' related experiences), and behaviours (observable changes in action and speech associated with whatever the neurobiology of these disorders happens to be). Each order of elements has a different history, and their evolution has been asynchronous; in fact, they only came together during the early part of the twentieth century. Since there is no reason to expect that this convergence is 'written in the nature of things', its explanation belongs more to history than to science. If the convergence hypothesis is correct, then those who believe that the history of the conditions now called mania and melancholia starts with the Greeks must be mistaken, for their anachronistic approach is, at its best, only chronicling the history of the words.

One of the problems confronting the historian is that the phrase 'affective disorders' refers to a family of subjective and objective behavioural disturbances. In current English-speaking psychiatry, for example, it names the depressive and manic syndrome, combinations thereof, and occasionally some of their accompanying anxiety symptoms.[144] As mentioned above, 'Affective' (the operative word), has itself a long and noble history and is part of a panoply of terms such as emotion, passion, feeling, sentiment, mood, affective equivalent, dysthymia, cyclothymia, dysphoria, etc. Although these terms name overlapping subjective states, they have different semantic provenance. Basically, it is unclear whether they refer to some fundamental unitary mental function or to combinations of functions.[145]

The affective disorders

Our current notions of depression and mania date from the second half of the nineteenth century and emerged from the transformation of the old notions of melancholia and mania. The ideological changes that made them possible included the availability of Faculty Psychology and of the anatomo-clinical model of disease, and the inclusion of subjective experiences into the symptomatology of mental disorders.[146] The concept of mania was first narrowed down, and the residue re-defined (under the influence of Faculty Psychology) as a primary disorder of affect and action. The pre-nineteenth century notion of melancholia was equally refurbished: this was facilitated by Esquirol's concept of lypemania which emphasized the affective nature of the disorder.[147] Once the right conceptual conditions were given, the new clinical versions of mania and melancholia combined into the new concept of alternating, periodic, circular or double-form insanity.[148] This process culminated with Kraepelin's concept of 'manic-depressive insanity' which included most forms of affective disorder under the same umbrella.[149]

The transformation of melancholia into depression

'Melancholia' wrote John Haslam in 1809: 'the other form in which this disease (madness) is supposed to exist, is made by Dr. Ferriar to consist in "intensity of idea". By intensity of idea I presume is meant, that the mind is more strongly fixed on, or more frequently recurs to, a certain set of ideas, than when it is in a healthy state.'[150] Haslam's perception was correct. Up to the period of the Napoleonic Wars, melancholia was but a rag-bag of insanity states whose only common denominator was the presence of few (as opposed to many) delusions. In practice, therefore, it is highly likely that it included cases of schizophrenia. Sadness and low affect (which were no doubt present in some cases) were not considered as definitory symptoms. Indeed, states of non-psychotic depression, of the type that nowadays would be classified as DSM IV 'Major Depressive Episode' would not have been called 'melancholia' at all. During the eighteenth century these states were classified as 'vapours',[151] 'spleen', or 'hypochondria', i.e. what Cullen called 'neuroses', and Sydenham and Willis, the previous century, had called 'nervous disorders'.[152]

The term 'depression'

To search for the origins of the term and the concept of 'depression' the historian does not need to go beyond the middle of the nineteenth century.[153] After the 1820s, conceptual changes determined that 'melancholia' could no longer be: 1. a subtype of mania, 2. a primary disorder of intellect, and 3. irreversible. What emerged from these changes was a form of partial insanity defined as a primary disorder of emotions whose features (clinical and aetiological) reflected loss, inhibition, reduction, and decline. Thus constituted, 'melancholia' was re-named 'depression', a term that had been popular in middle nineteenth century cardiovascular medicine to refer to a reduction in function.[154] The word was first used analogically as 'mental depression' but soon after the adjective 'mental' was dropped. By 1860, it appears in medical dictionaries: 'applied to the lowness of spirits of persons suffering under disease'.[155]

The first edition of Régis's *Manuel* defined depression as: 'the state opposed to excitation. It consists of a reduction in general activity ranging from minor failures in concentration to total paralysis.'[156] Physicians preferred the word depression to melancholia or lypemania, perhaps because it evoked a 'physiological' explanation. For example, Sir William Gull used it as early as 1868 in his article on 'hypochondriasis': 'its principal feature is mental depression, occurring without apparently adequate cause.'[157] By the end of the century, 'depression' was defined as: 'a condition characterized by a sinking of the spirits, lack of courage or initiative, and a tendency to gloomy thoughts. The symptom occurs in weakened conditions of the

nervous system, such as neurasthenia and is specially characteristic of melancholia.'[158] In his popular Manual, Savage defined melancholia as a 'state of mental
depression, in which the misery is unreasonable.'[159] Even Adolph Meyer cam-
paigned in favour of the new word.[160]

Thus constituted, depression was gradually enlarged by the addition of a number
of symptoms and states that ranged from stupor or 'melancholia attonita'[161] to
nihilistic delusions.[162] Kraepelin legitimized the term by using it in a adjectival
manner, and amongst the 'depressive states' he included melancholia simplex,
stupor, melancholia gravis, fantastic melancholia and delirious melancholia.[163] British psychiatry took longer to catch up, and continued treating the same group of
disorders as 'melancholia'; witness to this the famous 'Nomenclature of Diseases'
drawn up by a Joint Committee appointed by the Royal College of Physicians of
London in 1906 (see below).

There was, however, some disagreement concerning the clinical meaning of
the new melancholia (or depression). Because its symptoms were often found in
other insanities, a number of explanations were offered: 1. stage in the development of a unitary psychosis,[164] 2. separate disease, self-contained or part of a
cycle including euphorias and / or stupor,[165] 3. development of the subject's
personality,[166] i.e. an exaggeration of acquired vulnerabilities,[167] and 4. manifestation of a tainted pedigree.[168] These hypotheses were not considered as exclusive, and the manner of their combination engendered much debate. This is
partly explained by the fact that the logic of justification and falsification which
operated amongst nineteenth (and early twentieth) century alienists was based
on the marshalling of single cases and of counter-examples. Although the notion
of 'law of error' (Gaussian distribution)[169] was already available, it had not yet
penetrated the methodology of medicine. So, case reports exhibiting minor deviations from the idealized type created difficulty and forced alienists to declare
them as new forms.

In the eighth edition of his textbook, Kraepelin cut the Gordian knot by creating
an over-inclusive notion which comprised all forms of depression and mania, even
the notion of 'involutional melancholia'.[170] This omnibus concept was characterized
by: (a) a periodic course, (b) good prognosis, and (c) endogenicity (i.e. not related
to precipitants); all three criteria demanded standards of clinical description and
observation which at the time were difficult to achieve. They also led to surprising
conclusions, for example, that some paranoias, neurasthenias or (even) changes
in bowel habit (without other accompanying features) may be hidden forms of
manic-depressive illness.[171] These less recognizable Kraepelinian views are rarely
mentioned nowadays, perhaps because of selective reading: only those amongst his
clinical statements are quoted which remain intelligible to current psychiatrists.
In Kraepelin, the concept of affective disorder can be said to be at its most over-
inclusive: indeed, the history of the affective disorders after 1910 is no more than
the analysis of the fragmentation of the Kraepelinian notion.

Summary

Thus, in the period between Esquirol and Kraepelin seven assumptions accumulated in regard to the affective disorders:[172] 1. they were to be a 'primary' pathology of affect,[173] 2. had stable psychopathology,[174] 3. had brain representation,[175] 4. were periodic in nature,[176] 5. were genetic in origin,[177] 6. appeared in individuals with recognizable personality predisposition,[178] and 7. were endogenous in nature.[179] These beliefs originated from clinical observation, logical reasoning, and ideology, and not surprisingly, each has a different conceptual history.

The classification of the affective disorders

During the nineteenth century, the need to re-classify the affective disorders had various origins.[180] There was, first, the taxonomic impetus that affected the whole of medicine and the need to tidy up the nosology of psychiatry; there was also the influence of Faculty Psychology (the search for the primary disorders of affect) and the ever-looming presence of degeneration theory; and, finally, late in the century, there appeared the need to identify homogeneous clinical groups for neuropatholog-ical study, particularly in relation to the differential diagnosis between melancholia and dementia.[181]

The first point to make is that what was involved in the taxonomic drive was not just diseases changing pigeonhole. The magnitude of the transformation was so large that, without a metalanguage and a metaperspective, it cannot be fully appreciated.[182] From the vantage point of the twentieth century, pre-1800 concepts of insanity are only superficially intelligible. Up to the eighteenth century, insanity (lunacy, madness, vesania) was an opaque concept which predicated of the insane a state of *existence* rather than of mind.[183] The obvious problem with this view was to explain clinical remissions. For this, the notion of 'lucid interval' was created which accounted for 'normal' behaviour without abandoning the view that the person remained mad at a deep level.[184] This ontological belief is concealed from view by the fact that medical practitioners in earlier times 'contextualized' their description of madmen by talking about 'life-events', 'onset', 'lucidity', and specific individuals. Madness itself was only given a temporal context during the nineteenth century, when 'time' became, for the first time, a dimension of mental disorder.

Adding a time dimension rendered madness into a longitudinal process. This view achieved full development in the work of Kahlbaum,[185] and later in Wer-nicke[186] and Kraepelin.[187] The time dimension helped to deal with questions which had been unresolved up to the time of Kahlbaum such as what 'subsisted' or 'endu-red' or gave identity to mania, melancholia, and dementia: was it the symptoms themselves? The level of psychological energy (as, for example, in Griesinger)? The mental faculty involved (regardless of the symptoms)? The brain lesion? Due to the incipient state of neuropathology, first symptoms, and later faculties were chosen to play this ontological role. The problem with taking symptom combinations *prima facie* was that it led to a proliferation of new 'diseases'. So, faculties became popular as in the case of Esquirol's taxonomy; and in a way, we still have a classification based on the original disorders of intellectual, affective, and volitional functions.

But Kahlbaum first, and then Kraepelin (who followed him closely), postulated that to be considered a disease a symptom-cluster had to persist in time (i.e. had a course) and show brain representation. The first criterion was easier to comply with and drastic enough to reduce the number of insanities described. It was drastic enough in Kraepelin's hands to override clinical description and create two new super-diseases. But Kraepelin's nosology could not escape the curse of 'intermediate' cases, to the point that, as an old man, he grew sceptical and relinquished the dichotomy.[188] The taxonomic problem presented differently to the French for their psychiatry was under particular conceptual pressures such as that of degeneration theory.[189]

An important cause for this classificatory chaos was the failure of the anatomo-clinical model of disease which left alienists with mere symptom descriptions.[190] Phrensy, mania, melancholia, and dementia had been neatly defined at the beginning of the nineteenth century albeit on purely theoretical grounds.[191] In their effort to 'naturalize' madness alienists rejected these categories and only succeeded in causing their fragmentation. The gain, however, was that symptoms were for the first time independently 'observed' so that when new theoretical classifications of insanity were proposed[192] they were expected to tally with the reality of observation.

Nineteenth century France

During the first half of the nineteenth century classificatory fashions originating in France had a commanding influence on the rest of Europe. Pinel was perhaps the last great man to use melancholia and mania in the old, classical sense. Esquirol, Georget, Billod, Baillarger, Falret, Marc, Morel, Linas, Ritti, and Magnan, all implemented changes in these categories. Their work, however, had not yet been completed when the Kraepelinian view took France by storm splitting the ranks of her alienists.[193] Some, like Deny and Camus[194] supported the notion of an over-inclusive manic-depressive insanity; others stuck to the old views and the debate continued well into the 1930s.

PINEL Pinel defined melancholia as an insanity characterized by a circumscribed number of delusions (*délire exclusif*). His clinical conception of the condition, however, was wide: 'Melancholia frequently remains stationary for many years without its central delusion changing in character, and without causing much physical or psychological change. It can be seen in patients with this condition detained at *Bicêtre* for 12, 15, 20, or even 30 years, that they are still victims of the delusions that originated their admission . . . some having a more mobile character, and after observing the agitated behaviour of some lunatics, develop a manic state . . . others, after many years undergo a sort of internal revolution, and their delusions change. One of these patients, already advanced in age, had believed for years that he had been imprisoned by his parents who wanted his fortune; more recently, however, he began to fear that we wanted to poison him.'[195] Pinel included under melancholia all forms of chronic psychosis, including schizophrenia.

ESQUIROL AND *LYPÉMANIE* But this was soon to change. Under the influence of Faculty Psychology, and believing that melancholia was a primary disorder of emotions, Esquirol criticized the old usage: 'the word melancholia, consecrated in popular language to describe the habitual state of sadness affecting some individuals should be left to poets and moralists whose loose expression is not subject to the strictures of medical terminology.'[196] Prichard had a similar view,[197] and Rush, after criticizing Cullen's usage, advised against the use of the word 'melancholia' coining, instead, *tristimania*.[198]

But of all these new terms, it was 'lypemania' that survived the longest. Esquirol defined it as 'a disease of the brain characterized by delusions which are chronic and fixed on specific topics, absence of fever, and sadness which is often debilitating and overwhelming. It must not be confused with mania which exhibits generalized delusions and excited emotions and intellect nor with monomania that exhibits specific delusions and expansive and gay emotions, nor with dementia characterized by incoherence and confusion of ideas resulting from weakening.'[199] Esquirol even reported a clinical and epidemiological profile for the new disease: rates for lypemania were found to increase between May and August,[200] the age group most affected was that between 25 and 45,[201] and in 110 of 482 cases 'heredity' seemed to have played a role; common causes included domestic crisis, grief and disturbed relationships,[202] about a third of his cohort died, often of tuberculosis.

The term lypemania had its critics. Delasiauve called it too '*élastique* and apart from being less imprecise was no different in terms of content from the old term melancholia.'[203] Delasiauve was here referring to the fact that Esquirol had kept circumscribed delusions (a vestige of the old intellectualistic notion) as a *defining criterion*. Delasiauve was right for it is clear from studying Esquirol's case reports that lypemania included paranoid and delusional disorders.[204] Delasiauve suggested that the boundaries of lypemania be narrowed further to refer only to: 'an exaggeration and persistence of feelings of depression.'[205] The highest point in the history of lypemania was reached in the work of Billod who accepted that lypemania had to be defined on the basis of sad delusions and disordered affect, and suggested a four-fold classification: lypemania with sad delusions and sadness; sad delusions and no sadness; sad delusions and mixed or alternating affective disorder (this included the bipolar states); and no sad delusions and sadness. This contrived symmetry allowed the recognition of about sixteen subtypes. Some of these states have since disappeared (e.g. ironic or religious lypemania), others (e.g. hypochondriacal, stuporous, or irritable lypemania) are still found in current use under different names.[206]

The word 'lypemania' did not catch on in Germany, Austria, Switzerland or Great Britain, where the word 'melancholia' was maintained. Prichard paid no attention to the term nor did Griesinger who regularly quoted Esquirol.[207] Feucht-ersleben mentioned the term once, but did not acknowledge its origins; Bucknill and Tuke did, but continued using melancholia on the excuse that Esquirol himself had stated that the terms could be used interchangeably.[208] Lypemania is an example of what historians may want to call a 'bridge' category: it only served to catalyse the transition between the old notion of melancholia (as a primary disorder of intellect) to the new one (as a primary disorder of affect).

BAILLARGER, FALRET, AND THE COMBINED STATES In 1851, Jules Falret described, in one of his lectures at the *Salpêtrière*, a condition which he called *forme circulaire de maladie mentale*, consisting in 'a period of excitation followed by one of weakness ordinarily longer.'[209] In 1854, Baillarger read a paper before the *Académie de Médicine* reporting seven cases of what he called *folie à double forme* and which consisted 'in the succession of two regular periods, one of excitation and the other of depression.'[210] Few days after this paper had been read, Falret published the excerpt of his course including his earlier clinical description and claimed priority for the 'discovery';[211] two weeks after Baillarger's paper, Falret also managed to get time to read his own paper before *L'Académie de Médicine*.[212]

As Ritti showed in his monograph,[213] suggestions that patients may show com-bined depressive and manic periods were not new, and had been in the air for a long time. The issue of priorities cannot be resolved and is probably irrelevant. No doubt both Baillarger and Falret were talking about forms of manic-depressive ill-ness, as were others before, and indeed afterwards. For example, Billod, coined the term *à double phase*,[214] and Delaye and Legrand du Saulle, *folie alterne*.[215] However, the full concept of manic-depressive illness, as a separate illness, did not crystallize in France until 1883.

In 1880, and in an effort to solve the ongoing debate, *L'Académie de Médicine* decided to call for entries (as it had done before in relation to other clinical problems) on 'the form of insanity called circular, double-form, or alternating'. A. Ritti was awarded the first prize, and A.E. Mordret the second;[216] both monographs appeared the same year, and together created the conceptual basis for the disease that was to feature as the centrepiece in Kraepelin's manic-depressive 'circle'.

Cotard's syndrome

So-called *délire de Cotard* refers to a cluster of symptoms that may appear in the wake of severe melancholia. Of late, there has been renewed interest in the clini-cal[217–219] and neurobiological[220–222] aspects of this clinical phenomenon and hence it is important to trace its history. 'Nihilistic delusions' but not Cotard are mentioned in DSM IV;[223] neither term appears in ICD-10.[224] This section will review the original French sources for 'Cotard's syndrome' and its conceptual construction between 1880 and the First World War.

JULES COTARD   Jules Cotard was born on 1st June 1840 in Issoudun (France) and read medicine in Paris where he was a student of Broca and Vulpian; he became interested in the pathology of the nervous system whilst working under Charcot. His first substantial work was *Ètudes physiologiques et pathologiques sur le ramollissement cérébral*;[225] he obtained his doctorate in 1868 with an *Ètude sur l'atrophie partielle du cerveau*.[226] After seeing the great Lasègue interview a patient at the *Prefecture de Police*, he turned to psychiatry. In 1874, Lasègue introduced Cotard to Jules Falret, and these two men formed an enduring partnership at the Vanves asylum. His untimely death on 19th August 1889 followed an attack of diphtheria caught from his daughter.

Cotard was influenced by Condillac, Cabanis, Destutt de Tracy, Maine de Biran and Comte; and wrote on hypochondria, aboulia, and the 'psychomotor origin' of delusions.[227] At his funeral, Jules Falret described him as: 'a profound and original thinker, given to paradox, but guided by a robust sense of reality'.[228] This original bent of mind is illustrated in an early paper on *Folie*[229] where Cotard explored the difficulties posed by adopting ordinary terms into the scientific language of psychiatry, and rejected the principle of aetiological classifications of mental disorder.[230] Based on the belief that knowledge of the brain was insufficient to support causal explanations, he proposed a symptomatic classification.[231] Original thinking also led him to suggest that disturbances of affectivity might be 'the grounds on which delusions germinate'.[232]

On 28th June 1880, in a meeting of the *Societé Médico-Psychologique*, Cotard read a paper on *Du délire hypocondriaque dans une forme grave de la mélancolie anxieuse*[233] reporting the case of a 43 year-old woman who believed that she had 'no brain, nerves, chest, or entrails, and was just skin and bone', that 'neither God or the devil existed', and that she did not need food for 'she was eternal and would live for ever'. She had asked to be burned alive and had made various suicidal attempts.

Cotard was aware of the fact that similar cases had been described before and quoted Esquirol,[234] Macario,[235] Leuret,[236] Morel,[237] Krafft-Ebing,[238] and Baillarger,[239] the latter of whom had 20 years earlier reported similar cases in the context of general paralysis. Cotard diagnosed his patient as suffering from *lypémanie* (an Esquirolean category only partially related to 'psychotic depression episode' (see above).[240] Cotard explained that *délire hypocondriaque* resulted from 'an interpretation of pathological *sensations* often present in patients with anxious melancholia'. He suggested that a similar form of *délire* might have given rise to the myth of the 'wandering Jew'[241] and to cases of so-called *démonomanie*. He believed to have found a new subtype of *lypémanie* characterized by anxious melancholia, ideas of damnation or possession, suicidal behaviour, insensitivity to pain, delusions of non-existence involving the whole person or parts thereof, and of immortality. These were the original features of the complete Cotard's psychotic state (*délire de Cotard*).

Two years later, Cotard returned to the topic and introduced the term *délire des négations* (translated since then as *nihilistic delusions*): 'I would like to venture the term *délire des négations* to refer to those cases . . . in which patients show a marked tendency to denying everything'.[242] Carried to its extreme, this 'negating attitude' led the patient to deny the existence of self or world, and such delusions may be the only symptom left during the chronic state of melancholia. To make sense of this new symptom cluster in the context of French nosology, Cotard compared it with the *délire de persecution* (persecutory syndrome) which, since the time of Lasègue, had been central to French psychiatry.[243] In clinical practice, *délire des négations* may be found alone, as a manifestation of general paralysis, or associated with a persecutory syndrome.

In 1884, Cotard reported a case of melancholia with nihilistic delusions who complained of an inability to 'visualize the features of his children'. Recalling a case of Charcot's who had also 'lost the capacity to visualize absent objects', Cotard went on to suggest that nihilistic delusions might be secondary to a 'loss of mental vision', to an incapacity to evoke mental representations of objects not present to the senses.[244] Few days before his death he modified this view by suggesting that the primary disorder was a reduction in 'psycho-motor energy' (*la diminution de l'énergie psycho-motrice*) leading both to psychomotor retardation and loss of images (the latter causing the *délire des négations*).[245]

A digression is now required concerning the major difficulty posed by the translation of *délire*, which is usually rendered as delirium or delusion. These terms only manage to convey fragments of its French meaning. *Délire* is not a state of delirium or organic confusion (called in French *délire aigu*[246] and *confusion mentale*[247]) nor a delusion (called in French *idée or thème délirante*[248]): it is more like a syndrome that may include symptoms from the intellectual, emotional or volitional spheres.[249] Hence, translating *délire des négations* as nihilistic delusion gives the wrong impression (caused by the *intellectualistic* semantics attached to the term 'delusion' in English) that it exclusively refers to a 'thought'. As clearly described in his 1882 paper, Cotard never meant it to be a 'thought' but a symptom cluster. So, to talk about the delusion of being dead as Cotard's delusion,[250,251] makes little sense for *délire des négations* also entails the presence of anxiety, severe depression, and other attending delusions.

THE NAMING OF THE SYNDROME In 1893, Emil Régis coined the eponym *Cotard's syndrome*[252] and the term was made popular by Jules Séglas who reported the case of a man with 'intermittent anxious melancholia' with delusions of absence of organs, of negation, damnation, and immortality. In opposition to Cotard, Séglas proposed that nihilistic delusional states did not constitute a distinct clinical entity but only a severe form of anxious melancholia (*'une forme particulière de mélancholie anxieuse . . . une sorte d'aggravation de la maladie'*) (pp. 66–67).[253] Three years later, Séglas hypothesized that the condition was analogous to 'secondary paranoia', i.e. a terminal state of 'that clinical condition that foreign authors have called *Secündare Verrücktheit* (p. 419).[254] In later papers Séglas went on to classify nihilistic ideas according to whether their content involved the body; people and objects of the external world; or intellectual faculties and concepts (God, soul, etc.).[255,256] The extent of the denial might be partial or total and as reported by Baillarger,[257] the syndrome was occasionally associated with general paralysis, in which case, nihilistic delusions tended to be 'partial' involving ideas of non-existence or destruction concerning bodily organs. When associated with senile dementia, nihilistic delusions were episodic, fleeting and incoherent; and when associated with melancholia, they were total and systematized; Séglas considered the latter to be 'true secondary paranoia'.

Séglas believed that delusional ideas in general, and nihilistic ones in particular, should be classified according to origin (i.e. form) and not to content and suggested psychosensorial, affective and motor types.[258] He also hypothesized that at the basis of nihilistic ideas, there was a disturbance in 'mental synthesis' (as that causing depersonalization) leading to an inability to evoke images. Nihilistic ideas occurred in situations when the personality was modified by affective or motor disturbances (changes also central to melancholia).

Cristiani[259] supported the view that there was an association between Cotard's syndrome and chronic paranoia, and others followed this trend.[260,261,262,263] Anticipating modern views, Obici considered nihilistic delusions to be based on involutional and degenerative process, and made the important suggestion that they reflected the presence of an 'organic component'.[264]

THE FIRST CONTROVERSY (1892–1900) Soon after Cotard's death, the debate started on whether it had been his intention to describe a new disease or just a severe form of melancholia. Castin, Camuset and Charpentier (*inter alia*) believed the former, and Séglas, Régis, Toulouse, Pichenot, and Ballet the latter. Régis suggested a third interpretation, namely, that Cotard wanted to describe a 'syndrome', i.e. a symptom cluster which could also be found in mental disorders other than melancholia.[265] This view was to prove very influential.

The issue was debated at the third *Congrés de médicine mentale* (August 1892, Blois, France). To save the 'new disease' view, Falret distinguished between an 'essential' and a 'secondary' form of *délire des négations*, and stated that only the latter could appear in insanities other than melancholia;[266] he also agreed with Cotard's view that 'nihilistic delusions, like persecutory delusions, have a progressive course'.[267] Camuset, on the other hand, stated that the frequency with which nihilistic delusions were combined with ideas of possession, damnation, or immortality 'was not high enough' to constitute a separate syndrome; furthermore, because all patients with melancholia had 'negating attitudes' there was no reason to believe that nihilistic delusions *per se* had anything to do with prognosis.[268] Castin denied the existence of Falret's 'essential' form and also believed that what Cotard had described was just a collection of symptoms seen in a number of diseases.[269] Garnier, in turn, went as far as claiming that 'he had never seen a nihilistic delusion' of the type described by Cotard.[270] Charpentier stated that all nihilistic delusions were either hypochondriacal, melancholic or persecutory, and criticized Cotard for introducing a 'name' and not a disease.[271] De Cool also believed that nihilistic delusions could be found in most melancholic patients and were no different from ideas of guilt, ruin or damnation.[272] According to Arnaud, nihilistic delusions appeared in the wake of chronic melancholia, particularly in women between 50 and 60 years old, carrying a hereditary taint.[273] Trénel reported a case who also had grandiose ideas.[274] All in all, however, it was agreed that the *two defining elements* of the nihilistic delusions syndrome were anxious melancholia and systematized ideas of negation.[275]

THE SECOND CONTROVERSY (1900–1939) The categorization of the affective disorders changed during the early twentieth century;[276,277] not surprisingly, Cotard's syndrome was soon reported in relation to 'depression'[278,279,280] and 'manic-depressive illness'.[281,282,283,284] Reports of its association with general paralysis[285] and senile dementia[286] continued.

The syndromatic view predominated during this period. Deny and Camus divided Cotard's syndrome into a 'melancholic type' with nihilistic delusions referring to the patient's subjectivity and which were secondary to affective disorders; and a 'hypochondriacal type' where their content concerned the body, and which were primary ('primary paranoia').[287] Got considered Cotard's syndrome as a secondary delusion found in a subtype of anxious melancholia which he called 'pure melancholia' or 'symptomatic periodical insanity';[288] it was far more common in older age groups, although in the young it seemed to have a better prognosis; nihilistic delusions are even rarer in adolescents.[289]

Tissot suggested that nihilistic delusions resulted from the combination of an 'affective component' (anxiety) and an 'intellectual component' (the idea of negation), the former being considered as fundamental to distinguish 'true Cotard' from other nihilistic states.[290] Loudet and Dalke recognized non-systematized and systematized nihilistic delusions; the former were isolated, episodic, and could be found in general paralysis, alcoholic psychoses, and dementia; the latter (Cotard's syndrome), was characteristic of diseases such as anxious melancholia and chronic hypochondria; these authors also believed that there were 'complete' and 'incomplete' forms of the syndrome.[291] Obarrio *et al.* considered nihilistic delusions to be secondary to anxious melancholia.[292]

LATER DEVELOPMENTS Interest in the 'Cotard' state was renewed after the Second World War. For example, Perris suggested that Cotard's intention had been to describe a single symptom, a hypochondriacal delusion that occurred in anxious melancholia; he added, however, that it may be accompanied by 'disorders of sensation' and that it rendered the melancholia refractory to treatment; i.e. once the nihilistic delusion was established, it dominated the clinical picture and made it chronic.[293]

During this period the old syndromatic view[294,295] was also challenged by the view that it might, after all, be a different entity. For example, De Martis reported a case of a 38 year-old woman who after surgery showed a change in personality and after an initial period of anxiety developed ideas of negation of her body and of the world, ideas of enormity and of immortality; the author suggested that Cotard's syndrome may be a separate form of psychosis for the nihilistic delusions were structured from the start and had a chronic evolution unaltered by treatment; he further suggested that melancholia only triggered this condition in patients otherwise predisposed.[296] Enoch and Trethowan have written that it is 'justifiable to regard Cotard's syndrome as a specific clinical entity because it may exist in a pure and complete form, and that, even when symptomatic of another mental illness, such as endogenous depression, nihilistic delusions dominate the clinical picture'.[297]

Trémine has also considered Cotard's syndrome as a separate clinical entity which may develop in the chronic course of mental illness; but which 'was a reflection of the attitudinal changes brought about by chronic institutionalization'; he believed that Cotard's syndrome was a 'perfect illustration' of the decontextualized method of description employed in psychiatry during the second half of the nineteenth century.[298] A similar view about the role of institutionalization has been taken by Lafond[299] and also by Bourgeois who has claimed that Cotard's syndrome is a 'vestige of the asylums, and of the chronicity of the pre-therapeutic era'.[300] If so, it could be surmised that the 'therapeutic revolution' should have an important impact on its frequency;[301] this hypothesis, however, has not yet been tested. In a different vein, Joseph has described a case of a 30 year-old man with coexisting Cotard's and Capgras' syndromes and proposed that Cotard's syndrome was a distinct disorder because it might result from a specific parietal-lobe dysfunction.[302]

In summary, it would seem as if Cotard opted for the view that *délire des négations* was a sub-type of depressive illness. The debate on the nature of this clinical phenomenon that ensued after his death concluded that it was only a 'syndrome', i.e. a collection of symptoms that could be found associated with diseases such as agitated depression (anxious melancholia) or general paralysis. But it was also agreed that its central features were anxiety, delusions of negation, damnation and enormity. The syndromatic view predominated for more than 50 years until some authors began to suggest, based on the fact that the syndrome was clear-cut and stable, that it might constitute a different condition.

Nineteenth century Germany

It has been customary to accept the view,[303] started by Deny and Camus, that during most of the nineteenth century, the German contribution to the history of the affective disorders was negligible, and that it only became important after the work of Krafft-Ebing, Weygandt, Kraepelin and Dreyfus.[304] This view is anachronistic in that it judges 'importance' from the perspective of the present.

Under the influence of German Romanticism, writers such as Reil, Heinroth and Griesinger expressed views on the affective disorders which reflect the growing importance of 'affect' and 'passions' in the development of mental illness.[305] For example, Heinroth wrote: 'the origin of the false notions in patients suffering from melancholia . . . is being erroneously attributed to the intellect . . . here the intellect is not at fault . . . it is the disposition which is seized by some depressing passion, and then has to follow it, and since this passion becomes the dominating element, the intellect is forced by the disposition to retain certain ideas and concepts. It is not these ideas or concepts which determine the nature and the form of the disease.'[306] Writings by German alienists from this period also reflect an anti-Cartesian approach, for example, by classifying the insanities in terms of the 'single principle of cerebral development, both physical and psychological.'[307]

Griesinger

The concepts of melancholia and mania are difficult to elucidate in the work of Griesinger. In spite of his great influence and reputation, Griesinger had limited clinical psychiatric experience,[308] and hence based his definitions on borrowed cases and views. His beliefs on the mechanisms involved in the affective disorders came from various sources: (*a*) Herbartian associationism, which allowed him to identify 'the elementary symptoms (units of analysis) of insanity', (*b*) Broussais's notion of 'irritation' and his belief that mental disorder could result from increases or decreases in psychological energy or vitality, and (*c*) the 'unitarian' view, i.e. that there was one form of insanity which could change in its symptomatic expression through time.[309] Thus, although Griesinger's clinical description of melancholia has a 'modern' ring, it should not be forgotten that it belongs to a different conceptual world in which there were no independent psychiatric diseases but successive symptom clusters reflecting the oscillations of a vital principle.[310]

Kahlbaum

The views of Kahlbaum on melancholia and mania are confusing because he included both syndromes under the term *dysthymia* (which he attributed to Carl Friedrich Flemming).[311] In 1859, Flemming, one of the great leaders of German asylum psychiatry[312] published a book on *The Pathology and Therapy of the Psychoses* including a chapter on syndromes resulting from the primary disorder of the emotions.[313]

In 1863, Kahlbaum put forward an original classification, based on a longitudinal concept of disease.[314] The third group in this classification was the *Vecordias* (defined as idiopathic disturbances of mental life, with onset after puberty, and with more or less specific symptoms). These were sub-divided, according to Faculty

Psychology, into disturbance of intellect (*paranoia*), volition (*diastrophia*), and emotions (*dysthymia*). The latter included *dysthymia meläna* and *elata* according to whether there was a predominance of sad affect (*Vorwalten trauriger Affecte*) or elated affect (*freudiger Affecte*).[315] In regard to melancholia, Kahlbaum said: 'In our view melancholia is not a disease but a syndrome (*ein Symptomenkomplex*).'[316]

Krafft-Ebing

Krafft-Ebing is said to have used a 'modern voice' to define and classify melancholia and mania.[317] As Bercherie has noticed, Krafft-Ebing's taxonomic principles are based on a series of dichotomies.[318] Firstly, the psychoses are divided into those with and without intellectual retardation; then the latter into those with (organic) or without (functional) identifiable brain pathology; thirdly, the functional psychoses are split into those developing in degenerates (i.e. those with family loading of mental illness: psychoneurosis) and in 'normals'; finally, the psychoneuroses are divided into melancholia, mania, acute and hallucinatory insanity. Melancholia, Krafft-Ebing defined as a 'painful inhibition of psychological functions' and mania as an exalted facilitation. This classification reigned supreme in Germany until the time of Kraepelin.

Kraepelin and 'involutional melancholia'

Kraepelin's general views on manic-depressive insanity have been discussed above.[319] However, confusion remains in regard to the history of involutional melancholia.[320] Thus, let us first quote a standard definition: 'The term customarily refers to agitated depressions occurring for the first time in life after the age 45–50, in contrast to manic-depressive illness which manifest itself at an early age.'[321] The conventional story is that, up to the seventh edition of his textbook, Kraepelin considered involutional melancholia as a separate disease, and that when confronted by the evidence collected by Dreyfus,[322] he decided to include it, in the eighth edition, under the general heading of manic-depressive insanity.[323] Indeed, this account was first presented by Kraepelin himself: 'The fact that states of depression are specially frequent at the more advanced ages, had already before this forced the supposition on me, that the processes of involution in the body are suited to engender mournful or anxious moodiness; it was one of the reasons which caused me to make a special clinical place for a portion of these forms under the name melancholia. After the purely clinical foundations of this view were shaken by the investigations of Dreyfus, our representation also now lets the causal significance of age appear in a light somewhat different from my former view.'[324]

The story is, however, more complex and it is unlikely that the finding of Dreyfus alone caused Kraepelin's change of heart. For example, Thalbitzer claimed that his own work had also been influential.[325] In fact, in the eighth edition, Kraepelin abandoned not only involutional melancholia but the entire group of 'senile psychoses'. More to the point, the reasons which in the first place led him to consider involutional melancholia as a separate disease had been many: 'depression become more frequent with age, in older age groups psychomotor agitation was more frequent than retardation, outcome worsened with age, and melancholia often became complicated by 'mental weakness', that is cognitive impairment.'[326] In the eighth edition, twice did Kraepelin feel obliged to justify his change of opinion. First, he mentioned Dreyfus (see above); secondly, he stated that further experience had taught him that 'the arguments in favour of the separation of melancholia were not sound'[327] for 'dementias could be explained by the appearance of senile or arteriosclerotic disease; that other cases, after very long duration of illness, some of them displaying manic symptoms, had they still recovered. The frequency of depressive attacks in advanced age we have come to recognize as an expression of a general law which governs the change of colouring of the attack in the course of life. Lastly, the substitution of anxious excitement for volitional inhibition has proved to be behaviour which we meet with in advancing age in those cases also which decades previously had fallen ill in the usual form.'[328] This account was confirmed in his autobiography.[329]

Dreyfus and his monograph

By quoting Dreyfus in the eighth edition, Kraepelin burdened the young man (who was only 26 when he started the research) with the responsibility of having been the overt cause for his change of heart.[330] To test the hypothesis that involutional melancholia had a bad prognosis (i.e. did not recover), Kraepelin asked Dreyfus[331] to find out what had happened to all the cases he himself had diagnosed as 'melancholia' in 1892 (whilst he was head of the Heidelberg Clinic). At the time, 'melancholia' was used by Kraepelin as a shorthand for 'involutional melancholia'; the rest he called 'depressive states'.

Dreyfus completed the follow-ups in 1906, so the longest was about 14 years. He included 85 cases of which he described 44 in detail, sometimes transcribing daily medical entries from the index episode. In more than half of the total sample, Dreyfus managed personal follow-ups. Statistical analysis of Dreyfus's data[332] shows that only 43 subjects improved, and that the only significant correlation of outcome was with age! ($r = .30$; $p < .01$). When the sample is partialled out by sex, the correlation disappears for the males; in the females goes up to $r = .39$ ($p < .01$). The rate of recovery was higher for the younger group.[333] Thus, Dreyfus's conclusion that the natural history of involutional melancholia was no different from that of depression affecting younger subjects is not warranted by his own data (he did not include a control group). Indeed, he did not notice that, in his female patients, outcome was correlated with age.

The great synthesis suggested by Kraepelin in the eighth edition of his textbook created as many problems as it solved. Since the publication of his work, the history of the affective disorders in Europe and other parts of the world can be fairly described as attempts at solving the clinical problems and contradictions that it created.[334]

American views

The issue of involutional melancholia was also discussed in a meeting of the New York Neurological Society on 1st November 1904, with the participation of great men such as Dana, Starr, Collins, Meyer, Parsons and Diefendorf.

Dana reported a personal series of 400 cases of melancholia and divided them into two groups. One included cases with onset during 'involution or change of life'; this form was chronic and incurable, and was characterized by 'hypochondriacal and obsessive ideas, dysthesia, somatic delusions, hallucinations, self-accusations and at times suicidal ideas and impulses'.[335] A second group included cases starting in early life with no 'definite picture' which, according to Dana, Kraepelin might classify as manic-depressive. Dana believed that this latter group showed the clinical features of the 'involutional type' but nonetheless had a good prognosis. Dana's was not the first large American series of melancholics to be reported. Brush, from the Sheppard Asylum in Baltimore, had reported 100 cases of acute melancholia with high incidence of physical disease at the 1897 Meeting of the British Medical Association.[336] The same year, Weir Mitchell reported a series of 3000 cases of melancholia used to test the hypothesis that the disease was most 'apt to relapse in the spring or summer'. He found no evidence of seasonal changes.[337]

European views were predominant in the USA during this period. Smith Ely Jelliffe read a paper before the 66th Meeting of the American Medico-Psychological Association on 'Cyclothemia [*sic*], the mild forms of manic-depressive psychoses and the manic-depressive constitution' and not once quoted an American colleague. On these mild forms British psychiatrists had a great deal to say during the first 30 years of the twentieth century (see below).[338]

Nineteenth century Great Britain

Prichard

British psychiatric taxonomy took an important step forward in the work of James Cowles Prichard. Although influenced by French views, Prichard showed originality in spite of the fact that he did not have a great deal of clinical psychiatric experience.[339] Prichard classified melancholia as a subtype of 'moral insanity' (in fact, a disorder of the emotions): 'the faculty of reason is not manifestly impaired, but a constant feeling of gloom and sadness clouds all the prospects of life' 'this tendency to morbid sorrow and melancholy, as it does not destroy the understanding, is often subject to control when it first arises, and probably receives a peculiar character from the previous mental state of the individual.'[340] Following pre-nineteenth century views, mania was defined by Prichard as a form of 'raving madness' and included cases of acute psychotic mania, organic delirium and schizophrenia. Mania was for Prichard a harbinger for 'chronic and advanced states of madness'.[341]

Bucknill and Tuke

In their 'classification', Bucknill and Tuke limited themselves to listing psychiatric conditions. Melancholia and mania are described as separate entities, but not classified as subtypes of 'emotional insanity' (except the sub-syndrome that they called *melancholia without delusions*).[342] This listing of conditions without attempting to organize them according to some high level principle is a curious (and healthy) departure from contemporary fashion which, since the time of Pinel, and certainly of Esquirol, had dictated a threefold grouping for all insanities. Bucknill and Tuke listed six forms of melancholia: simple (non-psychotic), complicated (psychotic), acute, chronic, remittent and intermittent. Mania, in turn, was considered as a general form of madness, as Prichard had done before.

Maudsley

Maudsley's views on mania and melancholia, loosely follow the British tradition. He called melancholia 'insanity with depression' and made it tantamount to Bucknill and Tuke's 'simple melancholia' (i.e. non-psychotic depression). He also described a second group called 'melancholia with delusions' which more or less corresponds to the current concept of psychotic depression: 'in this form of depression the sad feeling is accompanied by a fixed sad idea or by a set of fixed sad ideas which crystallize, so to speak, out of or about it', 'out of the melancholic gloom emerge dimly and shape themselves by degrees positive delusions of thought.'[343] In this category he included melancholia with stupor, acute delirious melancholia, and hypochondriacal melancholia, and discussed symptoms such as suicide, homicide, and hallucinations.

Maudsley's analysis of mania was symmetrical to the one he afforded to melancholia. Mania was 'insanity with excitement' and included mania without delusion or simple mania where: 'there is an extraordinary excitement, without positive derangement, of feeling and thought: quickened thought flushed with elated and aggressive feeling,'[344] and 'recovery not taking place, what other issues has acute mania? The next most common event is that it becomes chronic, the excitement subsiding but the derangement continuing.'[345] Nodding in the general direction of the Continent, Maudsley concluded with regards to alternating recurrent insanity (*Folie Circulaire*): 'there is still one issue more of acute or rather subacute mania which it remains to take notice of – where it ends by being transformed, its seeming ending being but the beginning of an opposite – complexioned disorder. When the acute symptoms are past ... the patient falls instead into an abject melancholy depression.'[346]

The 1906 Nomenclature of Diseases

Towards the turn of the century, the pre-Kraepelinian view of melancholia and mania came to an end in Great Britain.[347] This was made official in the fourth edition of the *Nomenclature of Diseases* drawn up by the Joint Committee of the Royal College of Physicians of London[348] whose psychiatric members were George Savage and Percy Smith. 'Mania: Acute, recurrent and chronic' (145.) appears as a separate disorder including seven subtypes (a to g): 'hysterical, puerperal, epileptic, alcoholic, senile, from other acute and chronic disease or from injury, and delirious.' 'Melancholia: acute, recurrent or chronic' (146.) also appears under a different heading with seven sub-types (a to g): 'agitated, stuporous, hypochondriacal, puerperal, climacteric, senile, and from other acute or chronic disease or from injury.' Finally, 'Circular insanity, alternating insanity' (147.) is included without subdivisions. This classification lasted until the great British debate of the 1920s.

Aetiological views

Little has been written on late nineteenth century British aetiological views on the affective disorders. This section will limit itself to listing the most popular hypotheses. G.M. Robertson, then a senior assistant at the Morningside Asylum (later to become Professor of Psychiatry at Edinburgh), published in 1890 a provocative paper suggesting a 'modular' approach: 'what explanation is there of the existence of these symptoms of melancholia ... in answering this question we must know that we are investigating a function of an organ which has become diseased; the function being the production of depressed or painful emotion.'[349] Influenced by Darwin and Romanes, Robertson went on to identify a number of symptoms of melancholia (e.g. catalepsy) which he considered as the expression of vestigial behaviours.

Ten years later, John Turner asked another important question: 'very perplexing to the student of insanity is the question as to how states of exaltation or depression arise ... To what changes in the nervous system do they correspond? ... Are these changes localized in different parts of the nervous system in mania and melancholia?'[350] Turner decided against the modular view and adopted a Jacksonian stance:[351] 'whilst both melancholia and mania are associated with a dissolution of the nervous system, in the former case the reduction takes place along sensory lines of the reflex nervous arc, and in the latter along motor lines.'[352]

But, as mentioned above, the most accomplished paper on 'the cerebral localization of melancholia' was written by Bernard Hollander who, after reviewing the literature concluded that: 'a certain relation exists between the central area of the parietal lobe, namely, the angular and supramarginal gyri, and melancholic states of mind.'[353]

Great Britain and the Continent

It has been shown that, until the turn of the century, views on the affective disorders in France, Germany and Great Britain were more or less uniform. This is not very surprising as free communication existed between alienists from these nations.[354] Most European alienists shared the belief that mania and melancholia: (a) resulted from a primary pathology of the emotions, (b) could be combined in various ways, (c) resulted from cerebral disease, (d) were inherited, and (e) could recover. Kraepelin's synthesis, although resisted in France, reinforced this uniformity.

The commonality of views lasted well into the 1920s, when differences began to appear. The British continued worrying about clinical description, severity and classification; the French about inheritance and environmental triggers; and the Germans, influenced by Kretschmer's thinking, debated the question of constitution and personality factors. As an illustration of the debates that led to national differences, we shall explore the British debate on classification.

Early twentieth century Great Britain

During the 1920s, British views began to depart from those held in the Continent. This resulted from uncertainties concerning the nosological position of what was called 'neurotic, reactive, exogenous, psychogenic or constitutional' affective disorders. The view that these might need including with the rest of manic-depressive insanity was based on a number of arguments: (a) clinical observation, (b) challenge to Kraepelin's dichotomous view, (c) the growth of the psychodynamic hypothesis that there might be a 'continuity' between all forms of depression, and (d) the influence of Meyerian psychiatry.

As we have seen, during most of the nineteenth century the classification of mania and melancholia (whatever their definition) had not been difficult. Symptom pattern, presence or absence of delusions, course, and whether or not the two were combined provided sufficient taxonomic criteria. As we have also seen, cases requiring classification were collected from the severe end of the affective disorders (i.e. hospitalized patients). These classifications were, therefore, not encumbered by minor and non-psychotic affective disorders which, up to the First World War, were mainly seen in private consulting rooms[355] under the diagnosis of hypochondria, hysteria, neurasthenia, agoraphobia or psychasthenia. Indeed, clinical analysis of cases under these rubrics[356] shows that a good proportion would now be diagnosed as depressions and non-psychotic manic-depressive states. Apart from the social changes which led to differential patterns of care (e.g. the foundation of the Maudsley hospital with its emphasis on 'neurotic' out-patients), one of the factors in the rekindling of the classificatory debate in Great Britain was the dismembering of 'neurasthenia'; the reasons for this are beyond the scope of this book but suffice it to say that not all the cases released by this fragmentation could be fitted into its successor, that 'bridge' disease called psychasthenia.[357] These cases were to constitute the large group that Montassut called in his masterly monograph *constitutional depressions*.[358] In addition, the impact of psychodynamic ideas was beginning to be felt,[359] particularly in relation to mechanisms such as 'reactivity', and the issue of the relationship between personality and depression. A good illustration of this influence is to be found in the British debate over the clinical place of the minor or 'neurotic' depressions.

MAPOTHER In 1926, Edward Mapother, then superintendent of the Maudsley Hospital[360] presented a controversial paper at the Nottingham Meeting of the British Medical Association.[361] He stated that his problem was 'what meaning should be attached to the term 'manic depressive psychosis'. He believed that 'the range of the term was a matter of convention; at present there is no agreement, and no one with the authority to impose it.'[362] In a Meyerian fashion he continued: 'All would probably agree that under the heading are included cases of functional mental disorder which show as their predominant features one of a contrasting pair of anomalous types of reaction: '1. the depressive reaction, and 2. the manic reaction'. He asked whether all cases with these symptoms should be included or only some, as some 'cases merge into those where constitutional symptoms of one kind or the other are pretty constantly present'. With scepticism he added: 'it is unproven and improbable that any mental syndrome is due to a specific cause, and consequently there is no more likelihood of a constant course in mania or depression than in jaundice'.[363] He challenged the distinction between neuroses and psychoses which had 'really grown out of practical differences particularly as regards certification and asylum treatment', and concluded that, since a distinction could not be made, it was nonsense to try and differentiate between neurotic (anxiety neurosis) and psychotic depression.

E. Farquhar Buzzard, who was chairing, disagreed with the view that these two conditions could not be distinguished as did Thomas A. Ross, from the Cassel Hospital, who stated that: 'if Dr Mapother would carefully study mental states he would find that they would lead him to perceive fundamental differences between the psychoses and the psychoneuroses'[364] and added that these doubts originated from the fact that 'only a small section of the psychoneurotic group found their way to the Maudsley Hospital'!

Then, it was the turn of a young Scottish psychiatrist, working under Ross, called Gillespie,[365] who rose to say that he was surprised at Mapother's request that a 'meaning should be attached to the term manic-depressive psychosis' and that 'the failure [by Mapother] to mention clinical criteria he would have regarded as an accident, were it not for his later remark that details of mental state were utterly unreliable.'[366] 'This tendency more or less unconscious to depreciate clinical differentiation gave the key to Dr Mapother's subsequent surprising classification of all psychoneurosis as a subdivision of the manic depressive psychosis' 'the truth was that the latter was essentially a clinical conception, and that an attempt to define something that had been differentiated on purely clinical grounds in terms of the academic psychology after McDougall was likely to fail.'

Gillespie then flew his own colours: 'The task of psychopathology at present was not so much the discovery of a physical basis – that was not psychopathology, and smacked of the pseudo-physiologizing of the latter half of the nineteenth century – but the unravelling of the meaning and origin of mental symptoms as such ... it was to be regretted that Dr Mapother had made no mention of MacCurdy's work on the manic depressive psychosis ... [whose] work did much to upset what might be called the 'psychiatrist's fallacy' – that thought always followed emotion. Emotion probably more often followed thought.'[367] These statements by Gillespie, of importance to the history of the affective disorders in Great Britain, deserve further exploration.

GILLESPIE AND THE CAMBRIDGE CONNECTION Robert Dick Gillespie (1897– 1945) had trained under D.K. Henderson in Glasgow, and A. Meyer and C.P. Richter in Baltimore; after a meteoric career he succeeded Sir Maurice Craig at Guy's. In his relatively short life he wrote with originality on fatigue, sleep, hypochondria and depression. In 1926, there was a good reason for Gillespie to mention MacCurdy. In fact, these men were to collaborate between 1927 and 1929, whilst Gillespie held the Pinsent–Darwin Research Studentship in Mental Pathology at Cambridge.

MacCurdy (1886–1947) was a Canadian psychologist and psychiatrist[368] who first trained as a biologist at Toronto University, and then as a physician at Johns Hopkins. After doing postgraduate work in neuropathology under Alzheimer in Munich, he returned to New York as a psychiatric assistant to August Hoch.[369] It is suggested in this book that the change of heart on the nature of the affective disorders shown by Gillespie between the Nottingham debate and the publication of his own classical paper on the *Clinical differentiation of types of depression*[370] was due to MacCurdy's influence.

In this seminal paper, Gillespie reviewed the literature in detail, particularly the work of Kraepelin, Lange, Cimbal and Kretschmer, searching for depressive states that might be dependent on special features of personality or identifiable environmental factors. He also reported 25 cases which he classified into reactive (14), autonomous (7) and involutional (4). He stated that the three groups could be distinguished in terms of family history, symptoms, personality, and response to life events. These criteria, in fact, he borrowed from MacCurdy.[371] In view of this, Kendell's comment that Gillespie provided no 'justification for his assumption that classification on the basis of reactivity was more useful or more valid than that based on another criterion'[372] is, perhaps, harsh. Gillespie's paper must be read in conjunction with MacCurdy's book, where both conceptual and therapeutic justifications (not statistical, for at the time such an evidential methodology was not yet part of medicine) are provided.

BUZZARD AND THE 'MILDER FORMS' In 1930, Sir E. Farquhar Buzzard (knighted since chairing the BMA Nottingham meeting of 1926), returned to the issue of milder depressives without cyclothymia: 'We frequently see depressed patients who do not give this history of preceding elation or depression. A source of anxiety may be ascertained and its importance as an aetiological factor has to be measured. The sequence of events suggests that anxiety precipitated or caused depression.'[373] Buzzard identified some distinguishing features: 'Having referred to the difficulty of diagnosis in the milder forms – and the milder the form, the more difficult the diagnosis . . . let me emphasize those [clinical points] which I have come to regard as most helpful: 1. the type of depression, 2. the loss of all natural and accustomed interests, 3. the self-reproach, 4. the preservation of sleep, 5. the history of hypo-manic phase, 6. the coincident physical disturbances, and 7. the family history, particularly of suicide and alcoholism.'[374]

In the ensuing discussion H. Critchton-Miller 'regretted the title of the discussion . . . the term 'manic-depressive psychosis' may be correct enough for use in mental hospitals but it suggests too much. The term *cyclothymia*, on the other hand, covered the subject under discussion including the milder forms.'[375] He emphasized how important it was to know the subject's pre-morbid personality, and criticized Kretschmer's for his over-simplistic distinction between 'cycloids' and 'schizoids'. Crichton-Miller was interested in the 'physiological aspects' of the disease: 'In the first place periodicity appears to be a physiological rather than a psychological quality . . . in the second place there is great similarity between the euphoria of alcoholic intoxication and the exaltation of the cyclothymic . . . thirdly, there is similarity between the depression associated with chronic intestinal absorption (sic) and the depressed phase of cyclothymia . . . fourthly the commonest example of cyclothymia occurs in some women in relation to the menstrual cycle.'[376] He concluded that 'the problem is not one for the psychologist, but for the bio-chemist.'[377]

Next, George Riddoch emphasized stress and the psychological aspects of the disease, and Henry Yellowless felt that Kraepelin's taxonomy and psychology were out of date, and that the real clinical issue here was to differentiate the milder forms from neurasthenia; he concluded that they were talking about a physical disease and that psychological treatments were not indicated. W.R. Reynell agreed, and Helen Boyle (the only lady doctor to intervene in the debate) put forward an eclectic view based on Golla's endocrinological work (on thyroid disorder) and Stoddart's psychodynamic theory. E.B. Strauss, who had spent some time at Marburg working under Kretschmer (and whose translator into English he was to become), defended the views of his teacher, and emphasized the notion of 'reactive depression' which he defined as: 'a condition precipitated by an intolerable situation in the patient's life. It is allied to true neurasthenia, prison psychosis, and the like. Whether the condition is entirely exogenous or whether a current conflict stirs up and allies itself to unconscious mechanisms, may be debated by psychoanalysts.'[378]

The 'milder forms' in the Continent

A similar debate (although couched in different words) took place in France and Germany. It concerned the diagnosis and aetiology of the 'milder forms' of affective disorders. As mentioned above, the Kraepelinian synthesis had been based on the description of asylum cases, and had left out a large group of disorders composed of protracted griefs, dysphorias, minor depressions, anxiety disorders, and neurasthenias. Clinical decisions as to the nature of this group became important in the context of out-patient and private practice.

In comparison with his major contribution to the clinical and nosological aspects of the affective disorders, Kraepelin had been reticent on the role played by other modulatory factors, such as the 'personality'. On this the French were far more advanced.[379] After 1900, psychodynamic models and treatments became increasingly important: to these views, France was, perhaps, the most permeable of the three nations.[380] As has been hinted above, the breaking up of the old group of 'neuroses' (e.g. neurasthenia and psychasthenia)[381] set asunder a large number of clinical states which (as the British debate showed) began to be considered as the 'milder' forms of manic-depressive illness. To many, this solution was not satisfactory, as illustrated in the work of Courbon, Rouart, Benon, and Montassut.[382] The British debate flared up in the 1930s, as a result of the work of Aubrey Lewis;[383] this has been studied by Kendell[384] and is not treated further here.

Final summary

This section of the chapter has explored the origin of the 'depressive' states, and the way in which these were combined with mania by the middle of the nineteenth century. It has mapped the manner in which this process unfolded in German, French, and British psychiatry. Finally, it has studied the history of involutional melancholia and statistically evaluated the empirical evidence on which Kraepelin based his decision to include this syndrome under the heading of manic depressive insanity.

The relative unity of approach to melancholia and mania shown during most of the nineteenth century came to grief after the 1910s. The main factor responsible for this was the increase in the size and variance of the patient database: to asylum patients (with chronic and severe illnesses often complicated by physical disease) cases were added from private practice, out-patients, those released by the disintegration of the neurasthenia group, and those described as 'depressed' by the practitioners of psychoanalysis. During the 1920s, these 'milder' forms were diagnosed as manic-depressive, 'reactive', 'psychoneurotic' and 'personality' disorders. Current diagnostic categories have not yet fully escaped the influence of these early views.

ACKNOWLEDGEMENTS Dr Rogelio Luque, from Cordoba University, Spain, greatly helped with the writing of the section on Cotard's syndrome.

NOTES

1 pp. 63–66, Griesinger, 1867; Ribot, 1897; pp. 343–385, Bianchi, 1906; Bleuler, 1906; Chaslin, 1912.
2 By this is meant the description of signs and symptoms.
3 Bash, 1955; pp. 145–166, Schneider, 1959; pp. 108–117, Jaspers, 1963; pp. 65–76, Hamilton, 1974; pp. 232–247, Scharfetter, 1980; Berrios, On descriptive psychopathology, 1984.
4 Dodds, 1951; Landman, 1958; Pigeaud, 1981; Roccatagliata, 1973; 1981; *Colloque International De Bruxelles*, 1976; Simon, 1978.
5 Perkins has claimed that during the eighteenth century 'the scorn of the seventeenth century towards the passions was replaced by an exaltation of strong emotions. But reason was not abandoned and most characteristic eighteenth century thought combines the rational and the emotional.' p. 145, Perkins, 1969.
6 pp. 189–194, Luyendijk-Elshout, 1990; also pp. 7–39, Levi, 1964.
7 Mischel, 1973; Warren, 1921; Hoeldtke, 1967; Bricke, 1974.
8 Borgese, 1934; pp. 287–314, Lovejoy, 1936.
9 Ketal, 1975; Owens and Maxmen, 1979; Pollit, 1982. For the more general aspects of this problem see pp. 105–130, White, 1967; pp. 83–115, Ryle, 1949; also see Darwin, 1904; and illuminating essay by Browne, 1985.
10 Sartre, 1939; Bedford, 1964.
11 Thus, in addition to the re-adoption of the old terms mania and melancholia, new ones were coined such as *depression, affective equivalent* (Fonseca, 1963), *hysterical dysphoria* (Liebowitz and Klein, 1979), *alexythymia* (Lesser and Lesser, 1983, *dysthymia* (Akiskal, 1983), *aprosodia* (Ross and Mesulam, 1979), and *anhedonia* (Watson *et al.*, 1970; Harrow *et al.* 1977; Koh *et al.*, 1981) (see also Chapter 13, this book).
12 Rancurello, 1968.
13 Barrucand, 1967.
14 Schwartz, 1955.
15 Ellenberger, 1970.
16 Gelder, 1983; Erwin, 1978.
17 Kenny, 1963.
18 Schachter and Singer, 1962.
19 Ribot, 1897.
20 Donegan, 1968; Weiskrantz, 1968.

21 Bedford, 1964.
22 Ribot, 1897; Störring, 1907.
23 Krueger, 1928.
24 Mantegazza, 1878; Gruber, 1981; Darwin, 1872.
25 Deleule, 1969.
26 Ribot, 1897.
27 Leeper, 1948.
28 Ketal, 1975; Owens and Maxmen, 1979.
29 Bash, 1955.
30 Ryle, 1949.
31 Siomopoulos, 1983; Green, 1973.
32 Fellner von Feldegg, 1900; Gardiner, 1906; Washburn, 1906; Claparède, 1928; Beebe-Center, 1951.
33 Condillac, *Traité de Sensations*, 1947.
34 Dodds, 1951; Simon, 1972–3; Solmsen, 1983.
35 Lloyd, 1968; Fortenbaugh, 1975.
36 Gardiner *et al.*, 1937.
37 Reid, 1854.
38 Gardair, 1892; Monahan, (undated); Koninck, 1947; Simmonnet, 1983.
39 p. 344, Descartes, *The Passions of the Soul*, 1967; Kenny, 1968.
40 Weckowicz and Liebel-Weckowicz, 1982.
41 Büchner, 1897; Leary, 1978; Hilgard, 1980.
42 For example, Rousseau regarded the passions as natural depositories of goodness and as representing the purest side of man. Distortions in the understanding of man created by the 'civilized' intellect could only be corrected, according to him, by attending the call of the passions; Gardiner *et al.*, 1937; Riese, 1965. A direct consequence of this 'Copernican' change is the Romantic belief that man learns of certain concepts such as beauty from emotions and not from reason; that is, emotions have an 'epistemological' role (Abbagnano, 1961).
43 Fulcher, 1973.
44 Riese, 1960; Pigeaud, 1980.
45 Arbousse-Bastide, 1972. On Comte's personal experience with mental illness see Dumas, 1898.
46 p. 217, Lewes, 1878.
47 Saurí, 1969.
48 Tissot, 1865; Colonna d'Istra, 1913; Carlson and Dain, 1960; Bynum, 1964; Ey, 1978; Postel, 1979; Baguenier-Desormeaux, 1983.
49 p. 82, Esquirol, 1805.
50 Heiberg, 1927; Dodds, 1951; Drabkin, 1955.
51 Jackson, 1972; Kroll, 1973; Neugebauer, 1979.
52 *Colloque International de Bruxelles*, 1976.
53 Rosen, 1968; Jobe, 1976; MacDonald, 1981; Conry, 1982; Foucault, 1954; 1972; Saurí, 1969; Pigeaud, 1980; Saβ, 1983.
54 Balan, 1972; McMahon, 1976; Fischer-Homberger, 1979.
55 Starobinski, 1977.
56 Deerborn, 1937; Lewis, 1972.

57 Vol. 2, p. 97, Crichton, 1798.

58 Kageyama, 1984.

59 Dodds, 1951; Roccatagliata, 1973; Simon, 1978; Sarantoglou, 1980.

60 Heiberg, 1927; Drabkin, 1955; Berrios, On delirium, 1981.

61 Starobinski, 1962; Flashar, 1966.

62 *Colloque International de Bruxelles*, 1976; Jobe, 1976; Gangler-Mundwiller, 1979; Jackson, 1983.

63 Burton, 1883.

64 Jackson, 1980; MacDonald, 1981.

65 Evans, 1944.

66 Rosen, 1975; *Colloque International de Bruxelles*, 1976; Macdonald, 1981.

67 Jackson, 1983.

68 p. 78, Esquirol, 1976.

69 Heiberg, 1927; Drabkin, 1955; Roccatagliata, 1973; Simon, 1978.

70 Albrecht, 1970; Werlinder, 1978.

71 Klein, 1970; Brooks, 1976; see also Fodor, 1983.

72 Büchner, 1897; Leary, 1978; Hilgard, 1980.

73 Lantéri-Laura, 1970; Cantor, 1975; Cooter, 1979.

74 Hécaen and Lantéri-Laura, 1977.

75 Falret, De la non-existence de la monomanie 1864.

76 Esquirol, 1976; Kageyama, 1984.

77 p. 190, Heinroth, 1975.

78 Borgese, 1934; Lovejoy, 1936.

79 Boring, 1953; Danziger, 1980.

80 Barthes, 1972; King, 1968; Laín-Entralgo, 1978; López Piñero, 1983.

81 Berrios, Stupor: a conceptual history, 1981; Riese, 1960; Pigeaud, 1980.

82 Delacroix, 1924; Drevet, 1968.

83 Swain, 1978.

84 Bollote, 1973.

85 Riese, 1960; Pigeaud, 1980.

86 Rosen, 1964.

87 Kageyama, 1984. The History of *Délire exclusif* can be traced to earlier periods; for example, Hartley wrote: 'It is observed that mad persons often speak rationally and consistently upon the subjects that occur, provided that single one which most affects them be kept out of view' (p. 252, Hartley, 1834).

88 Walker, 1968; Jackson, 1983; Delkeskamp, 1977.

89 pp. 155–156, Pinel, 1809.

90 p. 3, Prichard, 1835.

91 p. 73, Heinroth, 1975.

92 Laín-Entralgo, 1978; López Piñero, 1983.

93 López Piñero, 1983.

94 Ackerknecht, 1967.

95 Pistoia, 1971; Lantéri-Laura, 1972.

96 Rochoux, 1842; Jacques, 1875; pp. 174–89, Rosmini, 1888; pp. 221–307, Höffding, 1892; Wundt, 1897.

 97 Delasiauve, Des diverses formes mentales, 1861; Soury, 1883.
 98 Noel, 1973.
 99 p 460, Rush, 1981.
100 Pinel, 1809.
101 Esquirol, 1805.
102 Delasiauve, 1851; Kageyama, 1984.
103 Feuchtersleben, 1847.
104 Broussais, 1828.
105 Laycock, 1840; pp. 76–107, Laycock, 1860.
106 Bucknill and Tuke, 1858.
107 Griesinger, 1867.
108 Falret, Le çons, 1854.
109 Falret, De la non-existence . . ., 1864; Falret, Discussion sur la folie
     raisonnante, 1866.
110 Morel, 1860.
111 Mackenzie, 1976.
112 Gardiner *et al.*, 1937.
113 Young, 1970; Hécaen and Lantéri-Laura, 1977.
114 Darwin, 1872; Gruber, 1981; Barnett, 1962.
115 p. 40, Coupland, 1892.
116 p. vii, Ribot, 1897.
117 p. 365, Morgan, 1903; see also Richards, 1977.
118 p. 174, Ziehen, 1909.
119 pp. 421–485, James, 1891; Gardiner *et al.*, 1937.
120 Tizard, 1959; Meyer, 1974.
121 Carpenter and Power, 1876.
122 Mairet, 1883.
123 Morel, 1866.
124 Hollander, 1901.
125 Berrios, On 'depressive pseudodementia', 1985.
126 Meyer, 1974.
127 Hécaen and Lantéri-Laura, 1977.
128 Rancurello, 1968; Brentano, 1973; Fancher, 1977.
129 Ward, 1889.
130 Green, 1973; Laplanche and Pontalis, pp. 13–14, 1973.
131 Green, 1973.
132 Fenichel, 1945.
133 Bleuler, 1906.
134 Bleuler, 1924.
135 Bianchi, 1906.
136 p. 84, Régis, 1906.
137 Jaspers, 1963.
138 Kraepelin, 1910–15.
139 pp. 1183–1185, Kraepelin, 1910–15.
140 pp. 1370, Kraepelin, 1910–15. In nineteenth century language,
     excitement and inhibition were considered as disorders of psychomotility
     and did not mean elation or depression, respectively.

141 Schneider, 1959. The idea of 'polarity' he borrowed from Max Scheler (1874–1928), his favourite philosopher.

142 Minkowski, 1966.

143 Bash, 1955.

144 Zerssen, 1988.

145 Berrios, On Psychopathology of affectivity, 1985.

146 Berrios, On Historical aspects of the psychoses, 1987; Berrios, On Melancholia and depression during the nineteenth century, 1988; Berrios, On Depressive and manic states during the nineteenth century, 1988.

147 Esquirol, 1820.

148 Foville, 1882; Ritti, folie à double forme, 1876; Mordret, 1883.

149 Kraepelin, 1921.

150 pp. 32–33, Haslam, 1809.

151 See, for example, cases in Cheyne, 1733.

152 Hare, 1991.

153 Jackson, 1986.

154 Berrios, On Depressive and manic states during the nineteenth century, 1988.

155 p. 264, Mayne, 1860.

156 p. 77, Régis, 1885.

157 p. 287, Gull, 1894.

158 p. 270, Jastrow, 1901.

159 p. 151, Savage, 1886. This text went through many editions, and was studied by countless clinical students.

160 Meyer, 1901.

161 Berrios, On stupor, 1981.

162 Cotard, 1882; Berrios and Lugue, 1995.

163 Kraepelin, 1921.

164 Griesinger, 1861.

165 Baillarger, 1854.

166 Montassut, 1938.

167 Freud, notes on a case of paranoia, 1963.

168 For example, Magnan and degeneration theory, see Saury, 1886.

169 Hilts, 1981.

170 Kraepelin, 1921.

171 Kraepelin, 1921.

172 Berrios 1985, 1987, 1988, 1988 (as per notes 145 and 146 above).

173 Bolton, 1908.

174 Foville, 1882.

175 Ritti, 1876.

176 Falret, mémoire sur . . ., 1854; Baillarger, 1854.

177 Foville, 1882.

178 Ritti, 1876.

179 Kraepelin, 1921; Chaslin, 1912.

180 Berrios, Historical aspects . . ., 1987.

181 Berrios, Depressive pseudodementia . . ., 1985; Dumas, 1894; Mairet, 1883.

182 By metalanguage is meant here a language of description capable of
     referring to first-order discourses as their primary object; by
     metaperspective is meant a notional observation vantage-point laying
     outside all temporal perspectives. Both notions are more *desiderata* than
     real options but serve to illustrate the difficulties involved in trying to
     explain, from within *the current nosological and taxonomic discourse*, what
     the perception of mental disorder was in earlier times.

183 By this is meant 'something' which, once acquired, was not susceptible to
     come and go. In other words, insanity seemed to lie outside time.

184 Haslam, 1809. There is also the oft-told anecdote of the lunatic who,
     after behaving rationally in front of the mob, was given his freedom
     against Pinel's advice. Once freed, he resumed his madness and had to be
     restrained. Although this is told to illustrate Pinel's great clinical acumen,
     the issue is, how did he know? My view is that he did not draw a
     conclusion based on probabilistic knowledge pertaining to a particular
     diagnosis; he simply based his prediction on the (ontological) belief that
     'once a lunatic always a lunatic'; and this is the nearest one can get to
     understanding pre-1800 views on madness.

185 Katzenstein, 1963.

186 Lanczik, 1988.

187 Berrios and Hauser, 1988.

188 Kraepelin, 1920.

189 Roubinovitch, 1896.

190 Berrios, Descriptive Psychopathology . . . 1984.

191 Pinel, 1809.

192 These were: a. total vs. partial, b. acquired vs. inherited, c. acute vs.
     chronic, d. anatomical vs. functional, e. reversible vs. irreversible,
     f. exogenous vs. endogenous, g. personality related vs not personality
     related, and h. form vs. content. In due course, the affective disorders
     were analysed *vis-á-vis* each of these dichotomies.

193 Ey, Les psychoses périodiques . . . 1954; Rouart, 1936.

194 Deny and Camus, 1907.

195 pp. 167–168, Pinel, 1809.

196 p. 148, Esquirol, 1820.

197 Prichard, 1835.

198 Rush, 1812.

199 pp. 151–152, Esquirol, 1820.

200 p. 159, Esquirol, 1820.

201 p. 161, Esquirol, 1820.

202 p. 166, Esquirol, 1820.

203 p. 382, Delasiauve, 1856.

204 p. 293, Sérieux and Capgras, 1909.

205 p. 384, Delasiauve, 1851.

206 Billod, 1856.

207 Griesinger, 1861.

208 p. 147, Feuchtersleben, 1847.

209 Falret, 1851.

210 Baillarger, 1854.
211 Falret, as per note 176, 1854.
212 Falret, see also charming piece by Pichot, 1995, 1854, as per note 176.
213 Ritti, 1883.
214 Billod, 1856.
215 Quoted in Ritti, 1883.
216 Mordret, 1883.
217 Förstl and Beats, 1992.
218 Greenberg *et al.*, 1984.
219 Campbell *et al.*, 1981.
220 Joseph and O'Leary, 1986.
221 Joseph, 1986.
222 Young *et al.*, 1992.
223 p. 377, American Psychiatric Association, DSM IV, 1994.
224 ICD-10, 1992.
225 Cotard and Prévost, 1891.
226 Cotard, 1891.
227 Cotard, 1891.
228 Falret, 1889.
229 Cotard, 1878.
230 Semelaigne, 1932.
231 Cotard, 1878.
232 Cotard, 1891.
233 Cotard, 1880.
234 Esquirol, Délire, 1814.
235 Macario, 1842.
236 Leuret, 1834.
237 Morel, 1853.
238 Krafft-Ebing, 1893.
239 Baillarger, 1860.
240 Berrios, On Melancholia and depression, 1988.
241 Meige, 1893.
242 Cotard, 1882.
243 Lasègue, 1884.
244 Cotard, 1891.
245 Cotard, 1891.
246 Ball and Chambard, 1881.
247 Chaslin, 1895.
248 Porot, 1975.
249 Garrabé, 1989.
250 Young, *et al.*, 1992.
251 Kearns, 1987.
252 Régis, 1893.
253 Séglas, 1884.
254 Séglas, 1887.
255 Séglas, 1889.
256 Séglas, 1897.

257 Baillarger, 1860.
258 Bercherie, 1980.
259 Cristiani, 1892.
260 Santangelo-Spoto, 1896.
261 De Sanctis, 1896.
262 Del Greco, 1896.
263 Giannelli, 1897.
264 Obici, 1900.
265 Régis, 1893.
266 Falret, 1892.
267 p. 391, Arnaud, 1892.
268 Camuset, 1892.
269 Ey, Délire de negations, 1950.
270 Garnier, 1892.
271 p. 390, Charpentier, 1892.
272 De Cool, 1893.
273 Arnaud, 1892.
274 Trénel, 1898.
275 Toulouse, 1893.
276 Berrios, On Melancholia and depression, 1988.
277 Berrios, On The psychopathology of affectivity, 1985.
278 Deny and Camus, 1906.
279 Blondel, 1912.
280 Revault D'Allonnes, 1923.
281 Blondel, 1912.
282 Rogues de Fursac and Capgras, 1912.
283 Vurpas, 1912.
284 Capgras and Daumezón, 1936.
285 Tissot, 1921.
286 Barbé, 1912.
287 Deny and Camus, 1906.
288 Got, 1912.
289 Dugas *et al.*, 1985.
290 Tissot, 1921.
291 Loudet and Martínez, 1933.
292 Obarrio *et al.*, 1932.
293 Perris, 1955.
294 Ahlheid, 1968.
295 Vitello, 1970.
296 De Martis, 1956.
297 p. 163, Enoch and Trethowan, 1991.
298 Trémine, 1982.
299 Lafond, 1973.
300 p. 1169, Bourgeois, 1980.
301 Bourgeois, 1969.
302 Joseph, 1986.
303 Bolton, 1908.

304 Deny and Camus, 1907.

305 Berrios, Psychopathology of affectivity, 1985.

306 pp. 190–191, Heinroth, 1975. Heinroth seems to be attacking views similar to those currently sponsored by the 'cognitive' theory of depression according to which negative cognitions lead to depressed mood.

307 Roubinovitch, 1896.

308 Wahrig-Schmidt, 1985. Griesinger was in his mid twenties when he wrote the first edition of his book on mental pathology and therapeutics.

309 Rennert, 1968.

310 Griesinger, 1861.

311 Kahlbaum, 1863; see also Bronisch, 1990.

312 Kolle, 1963.

313 pp. 56–80, Flemming, 1859.

314 Katzenstein, 1963.

315 p. 134, Kahlbaum, 1863.

316 p. 97, Kahlbaum, 1863.

317 Krafft-Ebing, 1879.

318 Bercherie, 1980.

319 Jackson, 1986; Rouart, 1936; Ey, Les psychoses périodiques, 1954.

320 Arnaud, 1899; Dana, 1904; Gaupp, 1905; Berger, 1907; Ducost, 1907; Phillips, 1912; Fishbein, 1949; Gibson, 1918; Treadway, 1913; Cordeiro, 1973; Ey, 1954.

321 p. 103, Post, 1965.

322 Dreyfus, 1907.

323 Kendell, 1968; Sérieux, 1907; Post, 1965; Jackson, 1986.

324 p. 169, Kraepelin, 1921.

325 p. 41, Thalbitzer, 1926.

326 p. 190, Kraepelin, 1921.

327 p. 191, Kraepelin, 1921.

328 p. 191, Kraepelin, 1921.

329 p. 74, Kraepelin, 1983.

330 Dreyfus, a Swiss psychiatrist, was born in Basle in 1879 and died in Zürich in 1957. He trained in Würzburg, Giessen and Heidelberg. In 1905, he came to work with Kraepelin in Munich. He then moved to Frankfurt where he was promoted in 1916 to a University Lectureship. He remained in this city until 1934, when he had to escape to Switzerland.

331 Dreyfus, 1907.

332 For details, see Berrios, On Affective disorders in old age, 1991.

333 Kraepelin, 1921; Brush, 1897.

334 Deny, 1909; Lange, 1928; Rocha, 1906; Soukhanoff and Gannouchkine, 1903; Rouart, 1936; Ey, 1954.

335 p. 1032, Dana, 1904.

336 Brush, 1897.

337 Mitchell, 1897.

338 Jelliffe, 1911.

339 Stocking, 1973.
340 p. 18, Prichard, 1835.
341 p. 79, Prichard, 1835.
342 p. 178, Bucknill and Tuke, 1858.
343 p. 188, Maudsley, 1895.
344 p. 234, Maudsley, 1895.
345 p. 262, Maudsley, 1895.
346 p. 276, Maudsley, 1895.
347 Bolton, 1908.
348 Royal College of Physicians of London, 1906.
349 p. 53, Robertson, 1890.
350 p. 505, Turner, 1900.
351 For an account of J.H. Jackson's views, see Berrios, On Positive and negative symptoms and Jackson, 1985.
352 p. 506, Turner, 1900.
353 p. 485, Hollander, 1901.
354 As evidence for this, see list of contributors in Tuke, 1892.
355 See, for example, Hopewell-Ash, 1934.
356 For example, 'cyclical neurasthenics'; see Sollier, 1893; Soukhanoff, 1909.
357 Janet, 1919.
358 Montassut, 1938.
359 Newcombe and Lerner, 1981.
360 Petrie, 1940.
361 Mapother, 1926.
362 p. 872, Mapother, 1926.
363 p. 872, Mapother, 1926.
364 p. 877, Mapother, 1926.
365 Henderson, 1945.
366 p. 878, Mapother, 1926.
367 p. 879, Mapother, 1926.
368 Banister and Zangwill, 1949.
369 McCurdy edited his classical book : Hoch A. *Benign Stupors*, 1921.
370 Gillespie, 1929.
371 MacCurdy, 1925.
372 p. 5, Kendell, 1968.
373 p. 881, Buzzard, 1930.
374 pp. 882–883, Buzzard, 1930.
375 p. 883, Buzzard, 1930.
376 p. 886, Buzzard, 1930. Crichton said this in spite of the reports to the contrary by Mitchell, 1897.
377 The term cyclothymia had been in use since the late nineteenth century, see Bagenoff, 1911; Jelliffe, 1911; Soukanoff, 1909; Deny, 1908.
378 p. 895, Buzzard, 1930.
379 See the magnificent books by Binet, 1892 and Ribot, 1884.
380 Hesnard, 1971.
381 Berrios, On Obsessional disorders during the nineteenth century, 1985.

382 Benon, 1937; Courbon, 1923; Rouart, 1936; Montassut, 1938.
383 Lewis, 1934; 1938.
384 Kendell, 1968.

CHAPTER 13

The anhedonias

The neologism *anhedonie*, coined by T. Ribot to name an 'inability to experience pleasure',[1] has not yet made it into the most recent French psychiatric diction-ary[2] nor does its English version feature in *OED*.[3] Its concomitant *concept* has merited both narrow ('blocking of the reward reinforcement of usually reinforcing stimuli')[4] and broad formulations ('loss of interest or pleasure in all or almost all usual activities and pastimes').[5] The *behaviour* to which anhedonia refers is not new: indeed, by the time of its coining it had already been reported in patients with 'melancholia' who were incapable of 'feeling joy any more'.[6] The *term* first took root in the psychoanalytic literature,[7] and in English-speaking psychiatry came into currency after 1979.[8] (The same holds true for France and Germany.)[9,10] Legitimated by DSM III[5] and recently by ICD-10,[11] anhedonia is now considered as a 'symptom' of two important clinical conditions (depression and schizophrenia). More empirical evidence is, however, required to confirm that the clinical *phenomena* in question are the *same* in both cases.

Anhedonia is a multivocal term. This partially results from the fact that the concept on which it is grounded is parasitical upon the ever changing definition of *pleasure*, i.e. of 'the *condition* of consciousness or *sensation* induced by the enjoyment or anticipation of what is felt or viewed as good or desirable; enjoyment, delight, gratification' (my italics).[3] However, because it is not even known whether 'there is something *fundamental which is common* to enjoying something, getting satisfaction out of something, being pleased at something, feeling good and so on' (my italics).[12] the definition of anhedonia is bound to be multiple and fuzzy. This state of affairs has also hampered the psychometry of anhedonia. Scale items vary in time span, quality of pleasure lost, culture and units of measurement.[13–19] Furthermore, it is known that subjects otherwise regarded as 'normal' may report an inability to 'enjoy' things.[20]

Matters historical

Classical beginnings

In the western world, conceptual analysis of the emotions has, in general, lagged behind that of the intellect.[21] Plato was one of the first to offer a 'psychological' (and intellectualistic) definition of pleasure: 'There being, then, three kinds of pleasure, the pleasure of that part of the soul whereby we learn is the sweetest, and the life of the man in whom that part dominates is the one most pleasurable'[22] Aristotle improved upon the Platonic view by adding to it dimensions such as duration and quality: 'This is why it is not right to say that pleasure is a perceptible process, but it should rather be called activity of the natural state . . .'[23]

From the start, pleasure seems to have been considered as a 'positive' experience, i.e. one resulting from the 'reading-off' of a mental content or *primordial soup*.[24] *Pari passu* with this positive definition, a negative one became available with Schopenhauer who defined pleasure as the absence of pain.[25] Another issue which prevents a clean definition of anhedonia is whether pleasure names a *specific* sensation or just a general quality attachable to any state of consciousness. In this regard, each emotion (or πάθος) has since Aristotle been measured against a yardstick of pleasure or pain so that 'one or the other of these opposites gives the basic feeling-tone to each emotion'.[26] Lastly, pleasure and pain are also believed to be essential forces in human motivation (i.e. human beings seek one and avoid the other): anhedonia might thus be expected to be accompanied by a reduction in the general energising of behaviour. It is not clear, however, whether this is always expressed in clinical practice.

Pre-nineteenth century vistas

In 1604, Thomas Wright discussed the motivational aspects of pleasure. In a section entitled 'the fixt motive to love is pleasure' he wrote: 'in all the sortes of men, and in all sortes of beasts, I daily and hourly discover, an insatiable desire of delight'[27] Hobbes[28] re-contextualized the analysis of pleasure. For him, sensual pleasures were not a good guide to prudent living: 'pleasure therefore is the apparence or sense of good; and molestation or displeasure, the apparence, or sense of Evill. And consequently all Appetite, Desire and Love, is accompanied with some Delight more or less . . . some arise from the sense of an object Present; And those may be called *Pleasures of Sense* . . . others arise from the Expectation, that proceeds from foresight of the End, or Consequence of things; whether those things in the Sense Please or Displease: And these are Pleasures of the Mind of him that draweth those consequences' (italics in original).[29]

As Fraser noted: 'Pleasure and pain play a supreme role in Locke's ethical system, as motives for conforming to moral relations, [for according to him] if men were destitute of all capacity for pleasure and pain, human life would be transformed'.[30] Locke wrote: 'Amongst the simple ideas which we receive both from sensation and reflection, pain and pleasure are two very considerable ones . . . these, like other simple ideas, *cannot be described, nor their names defined*; the way of knowing them is, as of the simple ideas of the senses, only by experience . . . by pleasure and pain, delight or uneasiness, I must all along be understood (as I have above intimated) to mean not only bodily pain and pleasure, but whatsoever delight or uneasiness is felt by us, whether arising from any grateful or unacceptable sensation or reflection' (my italics).[31]

David Hartley offered one of the earliest neurophysiological models of pleasure and acted as a bridge between Locke and the nineteenth century. According to his doctrine of 'vibrations', pain and pleasure ranged along a continuum: 'In like manner the pleasures of an agreeable warmth, and the refreshing coolness, when we are hot or cold, respectively, of gentle friction and titillation, leave traces of themselves, which by association are made to depend upon words, and other symbols'.[32] Battie, a follower of Hartley, considered that all sensations were accompanied by 'pleasure' or 'uneasiness';[33] and also described 'anxiety' ('sensation too greatly excited by real objects') and 'insensibility' ('sensation not sufficiently excited by real objects') the former preceded madness, and the latter was its conclusion.

The Swiss Bonnet also offered an original account. In his *Essai de Psychologie* he proposed three types of pleasure and pain: 'there are [those] which are purely physical and somatic and which relate to the lower aspects of the soul, the sensitive faculty. There are others which are spiritual, and which relate to the superior part of the soul, namely understanding and reflection. Lastly, there are combined (*mixtes*) states such as the pains and pleasures of the imagination. The physical pleasures are predominant during infancy, the mixed ones in adolescence, and the spiritual ones only become available during the reign of reason'.[34]

The nineteenth century

At the beginning of the nineteenth century, views on the nature of pleasure began to follow diverging routes. Thomas Reid[35] and Dugald Stewart[36] (who were more influential in France than England) developed a 'psychological' perspective, continued by writers such as Alexander Bain. A 'clinical' perspective, on the other hand, appeared later in the century mainly focusing on failures to experience pleasure.

THE PSYCHOLOGICAL BACKGROUND Reid and Stewart dedicated less time to emotions and feelings (including pleasure) than Brown and Hamilton, late members of the 'Scottish' school. Whilst Brown held the conventional view that pleasure and pain were polar opposites,[37] Hamilton imaginatively contrasted cognitions and feelings: whilst the 'peculiarity of cognition was objectification' in the case of feelings, on the 'contrary, consciousness does not place the mental modification or state before itself; it does not contemplate it apart, – as separate from itself, – but is, as it were, *fused into one*. The peculiarity of feeling, therefore, is that there is nothing but what is *subjectively subjective*; there is no object different from self, – no objectification of any mode of self. We are, indeed, able to constitute our states of pain and pleasure into objects of reflection, but in so far as they are objects of reflection, they are not feelings, but only reflect cognitions of feelings' (my italics).[38]

Hamilton's view of pleasure is relevant to the reporting of anhedonia, for patients are expected to describe the absence of a state which, according to Hamilton, is 'fused' with their consciousness. In trying to do so, subjects distance themselves from their feelings and end up providing *examples* of 'lack of enjoyment'. The problem here is that the choice of these *specific objects and situations* is controlled less by the extent or quality of the actual drop in 'pleasure' (which is what the clinician wants to capture if he/she is to differentiate, say, between the anhedonia of depression and of schizophrenia) than by external contingencies and conceptual frames.

Not all French views on pleasure followed Scottish philosophy.[39] Following the spiritualist philosophy of his time, Garnier[40] proposed another classification: the *general* category of sentiments was first to be divided into feelings (*affections*) and affective tendencies (*tendances affectives*); then the former was divided into pleasure and pain and other emotions, and the latter into inclinations and passions.[41] Likewise, Ribot started his own physiological approach to pleasure: this proved the most influential.[42]

Another nineteenth century debate relevant to the concept of anhedonia relates to the putative difference between 'sensations possessing an affective tone (*betönte Empfindungen*) and feelings proper'.[43] Kant had expressed the view that 'no feeling existed which [was] not ascribable to some object, and consequently which [was] not connected to sensations and presentations'. Herbart, in turn, divided feelings into 'those which depended upon the nature of what is felt and those which depend upon accidental mental conditions',[44] that is, resulted from sensations or from a 'reciprocal action of presentations', respectively. Different from the 'classical view' (that only considered lower and higher forms of pleasure), this new approach distinguished between 'feelings proper' and general sensations with a secondary 'feeling tone'. This dual notion can also be found in Ribot who separated lack of feeling caused by 'anaesthesia' (i.e. absence of pleasure *sensations*) from lack of feeling resulting from failure in *higher* (perhaps cognitive) mechanisms involved in the construction of pleasure.

Of Alexander Bain, Ribot[45] once said that 'were his Scottish teachers to come to life, they would not disavow him'. Between 1859 (first edition)[46] and 1875 (third edition)[47] of his *The Emotions and the Will*, Bain changed his definition of feeling. In the first, he had written: 'The fact or property named feeling is totally distinct from any physical property of matter . . . We observe in a living being a large assemblage of those so-called material qualities; but the property named feeling, or conscious- ness, belonging to men and animals, is distinct from any of these – being an ulti- mate, or irreducible, manifestation, the basis of the great superstructure known as the Mind'.[46] Sixteen years later, he stated: 'feeling comprises all our pleasures and pains, together with states that are indifferent as regards pleasure or pain and are characterised simply as Excitement'.[47] And then, in a classical article in *Mind* (and at his most physiological): 'a theory of pleasure and pain is wanting if it does not somehow introduce us to the very great variety of modes of both the one and the other. The science of the human mind is incomplete, so long as it fails to classify our hedonic states according to the closeness of their similarity. The division of our susceptibilities according to our known sense organs is one obvious mode of effecting such a classification'.[48]

Wundt's views are far less physiological: 'in all these cases we see that the feeling of pleasure, which is bound to certain sensations and ideas, is purely subjective. It is an element that is not dependent upon the impression itself, but also and always and most of all dependent upon the subject receiving the impression'.[49]

PSYCHOPATHOLOGICAL ANTICIPATIONS Early reports of patients showing fail- ure of 'pleasure function' are scanty, and as a rule, unaccompanied by theoretical discussion. For example, Haslam wrote that: 'in [some young patients] *sensibility* appears to be considerably *blunted*; they do not bear the same affection towards their parents and relations; they become unfeeling to kindness, and careless of reproof. To their companions they show a cold civility, but take no interest what- ever in their concerns' (my italics).[50] It is unclear whether Haslam was referring to emotional responsiveness or to a general decline in psychosocial competence.

'Physical insensibility' was the main feature of Esquirol's *lypémanie*: 'sensation, concentrated in an only object, seems to have withdrawn all the organs; the body remains impassive to any impression'.[51] One of Esquirol's patients wrote: 'Sur- rounded by all that can render life happy and agreeable, still to me the faculty of enjoyment and of sensation is wanting – both have become physical impossibilities . . . I cover them [my children] with kisses, but there is something between their lips and mine; and this horrid something is *between me and all the enjoyments of life* . . . The functions and acts of ordinary life, it is true, still remain to me; but in every one of them there is something wanting – to wit, the sensation which is proper to them, and the pleasure which follows them . . . Each of my senses, each part of my proper self, is as it were separated from me and can no longer afford me any sen- sation; . . . it seems to me that I never actually reach the objects which I touch. . . .

I feel well enough the changes of temperature in my skin, but I no longer experience the internal feeling of the air when I breathe' (my italics).[52] (Griesinger gives no reference for this quotation, which I have been unable to find in Esquirol's works.) The view that lack of sensitivity is a feature of *lypémanie* lasted well into the second half of the century; for example, Calmeil stated that in lypemanics 'the affective sensibility is flattened', and that 'the real world, the world of the past times, has now little interest' for them.[53]

Bucknill and Tuke also believed that 'young [melancholic] men and women may be thus affected; ceasing to be interested in any occupations; averse to going out or into society, and, in all the chances of life, neither rejoicing nor sorrowful, neither hopeful nor anxious'. These authors asserted that 'an aversion to human society, a desire for solitude, and a repugnance to the pleasures of the world, constitute the very essence of all melancholy'.[54]

Amongst the 'anomalies of emotion', Griesinger described a 'continual dissatisfaction with the external world' and 'abnormal states of emotional dullness (*Gemüths-stumpfheit*), and even of total loss of emotions (mood?)' (*völligen Gemüthlosigkeit*) (pp. 66–67).[52] He related these to the 'anaesthesia of the insane', which he divided into those related to the body (i.e. with a central basis) and those 'related to the intellectual, most inward, act in sensation' (p. 82).[52] To explain the latter, Griesinger described a normal reaction to painful emotions, in which 'the external world appears to have become suddenly cold and strange' and 'nothing can now excite in us a lively impression'. For him 'an analogy may be seen between these latter states and the complaints of melancholics, as their intensity, their duration, and their want of mental motive, urge the patient openly to complain of such changes in his power of receiving impressions' (pp. 82–83).[52] He named this reaction 'mental anaesthesia': 'the patient can no longer rejoice in anything, not even the most pleasing' (p. 223).[52] It is not clear whether 'mental anaesthesia' was a trait or state as in Griesinger's writings *Gemüth* refers both to a temporary feeling (emotion) and to a more lasting affective state (mood).

Likewise, in 1895, Séglas described apathy and indifference to all sensations in patients with non-psychotic depression.[55]

Ribot Théodule Armand Ribot (1839–1916) was one of the most important French philosopher–psychologists of the second half of the nineteenth century. He rejected the overt metaphysical aspects of French psychology and the view, originated with Maine de Biran and Jouffroy that 'the mind (or soul) has immediate knowledge of itself'. He believed that facts about the mind could only be discovered by experimental work, and endeavoured to bring together the organicism of Cabanis, Destutt de Tracy, Bichat and Ampère, the empiricism of English psychology, Darwinism, the experimentalism of the new German physiology, and the clinical and theoretical discoveries of Magnan, Ball, Luys, Voisin, Robin, and Jackson. He had the support of great men such as Taine, Charcot, Liard and Renan and in 1885 became professor of Experimental Psychology at the University of Paris and in 1888 was given the chair of comparative and experimental psychology at the *Collège de France*. In 1876 he founded the famous *Revue Philosophique de la France et de l'Ètranger* which he edited until his death. From this position he exercised an enlightened control upon French psychology and counted amongst his disciples men of extraordinary vision such as Janet, Dumas and Paulhan. His contribution has been divided into three periods, marked by different interests and intellectual influences.[56,57]

In 1875 he published the first edition of *La Psychologie Anglaise Contemporaine* (*École Expérimentale*), where he introduced his contemporaries to the work of Hartley, the Mills, Spencer, Bain, Lewes and Bailey. In its important introduction, Ribot planned out a new course for French psychology and for himself.[45] The new psychology was to study the laws governing human and animal behaviour both under normal and pathological conditions. An admirer of John Locke, he never abandoned associationism and inductivism. However, Ribot also believed that psychology had to be based on physiology for that was the only way of subjecting behaviour to the general laws of nature.

La Psychologie des Sentiments, the book where Ribot coined the term *anhedonie* belongs to the *second* stage of his career, and was first published in 1896. A. Binet called it 'the most important of Ribot's works' but did not comment upon the coining of anhedonia.[58] Ribot started by complaining that the emotions had so far 'exerted only a moderate seduction upon workers' (p. v) and that publications in that field were 'less than the twentieth part' of the total for all psychology. He put this down to the 'prejudice which assimilates emotional states to intellectual states, considering them as analogous, or even treating the former as dependent on the latter'. To this view he opposed a 'physiological approach' according to which states of feeling 'are primitive, autonomous, not reducible to intelligence, able to exist outside it and without it' (p. vi). The book opened up with a Darwinian analysis of 'the evolution of the affective life' and included sections on the 'general' and the 'special' psychology of emotions. Chapter 3 of section 1 concerned pleasure. After complaining of the scanty nature of data on the psychology and physiology of pleasure, Ribot dismissed the view that it was a phenomenon opposed to pain (or grief) and agreed with Wundt's definition (see above). He also rejected the hypothesis that pleasure was just a 'sensation' as proposed by Nichols in America and Bourdon in France for there were 'neither special nerves nor special organs' for pleasure. He saw it as a *complex* state: 'whether the point of departure is a physical excitation, a representation, or a concept, two distinct events take place, as in the case of grief: on the one hand an internal state of consciousness, which we describe as agreeable; on the other a bodily external condition . . .' (p. 51).

Based on a paper by George Dumas published the same year (*Recherches Expérimentales sur la Joie et la Tristesse*), Ribot supported a version of the Lange's theory of emotions. He thus considered pleasure to be 'an additional phenomenon, a symptom, a sign, a mark, denoting the satisfaction of certain tendencies [which] cannot be regarded as a fundamental element of the life of the feelings' . . . 'like pain, pleasure is separable from the complex of which it forms part, and under certain abnormal conditions may totally disappear. Anhedonia (if I may coin a counter-designation to analgesia) has been very little studied, but it exists. I need not say that the employment of anæsthetics suppresses at the same time pain and its contrary; but there are cases of an insensibility relating to pleasure alone' (p. 53). Anhedonia might be seen in a variety of 'organic' situations (e.g. medullar injuries, liver disease, etc.) and also in 'cases of profound melancholia'; Ribot listed examples for both conditions taken from reports by Brown-Séquard, Fonssagrives, Cros, and Esquirol.

Other French writers For a while it seemed as if the term and concept of anhedonia might take off. In 1899, G.L. Duprat, in his book on *l'Instabilité Mentale* wrote: 'severe instability leads to analgesia and *anhedonia*, that is, morbid indifference. This depends not so much on the actual intensity of the stimuli but above all on the aptitude of the subject to experience both the subjective and physiological changes'[59] And in 1903, Pierre Janet reported the case of a woman with 'extraordinary indifference' to both pain and pleasure'.[60]

Twenty years later, A. Deschamps took up the notion again: 'It can also be said that the severely asthenic show an absence of pleasure, what has been called anhedonia. A sign of improvement in the asthenic is that the sensation of pleasure returns to normal'.[61] It would seem that, at least in these writers, anhedonia was linked up to conditions allegedly resulting from disorders of psychological balance and energy. After the First World War these conditions all but disappear and with them the notion of anhedonia.[62–66]

Non-French writers

At the very end of the nineteenth century, Bevan Lewis wrote: 'In simple pathological depression the patient exhibits a growing indifference to his former pursuits and pleasures: the ordinary duties of life and business become irksome and devoid of interest . . .and the *environment fails to call up pleasurable associations*'. (my italics).[67] In his Gifford Lectures, William James distinguished between 'state' anhedonia: the 'passive joylessness and dreariness' of some forms of 'pathological depression' or the 'temporary condition connected with the religious evolution of a singularly lofty character' and 'trait' anhedonia: 'some persons are affected with anhedonia permanently . . . the annals of suicide supply such examples . . .'.[68] Perhaps autobiographically,[69] he also reported that a: 'prolonged seasickness will in most persons produce a temporary condition of anhedonia'.[68]

Lastly and on pleasure, Angell stated: 'Theories of the general nature of the hedonic or pleasure-pain consciousness . . . deal, mostly without sufficient discrimination, with three relatively distinct problems: (1) psychophysiological (the organic correlate of hedonic states); (2) psychological (the place of pleasure and pain in the development of conscious process); (3) genetic or biological (the origin and evolutionary significance of hedonic consciousness together with its organic correlate)'.[70]

KRAEPELIN AND BLEULER These authors viewed the *concept* of anhedonia (they did not use the *term*) as a deterioration of emotional life. Kraepelin wrote: 'The singular indifference of the patients towards their former emotional relations, the extinction of affection for relatives and friends, of satisfaction in their work and vocation, in recreation and pleasures, is not seldom the first and most striking symptom of the onset of disease (dementia praecox). The patients have no real joy in life, 'no human feelings'; to them 'nothing matters, everything is the same'; they feel 'no grief and no joy', 'their heart is not in what they say'. A patient said he was childish and without interest, as he had never been before. Another said that nothing gave him pleasure, he was sad and yet not sad'.[71] Loss of pleasure and interest, and the annihilation of emotional activity were aspects of his wider concept of 'indifference'.

Bleuler shared the view that in schizophrenia there was: ' . . . an indifference (*Gleichgültigkeit*) to everything, to friends and relations, to vocation or enjoyment, to duties for rights, to good fortune or bad'[72] Bleuler referred to 'indifference' as an *äußere Signatur* and used the term *Gleichgültigkeit* instead *of Gemütlosigkeit* or *Gefühlslosigkeit* which would have perhaps made stronger reference to the patient's subjectivity.

JASPERS AND KRETSCHMER Jaspers returned to the old distinction between 'feelings' and 'sensations': The former were 'states of the self (sad or cheerful)' and the latter 'elements in the perception of the environment and of one's own body (colour, pitch, temperature, organic sensations)'.[73] Pleasure was not a sensation but a feeling: it is 'an experience of harmonious biological function, of general wholesomeness and success, of a capacity to linger over things; pleasure also lies in psychic equilibrium and well-being'. The loss of pleasure is part of 'apathy' (he did not mention the term 'anhedonia') where 'the patient is fully conscious and orientated, sees, hears, observes and remembers, but he lets everything pass him by with the same total indifference; happiness, pleasure, something positive in which he is involved, danger, sorrow, annihilation are all the same. He remains dead with wakeful eyes'. (On the concept of apathy see Franck.)[74]

'Apathy' is to be differentiated from the 'feeling of having lost feeling' (*Das Gefühl der Gefühl* (p. 93) in which 'patients complain that they no longer love their relatives, they feel indifferent to everything. Food does not gratify . . . All sense of happiness has left them. They complain they cannot participate in things, they have no interest'.[75] This complaint can be seen in patients with periodic psychoses and depression.

Kretschmer suggested that the 'autistic component' of what he had labelled the 'predominantly anaesthetic schizoid temperament' was 'unfeelingness, lack of affective response to the world about him, which has no interest for his emotional life, and for whose own rightful interest he has no feeling'.[76]

Psychoanalytic views

To Freud, 'hedonic (pleasure) regulation' was a prime motivational agent. He believed that neurotic conflict led to a loss of capacity for enjoyment which covaried with the amount of energy available, in other words, individual differences were quantifiable.[77] Although Freud did not use the term anhedonia, he commented upon the diminished capacity for pleasure and sexuality seen in some patients with psychoses – most notably, Schreber.[78]

The term *anhedonia* re-appeared with Myerson,[79] Menninger and Glauber. Myerson was the first to propose a developmental model reporting that an early feature of anhedonia in the 'lives of many housewives' was an 'inability to become pleasurably interested in anything'. He described an 'anhedonic syndrome' as a feature of certain neuroses and of depression:[80] 'The term 'constitutional anhedonic personality' is here used to designate individuals who, from the earliest period of their lives, have shown impairment amounting to serious deficit in the important drives or desires of life, with a correspondent failure in satisfaction ... The anhedonic syndrome is manifested, first, by the disappearance or the impairment of the appetite for food and drink and failure in the corresponding satisfactions. ... Secondly, there is a failure in the drive or desire for activity and the corresponding satisfaction. ... Thirdly, the appetite or desire for rest and the satisfaction of recuperation are also involved in the anhedonic syndrome. The tired feeling ... may be supplanted by a final absence of the feeling of fatigue. ... Fourthly, the sexual drives and satisfactions are conspicuously altered in the acquired anhedonic states. ... Finally, the social desires and satisfactions, which belong indissolubly to the nature of the herd animal known as man, become disorganized, deficient and even destroyed ... The difference between anhedonia and the acquired anhedonic states is that the individual has shown impairment of all these drives from the earliest days of his life, or, if all the drives have not been deficient, some have been conspicuously impaired or deficient from childhood on. Such individuals go through life without experiencing real hunger for food. ... The term constitutional, it must be noted, is here declared to be not necessarily hereditary. The constitution can be altered by environmental forces operating at an early period of life'.[81] In suggesting that anhedonia may lead to a form of 'withdrawal psychosis',[82] Myerson anticipated both Rado[4] and Meehl,[83] considered by many as the most influential psychodynamic authors in this field.

Menninger viewed anhedonia as a symptom of 'neurotic martyrdom',[84] and Glauber recognized a 'primary form of anhedonia' showing 'clinically as a chronic state of lack of conscious pleasure – distinct from psychological states having a quality of painfulness often punctuated by acute anxiety, unconsciously utilized to re-establish the chronic state whenever its maintenance is threatened by pleasure or by depression.' This specific form of anhedonia was characteristic of 'schizoid personalities' and was either 'a chronic state or experienced transiently as a strong reaction to a painful frustration; in both there is indifference to objects, absence of closeness and feeling of emptiness'.[85]

Anhedonia and schizophrenia

More recent views on anhedonia are mostly based on the theoretical framework developed by Rado, Meehl and Klein. Their ideas have been so powerful that little effort has been made to re-think the concept anew by linking it, for instance to the current debate on the nature of pleasure.

For Rado,[4,86,87] the so-called 'schizotype' resulted from an interaction between an inherited predisposition to schizophrenia ('anhedonia') and the environment. Such predisposition led to a 'blocking of the reward reinforcement of usually rein-forcing stimuli'. Pleasure was an 'essential enzyme' (p. 277)[4] whose absence impaired sexual functioning and undermined self-confidence, social interest, and the 'welfare emotions' of love, joy, pride, and affection. Unable to experience such pleasures, the schizophrenic becomes flat and apathetic, and lacking the drive to pursue rewarding activities, he withdraws or embarks in deviant behaviours.

Arieti put forward the view that anhedonia was a defence mechanism.[88] Based on the observation that in recent times the behaviour of subjects with schizophrenia seems to have been modified by 'marked changes in the sociocultural environ-ment'[89] this author criticised Rado's theory: 'In previous times most patients inhibited or repressed their sex life to such an extent that they were considered by Rado and Daniel[86] to be *unhedonic*; that is, they were considered unable to experi-ence pleasure, sexual or otherwise. Now many of them tend to follow heterosexual, homosexual, or exhibitionistic impulses';[90] 'some psychiatrists, who believe strongly in Rado's theory of anhedonia, are sceptical when former schizophrenics report full sexual gratification. These therapists are inclined to believe that the orgasm did not really take place, but was a fantasy of the patient. Maybe the patient is hallucin-ating again. My clinical experiences with former schizophrenics have convinced me that this is nonsense'.

Meehl, in turn, proposed that the 'schizotypal personality organisation' resulted from an interaction between a defect in neural integration (schizotaxia) and adverse social learning.[91] Anhedonia was detectable by assessing: 'situational independence, absence of interfering affect or content, pervasiveness of pleasure deficit, self-descriptions of anhedonic, and no spontaneous report of pleasure, among others'. Meehl conceived of 'low hedonic capacity' or 'joylessness', as a higher-order, dimen-sional disposition of polygenic origin important to the development of both schizo-phrenia and depression; 'hedonic capacity', in turn, was a positive personality attri-bute (the 'pleasure parameter') normally distributed in the population.[92] Reduced hedonic capacity was a heritable trait of schizophrenia. The term 'hedonic' was chosen to highlight the fact that it was a positive attribute, power or disposition, that manifested itself by degrees; in this sense it was not always 'pathological'. Hedonic impairment was not pathognomonic of schizophrenia but its presence increased risk in those genetically predisposed.[93]

Anhedonia and depression

For Klein, one of the pathognomonic features of 'endogenomorphic depression' was: 'a sharp, unreactive, pervasive impairment of the capacity to experience pleasure or to respond effectively to the anticipation of pleasure'.[94] Later on, the same phenomenon was redefined as 'a phasic, temporary, severe lack of present or anticipated satisfaction associated with the conviction that one cannot perform adequately' and regarded as a trait common to all depressive states which was 'embedded within several psychopathological constellations, and it is the nature of the associated findings that in large measure determines both the prognosis and treatment course'.[95] Anhedonic depressions showed a favourable response to tricyclic antidepressants and might reflect a specific disorder in the central nervous system; in these patients, the capacity to experience pleasure improved before other symptoms. In 1987 (and going back to the Aristotelian distinction) Klein distinguished between 'consummatory pleasure' (linked to biological drive reduction) and 'appetitive pleasure' (linked to pleasurable activities). Deficits in consummatory pleasure were accompanied by an absence of appetitive pleasure, and this was characteristic of 'endogenomorphic' depression.[96]

There is wide agreement that anhedonia is a symptom of depression.[97-101] Beck has also noticed that 'the emphasis placed by some of the patients on loss of satisfaction gives the impression that they are especially oriented in their lives toward obtaining gratification. Whether or not this applies to the pre-morbid state cannot be stated with certainty, but it is true that, in their manic states, the feverish pursuit of gratification is a cardinal feature'.[97] This author includes loss of interest in sex, food, other people, etc. amongst the vegetative and physical manifestations of depression. More recently, those supporting a 'cognitive model' have proposed that anhedonia results from a failure in the capacity for reinforcement.[102-104]

Clinical phenomena redolent of anhedonia have been frequently reported. For example, Kräupl Taylor wrote on 'essential hypomelancholic symptoms': 'there is usually a decrease in mental and physical activity, in self-confidence and in the enjoyment of pleasure. The patient lacks energy and initiative in general'.[105] Sifneos[106,107] has suggested that anhedonia represents an irreversible global diminution of affective capacity and that all alexithymic patients exhibit anhedonic features. Interestingly, however, not all anhedonic patients are alexithymic. Nelson *et al.* have proposed that 'lack of reactivity or inability to experience pleasure is a 'necessary symptom for the diagnosis of melancholia';[108] and Akiskal and Weise have defined dysthymia as "a chronic state of depressive anhedonia, so chronic that it can be considered a trait – in brief, a 'personality'.[109]

The *concept* of anhedonia was considered by DSM-III (1980) as a *necessary* (but not sufficient) criterion of melancholia: 'lack of pleasure in all or most all activities, lack of reactivity to usually pleasurable stimuli'. DSM-III-R[110] and DSM-IV have dropped the qualification of 'necessary' although anhedonia remains as a 'chief' symptom of major depression. Two specifiers appear in DSM-IV: 'With Melancholic Features' can be added to the diagnosis of Major Depression if there is 'a near-complete absence of the capacity for pleasure, not merely a diminution';[111] and the *term* anhedonia, defined as 'a loss of interest or pleasure' appears as a negative 'symptom' (not a criterion) of schizophrenia in the section dedicated to 'Associated Features and Disorders'. Under the construct 'somatic depression', ICD-10 includes a reference to loss of interest or in the capacity for pleasure. These considerations bring this historical study uncomfortably close to the present.

Conclusions

The understanding of anhedonia requires that the history of the word, concept, and behaviour are investigated separately. The word was coined by Ribot and this fact is only important in as much as the great French psychologist also developed an accompanying concept. Concepts of anhedonia, in turn, have always been dependent upon on-going definitions of 'pleasure'. This has rendered them unstable as the latter undergo periodic change. As Edel has written: 'the variety of approaches to pleasure and happiness in the historical career of the concepts makes isolation to any one perspective no longer plausible. The linguistic–analytical study brings a greater appreciation of the complexity of the phenomena . . . and a full scientific study can no longer limit itself to physiological bases, but must now embrace genetic and functional aspects on all levels.'[112] Lastly, the fact that behaviours involving deficits in a putative unitary 'capacity to experience pleasure' have been known for a long time (regardless of what term they travel under or by which concepts they were being explained) suggests that the clinical phenomenon may be the expression of a biological defect.

The conceptual and historical analysis of anhedonia helps to understand why this clinical phenomenon has resisted adequate definition and measurement, and why the clinical assumption is still made that complaints of inability to experience pleasure as found in depression, schizophrenia, substance-related disorder or anxiety refer *to the same* (or very similar) biological phenomena. That this assumption is unwarranted can be seen from the fact that pleasure is a hierarchical concept whose mechanism can be disabled at various levels, each having a different biological representation. Whether a more detailed analysis of the phenomenology of anhedonia will be able to determine at what level the deficit occurs is an empirical question, but one which requires that a conceptual frame is available. The historical analysis offered in this chapter is the first step in that direction.

ACKNOWLEDGEMENT Dr José Olivares from Vigo, Spain, greatly helped in the writing of this chapter.

NOTES

1 Ribot, 1897.
2 Postel, 1993.
3 *Oxford English Dictionary*, 1993.
4 p. 276, Rado, 1956.
5 p 214, APA, DSM III, 1980.
6 p. 37, Clouston, 1887.
7 Watson *et al.*, 1970.
8 Snaith, 1993.
9 Loas and Pierson, 1989.
10 Cohen, 1989.
11 ICD-10, 1992.
12 p. 341, Alston, 1967.
13 Cautela and Kastelbaum, 1967.
14 MacPhillamy and Lewinsohn, 1974.
15 Fawcett *et al.*, 1983.
16 Watson *et al.*, 1970.
17 Chapman *et al.*, 1976.
18 Mishlove and Chapman, 1985.
19 Kazdin, 1989.
20 Olivares and Berrios, 1995.
21 Berrios, Psychopathology of Affectivity, 1985; also see chapter 12, this book.
22 Book IX, § 583, Plato: Dialogues, 1961.
23 Book VII, 12, § 1153*a*, Aristotle: Nicomachean Ethics, *The Complete Works*, 1984.
24 Berrios and Marková, 1995.
25 Schopenhauer, 1950.
26 p. 233, Tracy, 1969.
27 p. 203, Wright, 1604.
28 Sorell, 1986.
29 p. 122, Hobbes, 1968.
30 p. 302, Footnote 1, Fraser, 1959.
31 Book II, Chapter 20, Locke, 1959.
32 p. 92, Hartley, 1834.
33 p. 27, Battie, 1758.
34 pp. 185–186, Bonnet, 1783.
35 Reid, 1854.
36 Stewart, 1818.
37 pp. 102–103, Brown, 1828.
38 p. 432, Hamilton, 1859.
39 Boutroux, 1908.

40 Garnier, 1852.
41 Lalande, 1976.
42 pp. 419–422, Dumas, 1923.
43 p. 185, Villa, 1903.
44 p. 76, Herbart, 1895.
45 Ribot, La Psychologie Anglaise, 1896.
46 p. 3, Bain, 1859.
47 p. 3, Bain, 1875.
48 p. 222, Bain, 1903.
49 pp. 52–53, Wundt, 1912.
50 pp. 64–65, Haslam, 1809.
51 p. 204, Esquirol, 1838.
52 cf. pp. 218–219, Griesinger, 1861.
53 p. 545, Calmeil, 1869.
54 p. 148; p. 159, Bucknill and Tuke, 1858.
55 p. 288, Séglas, 1895.
56 Janet, 1916.
57 Benrubi, 1933.
58 Binet, 1896.
59 p. 154, Duprat, 1899.
60 p. 31, Raymond and Janet, 1911.
61 p. 131, Deschamps, 1919.
62 E.M.C. *Psychiatrie*, 1987.
63 Ey *et al.*, 1978.
64 Porot, 1975.
65 Koupernik *et al.*, 1982.
66 Lemperiere, 1983.
67 Bevan-Lewis, 1899.
68 pp. 145–147, James, 1903.
69 p. 215, Perry, 1936.
70 Angell *et al.*, 1901.
71 p. 33, Kraepelin, 1919.
72 pp. 47–48, Bleuler, 1911.
73 p. 109; p. 317, Jaspers, 1963.
74 p. 78, Franck, 1875.
75 p. 93, Jaspers, 1948.
76 p. 162, Kretschmer, 1936.
77 Freud, Introductory lectures, 1963.
78 Freud, Notes on a case of paranoia, 1963.
79 Myerson, 1920.
80 Myerson, 1923.
81 Myerson, 1944.
82 Myerson, 1946.
83 Meehl, 1962.
84 Menninger, 1938.
85 Glauber, 1949.
86 Rado, Psychoanalysis of behaviour, 1956.

 87 Rado, 1960.
 88 Arieti, 1960.
 89 p. 46, Arieti, 1974.
 90 p. 46, Arieti, 1974.
 91 Meehl, 1962; 1974; 1975.
 92 Peterson and Knudson, 1983.
 93 Meehl, 1987.
 94 p. 175, Klein, 1974.
 95 Klein *et al.*, 1980.
 96 Klein, 1987.
 97 p. 18, Beck, 1967.
 98 Beck, 1974.
 99 Lazarus, 1968.
100 Seligman, 1974.
101 Lewinsohn, 1974.
102 Ferster, 1966.
103 Costello, 1972.
104 Akiskal and McKinney, 1972.
105 p. 141, Taylor, 1966.
106 Sifneos, 1967.
107 Sifneos, 1987.
108 Nelson *et al.*, 1980.
109 Akiskal and Weise, 1992.
110 APA, DSM III-R, 1987.
111 p. 383, APA, DSM IV, 1994.
112 p. 387, Edel, 1973.

PART IV

Volition and action

CHAPTER 14

The will and its disorders

The 'will' no longer plays a role in psychiatry and psychology. A hundred years ago, however, it was an important descriptive and explanatory concept, naming the human 'power, potency or faculty' to initiate action. At the end of the nineteenth century, it came under attack:[1,2] 'the domain of the voluntary, *reified under the name of will* in popular language was adopted by the primitive psychology of faculties'. (my italics)[3] Experimentalism, psychoanalysis and behaviourism accelerated its fall, and by the end of the First World War, the will was no longer a fashionable concept.[4,5] This created a conceptual vacuum in the 'domain of the voluntary' which has since been unsatisfactorily filled by notions such as 'instinct',[6] 'drive',[7] 'motivation',[8] 'decision-making',[9] and 'frontal lobe executive'.[10] The decline of the will also led to neglecting the study of aboulia, impulse, agoraphobia, and obsession as 'pathological disorders of the will'. This chapter deals with the history of these disorders.

Will before the nineteenth century

The meaning of will was constructed in Classical times as a semantic blend of *impulse, instinct, tendency, desire, objective* and *inclination*. The Greeks, however, did not have a *separate* notion of the will and considered human action as being closely integrated with the intellect and the emotions: thus, Plato believed that desires or appetites (*orexis*) were related to sensations, whilst the will (*boulesis*) was linked to reasons and thoughts: 'of our unnecessary pleasures and appetites there are some lawless ones, I think, which probably are to be found in us all, but which, when controlled by the laws and the better desires in alliance with reason, can in some men be altogether got rid of'.[11]

Aristotle, on the other hand, did not 'seem to have been much interested in will and emotion'.[12] Nonetheless, he proposed that appetite and will were involved in action: 'Beyond these again is the appetitive part, which in both definition and capacity would seem to be different from them all. And it is surely unreasonable to split it up; for there is will in the calculative, and desire and passion in the irrational part; and if the soul is divided into three, appetite will be found in each'.[13] Therefore, as compared with sheer appetites, the will was a rational, calculative activity.[14] From this period on, and based on the belief that volitions are governed by the intellect, a view of the will as a 'rational appetite' has predominated.[15] This view can be found as late as Kant: 'The will is conceived as a faculty of determining oneself to action in accordance with the conception of certain laws'.[16]

In opposition to the integrative view developed by the Greeks, the Judeo-Christian tradition made the point of distinguishing between a deliberative, decision-making faculty and an executive faculty (the will).[17] For example, St Augustine suggested that the will was an independent power,[18] and John Duns Scotus viewed it as the motor of all mental faculties.[19,20] The Judeo-Christian tradition lasted into the Modern era when John Locke was able to steer a middle course: 'This power that the mind has thus to order the consideration of any idea, or the forbearing to consider it; or to prefer the motion of any part of the body to its rest, and vice versa, in any particular instance, is that which we call will. The actual exercise of that power, by directing any particular action, or its forbearance, is that which we call volition or willing'.[21]

Hume was happy to emphasize the 'subjectivity' of the notion: 'by the will, I mean nothing but the internal impression we feel and are conscious of, when we knowingly give rise to any new motion of our body, or new perception of our mind'.[22] This subjectivism was taken further by Condillac: 'we understand by will the absolute desire that whatever we wish is within our reach'.[23] Such absolute desire was, however, learned: 'The memory of having satisfied some of its desires makes the statue [a thought experiment used by Condillac to explain how psychological functions were acquired] feel that it might be able to satisfy new ones, particularly because unaware of potential obstacles, it is unable to see why new desires cannot be satisfied in the same way as old ones'.[24] But as Boas was to notice, there was a flaw in this argument: 'But after Condillac had broken down our ideas into the sensory elements which gave rise to them, the problem arose as to how they were combined into new syntheses. It was clear, for instance that such phenomena as abstract or general ideas and as the association of ideas in memory could not be explained by the soul's activity, for the Condillacist technique eliminated the possibility of the soul's doing anything'.[25]

Volonté was defined in the French *Encyclopédie* as: 'the effect of the impression of an object present to our senses or reflection, in consequence of which we are attracted by it as something good, or are repelled as something bad . . . thus, there is always an object in the willed action of the will.';[26] and *volition* as: 'an act of the mind knowingly exerting that dominion it takes itself to have over any part of the man, by employing it in, or withholding it from any particular actions. And what is the will, but the faculty to do this?' Reflecting contemporary empiricist beliefs, the *Encyclopédie* iterated Condillac's notion that the 'force' of the will originated in the object or sensation itself, and quoted John Locke[27]

During the nineteenth century there was a further reaction against the view that the will could be reduced to other mental functions. For example, a strong 'voluntarist' philosophy appeared in the work of Maine de Biran who proposed to replace *cogito ergo sum* by *volo ergo sum*. As Drevet has written: 'The real oppositions between Maine de Biran and Descartes are implicit. First of all, the self of 'I think' is no longer the self of Maine de Biran who will say 'I want' or 'I try''.[28,29]

France and the Scottish philosophers

The French reaction against Condillac and Locke was inspired by Thomas Reid and Dugald Stewart whose version of Faculty Psychology revolved around the notion of 'mental power'.[30,31,32] Maine de Biran, Laromiguère, Royer-Collard, Cousin and Garnier developed a spiritualist philosophy which encouraged the revival of the will.[33] Thus, Maine de Biran[34] criticised Condillac's associationism,[35,36] proposing instead a form of metaphysical and psychological 'voluntarism'.[37] A similar view was taken by Laromiguère,[38] whose ideas influenced alienists such as Esquirol (who had been his student), Royer-Collard, Cousin, and Paul Janet, and through them, most of nineteenth century French psychiatry.

THOMAS REID Reid dedicated a full essay to the will: 'every man is conscious of a power to determine, in things which he conceives to depend upon his determination. To this power we give the name of will; and, as it is usual, in the operations of the mind, to *give the same name to the power and to the act of that power*, the term will is often put to signify the act of determining; which more properly is called volition' (my italics).[39] Reid advised that the defining features of the will should be obtained from introspective analysis: (*a*) every act of will must have an object, (*b*) this must be some action of our own, (*c*) it must be believed to be within our power, (*d*) 'volition is accompanied with an effort to execute that which we willed', and (*e*) there must be something 'in the preceding state of the mind that disposes or inclines us to that determination'.[40]

Reid warned that although: 'the faculties of understanding and will [were] easily distinguished in thought, [they were] rarely, if ever, disjointed in operation. In most, perhaps in all the operations of the mind for which we have names in language, both faculties are employed, and we are both intellective and active'[41] Lastly, acts of will could be long-lasting: 'this deserves the more to be observed, because a very eminent philosopher [Hume] has advanced a contrary principle; to wit, that all the acts of the will are transient and momentary'[42]

THOMAS BROWN Whilst Dugald Stewart mostly followed Reid, Dr Thomas Brown, the third important member of the group, initiated a revisionist drive later completed by William Hamilton. Based on the view that the will was an all-pervasive mental function, Brown rejected earlier approaches: 'the division of the mental phenomena into those which belong to the understanding and those which belong to the will, seems, therefore, to be as faulty as would be the division of animals into those which have legs and those which have wings; since the same animals might have both legs and wings'.[43] Brown disagreed with the division of mental powers into intellectual and active on the grounds that intellectual phenomena were also active: 'So little, indeed, are the intellectual powers opposed to the active, that it is only when some intellectual energy co-exists with desire, that the mind is said to be active'[44] 'To will, is to act with desire; and unless in the production of mere muscular motion, it is only intellectually that we can act. To class the active powers, therefore, as distinct from the intellectual, is to class them, as opposed to that, without which, as active powers, they cannot even exist'.[45]

Brown endeavoured to reduce will to desire: 'Under Brown's analysis, mystery vanished from the will: will is an amalgam of desire and the belief that one has it in one's power to realize the desire; there is no further, indefinable operator in our voluntary actions'.[46,47]

Faculty Psychology in Britain
In Britain, phrenology represented the anti-associationistic reaction and encouraged a new theory of alienism.[48] For example, the work of Sir Charles Bell on the sensory and motor divisions of the nerves, and of Marshall Hall on reflex action, were interpreted as supporting the existence of individual and localizable nervous functions, and thereby, Faculty Psychology.

In Britain, the will also played a role in wider debates. Macaulay, Carlyle, Froude, and Smiles believed that the expansion of the British Empire had been due less to intellectual prowess than to control of the emotions and mastery of the will. Even men less prepared to extol the virtues of the Empire, such as Arnold, Mills, Newman, Bagehot, Morley, and Stephens, believed that one of the strong points of the English public school system was the education of the will. The will was thus a central concept in education, the self-help creed, and forensic medicine.

Nineteenth century theories of the will
The concept of the will was also central to nineteenth century philosophy of mind, psychology, and alienism.[49] Human beings were believed to be endowed with a discrete power or faculty of willing which embodied their essence as persons: 'it seemed to many in the nineteenth century that the human mind harboured deep and natural desire-like forces ("will", so called) comparable to the forces that were being tamed in the environment "without"'.[50] Nineteenth century views on the will were modelled upon the new physical notions of force and energy.[51]

According to whether the will was considered as subordinate to other mental powers or not, nineteenth century views are divided into *reductionist* (intellectualist, sensualist, and physiological) and *non-reductionistic*, (the strongest amongst the latter being the metaphysical version of Schopenhauer).[52] Nineteenth century psychopathological thinking dictated that, if the will was an autonomous mental function, it should also be subject to disease.[53,54] The 'pathological disorders of the will' opened up a new field of inquiry in psychological medicine, and brought alienists into occasional conflict with lawyers as some 'criminal' behaviours were reinterpreted as disorders of the will.[55]

REDUCTIONISTIC THEORIES George Combe, a phrenologist (and faculty psychologist), sponsored an intellectualistic view: 'will is a peculiar kind of mode of action of the intellectual faculties, different from perception and judgement it results from the decision and resolution of the understanding or intellect to follow a certain course of action prompted by the propensities, by the sentiments, by both acting together, or by external compulsion'.[56] Herbart, an associationist thinker, propounded that the will could be defined as an 'effort' caused by a 'presentation' (i.e. a sensation or simple element of consciousness) to maintain itself in place and prevent other presentations from overcoming it'.[57] The will (like feeling) was a 'moment in the life of a presentation'; the driving force of the will was 'borrowed' from external stimuli.

The view that the will was a form of 'reflex action' was developed in Britain. Charles Bell distinguished between anterior (motor) and posterior (sensory) nerves in the spinal chord, and suggested that this division might provide a model for the will. Marshall Hall also saw reflex actions as inchoate expressions of will. This physiological view, however, did not conform with introspective analysis which identified a conscious component of 'wanting'; henceforth, attempts were made to find the 'higher' components of 'unconscious cerebration'.[58] Bain suggested another 'conscious' control: 'the will, volition, or voluntary action is, on the outside, a physical fact; animal muscle and the nervous stimulation is one of the mechanical prime movers; the extension and improvement of our voluntary power is one large department of our education in the will, altogether, I reckon up three elements: two primitive, instinctive, or primordial, and the third a process of education.'[59,60] For Bain, 'the vital difference between belief and conception, between memory and imagination, lay in the dependence of belief and memory on the will, in that the action of the latter determined the nature of the real world'.[61] J.H. Jackson believed that will was only a 'name invented by men for different aspects of the ever present and yet always changing latest and highest mental state which in their totality constitute what we call consciousness'.[62] Like the latter, the will was diffusely localized in the cortex, and the highest motor centres were sited in the corpus striatum.

In 1873, Ribot wrote: 'When we compare two analysis of the will, one written by Mr Mill, the other by Mr Bain, with an interval of thirty years between them; when we see how far the last surpasses the first in the amount of facts observed in precision, in descriptive exactitude, we are forced to conceive a good opinion of the experimental method in psychology'.[63] At the end of the century, however, Bain's model came under attack.[64] The conflict arose from an ambiguity in the concept of 'volition' which seemed to comprise both the idea of an 'internal', thought-guiding activity and of an external component manifesting itself in actual motor behaviour.[65] Whilst evolutionism easily explained the presence of behaviour (as a useful adaptation), there were difficulties to explain the existence of the internal element. Some, like Müsterberg believed that volitions were 'complexes of feelings' for which there was not explanation.[66] To this was added the failure by researchers to identify specific motor centres responsible for volitional function. By the turn of the century, this failure led to a 're-psychologisation' of the will.

To explain the will, other thinkers resorted to functions other than the intellect. Brentano propounded that will was subordinated to the feelings;[67] and Münsterberg reduced it to 'ideo-emotional units'. Upham, returning to the Greeks, proposed a 'systemic' approach according to which all mental power acted in unison and depended upon each other: 'It is not to be inferred, when we speak of one part of the mind in distinction from another, and of passing from one part or power to another, that the mind is a congeries of distinct existences, or that it is, in any literal and material sense of the terms, susceptible of division'. The will was conceived of as an 'executive function' of the brain, not as a faculty: 'The term will merely embodies and expresses the fact of the mind's operating in a particular way'.[68]

NON-REDUCTIONISTIC THEORIES The view that the will was an autonomous, irreducible power of the mind was also popular during the nineteenth century; for example, Garnier wanted to *d'établir la multiplicité des facultés*. Faculties (or powers) were specialized mechanisms of the mind that caused the phenomena of the soul.[69] Will was the faculty that produced volitions: 'The will is, therefore, a separate faculty, and not, as others claim, the mode of expression of the other faculties'.[70] Garnier opposed the view that the will was abolished in insanity: 'The madman has lost neither intelligence nor will; it is not a volitional failure that marks the difference between the normal and the madman'.[71]

Later, Höffding was to write: 'if anyone of the three species of conscious elements is to be regarded as the original form of consciousness, it must evidently be the will'.[72] William James also warned against reducing will to feelings: 'the only ends which follow immediately upon our willing seem to be movements of our own body. Whatever feelings and havings we may will to get, come in as results of preliminary movements which we make for the purpose'.[73] Wundt defended a 'voluntaristic psychology' based on the assumption that 'psychology refuses to accept any attempts to *reduce volitions to idea, and at the same time emphasizes the typical character of volition*, for of all psychological experiences, volitional acts are universally recognized as primary occurrences made up of a series of continual changes in quality and intensity' (my italics).[74]

But as Sully put it, all these views were based on introspective analyses: 'no actions of the organism which are carried out unconsciously can fall under the head of conation, seeing that, according to our definition of mind they lie outside the properly psychological domain altogether . . . it seems best, on the whole, to make the terms conation and volition comprehensive enough to include all actions which have a conscious accompaniment, and which we will henceforth mark of as 'psychical actions'.[75]

Summary

Since classical times, and up to the end of the nineteenth century, the will (as a philosophical and psychological concept) has been central to western thinking. The Judeo-Christian view that the will constituted an autonomous mental function predominated over the older Greek one that action was fully integrated with feelings and intellect. During the late part of the nineteenth century, the view of the will as an independent faculty of the mind came under attack, and its decline was accelerated by attacks from psychoanalysis and behaviourism.

During the nineteenth century the view that the will was an independent mental function was also popular, and clinical phenomena such as aboulia, impulses and obsessions were conceptualized as resulting from pathological changes of the will. At the turn of the century, these disorders were set asunder by the decline of the will as a descriptive and explanatory concept. Their history will now be told in some detail.

The pathology of the will

The idea that mental health depended upon the free exercise of the will can already be found in late eighteenth century psychiatric writings. For example, in the *Magazin zur Erfahrungsseelenkunde*, Maimon wrote: 'The health of the mind consists in that state in which the will is free and can exercise its function without obstacle. Any state in which this does not obtain can be considered as a disorder of the mind'.[76,77] The greatest sponsor of the pathological disorders of the will during that period was, however, Matthey.

André Matthey

This great Swiss physician proposed the first classification of the disorders of the will. The *Pathomanies* were 'perversions of the will and of the natural inclinations (*penchans*) without obvious impairment of the intellectual functions'. The pathomanias were subdivided into four 'species'. The impulsions without madness (*fureur sans délire*) were 'unwilled impulses to commit acts of ferocity or anger without madness' and were subdivided in *tigridomanie* or the 'irresistible inclination to spill the blood of fellow creatures without reason or mental illness' and *Folie raisonnante* in which 'there was aggression against inanimate objects.' *Uiophobie* was an 'irresistible aversion or antipathy towards one's own children'. *Klopémanie* was 'an irresistible impulse to steal without being poor or to embark in shameful acts'. And *mélancolie suicide*, was a 'tendency to suicide without madness' recognized in three subvarieties: tedium of life (*ennui*) without 'manifest alteration of organic or psychological functions' (*melancolia anglica* of Sauvage); acute reactions to strong emotion; and suicidal behaviour complicated by hypochondria but without madness.[78] Important French clinical categories, developed late in the century, can be traced back to this seminal work. By bringing together behavioural phenomena whose only 'family resemblance' was that of involving unexplained or bizarre actions, and by attributing this to a common pathology, Matthey created the concept of 'disorder of the will'.

Heinroth

For Heinroth, will was that part of the mental machinery that brought us nearer to God: 'A man's will, like his spirit, has its roots in the Eternal being. The will is a certificate of our divine origin'.[79] It was 'a truly creative element' as long as 'it was fused with and permeated by reason.' Failures in such fusion would cause havoc in mental life: 'wherever the capacity to choose fails to obey reason, but follows unrestrained desires, it degenerates into unrestrained passion, into a savage impulse of destruction'[80] This view led Heinroth to conflate clinical and moral states, the latter related to the classical notion of *akrasia* or 'weakness of the will'.[81,82]

Heinroth rejected old explanations for impulsive rage such as 'bile or worms or a hundred other irritations' and re-defined the semantics of voluntary action: 'there are many involuntary movements, but not a single involuntary action, for action cannot be imagined without willing. But there is such a thing as a forced, unfree volition, that is, a volition which acts under the influence of a blind, powerful stimulus.' This happened when 'the will separated itself from reason and was no longer determined by feeling or intellect'.[83] Overexcitement of the will led to rage; apathy was the opposite: 'it was nothing but exhaustion of the power of self-determination caused by organic weakness, which in turn, is caused by inertia and an enslavement of the will'.[84] Heinroth made use of organic explanations, but like many of his successors, he also felt that the ultimate causes of mental illness were psychological.

Esquirol

Esquirol discussed pathological changes of the will in relation both to insanity in general, and to *monomanie*, a clinical category of his own creation. In regards to insanity he wrote: 'In some cases of insanity, man loses his will and is no longer the master of his acts. The insane may be controlled by his ideas and impressions and is condemned to do things he knows to be wrong ... these irresistible acts or automatic determinations as have been called by some authors, are independent of the will'.[85] The will might be affected in various mental conditions. For example, in *lypémanie* (depression), it was inflexible, i.e. nothing will change their delusions; or it may be abolished and 'impotent to execute'.[86] The subject with dementia was also affected by a weakening of the will and 'had no desires, aversions, hates'.[87]

Monomanie was a 'chronic brain disease, without fever, characterised by a lesion of either the intelligence, affect or will' thereby giving rise to *monomanie intellectuel*, *affective* and *instinctive*, respectively. In the latter 'the will was impaired. The patient carried out acts which his reason and affect had not determined, that his conscience rejected, and that his will could not prevent; actions were involuntary, instinctive and irresistible'.[88] Influenced by French spiritualist Roman Catholic philosophy, Esquirol differentiated between a stage of reasoning and moral decision-making and volition proper. In *monomanie instinctive* the disorder of the will was *primary*, in other *monomanies* such as *lypémanie* it was secondary to delusions or changes in mood. For example, Mlle F., a case with obsessions, Esquirol diagnosed as a volitional disorder.[89]

During the second half of the nineteenth century, Prosper Despine denied the existence of 'volitional monomania': 'this form of insanity, or rather of mental alienation without insanity cannot manifest itself in a man when his brain is healthy ... for in health there cannot be irresistible instincts (*penchants irrésistibles*) that can be stronger than the will'.[90]

Marc

Whilst Hoffbauer, the other great early nineteenth century writer on the forensic aspects of insanity, made no mention of disorders of the will and emphasized, in a Platonic fashion, the 'anti-social implications of the disorders of intellect and affect',[91] Marc discussed primary and secondary disorders of the will: 'If it is admitted that the will may become disordered, it may be found in conditions which are primitive or consecutive and in varied degrees'.[92] Secondary lesions of the will resulted from imperfection of the intellect (delusions). He accepted Esquirol's category of instinctive monomania in which bad acts followed disturbance of the volitional faculty.

Billod

The most important writer on the diseases of the will to appear after Matthey was Ernest Billod. Follower of the philosophical eclecticism of Victor Cousin, this great and controversial alienist trained under Ferrus and Voisin, and held rigid views on matters clinical to the point that he was sacked from the Bois asylum for pursuing an admission policy that led to severe overcrowding. He also became the self-styled champion of pellagra whose prevalence in mental hospitals he is likely to have exaggerated.[93] Early in his career, he was an enthusiastic follower of *la méthode psychologique* propounded by Falret the elder, according to which the behaviour of the insane was best studied in terms of normal psychology.[94]

In his seminal paper on the diseases of the will, Billod starts by complaining that 'recent work has been mostly on disorders of attention and affect and has neglected those of the will'.[95] This was due to the fact that 'for most people will is not a faculty different from thinking or affect; for others it is simply the power that carries out (rather than generates) the volition'.[96] Disorders of the will involved: (*a*) the creation, deliberation, and determination of volitions, and (*b*) the will as such. There were also disorders consequent upon the execution of a volition. Only those involving the 'will as such' could be called 'primary' and were sub-divided into states where the will was either weak or exalted. There were also secondary alterations and distortions of volition. *Lypémanie* (depression) and *manie* gave rise to opposite disorders: 'I believe that in *lypémanie*, the will is depressed, and in mania excited'.[97]

In regard to the states of increased and decreased will power, Billod wrote: 'There is, I believe, a *genius* of the will as there is one of intelligence, and also an *idiotism* of one as of the other. Each of these states can exist in isolation'.[98] The strength of the will depended on the state of other mental faculties. According to what Billod called the *effet de bascule* when volition decreased, the strength of other faculties would increase. He concluded that: 'disorders of the will should be as well known as those of intelligence and affect'.[99]

Griesinger

Griesinger included the disorders of the will with those of the intellect. Will was the result of ideas influencing muscular movements: 'If the known and definite presentations (*Vorstellungen*), by being united to the impulses of movement exercise an influence upon the muscular movements, this is called will'.[100] The will was but a 'hierarchy of reflex actions' under the control of consciousness.

In the insane, the disturbances of the will ranged from 'total absence of volition' to increase in power: 'Weakness of the will may result from incapacity to reach conclusions which may be due to troubles in perception or to the lack of a strong ego (*Mangel eines gehörig kräftigen Ich*) . . . these states manifest themselves in passivity and apathy, or in great hesitation and irresolution . . . and are frequent in the stage of melancholia'.[101] Increases in the power of the will 'take the form of inordinate desire, a thirst for action, a passion for making plans . . . and a pathologically increased sense of the self. This can be seen in the so-called partial insanity (*Wahnsinns der Fall*)'.[102] (The latter category was equivalent to Esquirol's volitional monomania but Griesinger did not refer to this possibility.)

Ribot

No work on the will and its disorders is better known than Ribot's.[103] Published in 1883, it eclipsed A. Herzen's *Analisi Fisiologica del Libero Arbitrio Umano*, which had been available in three languages since ten years earlier.[104] Ribot's book was followed by others but no one achieved its popularity: see, for example, Friedrich's *Die Krankheiten des Willens*,[105] Maudsley's *Body and Will*,[106] Allier's *Les Défaillances de la Volonté*[107] and Bertrand's *La Psychologie de l'Effort*.[108]

Ribot's work is the point of convergence of positivism, anti-metaphysical psychology, Spencerian evolutionism, and clinical analysis.[109] He conceived of 'volitions' as facts and avoided becoming entangled in the question of free will: 'as a mental act (*état de conscience*), volition is no more than an affirmation or a negation. It is analogous to judgement'.[110]

Will is envisaged as a psychophysiological phenomenon subject to the laws of evolution; it includes tendencies[111] toward action or inhibition which are responsive to external influences. Ribot considered *character* (on the history of this notion see[112]) as the ultimate source of the will.[113,114] Volition was the last link in a chain whose origin was the 'simple reflex' and which included: (*a*) a primordial automatic activity, invariable and unconscious, (*b*) the growth of individual appetites, desires, feelings, and passions, and (*c*) ideomotor acts that reach the status of 'perfect volitions'. By themselves, volitions cannot produce action or inhibition: 'the volitional act has two elements: a conscious state, impotent to start anything and the organic machinery that alone has the power; these two components may become dissociated'.[115]

Disorders of the will may result from a lack or an excess of impulsion. *Aboulia* results from the former mechanism and in its pure form shows little or no involvement of other faculties; other conditions resulting from a lack of will were *agoraphobie* where the 'weakness of the will originates from a feeling of fear',[116] *folie du doute*, where 'hesitation and impotence of will are extreme', and the so-called psychical *paralyses*, due to an 'inertia of the motor images which were indispensable for the carrying out of an intended movement.' In the disorders of excessive impulsion, the power to 'control' and to 'inhibit', which is the highest in the structural evolution of will, is impaired. In addition, there might be a predominance of 'instincts' caused by a concomitant poverty of intellectual functions. Ribot included in this group disorders such as kleptomania, pyromania, suicidal mania, etc.

Aboulia

By the turn of the century, aboulia had been defined as a 'loss, lack or impairment of the power to will or to execute what is in mind. In this condition there is no paralysis or disorder of the muscular system, and frequently there is no lack of desire or of realisation of the end sought; but the transition from motive and desire to execution becomes abnormally difficult or impossible'.[117] Clinical examples also included 'made' actions, obsessional paralysis, and melancholia. Aboulia was also defined as 'a form of insanity characterized by inability to exert the will; other faculties, it is alleged, not being of necessity affected'.[118] Nineteenth century accounts of aboulia were clearer than current ones.[119]

The term *Abulie* can be found in clinical use as early as 1847.[120] By 1858 it appeared in medical dictionaries: 'Absence of will, type of insanity in which this symptom is dominant'.[121] The corresponding behaviour was first described by Billod[122] and then by Guislain: 'Patients are able to want mentally, according to the rules of reason, they can experience the wish to do, but are unable to act accordingly. They want to work but cannot, they have not got the power (*ils n'en ont pas le pouvoir*).[123] Ribot believed that in aboulia the muscular system, mechanisms for automatic activity, intelligence and capacity to conceive objectives were normal; it was, therefore, a 'pure disease of the will' in which the capacity for action was abolished and which reduced sufferers to being 'a pure intellect'.[124] Two pathogenic mechanisms might be involved: weakness of the commands sent to the motor centres or dysfunction of the centres themselves; Ribot favoured the former.

Not everyone agreed. Langle[125] suggested that aboulia resulted from exaggerated 'inhibition'.[126,127] Cotard attacked this view and offered another model according to which the mind included a self and a non-self: aboulia resulted from pathology of the self whereas 'inhibition' could only affect the non-self.[128]

Aboulia became a popular term, and ways of educating the masses were suggested (by Payot and others) to 'combat the evil of aboulia amongst students and other intellectual workers.'[129] At a more scholarly level, and in addition to aboulia, Lapie described the *paraboulies*, i.e. states of perversion of the will which led to crime.[130] The relationship between automatic behaviour, reduction in psychological 'tension' and aboulia was discussed by Janet who made aboulia one of the symptoms of psychasthenia.[131,132]

During this period, the most important book on the association between psychological automatism, suggestion, and will was Paulhan's.[133] During the late 1890s, the view that aboulia was a primary disorder of the will began to give way, particularly amongst those practising 'psychotherapy'. Both at the Tolouse and Brussels meetings, Hartenberg and Valentin propounded that the emotions played a central role in aboulia for which: 'the treatment of choice is moral treatment. By this we understand psychotherapy . . . we employ therapeutic suggestion to deal with three elements: the idea (intellectual element), the emotive state (affective element) and the association between the two'.[134]

'Impulsion' *and the will*

During the nineteenth century, the *concept* of *impulsion* was used to refer to all manner of paroxysmal, stereotyped, and (apparently) *involuntary* actions.[135] The actual *word* had been imported into the French language from mechanics;[136] its 'explanatory' force, however, derived from allusion to vestigial behaviours, drives, cravings, and appetites all of which were believed to escape the control of the will.

By the 1860s, *impulsion* was caught in two dichotomies: it was used both as a description and as an explanation, and it was considered at the same time as being both internally generated and as a reaction to external events. The 'endogenous' view was the first to appear;[137,138] indeed, cases of what later was to be called *impulsive or instinctive insanity* had already been described by Pinel as *manie sans délire*[139] and by Georget as *impetuosité de penchans*.[140]

Dagonet imposed order in the field and defined impulsion as 'an irresistible and involuntary act, that imposed itself upon the mind just as did hallucinations'.[141] His views are, however, tinged by religious and moralistic connotation. Less obviously religious was Magnan who believed that impulsions resulted from a combination of 'a rapid explosion of energy and a lack of volitional control and vigilance': 'Impulsion is a mode of cerebral activity forcing actions that the will cannot prevent'.[142]

Considering this view as 'simplistic', Bourdin suggested a four-fold division: impulsions could be conscious, unconscious, false, and combinations thereof. Conscious impulsions were secondary to obsessions; unconscious impulsions followed fleeting ideas and left no memory (as in epilepsy); pseudo-impulsions resulted from the acting out of a delusion or a hallucination and were typical of insanity; and mixed impulsions were seen in hysterical insanity.[143] In the work of Bourdin, impulsions lost most of their moral connotations and mysterious irresistibility and became incorporated into the field of mental disorder. Pitres and Régis completed this process: 'impulsions have no special aetiology and their cause merges with that of insanity . . . impulsivity is a return to elementary reflex action which betrays a form of inferiority, whether innate or acquired'.[144]

Dagonet, however, saw fit to resuscitate the notion of 'impulsive insanity' (*folie impulsive*) under which he included phobias, homicidal and suicidal tendencies, manic behaviour, hypochondriacal preoccupations, and epileptic seizures.[145,146] He concluded that any subject suffering from insanity might show *impulsions violentes, irresistibles* which could be primary or secondary to delusions, emotions or hallucinations, and which led to a 'failure of the will'.[147] A disorder redolent of obsessional illness was also included: 'the more one tries to discard the idea, the more it becomes imposed upon the mind, the more one tries to get rid of the emotion or tendency, the stronger it becomes'.[148]

Obsessions and the will

During the nineteenth century, obsessions were variously explained as intellectual, volitional and emotional disorders; in the event, the third of these views predominated and with minor change has lasted to this day.[149] Aboulia and obsessions were closely associated in the work of Janet, e.g. his 'psychasthenic' patients were described as suffering from both.[150]

The aftermath

After the turn of the century, the number of papers discussing the will and its disorders shows a decline. There has been little research into the causes of this important change but there is no reason to believe that it was occasioned by some crucial piece of empirical research showing that the will 'did not exist' or that it was a useless or unwieldy concept. (Will-related concepts are currently discussed as the 'philosophy of action'.[151-153]) The more likely explanation is that the will became a casualty of fashion, and of the anti-will view entertained by psychoanalysis and behaviourism. To its decline also contributed the anti-rationalism and pessimism that appeared in the wake of the First World War and the acceptance of mechanistic and neurological explanations for the disorders of motility (e.g. tics, forced movements, stereotypes, etc.) seen after the epidemics of encephalitis lethargica.

The decline of the will left psychiatry without a model to account for the pathology of action. Some of the disorders once associated with the will have been reconceptualized away (e.g. obsessions), others (e.g. impulse) remain unexplained, yet others (e.g. aboulia) have been quietly dropped out of circulation. Categories such as lack of 'motivation' or disorders of 'drive' and 'desire' are not more illuminating than the old term disorder of the will. The fashionable neuropsychological notion of 'frontal lobe executive' is not free from the very same conceptual objection (regression *ad infinitum*) that once was considered as fatal to the concept of will.

It is suggested here that the current interest in a 'modular approach' to symptoms and mental functions should encourage researchers to study the psychology of action. The fact that cognitive models may be easier to develop than those pertaining to volition should not be an excuse, as the disorders of the will remain central to psychiatry (as seen, for example, in personality disorders, chronic fatigue syndromes and forensic psychiatry).

ACKNOWLEDGEMENT Dr Margaret Gili from Marjorca University greatly helped in the writing of this chapter.

NOTES

1 Bradley, 1902.
2 Tawney, 1903.
3 p. 470, Piéron, 1968.
4 Foulquié, 1972.
5 Irwin, 1942.
6 Hartmann and Witter, 1966.
7 Woodworth, 1918.
8 Hinde, 1960.

9 Edwards and Tversky, 1967.
10 Passingham, 1993.
11 Republic, 571*b*, p. 798, Hamilton and Cairns, 1973.
12 p. 7, Hett, 1986.
13 De Anima, 432*b*, 5, p. 183, Hett, 1986.
14 Kenny, 1979.
15 Abbagnano, 1961.
16 p. 45, Kant, 1909.
17 Charlton, 1988.
18 Dihle, 1982.
19 Wolter, 1986.
20 Hoeres, 1962.
21 Book II, Chapter XXI, Para 5, Locke, 1959.
22 Book II, Part III, section I, p. 399, Hume, 1888.
23 Part I, section III, Para 9, Condillac, 1947.
24 Part I, section III, Para 9, Condillac, 1947.
25 p. 10, Boas, 1929.
26 p. 10, Diderot and D'Alembert, 1753.
27 See Book II, Chapter XXI, Para 15, in Locke, 1959; Condillac, 1947.
28 p. 58, Drevet, 1968.
29 see also: pp. 81–104, Moore, 1970.
30 Rullier, 1815.
31 Brooks, 1976.
32 Spoerl, 1936.
33 Boutroux, 1908.
34 Moore, 1970.
35 Le Roy, 1937.
36 Mondolfo, 1924.
37 Maine de Biran, 1929.
38 Taine, 1901.
39 Essay II, Chapter 1, Reid, 1854.
40 pp. 59–64, Reid, 1854.
41 Essay II, Chapter 3, Reid, 1854.
42 Essay II, Chapter 4, Reid, 1854.
43 p. 98, Brown, 1828.
44 p. 99, Brown, 1828.
45 p. 99, Brown, 1828.
46 p. 402, Grave, 1967.
47 see also: Grave, 1960.
48 Cooter, 1976.
49 Smith, 1979.
50 p. xxii, O'Shaughnessy, 1980.
51 O'Shaughnessy, 1980.
52 Safranski, 1991.
53 Buchan, 1812.
54 Matthey, 1816.
55 Smith, 1981.

56 p. 141, Combe, 1873.
57 pp. 200–201, Villa, 1903.
58 Walshe, 1957.
59 Bain, 1875.
60 Bain, 1866.
61 p. 45, Greenway, 1973.
62 p. 199, Jackson, 1932.
63 p. 76, Ribot, 1904.
64 James, 1891.
65 Bastian, 1892.
66 Münsterberg 1898.
67 Brentano, 1973.
68 p. 483, Upham, 1886.
69 p. 61, Garnier, 1852.
70 p. 74, Garnier, 1852.
71 p. 47, Garnier, 1852.
72 p. 99, Höffding, 1892.
73 p.486, James, 1890.
74 p. 18, Wundt, 1897.
75 p. 172, Sully, 1892.
76 p. 9, Maimon, 1792.
77 Förstl *et al.*, 1991.
78 pp. 146–147, Matthey, 1816.
79 p. 227, Heinroth, 1975.
80 p. 228, Heinroth, 1975.
81 Charlton, 1988.
82 Urmson, 1990.
83 p. 228, Heinroth, 1975.
84 p. 229, Heinroth, 1975.
85 p. 6, Esquirol, 1838.
86 p. 208, Esquirol, 1838.
87 pp. 45–46, Esquirol, 1838.
88 p. 332, Esquirol, 1838.
89 Berrios, On Obsessive–compulsive disorder, 1989.
90 p. 486, Despine, 1875.
91 Hoffbauer, 1827.
92 p. 86, Marc, 1840.
93 Ritti, 1900.
94 Billod, 1855.
95 p. 15, Billod, 1847.
96 p. 17, Billod, 1847.
97 p. 195, Billod, 1847.
98 p. 194, Billod, 1847.
99 p. 202, Billod, 1847.
100 p. 41, Griesinger, 1861.
101 pp. 75–76, Griesinger, 1861.
102 p. 76, Griesinger, 1861.

103 Ribot, 1904.
104 Herzen, 1880.
105 Friedrich, 1885.
106 Maudsley, 1883.
107 Allier, 1891.
108 Bertrand, 1889.
109 pp. 150–153, Boutroux, 1927.
110 p. 29, Ribot, 1904.
111 Ribot, 1915.
112 Berrios, On European views on personality disorders, 1993.
113 Ribot, 1892.
114 Ribot, 1896.
115 p. 151, Ribot, 1904.
116 p. 56, Ribot, 1904.
117 p. 816, Jastrow, 1901.
118 p. 51, Tuke, 1892.
119 Förstl and Sahakian, 1991.
120 Leubuscher, 1847.
121 p. 7, Littré and Robin, 1858.
122 Billod, 1847.
123 p. 144, Guislain, 1852.
124 pp. 49–50, Ribot, 1904.
125 Langle, 1886.
126 Brown-Séquard, 1889.
127 Smith, 1992.
128 Cotard , 1891.
129 Payot, 1931.
130 Lapie, 1902.
131 Janet, 1898.
132 Janet, 1919.
133 Paulhan, 1903.
134 pp. 45–46, Hartenberg and Valentin, 1897.
135 Berrios, On Obsessions, 1989.
136 Littré, 1877.
137 Dagonet, 1870.
138 Porot, 1975.
139 Pinel, 1809.
140 Georget, 1820.
141 p. 17, Porot, 1975.
142 p. 218, Bourdin, 1896.
143 pp. 238–239, Bourdin, 1896.
144 p. 208, Pitres and Régis, 1902.
145 Dagonet, 1870.
146 Baldwin, 1901.
147 p. 15, Dagonet, 1870.
148 p. 20, Dagonet, 1870.

149 Berrios, On Obsessions, 1989.
150 Janet, 1898; 1919.
151 Kenny, 1963.
152 White, 1968.
153 Moya, 1990.

CHAPTER 15

Feelings of fatigue

Feelings of fatigue can be found in association with a number of physical and psychiatric conditions, and form part of the experiential meaning of technical and vulgar terms such as asthenia, anergy, tiredness, weariness, languor, lassitude, depression, melancholia, acedia, apathy, inertia, aboulia, lethargy, exhaustion, vecordia, tediousness, ennui, debility, lack of vitality, lack of vigour, pusillanimity, adynamia, boredom, feebleness, failing of strength, hyperaesthesis, irritability, anhedonia, 'being out of sorts', 'out of being', 'feeling knackered', and 'down in the dumps'.

Before embarking on the history of these phenomena, the semantic field of 'feelings of fatigue' and cognate terms must be clarified; to do so five questions may be asked. The first is whether such terms have a common denominator; it would seem that they do partake in a 'primary sensation' conferring upon them a sort of 'family resemblance'.[1] The second question is whether such common sensation is distinctive enough to be differentiated from others such as mild pain; it will be shown that feelings of fatigue have been historically considered as a primary experience. The third question is whether it is distinctive enough to be recognized even when not accompanied by its usual causal associations, e.g. when experienced in situations not preceded by exertion; clinical observation shows that subjects respond with alarm to the presence of feeling of fatigue when it appears 'unexplained'. The fourth question is whether this unexplained feeling of fatigue is phenomenologically identical to that experienced after exercise; the answer to this question must be sought in empirical research. The fifth question is whether it is likely that the feeling of fatigue will be related to a common neurobiological structure or mechanism, for example, to putative 'fatigue receptors' whose activation by exogenous or endogenous agonists might trigger the experience.[2]

Mosso

Fatigue, as opposed to feeling of fatigue, was well studied during the nineteenth century as attested by the classical book by Angel Mosso,[3] a disciple of Hugo Kronecker in Leipzig. Kronecker worked on the muscle of the frog, and like other physiologists of the period (Ludwig, Schmidt, Aducco, Maggiora), was interested in the 'laws of fatigue'.[4] This mostly animal work was based on the measurement of muscle performance by means of dynamometers and myographs and did not include the assessment of 'feeling of fatigue'. But Mosso endeavoured to develop a unitary view of fatigue that included both its physical and intellectual (mental) aspects. Whilst doing so he pondered over the feeling of fatigue: 'Humboldt, when showing how the living environment can enrich language, tells us that the Arabs have more than 20 words for the desert. But we have only one term for fatigue. The reason for this is easy to understand as fatigue is too featureless an internal sensation to distinguish its varieties.'[5] Mosso was well aware of the difficulties involved in the description of primary sensations: 'what fatigue, pleasure, hunger, or thirst means can be *understood* and their intensity qualified by the use of adjectives, but such descriptions cannot compete in precision with the image that the desert impresses on us.'[6] Mosso explained this by referring to the vagueness of proprioceptive sensations: 'Fatigue, which can be considered as a sort of poisoning, can alter the composition of the blood and biological homoeostasis, however we just feel it as a vague sensation of tiredness.'[7]

Since the work of Mosso, and later of the French School,[8] the belief emerged that intellectual (mental) fatigue reflected a decline in the energy metabolism of neurons, and that behavioural and cognitive variables covaried with it.[9] Mosso's views on the vagueness and inaccessibility of the feeling of fatigue remained influential. For example, MacDougall[10] suggested that 'a sharp distinction must be drawn between objective and subjective exhaustion, between fatigue (*Ermüdung*) and weariness (*Müdigkeit*).'[11] He defined weariness as: 'a superficial fact of attention, which may appear, disappear and reappear many times in a day, [it] can be induced in a fresh subject by dull work, monotony, stale familiarity, [it] can abate as fatigue increases; weariness is a fluctuating personal attitude which is *scarcely susceptible of record in any form*.'[12]

Ioteyko

Mosso also influenced the work of Josefa Ioteyko whose research on fatigue started with her doctoral thesis of 1896 on 'fatigue and muscle respiration'. By the time her great book on fatigue[13] appeared she had already moved from Brussels to Paris, and completed about ten important research publications. Ioteyko considered the feeling of fatigue as a separate albeit vague experience, and justified its inclusion in evolutionary terms: 'in higher species, particularly in man, a third condition is essential to define fatigue: this is a sensation of "malaise" known as feeling of fatigue.'[14] Others took a more 'composite view' of its nature: 'feeling of fatigue is not a simple act, but a psychological state made out of a number of simpler elements which include changes in affect or sentiment corresponding to obscure and sometimes subconscious tactile and muscular sensations. Feeling of fatigue is but a form of *coenesthesia*.'[15]

Other researchers

Views like these precluded the development of an adequate phenomenology of the feeling of fatigue and effectively put it beyond the reach of measurement. MacDougall himself suggested that: 'in the study of fatigue we have to seek for the phenomena of actual reduction in capacity for productive work; and from its effects we must discriminate the factors of interest and weariness.'[16] But since weariness did not hold a linear, or monotonic correlation with fatigue, then studying the latter threw little light on the feeling itself.[17]

A second line of research into fatigue during the nineteenth century related to the concept of intellectual fatigue amongst school children, and to its relevance to teaching methods. Kraepelin,[18] Ebbinghaus,[19] and Griesbach did much of the earlier work in this area. By the end of the century, however, MacDougall[20] was able to celebrate the fact that schoolmasters, such as Kensies[21] and Wagner[22] had showed interest in this type of work. Most of this research was based on the 'work curve' paradigm developed by Kraepelin[23] and later completed by Pauli and Arnold.[24]

Early work on the objective aspects of fatigue was marred by a conceptual confusion that impeded comparison of results: for some fatigue was the *correlation* between stress (and other independent variables) and the dependent variables; for others, it was the *effect* itself.[25] The analysis of feeling of fatigue, on the other hand, was caught up in the debate as to whether it was a truly *primary* experience or an introspective reading of *peripheral* sensations (à la James–Lange).[26] A third view was a compromise according to which feeling of fatigue interacted with the peripheral sensation.[27]

After the Second World War, Bartley and Chute[28] suggested that the 'experience of fatigue' might be evaluated by 'psychological methods'. Even then, they did not include amongst these methods the measurement of the feeling of fatigue. Pierre Bugard[29] in a book which can be said to represent the culmination of the old approach, dedicated little space to feeling of fatigue, in spite of the fact that he echoed Coirault's view that 'fatigue is an state of nervous suffering, which, together with insomnia, constitutes the common denominator of the prodromal phase of many mental diseases.'[30] Bugard considered visual and sensory changes as the best indicators of central nervous system fatigue.[31]

In the realm of psychopathology, however, emphasis was definitely put on the feeling itself. Thus, early in the twentieth century fatigue was defined as 'lassitude or weariness resulting from either bodily or mental exertion'[32] and Jaspers himself called for a distinction between objective and subjective fatigue (feeling of weariness or fatigue).[33] A reason for this was that alienists were forced to pay attention to the phenomenon: since late in the nineteenth century, a population of subjects had appeared whose complaint was unexplained feeling of fatigue. This created the need to develop techniques that might differentiate simulators from real patients.[34]

Feeling of fatigue and related experiences in psychopathology

During the late nineteenth century, information on feeling of fatigue can be found in writings on 'nervous prostration' and neurasthenia.[35] The latter category, supported by a newly developed theory of functional nervous disorder,[36] became a fashionable diagnosis in the hands of writers such as G.M. Beard[37] and engulfed those functional disorders that had feeling of fatigue as one of its symptoms.[38]

The concept of neurasthenia was the final stage in the evolution of 'asthenia' an old and noble notion that, during the late eighteenth century, had played an important role in the constitution of Brunonianism. Brown wrote: 'Asthenic disease is an state of the living body characterized by a weakening, occasionally disordered, of all functions.'[39] All asthenic diseases were not, of course, accompanied by fatigue;[40] some included states of defective excitation that distorted their symptomatology; others, like emaciation or extenuation did, however, include feelings of fatigue.[41] By the end of the nineteenth century 'asthenia' had lost its theoretical role and become the plain name for 'lack or impairment of strength.'[42] Tuke did not even include the term in his Dictionary.[43]

A derivative category was 'adynamia' defined as 'a state of impotence and lack of force of the organism.'[44] It soon also became a hypothetical construct: 'strictly speaking, adynamia accompanies all diseases ... adynamia is little else than an appearance, a phenomenon which can be attached to different diseases ... pathologists conceive of it as a direct reduction in vital force or in the functional rhythms, as a form of asthenia.'[45] Adynamias could result from excessive or insufficient stimulation.

Irritability

Another related category was irritability, still defined during the middle of the nineteenth century in the same way as Von Haller[46] had done a century before: 'a property peculiar to muscle substance by which it contracts on the application of stimuli.'[47] Glisson had first used the term irritability during the seventeenth century to name a property of body fibres independent of consciousness and of the nervous system.[48] This concept (together with sensibility) underwent elaboration during the following century, and in its British version (particularly in the hands of Cullen and Whytt) it came to be related to the nervous system. In the end, both concepts were to become properties of the cell.[49] Irritation, a modality of irritability, played an important role in the development of the concept of neurasthenia, via the mediating notions of nervous and spinal irritation.[50] Asthenia, now defined as 'a state of spinal nervous exhaustion caused by excessive irritation following over-stimulation'[51] reappeared as one of the forms of presentation of the spinal irritation syndrome, and was called 'spinal neurasthenia'. Beard extended the concept and explanatory mechanism from the spinal cord to the brain. In 1887, Charcot legitimatized neur-asthenia as a 'major neurosis' but proposed a narrow view of the disorder.[52] This allowed him to say that neurasthenia and hysteria could be found combined.[53]

Neurasthenia and psychasthenia

Fatigue and feeling of fatigue were central symptoms of neurasthenia. For example, Savill included 'mental exhaustion and inability to think and study . . . easily tired, easily startled, state of debility and exhaustion,'[54] and Cobb supported this view in one of the last great books to be published on the subject.[55] Fatigue and feeling of fatigue were, however, also present in other *psychonevroses*. Dubois, one of the most important writers on these group of disorders, showed much interest in *fatigabilité* (feeling of fatigue) a term which, he complained, was not in the French dictionary, and which named a 'gradual diminution of functional power, a difficulty to persist on the task at hand . . . etc.'[56] He quoted Tissi's work on cyclists, and agreed that fatigue could lead to 'transient, experimental psychosis.'[57] He also quoted Féré's work on the mental symptoms of fatigue.

According to Féré, fatigue after severe exercise produced similar symptoms to those exhibited by neurasthenics.[58] These included nihilistic and paranoid ideas, selfish attitudes, re-kindling of obsessional thoughts and compulsions, and depression.[59] Féré linked proneness to fatigue[60] with the theory of degeneration,[61] and saw an association between tendency to nervousness and high arousal.[62] Heckel wrote at length on the complex interaction between the feeling of fatigue and psychiatric symptoms[63] and so did Spanish writers: 'the subject presents depression and apathy, there is a weakness of the will, and sometimes aboulia, there are illusions and increased susceptibility to suggestion.'[64]

Fatigue and feelings of fatigue also featured prominently in the notion of 'psy-chasthenia', a fragment of the old neurasthenia concept.[65] The creation of psychas-thenia, as Cobb[66] noticed, was a reaction against the 'organic' view of neurasthenia: 'it is small wonder that a reaction to this view should set in, and a school arise which loudly declaimed the opposite – namely, that neurasthenia was caused by abnormal mental processes, which produced the disorder by means of mental mech-anisms; the work of Janet marked the first step towards the recognition of the psychical etiology of this disease.'[67]

Janet wrote: 'tiredness and a horrible sense of fatigue is caused in psychasthenics by the least physical or psychological effort[68] . . . fatigue rapidly affects sensations and perceptions, intellect and movement.'[69] One of his patients complained of 'a blanket of fatigue falling over me'. The concept was based on the view that in psychasthenics there was a drop in psychological energy leading to a 'loss of the sense of the real', a 'feeling of incompletion', and obsessions, compulsions and phobias.[70]

Neurasthenia and psychasthenia were themselves broken up and disappeared after the Great War. The feelings of fatigue were set asunder and became incorpor-ated into conditions such as anxiety and the affective disorders.[71]

Ribot, Dechamps, and feelings of fatigue

Ribot expressed much interest in the experiential quality of the feeling of fatigue which he considered as an internal sensation similar to hunger and disgust. By means of a survey he identified various 'modes' of presentation: 'some feel it in the muscles; others mentally: muscular twitchings in the calves of the legs, the eyes feel swollen, a feeling of relaxation, slowness of movement, general lassitude of a diffuse kind, mental weariness, heavy feeling in the brain' 'although all the responders could revive their feelings of fatigue, some did so with difficulty.'[72]

More important than Ribot's was Dechamps's work as he was one of the first to notice that fatigue and feelings of fatigue did not often 'correlate';[73] thus, in diseases such as tabes or chorea, feelings of fatigue 'were not experienced even after severe work' whilst in neurasthenia, feelings of fatigue 'were intense without having done any work'. For Dechamps fatigue 'resulted from chemical and anatomical changes', whilst feelings of fatigue from the 'synthesis of tactile sensations, both peripheral and internal (*coenesthesia*).'[74]

Anhedonia

Anhedonia was a term coined by Ribot:[75] 'like pain, pleasure is separable from the complex of which it forms part, and under certain conditions may totally disappear. Anhedonia (if I may coin a counter-designation to analgesia) has been little studied but it exists.'[76] The new symptom was then incorporated by Kraepelin and Bleuler into the symptomatology of depression and schizophrenia.[77]

Phenomenology of the feeling of fatigue

Feelings of fatigue remain a poorly defined experience, whose recognition may even vary according to cultural background.[78] This is so because the term is ambiguously poised in regard to its referent: when used in the first person (i.e. 'I feel fatigued') it names an experiential state; when in the third person (i.e. 'He is fatigued') it must include reference to objective signs of fatigue. Furthermore, it is unclear whether the experience is primary or a composite feeling–state; or whether its somatic accompaniments (e.g. breathlessness, nausea, muscular tiredness, aching, etc) are all part of the concept. If, like pain, the feeling of fatigue names a primary feeling–state[79] then it could be hypothesized that it is the same for all clinical situations: in other words, the fatigue of Addison's disease should be the same as that of multiple sclerosis, depressive illness, neoplasm, anxiety disorders, myalgic encephalomyel-itis,[80] or glandular fever. This question can only be answered by empirical research. A good instrument for its assessment, however, will be difficult to construct.[81] The semantic structure from which the scale items will have to be drawn[82] is a complex one and includes sensory, emotional, cognitive and evaluative components. In prac-tice, this means that the feeling of fatigue, like fatigue itself is a multi-dimensional state.[83] To avoid undue contamination from organic symptoms or proprioceptive information, such a scale will have to be based on the psychological attributes of the experience.[84]

Thus, the first stage in the identification of the semantic construct of the feeling of fatigue will have to tease out at least four meanings: 1. Feeling of fatigue following work where the experience is fully explained by the antecedent and is associated with the cognition of not wanting to continue performing. This constitutes the typical, anchor meaning; 2. Premature feelings of fatigue which obtain when the experience is reached too quickly, or when recovery takes too long, 3. Unexplained feelings of fatigue where the experience causes alarm because there is no relevant antecedent; it may also be accompanied by feeling like not starting any task. This meaning is common in relation to physical and psychiatric disease; and 4. Feeling like not embarking on any activity which occurs in the absence of a feeling of fatigue (e.g. anhedonia, aboulia, inertia, lack of drive, amotivation, mild irritability, lack of concentration, boredom, and the 'can't be bothered' feeling).

There has been a tendency to lump all these states together but they generate different questions and need to be separated; they might also lead to varied predictions in regard to correlations with objective measures of fatigue and symptoms belonging to the background disease.

NOTES

1 Wittgenstein, 1967.
2 Bugard, 1960.
3 Mosso, 1903. Angel Mosso (1846–1910) was an Italian physician, archeologist and inventor of physiological instruments, who from 1876 held the chair of physiology and therapeutics at the University of Turin. He was a founder, together with Emery, of the famous *Archives Italiennes de Biologie*, an Italian journal published in French. He was interested in cardiovascular and exertion physiology and wrote more than 25 books on related topics (for more details see Anonymous, Mosso, 1923).
4 Kronecker, 1871.
5 p. 119, Mosso, 1903.
6 p. 119, Mosso, 1903.
7 p. 121, Mosso, 1903.
8 Féré, 1903.
9 Baldwin, 1901.
10 MacDougall, 1899.
11 p. 204, MacDougall, 1899.
12 pp. 204–205, MacDougall, 1899.
13 Ioteyko, 1920.
14 p. 7, Ioteyko, 1920.
15 p. 377, Anonymous. Fatiga, 1921.
16 p. 205, MacDougall, 1899.
17 MacDougall, 1899, see also Garth, 1918.

18 Kraepelin, 1898.
19 Caparrós, 1986.
20 MacDougall, 1899.
21 Kensies, 1898.
22 Wagner, 1898.
23 Kraepelin, 1902.
24 This methodology of analysis did not include the feeling of fatigue; in general, the history of fatigue in education falls beyond the scope of this chapter.
25 Gubser, 1972.
26 pp. 93–94, Ioteyko, 1920; Poore, 1895.
27 Waterman, 1909.
28 Bartley and Chute, 1947, see also 1952 Proceedings of Symposium on Fatigue held by the *Ergonomics Research Society* (Floyd and Welford, 1953).
29 Bugard, 1960.
30 pp. 6–7, Bugard, 1960.
31 Bugard, 1960.
32 *OED*, second edition.
33 p. 206, Jaspers, 1963.
34 p. 207, Jaspers, 1963.
35 Deusen, 1869.
36 López Piñero, 1983; Chatel and Peel, 1970; Carlson, 1970; Gosling, 1987.
37 Di Mascio, 1986; Sicherman, 1977.
38 Cowles, 1893; Savill, 1906; Dubois, 1905; Cobb, 1920.
39 p. 79, Brown, 1800; Risse, 1970.
40 A useful offshoot of Brunonianism was the rejection of bleeding as a treatment for asthenic diseases (see p. 104, Brown, 1800).
41 p. 81, Brown, 1800.
42 Baldwin, 1901.
43 Tuke, 1892.
44 Fabre, 1840.
45 p. 91, Fabre, 1840.
46 Neuburger, 1981.
47 Mayne, 1860.
48 Temkin, 1964.
49 Albarracín Teulón, 1983; Hall, 1969.
50 pp. 64–76, López Piñero, 1983.
51 p. 73, López Piñero, 1983.
52 p. 59, Charcot, 1987.
53 pp. 127–142, Charcot, 1971.
54 pp. 48–49, Savill, 1906.
55 p. 22, Cobb, 1920.
56 p. 139, Dubois, 1905.
57 p. 139, Dubois, 1905.
58 Féré, 1903; 1899.
59 pp. 139–140, Féré, 1899.
60 pp. 168–172, Féré, 1903.

61 Danion *et al.*, 1985; Hermie, 1986; Wettley, 1959; Dowbiggin, 1985.

62 p. 185, Féré, 1903.

63 pp. 215–218, Heckel, 1917.

64 pp. 366–367, Anonymous, Fatiga, 1921.

65 Berrios, On Obsessional disorders during the nineteenth century, 1985; Raymond, 1911; Blumer, 1906.

66 Cobb, 1920.

67 p. 352, Cobb, 1920.

68 p. 347, Janet, 1919.

69 p. 348, Janet, 1919.

70 pp. 173–174, Berrios, Obsessional Disorders. . ., 1985.

71 Berrios, On Melancholia and depression during the nineteenth century, 1988.

72 p. 147, Ribot, 1897.

73 Deschamps, 1919.

74 p. 114, Deschamps, 1919.

75 Ribot, 1897; see Chapter 13, this book.

76 p. 58, Ribot, 1897.

77 Loas and Pierson, 1989.

78 Kleinman, 1986.

79 Bech, 1987.

80 Behan *et al.*, 1985; Anonymous. Epidemic myalgic encephalomyelitis, 1978.

81 Muscio, 1921.

82 Grayson, 1988; Osterlind, 1983.

83 Wells, 1908.

84 Bartenwerfer, 1960; Marek *et al.*, 1988.

CHAPTER 16

Catalepsy, catatonia and stupor

The nineteenth century concept of 'disorder of motility' is one of the most difficult to grasp from the perspective of today. This tells much about the role of ideology and metaphor in descriptive psychopathology. For what might have in common clinical states as diverse as stupor, akinesia, catalepsy, psychomotor retardation, agitation, impulsions, bradyphrenia, parkinsonism, dyskinesias akathisia, grimacing, mannerisms, posturing, stereotypies, soft neurological signs, tremors and tics except, perhaps, the fact that they all refer in a general way to human movement? Confronted with such a list, the neurologist of today might respond as he would to a medieval bestiary, i.e. with amused disbelief. Of the old disorders of motility he will say that they are either involuntary movements of basal ganglia origin or psychogenic disorders, i.e. 'voluntary' movements pretending to be otherwise.

Unfortunately, things are not as simple as this. For what is the status of catatonia or depressive stupor? Are they basal ganglia phenomena? Are they just 'psychogenic' states under the patient's control? Is it that he cannot move or that he does not want to? Should the complaint that he cannot move ever be taken seriously? On the other hand, is the 'cannot' of stupor analogous to the 'cannot' of hysterical paralysis? Where are the empirical answers to these questions? Should we accept Ajuriaguerra's 'psychomotor syndromes',[1] or Hunter's 'brain disease' view,[2] or Marsden et al.'s 'areas of common interest',[3] or the 'conflict of paradigms' view?[4] One approach to these complex issues is historical analysis, i.e. the going back in time to a period when dichotomies such as voluntary–involuntary, cortical–sub-cortical, and organic–psychogenic had not yet been invented.

The first issue in regard to abnormal movements concerns the ascertainment of 'voluntariness'. Nineteenth century alienists were fully aware of the difficulties involved. For example, Griesinger wrote: 'in cases of obstinate mutism (*Stummheit*), which sometimes goes on for ten years or longer, we must first of all discover whether the patient does not want to speak or *cannot speak* (as in chronic catalepsy, deep melancholia, stupor or dementia) (*chronisch-cataleptische Zustände, tiefe Melancholie, Stupor, Blödsinn*).'[5] Thus, whilst Griesinger believed that, in the latter conditions, the patient *cannot* act, many nowadays will say that he does not want to. Likewise, Griesinger attributed an inordinate number of motor disorders to insanity: some, like pupillary asymmetries, true paralysis, and seizures are easy to re-classify as 'neurological' (after all, his subjects had been recruited in a period when neurology and psychiatry had not yet been separated). Others, such as catalepsy, stupor and mannerisms were as much a problem for him as they are to us. Few had the faith of Luys, the great French alienist, who had a physiological view of the will and hence found no difficulty in conceiving of all motility disorders as the expression of mental disorder.[6]

Catalepsy

The word catalepsy is almost as old as the behaviours it was coined to refer. The more so to wonder at the fact that this dramatic clinical phenomenon is no longer seen in clinical practice.[7] In its complete form, catalepsy included a full and sudden motor paralysis, with normal or increased muscle tone, total sensory disconnection with anaesthesia and analgesia, passive posturing (i.e. the subject would remain in any position set by the examiner), and total amnesia for the event. The attack would last from minutes to a full day, come unannounced or heralded by prodromal experiences very similar to a panic attack.[8] Catalepsy might be unilateral or bilateral,[9] primary (idiopathic, simple, franc) or secondary (complicated); the former occurring in apparently normal subjects and tending to be complete and of shorter duration; the latter occurring associated with hysteria, ecstasy and somnambulism, and tending to incompletion and long duration.[10] Students, members of religious orders, and the military were said to be prone to the disorder.[11] Catalepsy was different from hysteria and from simulated disorders. During the nineteenth century, the debate was on whether catalepsy was a symptom[12] or a disease.[13] By the time Axenfeld wrote his treatise the condition was becoming *'très rare, d'une nature énigmatique'*; he considered tension, abolition of sensation, and resistance to fatigue as its pathognomonic features.[14]

British writers had a slightly different view. Copland wrote: 'catalepsy and ecstasy, although treated of by some writers as distinct affections, generally present very nearly the same pathological conditions, as respects the presumed states of circulation in the brain.'[15] Tuke defined catalepsy as a neurosis, frequent in women, and characterised by 'the patient's inability to change the position of a limb, while another person can place the muscles in a state of flexion or contraction as he will.' He suggested that the attack of catalepsy was due to 'erethism of the cerebral substance and engorgement of the blood vessels,[16] involving pressure on that part of the brain which is the seat of intelligence, and the origin of the motor and sensory nerves.'[17] British clinical students were still being taught at the turn of the century that 'one of the characteristic symptoms of this condition was muscular rigidity. I have rarely met with this condition in a very fully developed form, but at the same time it is rare to be without some case of partial catalepsy in Bethlem.'[18]

Changes began to appear in the conceptualisation of catalepsy early in the twentieth century, for example White wrote: *'Suggestibility* may be said to be the exact opposite of negativism. The patient's reactions are determined by impressions or suggestions derived from others. it is manifested in various ways. In extreme cases the patient resembles a clay figure; the limbs can be placed in any position and are there retained indefinitely. This condition is designated as catalepsy or *flexibilitas cerea*.' [19] The view that suggestion was the central mechanism of catalepsy originated from the work of Babinski who, in a famous session of the *Société de Neurologie* of Paris in 1901, presented his revisionist definition of hysteria and proposed that it was a *pithiatic* clinical phenomenon, i.e. one which could be treated by persuasion and suggestion.[20] This view was far more popular amongst psychiatrists than neurologists.[21]

White's definition of catalepsy no longer assumes a 'disease view' nor does it rely on Petetin's popular 'blood-supply' mechanism. To understand this shift we must go back a few years to explore Charcot's views on hysteria and catalepsy. Charcot started his research into hysteria and epilepsy by chance. The old Sainte-Laure wards, where hysterical, epileptic and insane patients were kept (and that had once belonged to Delasiauve) had fallen into disrepair and the Administration of *La Salpêtrière* decided to move all patients with 'attacks' to a new ward which, by right, was offered to Charcot as the senior physician.[22] Trillat has perceptively commented on the clinical biases that the mixture of patients was to create,[23] one such was Charcot's *hystéro-épilepsie*.

From the point of view of this chapter, attention must be given to the way in which Charcot's concept of hysteria engulfed the phenomenon of catalepsy. In 1878, Charcot published a paper in *Le Progrès Médical* entitled *Catalepsie et somnambulisme hystériques provoqués* reporting the use of hypnosis in two female patients (Louis and Alphonsine) and the induction of catalepsy by means of a bright light. Furthermore, catalepsy could be changed into lethargy by closing the subjects's eyelids.[24] In Charcot's school, hypnosis and hysteria are found 'intimately linked.'[25] But catalepsy was also considered as a marker of depth of suggestion by the Nancy school (Bernheim's 'catalepsy by suggestion').[26] In the Breslau school, Heidenhain likewise considered the hypnotic state as 'catalepsy artificially produced.'[27]

By the end of the First World War, the notion of primary catalepsy had gone, and the 'secondary' type was considered as a hysterical symptom, no longer related to the real nervous system.[28] Effort were made to develop an animal model, and cats were reported showing irreversible 'catalepsy' after lesions around the mamillary bodies.[29] By the end of the second World War reports of the symptom in humans had become rare. In a recent textbook of descriptive psychopathology the term has disappeared from the list of contents altogether.[30] Catalepsy is no more.

Catatonia

Catatonia, whether considered as a disease or a syndrome has also become rare in the psychiatry of the advanced countries. Reasons for this are mostly unknown although it is unlikely that social factors are the only ones at play. Catalepsy and catatonia seem related in the sense that the latter is likely to be a genuine psycho-motor disorder whilst the former might have been its 'psychogenic' phenocopy. By the same token, what used to be called 'complicated catalepsy', i.e. a disease lasting for months and accompanied by hallucinations and delusions, is likely to have been true catatonia.

Catatonic behaviour existed before the term was ever coined by Kahlbaum, for example, one such case was reported by Morel in 1852 and 8 years later named *démence précoce*. On the other hand, as it is often the case with the *editio princeps* for any disease, few of Kahlbaum's clinical descriptions can be said to be 'typical' of what was later to be known as 'catatonia' (see Tables 16.1, 16.2). In the late 1890s, Kraepelin subsumed catatonia under the category of dementia preacox;[31] but soon after, reports appeared that catatonia was also seen in manic depressive insanity, and during the early 1920s, encephalitis lethargica was shown to be complicated by similar behaviour; neuroleptics and other drugs have also been found to cause catatonia-like states. Reduced to a syndrome, catatonia limped along until it began to disappear in the developed countries after the 1940s; however, cases are still seen in third-world countries.

Kahlbaum

There is a difference between what Kahlbaum actually described and what he thought he was describing at the time. It is difficult to account for the difference without first mentioning his nosological ideas. Kahlbaum was not particularly interested in collecting a group of disorders with a common brain lesion. In relation to the neuropathological 'zeal' of other alienists he wrote: 'This work produced much valuable material but contributed nothing to the basic views on the origin of mental illness or on the anatomical locus of their diverse and significant manifes-tations; the view is now spreading that only *comprehensive clinical observation* of cases can bring order and clarity into the material . . . it has now been recognized that it is futile to search for an anatomy of melancholy or mania, etc. because each of these forms occurs under the most varied relationships and combinations with other states, and they are just as little the expressions of an inner pathological process as the complex of symptoms call fever . . . how wrong it inevitably was to expect pathological anatomy alone to reform the obsolete psychiatric framework.'[32] These major words were as valid then as they are now. Kahlbaum was, in fact, proposing a Copernican revolution: it was yet Utopian to rely on brain lesions to generate a classification of diseases, psychiatrists needed to map, better than ever before, the presentation of mental disease.

This is precisely what he tried to do in his monograph on catatonia. The German version of the term, *Spannungsirresein*, enshrines the central feature of the disorder. Such cases Kahlbaum had already presented to his colleagues twice before.[33] How-ever, since 'no special report had been published of either meeting, it was not surprising that my data on catatonia are incompletely known and understood.'[34]

Table 16.1.

Age	31 (SD = 8)
Sex	male = 18 / female = 7
	missing = 1
Duration of illness	29 (SD = 29)
(in months)	(range = 1 to 84)
Depression at onset	12
Neurological signs	11
Epileptic seizures	9
Masturbation as cause	3
Posturing	12
Flexibilitas Cerea	9
Hallucinations	11
Delusions	7
Verbigeration	7
Outcome	improved 8
	chronic or dead 8
	missing data 10

In the 1874 monograph he tried to 'describe a disease pattern which has somatic components expressed in muscular symptoms (*Muskuläre Symptome*) . . . which play an essential role in the definition of the disease (*eine wesentliche Bedeutung für die Gestaltung des ganzen Krankheitsprocesses*).'[35] His disease, he felt, had already been anticipated in the old notion of *melancholia attonita* which 'may be described as a state of motionless mutism, rigid face, eyes looking at the distance, lack of movement or reaction to stimuli, there may be flexibilitas cerea as in catalepsy . . . the obvious association of this illness with muscular symptoms has been neglected.'[36] Thus, Kahlbaum tried to extricate from the large mass of 'melancholic stupors' a sub-group with cataleptic features which were not necessarily depressed and presented delusions. Some patients showed 'verbigeration': 'a psychopathological phenomenon during which the patient appears to make a speech composed of repeated and meaningless words and sentences.'[37]

A statistical analysis of Kahlbaum's cases shows that he reported 26 cases altogether, of which case 15 was very incomplete, case 16 was a 44 year-old woman with tuberculosis who died soon after, case 17 a man with peritonitis and terminal delirium, case 18 another 26 year-old consumptive, and cases 22 to 25 all had general paralysis of the insane, and died of it. The results of the analysis are as shown in Table 16.1.

Table 16.2.

Factor 1 ('Neurological') (variance = 29%)	
Duration	.64[a]
Neurological	.71
Seizures	.80
Hallucinations	.71
Factor 2 ('Psychotic depression') (Variance = 22%)	
No neurological	.58
Hallucinations	.37
Delusions	.93
Verbigeration	.93

[a]Loadings for the variables.

No differences between males and females was found on any of the listed symptoms; a robust correlation, however, existed (r = .56, p < .01) between age and flexibilitas cerea (i.e. the younger the patient the higher the chance of the symptom being present). Exploratory factor analysis (to identify a factor that might be recognized as a 'catatonic syndrome') was carried out. Two factors accounting for 51% of variance were extracted but posturing, flexibilitas cerea and verbigeration behaved orthogonally, suggesting that no 'catatonic' factor seems to be present in Kahlbaum's original cases (see Table 16.2).

Kahlbaum's cases included two types: clear *organic deliriums* who might have shown fleeting psychomotor disorders, but which had little to do with the disease he wanted to represent; and a smaller group of *psychotic depressives* some of which had 'catatonic' features. Neither groups supports his idealized definition: 'catatonia is a brain disease with a cyclical, alternating course, in which the mental symptoms are, consecutively, melancholia, mania, stupor (*Stupescenz*), confusion (*Verwirrtheit*) and eventually dementia (*Blödsinn*). One or more of these symptoms may be absent from the series of psychological symptom clusters (*psychischen Gesammtbildern*).[38] In addition to the mental symptoms, neurological motor and convulsions (*Krampfes*) are also essential signs.

The result of this analysis is at variance with the commentaries of some American writers[39] and more specifically with the factor structure of catatonia described by Abrams *et al.*[40] But it is, however, in agreement with the conclusions of Séglas and Chaslin[41] of over a hundred years ago, and of Pauleikhoff more recently, although neither carried out a statistical analysis of Kahlbaum's cases.[42]

Stupor

Stupor names a symptom complex whose central feature is a reduction or absence of relational functions (i.e. action and speech). The stuporous patient emanates an eerie feeling of remoteness, and both spontaneous and reactive behaviour may be involved. Stupor and cognate states have been reported to be associated with catatonia,[43] mania,[44] depression,[45] hysteria,[46] sudden emotional stress,[47] acute confusional state,[48] mid-line brain lesions,[49] frontal lobe atrophy,[50] epilepsy,[51] migraine,[52] diffuse brain damage,[53] apallic syndrome,[54] Parkinson's syndrome,[55] idiosyncratic response to sodium valproate,[56] cycloid psychoses,[57] bulbocapnine intoxication,[58] neuroleptics,[59] and encephalitis.[60] Operational definitions have been offered for both 'psychiatric' (functional)[61] and 'neurological' (organic)[62] forms of stupor but it is unclear whether these have in common any relevant clinical feature.

Since the turn of the century, the predominant view has been that 'functional' stupors are 'psychogenic' or 'secondary'[63] whereas 'neurological' ones are states of behavioural disorganization resulting from organic pathology.[64] This distinction has no heuristic value as little is known on the neurophysiology of psychiatric stupors. This may be due to various reasons. Firstly, 'motility' and 'consciousness', the two concepts in relation to which stupor has been defined, remain opaque to analysis. Secondly, psychiatric stupors have become infrequent and no adequate case databases seem to exist. Thirdly, psychiatric stupor is a transient phenomenon and a medical emergency so that it is not often accessible to complex neurobiological research. Fourthly, the available terminology to describe all states of reduced behavioural output remains inadequate.[65] Finally, the history of stupor has been much neglected.[66]

The history of the word

The word stupor (*Benommenheit, Stumpfsinn*) (*stupeur, stupidité*) derives from the Latin root *stuporem* which means 'numbness', 'dullness', 'insensibility'.[67] *Stumpfsinn* derives from the old high German word for 'blunt'.[68] Hobbes asked 'for what is stupor but that which the Greeks call 'anaesthesia', that is, a cessation from the sense of other things?'[69] From Classical times the term has meant 'non-responsiveness' due to a 'numbing' of the senses. The Latin term itself comes from the Sanskrit *stumbh* (to be stunned), which expanded the earlier descriptive stem *stna* (motionless).[70] Neurological usage is, therefore, closer to etymology. By insisting upon the presence of clear consciousness, psychiatrists have strained the semantic boundaries of the term stupor and raised important issues such as why does the patient choose to remain unresponsive when, in fact, he has intact awareness. Explanations based on pathology of volition, unconscious inhibition and delusional control have been offered to account for this phenomenon.

Synonyms and cognate phenomena

The psychiatric literature has referred to stupor or stupor-like states by such categories as: *stupidité*,[71] *démence aiguë*,[72] *melancholia attonita*,[73] *catalepsie*,[74] *Stumpfsinn*,[75] anergic and delusional stupor,[76] torpor,[77] psychocoma,[78] *Verwirrtheit*,[79] stares, *Irrfühlen, phrénoplexie, extase*,[80] stupemania,[81] *confusion mentale primitive*,[82] *Benommenheit, Akinesis*,[83] benign and malignant stupor,[84] hypobulic state,[85] and restlessness.[86]

Cognate neurological states characterized by a severe reduction in relational function resembling stupor are: apallic syndrome,[87] akinetic mutism,[88] parasomnia,[89] anoetic syndrome,[90] lucid stupor,[91] hypersomnia,[92] *stupeur hypertonique post-traumatique*,[93] coma vigile,[94] *vita reducta*,[95] coma prolongé,[96] post-traumatic catatonia,[97] persistent vegetative state,[98] locked-in syndrome, acute global aphasia,[99] and amentia.[100]

History of the concept

In Greek and Roman medicine the clinical state to which stupor currently refers was included in the class of 'behavioural unresponsiveness'. Greek writers referred to this group as morosis,[101] lethargus, carus, agrypnos, coma, and catalepsis.[102] Lethargus meant for Aurelianus a state that was 'neither a deep sleep nor a delirium, but rather a torpor (numbness) with reduction of all physiological function'.[103] Catacho was defined by Filippo de Cesarea as 'emptiness of the spirit with immobility of the body'.[104] Galen distinguished two types of coma: a deep sleep with eyes closed, and another with eyes open (*agrypnos coma, coma vigilante*).[105] Latin writers used terms such as *mentis consternatio, hebetudo* and *stupiditas* to refer to similar mental states.[106] Enshrined in Galenic medicine these views survived well up to the sixteenth century. In 1583, Barrough wrote: 'catoche or catalepsis in Greeke . . . in English it maie be called Congelation or taking . . . it is a sodaine detention and taking both of mind and body, both sense and moving being list, the sicke remaining in the same figure of bodie wherein he was taken, whither his eyes be open or shut.'[107] Bayfield iterated this view a century later.[108] In his *Praxeos Medicae*, Felix Platter included a chapter on 'Mentis consternatione' which he divided into: post-prandial somnolence, inebriated or alcoholic torpor, delusional stupor, demonic stupor, stuporous torpor, apoplectic stupor, epileptic stupor, cataleptic stupor, ecstatic stupor, and stupor with preservation of movement.[109] Some of these states are redolent of catatonic or depressive stupor.

Erasmus Darwin subdivided the stupor-like states into categories such as stupor, lethargus, catalepsy and torpor in order to fit them into his own classification of disease of irritation (stupor and torpor), volition (catalepsis and lethargus), sensation and association.[110] Conceptually, these views depended upon the hypothesis that stupor was due to numbness. A good illustration of this is Turnbull's definition of stupor as 'a numbness in any part of the body, whether occasioned by ligatures obstructing the blood's motion, by the palsy or the like.'[111]

Nineteenth century and after

The history of stupor can be divided into four periods. During the first, which goes from the beginning to the 1830s, stupor-like states were described in behavioural terms and non-responsiveness was assumed to result (as it had been in earlier centuries) from 'numbness' of the senses. The second period, covering the next two decades, is characterized by the inclusion of subjective, experiential elements to the definition and analysis of stupor. The third, which reaches the 1890s, saw the development of an 'interactional' view according to which symptoms of stupor such as negativism and echo phenomena were considered as meaningful behavioural exchanges; in other words, the 'psychologization' of the 'psychiatric' stupors achieved completion. The fourth period covers up to the present day, and is characterised by attempts to analyse stupor as a primary motor disorder and as a stereotyped, vestigial behavioural programme.

THE FIRST PERIOD Pinel did not separate stupor from *idiotisme* but reported a form of the latter caused by 'strong and unexpected emotions'. 'Oversensitive individuals may show a suspension of psychological function as the result of sudden emotional shock . . . they may remain in this state for months or years . . . showing lack of expression, fixed gaze, immobility, muteness and disregard for food.'[112]

Esquirol separated 'dementia' from 'idiotisme', defining the former as 'a form of insanity where ideas, emotions and volitions are affected; it is characterized by the weakening and obliteration of intellectual, emotional and volitional faculties.'[113] Dementia could be acute and chronic; *démence aigue* was a transient state, with sudden onset, that resulted from a host of organic and psychological causes. For example, there was the case of a man who oscillated between agitation and stupor: 'he would hold his head down with a fixed and empty gaze and total indifference to his surroundings. He would remain motionless wherever he was left, dribble from mouth and nose and be incontinent of urine. He would clench his teeth when forced to drink.' During lucid intervals the patient would report 'inability to move' and being 'too weak to start any action' during the attacks.[114]

Georget classified 'stupidity' as the fourth genre of insanity and believed that the cognitive faculties might be predominantly involved: 'acquired absence of cognitive function, whether due to lack of mentation or inability to manifest it.' Emphasis on the intellectual faculties led him to accept introspection as a source of symptoms: '*Aliénés stupides* are in a state of psychological annihilation, indifference to their surroundings and insensitivity to stimulation . . . only after remission their real mental state can be known.' 'The mental content experienced by these patients is delusional in nature and suggests that stupidity is different from idiotism and dementia.'[115] Georget died young, and this view was developed by Baillarger 20 years later.

The most important work on *stupidité* during this period was that by Étoc-Demazy. Based on ten cases (two borrowed from Georget), this great alienist identified the fundamental features of stupor. Four cases recovered and two (5 and 6) are vivid descriptions of the syndrome that was later to be called 'catatonia'. Ètoc-Demazy agreed with Georget that a retrospective analysis of the mental state was essential for differential diagnosis. Post-mortem of four cases seemed to show 'typical' brain lesions (likely to have been non-specific terminal brain changes). The four conclusions he drew are important to the history of stupor: 1. 'stupidity' is not a genre of insanity but a complication of mania or monomania,[116] 2. symptoms evolve in two stages (diminution of cognition and suspension of relational functions), 3. the symptoms themselves cannot predict duration or outcome, and 4. *stupidité* and *démence* are different syndromes.[117]

THE SECOND PERIOD After the work of Georget and Ètoc-Demazy, the 1840s witnessed the development of a diagnosis of stupor based on subjective experience. Based on 18 cases (8 his own, 2 borrowed from Georget, and 8 from Étoc-Demazy) Baillarger challenged the view that *stupides* were devoid from mental experiences and proposed that these symptoms should be included in the diagnosis. He can be said to have developed the first 'psychiatric' conception of stupor, of which depressive stupor (*melancholia attonita*) was the paradigm. He suggested that stupor was different from catalepsy but three of his cases seemed (in retrospect) typical catatonic stupors with catalepsy. Like others during this period, he included stupor under *lypémanie* (Esquirol's name for major depressive illness). Baillarger's conclusions summarize well the fundamental changes he suggested: 1. stuporous patients experience delusional experiences which they recollect after improvement, 2. these delusions are depressive in nature, and may contain suicidal ideation, 3 illusions and hallucinations are present and transport the patient to a world of fantasy, 4. 'stupidity' is an advanced state of depression, and 5. 'stupidity' is analogous to dreaming.[118]

But stupors could also be found with little or no delusional and hallucinatory experiences. These did not fit into Baillarger's restricted definition and Ball decided to call them 'cerebral torpor' which he characterized as having empty inner life, hypokinesis, mutism, reduced cognition, good prognosis, and either psychological or organic origin; they were, in fact, more frequent than Baillarger's florid form.[119] Based on this analysis, Ritti suggested the existence of melancholic and symptomatic stupors; the former was similar to Baillarger's type; the latter was a rag-bag of states such as organic commas and catatonias.[120]

The predominance of French sources during this period reflects the historical fact that the debate on stupor took place in that country. German views only came to the fore after Griesinger who, in the second edition of his book, included a section on 'melancholia with stupor' and criticized the term *stupidité*. His analysis was influenced by the theoretical view that there was an 'insanity consisting in the

morbid production, governing and persistence of emotions and emotional states'
and another 'consisting in disorders of the intellect and will which do not proceed
from a ruling emotional state.'[121] Griesinger described two types of 'melancholic
stupor' (*Schwermuth mit Stumpfsinn*): one with rigidity, catalepsy, negativism, clouding, incontinence and fantastic hallucinatory and delusional experiences, and
another which was like a 'a half-sleeping state without distinct dreams or
hallucinations', abulia and melancholia, and which could be confused with
dementia. It is tempting to see here an early distinction between the catatonic and
depressive forms of stupor.

Debate on whether 'melancholia with stupor' or *melancholia attonita* constituted
a form of depression (as Baillarger suggested) continued well into the second half
of the century. and culminated in Kahlbaum's proposal of 1869 and 1874 that
such condition was, in fact, the first stage of 'vesania catatonica'.[122] By this period,
however, the view that consciousness could itself become disordered started to gain
currency, and Krafft-Ebing was able to re-define stupor as an 'elementary disorder
of consciousness' found in association with many conditions, and to sub-divide it
into *melancholia attonita* and *Stupidität* or 'curable dementia'.[123]

British views Up to this period, British psychiatry had simply echoed Continental
views. However, in the second volume of the *Asylum Journal*, Monro described 'cataleptoid insanity': 'some patients stand in apparently profound sopor; their eyes are
glued down or else staring open in a fixed manner, the skin is cold and clammy,
you speak to them, they will not answer, you offer them food, they will not eat.
They, indeed, are most unwilling to move from the spot which they have taken
up; the state of the intellect in these cases is often hard to arrive at; sometimes
when you lay hold suddenly of such a patient you may shake him out of the stupor,
and you find that his mind is by no means lost, that he has a clear perception of
all that has been going on even during the trance.'[124] Monro rejected the term
'acute dementia', and considered his description as a separate form of insanity.
Kahlbaum did not refer to this article in his 1874 monograph on catatonia.

In an early paper, Maudsley summarized views on the distinction between *melancholia attonita* and 'the stupor of actual dementia'; it is clear from his description,
however, that 'catatonic' stupors were included in both groups.[125] Maudsley supported a syndromic view 'stupor is no more than a descriptive name comprehending
different forms of mental disorder.'[126] By far the most important British work on
stupor during this period is Newington's who borrowed much from Dagonet's paper
of two years earlier. Based on a study of 12 female cases from the Royal Edinburgh
Asylum, Newington distinguished an anergic and a delusional form of stupor which
he proposed instead of the older forms 'acute dementia' and 'melancholic stupor',
respectively.[127] It has been suggested that Newington's groups refer to catatonic
(malignant) and depressive (benign) stupor, respectively.[128] This is unlikely to be
so as the median age for his 'depressive' stupors was under 22 (too young for this

complication) and many showed 'catatonia-like' states. Furthermore, Newington's clinical criteria often did not apply to his own cases: realizing this, he claimed that sometimes the 'original delusional form was, as it were, masked by the anergic form'. Criteria for anergic stupor were: strong heredity, sudden onset, cognitive impairment, amnesia for the event, flattened emotion, absence of volition, 'cataleptoid condition' (à la Monro), tendency to emaciation, cyanotic appearance and incontinence; criteria for delusional stupor were: strong heredity, insidious onset, rich subjective experiences, memory for the event, evidence of fear or grief, eyes fixed or obstinately closed, negativism, posturing, insensitivity to pain, insomnia and constipation. It seems clear that Newington's clinical syndromes cut across the catatonic-depressive stupor distinction.

This confusion was not lost to Clouston who subdivided stupor (which he called *psychocoma*) into melancholic, anergic, secondary, general paralytic, and epileptic. His anergic stupor (wider than Newington's) corresponds well to the catatonic stupor of later authors.[129] Tuke was more specific in his criticism of Newington: 'of one thing there can be no doubt, that the delusional stupor of today may be the anergic stupor of tomorrow . . . There are cases in which the ablest alienist is unable to decide whether the mind is what the outward expression would lead us to infer – a complete blank – or the seat of such intense depression and painful delusion as only to simulate dementia. Mental stupor may be applied to cover both conditions.'[130] Dealing with the catatonic form, Whitwell attempted an aetiological analysis and saw stupor as a form of 'dystrophoneurosis', i.e. of brain malnutrition.[131] Savage still used 'melancholia with stupor' and 'acute primary dementia with stupor' (in the latter, 'delusions render the patient statuesque') and proposed that the presence of amnesia for the event should be used to differentiate the two forms of stupor, the melancholic being accompanied by recollection of painful experiences.[132] Bernard Hollander dealt with stupor both under 'melancholia' and 'primary dementia', and followed Savage's clinical groups.[123]

THIRD PERIOD Up to this point, the symptoms of stupor suggested a division between those related to melancholia (florid subjective symptoms) and catatonia or 'primary or acute dementia' (inhibition of function). The third period in the history of stupor unfolded against the Kraepelinian separation between dementia praecox and manic depressive insanity which demanded a final re-alignment of the clinical forms of stupor. More importantly, this period witnessed the development of psychodynamic ideas and a re-analysis of some of the features of stupor (e.g. negativism, echo phenomena) in terms of interactions or 'communications' between patient and environment. This view was suggested by Kraepelin himself.

Kraepelin In the sixth edition of his textbook, Kraepelin started bringing together various insanity states under the name of dementia praecox, and separating the latter from manic-depressive insanity. This offered him a way of sub-dividing stupors into catatonic, manic, depressive and hysterical. Stupor followed the period of excitement in catatonic insanity: 'The patients become quiet, shy, monosyllabic . . . stare fixedly in front of them . . . all independent volitional expression is silent; speech, the taking of food, intercourse with the surroundings.' It was in this context that Kraepelin mentioned *external* influences: 'The behaviour of the patients towards external influences shows, however, certain differences, which indeed are subject to much variation.' Echolalia, echopraxis and continuous imitation of movement were elicited by external influences; and so were sudden interruptions and reversals, refusal of verbal answers, communication by writing, etc. Kraepelin found that, during these situations, stuporous patients often monitored their surroundings. However, because 'consciousness was for the most part clouded . . . it was often difficult to obtain a reliable account of the real substance of their recollections.'[134] On the other hand, manic stupors followed 'mixed states': 'Patients are usually quite inaccessible, do not trouble themselves about their surroundings, give no answer . . . not infrequently catalepsy can be demonstrated.' The patients 'often have a quite accurate recollection of the time that has elapsed but are totally unable to explain their singular behaviour.'[135] Depressive stupor constituted for Kraepelin the highest degree of 'psychic inhibition'. Patients were 'deeply apathetic, no longer able to perceive the impressions of the surroundings and to assimilate them . . . occasionally it can be recognized that the inhibition of thought is slighter than the volitional disorder . . . sometimes they display catalepsy and lack of will power, sometimes aimless resistance to external interference . . . they are unable to care for their bodily needs . . . now and then periods of excitement may be interpolated . . . after the return of consciousness, which usually appears rather abruptly, memory is very much clouded, and often quite extinguished.'[136] For all the elegance of Kraepelin's clinical descriptions not enough differential criteria were provided to separate the three forms of stupor; thus, decisions as to what type of stupor was in hand had to emanate from knowledge of the patient's past history.

Bleuler also supported an interactional view of stupor, and illustrated this by quoting a case[137] who would give up his mutism when asked questions relevant to his delusions; he also made the point, often repeated since, that visits from relatives may bring patients out of their stupor and that 'last minute answers' are common amongst stuporous catatonics. Bleuler, however, insisted on a more specific usage of 'stupor' in relation to catatonia: 'It has been claimed that many catatonics are in a stuporous condition', but 'if we use stupor in Ziehen's sense (i.e. aprosexia,[138] inhibition of cognitive function and immobility) only few catatonics (those with *Benommenheit*) are actually stuporous.'[139] This tendency to over-diagnosis Bleuler explained on the basis that 'akinetic catatonics are hyporeactive to their environment'. Years later, he was to iterate this syndromic view: stupor may follow 'maximal apathy, inhibitions, obstructions, over-powering through fright or anxiety and cerebral torpor of any kind.'[140]

The question of the 'pseudo-reversibility' of stupor – hinted at by Bleuler – has not been solved to this day in spite of a later suggestion that it was a 'disorder of action and not of motorium.'[141]

Hoch and Kretschmer Hoch's classical book on benign stupors was published in 1921. Written in the Meyerian tradition, this work studied 25 cases in terms of seven criteria: poverty of affect, inactivity, catalepsy, negativism, thinking disorder, ideational content, and physical peculiarities. 'Partial' and 'complete' stupors were identified, those appearing in the context of manic-depressive psychosis were benign; the converse was true for stupor accompanying dementia praecox. Hoch offered a 'psychological' explanation, and saw stupor as a reaction consisting in 'levels of regression' which could reach 'ideas of death', 'negativism' and 'total lack of mentation'. Hoch's clinical sub-division did not work, for, on follow-up, Rachlin found that 10 out of the 13 cases of 'benign stupor' had developed catatonic schizophrenia.[142]

Kretschmer explored stupor in terms of his 'hypobulic mechanism'. In normal individuals, these vestigial mechanisms are under the control of higher 'phylogenetic levels'; in hysteria and schizophrenia: 'we actually find in the same symptom complexes, which reveal atavistic imaginal processes, certain psychomotor peculiarities that can again be parallelled by phylogenetically earlier states in the development of expressional functions . . . In addition to the hysterical attack there are other motor protective and defence mechanisms . . . such as limping, feigning death, and so on. The same reactions are common to many animals as instinctive dispositions. Stupor, motor rigidity with or without functional anaesthesia, are common features of catatonia and hysteria.[143]

The third period in the evolution of stupor is, thus, characterized by the appearance of the interactional view first sponsored by Kraepelin and Bleuler. This was widened into a general view of stupor as resulting from psychological inhibition or regression, as illustrated by the work of Hoch and Kretschmer. This was to overshadow earlier Wernickian notions of stupor (and other movement disorders in psychiatry) as primary disorders of motility.[144]

FOURTH PERIOD The decline of the psychodynamic view, and the growth of experimental research, led to a revival of organic and ethological views of stupor, and a return to the Wernickian concept of disorder of motility. Since early in the century, a number of reports suggested that chemical or anatomical lesions to certain brain sites might cause cataleptic states.[145] Related clinical states such as subcortical dementia[146] and the forms of stupor found in association with catatonia, normal pressure hydrocephalus, and Parkinsonism following encephalitis lethargica[147] seem to inculpate the basal ganglia[148] and their frontal circuits as a potential site for the disorders of motility.

Another source of evidence originated from behavioural and neurochemical studies of the phenomenon of 'tonic immobility', 'animal hypnosis', 'freezing reaction' or 'trance state'. This stereotyped, hard-wired behavioural response, may occur naturally or be experimentally produced in small birds, mammals and reptiles[149] and consists in sudden obliteration of movement and action in response to a threatening stimulus. It may last from minutes to hours and has been described as the final stage in the fear response against predation.[150] The duration and quality of this state may be prolonged by LSD-25, chlorpromazine in large doses, adrenaline, morphine, physiostigmine, monoamine oxidase inhibitors and tryptophan; and shortened by imipramine, serotonin, D-amphetamine, chlorpromazine in small doses of scopolamine.[151] Only some of these compounds have so far been tried in the treatment or experimental manipulation of human stupor. Tonic immobility may prove to be a useful animal model if the hypothesis is accepted that human stupor is also the expression of a vestigial form of behaviour triggered by psychological or organic noxae. A hypothesis of this kind would encourage the search for neuro-physiological and neuro-chemical explanations and move away from the purely psychogenic, 'voluntaristic' view of stupor which has so far proved to be heuristically sterile.

NOTES

1 Ajuriaguerra, 1975.
2 Hunter, 1973.
3 Marsden *et al.*, 1975.
4 Rogers, 1985.
5 p. 107, Griesinger, 1861.
6 pp. 166–167, Luys, 1881. For a discussion of the history of the physiology of will acts and motor behaviour, see Jeannerod, 1983.
7 Mucha, 1972. Mucha has suggested that catalepsy was eventually reinterpreted in organic terms. This is only partially true for such cases have also disappeared from medical and neurological practice.
8 Linas, 1877.
9 Georget, 1834.
10 Linas, 1877.
11 Linas, 1877.
12 Falret, 1857.
13 Linas, 1877.
14 pp. 908–919, Axenfeld, 1883.
15 p. 290, Copland, 1858.
16 This was a repetition of Petetin's view of a century early. Jacques Henri Desiré Petetin (1744–1808) trained at Montpellier and practised in Lyon. He started as a critic of the doctrine of animal magnetism but later became a convert. The book on which he discusses his blood supply theory is: *Mémoire sur la Découverte des Phénomènes que Présentent la*

catalepsie et le somnambulisme, 1787. Georget also championed this view during the nineteenth century.

17 pp. 184–185, Tuke, 1892.

18 pp. 181–182, Savage, 1886.

19 p. 66, White, 1913.

20 Babinski, 1934.

21 In 1908, two sessions of the *Société de Neurologie* in Paris were dedicated to discussing Babinski's notion of *pithiatisme*. Most of the great men of the time such as Raymond, Dejerine, Pitrés, Janet and Crocq spoke against it, see *Discussion sur L'Hystérie*, 1908.

22 Marie, 1925.

23 Trillat, 1971.

24 Charcot, 1886. The reverse phenomenon was also reported, namely, that catalepsy could be provoked by opening the subjects' eyelids (p. 174, Bourneville and Regnard, 1873–1880).

25 p. 57, Barrucand, 1967.

26 Bernheim, 1917.

27 Heidenhein, 1899.

28 pp. 440–442, Anonymous, On Catalepsia, 1921.

29 Ingram *et al.*, 1936.

30 Sims, 1988.

31 For general histories of catatonia, see Meyer, 1899; Arndt, 1902; Mickle, 1909.

32 p. 2, Kahlbaum, 1973.

33 Kahlbaum, 1870.

34 p. 6, Kahlbaum, 1973.

35 p. 4, Kahlbaum, 1874.

36 p. 5, Kahlbaum, 1874.

37 p. 39, Kahlbaum, 1874.

38 p. 87, Kahlbaum, 1874.

39 There is also much confusion in the literature about this, and descriptions such as 'brilliant' (p. 315, Morrison, 1974) abound. Others state that a 'careful examination' of Kahlbaum's catatonia reveals . . . a cyclic, alternating disease' (p. 218, Magrinat *et al.*, 1983).

40 Abrams *et al.*, 1979. In more recently diagnosed catatonics these researchers found Factor 1: mutism, negativism, stupor; Factor 2: mutism, stereotypy, catalepsy, automatic obedience.

41 Séglas, 1890.

42 pp. 494–495, Pauleikhoff, 1969.

43 Kahlbaum, 1874.

44 Kraepelin, 1921.

45 Baillarger, 1843; Hoch, 1921.

46 Kretschmer, 1934; Neustatter, 1942; Gómez, 1980.

47 Weitbrecht, 1968; Garmany, 1955.

48 Hoenig *et al.*, 1959.

49 Cairns *et al.*, 1941.

50 Ruff and Russakoff, 1980.

51 Herman *et al.*, 1942.
52 Lee and Lance, 1977.
53 Plum and Posner, 1972.
54 Peters, 1977.
55 Economo, 1931; Critchley, 1929.
56 Sackellares *et al.*, 1979.
57 Leonhard, 1979.
58 Jong, 1956.
59 Baruk, 1958.
60 Raskin and Frank, 1974.
61 Wing *et al.*, 1974.
62 Plum and Posner, 1972.
63 Scharfetter, 1976; Lishman, 1978; Alonso Fernández, 1977; Searles, 1952.
64 Plum and Posner, 1972.
65 Bash, 1955.
66 Zilboorg, 1941; Ackerknecht, 1957; Alexander and Selesnick, 1966; Baruk, 1967; Leibbrand and Wettley, 1961.
67 Lewis and Short, 1879.
68 Walshe, 1951.
69 Hobbes, quoted in *OED*.
70 Littré, 1878.
71 Georget, 1820.
72 Esquirol, 1838.
73 Baillarger, 1843.
74 Falret, 1857.
75 Griesinger, 1861.
76 Newington, 1874.
77 Ball, 1881.
78 Clouston, 1887.
98 Wille, 1888.
80 Dagonet, 1872.
81 Whitwell, 1889.
82 Chaslin, 1892.
83 Wernicke, 1906.
84 Hoch, 1921.
85 Kretschmer, 1934.
86 Meduna, 1950.
87 Kretschmer, 1940.
88 Cairns *et al.*, 1941.
89 Jefferson, 1944.
90 Duensing, 1949.
91 Ajuriaguerra *et al.*, 1953.
92 Facon *et al.*, 1958.
93 Fishgold and Mathis, 1959.
94 Mollaret and Goullon, 1959.
95 Masshoff, 1963.

 96 Vigoroux, 1964.
 97 Jellinger *et al.*, 1963.
 98 Jennett and Plum, 1972.
 99 Plum and Posner, 1972.
100 Hartmann and Schilder, 1924.
101 Ritti, 1883.
102 Siegel, 1973.
103 Siegel, 1973.
104 Roccatagliata, 1973.
105 Siegel, 1973.
106 Ritti, 1883.
107 Barrough, 1583.
108 Bayfield, 1663.
109 Platter, 1602–1603.
110 Darwin, 1796.
111 Middleton *et al.*, *c.*1780.
112 Pinel, 1809.
113 Esquirol, 1838.
114 Esquirol, 1838.
115 Georget, 1820.
116 'The symptoms of stupidity vary according to the type of insanity affecting the individual. It is a syndrome that, like paralysis, superimposes itself upon many conditions': Ètoc-Demazy, 1833.
117 After Ètoc-Demazy, 'stupidity' named a state of unresponsiveness, accompanied by cognitive and motility disorders complicating mental or physical disease (Dagonet, 1872). His view that the symptomatology of stupor is not very helpful in predicting outcome was also influential.
118 Baillarger, 1843. The view that stupidity might be associated with oniric activity was not accepted, and some like Guislain and Morel clung to the idea that 'suspension' of function was 'pathognomonic' of stupor. Marcé and Aubanel supported Baillarger in believing that stuporous patients experienced a rich and often terrifying inner life. The debate continued in French psychiatry well into the second half of the century, as may be seen from the proceedings of the *Société Médico-Psychologique*, 1869; Dagonet, 1876; Ritti, 1883.
119 Ball, 1881.
120 Ritti, 1883.
121 Griesinger, 1861.
122 Mora, 1973; Llopis, 1954.
123 Krafft-Ebing, 1893.
124 Monro, 1856.
125 Maudsley, 1866.
126 Maudsley, 1895.
127 Newington, 1874.
128 Hoch, 1921.
129 Clouston, 1887.
130 Tuke, 1892.

131 Whitwell, 1889.
132 Savage, 1886.
133 Hollander, 1912.
134 Kraepelin, 1919.
135 Kraepelin, 1921.
136 Kraepelin, 1921.
137 The case was taken from Riklin, 1906.
138 Aprosexia meant for him impaired attention.
139 Bleuler, 1911.
140 Bleuler, 1924.
141 Strauss and Griffith, 1955.
142 Rachlin, 1935.
143 Kretschmer, 1934.
144 Ajuriaguerra, 1975; Sarró Burbano, 1960.
145 For example, cataleptic state produced by morphine in rats (Mavrojannis, 1903); bulbocapnine (Jong de, 1956); neuroleptics (Baruk *et al.*, 1958; Gelenberg and Mandel, 1977); endorphins (Bloom *et al.*, 1976); reserpine and α-methyl-*p*-tyrosine in rats and monkeys, and its antagonism by L-dopa (Bédard *et al.*, 1970; Carlsson *et al.*, 1957). Likewise, similar states may be obtained after inflicting lesions in cats in the transition between mid- and fore-brain (Ingram *et al.*, 1936); space occupying lesions in related areas in humans (Cairns *et al.*, 1941); in the residual stages of the apallic syndrome (Peters, 1977).
146 Albert, 1978.
147 Economo, 1931.
148 Hassler, 1978 was one of the earliest to describe an arousal or alerting function associated with the basal ganglia.
149 Gallup and Maser, 1977.
150 Ratner, 1967.
151 Gallup and Maser, 1977.

CHAPTER 17

Tremor, rigidity, akathisia, and stereotypy

Whilst stupor is the paradigm case for the motility disorders, parkinsonism represents the best example of symptomatology of the basal ganglia. This section explores its history both in its relationship to Parkinson's disease (PD) and to other clinical situations. The view that PD is but a collection of disorders variously sharing features such as tremor, rigidity, akinesia, and dysautonomy is becoming fashionable.[1] Since the last century, this syndrome or 'construct' has been called parkinsonism[2] and is now known to result from damage to pigmented cells in the substantia nigra and sympathetic ganglia. When the cause is unknown the syndrome is called 'idiopathic'[3] or Parkinson's disease proper; however, there is no evidence that this group – defined by exclusion – is homogeneous.[4] It could be said that PD is a prototypical construct kept alive by alternatively defining it on the basis of clinical presentation or neuropathological marker (Lewy bodies). Unfortunately, the two definitions do not match: some with the symptoms do not have Lewy bodies, many with the latter do not have the disease.

This makes PD into an interesting historical subject as it offers the possibility of separately studying the history of terms (Parkinson's disease, paralysis agitans, etc), behaviours (tremor, akinesia, rigidity), and concepts and hypotheses. It also offers an opportunity to understand the way in which during the nineteenth century diseases were taken over by medical specialisms. This is the case with PD which, in spite of its clear psychiatric component, has been firmly kept within neurology. Indeed, to maintain the status quo, such component was for a long time either denied or played down.

Paralysis and *scelotyrbe* during the eighteenth century

It would be difficult to understand the contribution of James Parkinson (after whom the disease was named by Charcot in 1862) without knowing of the medical concepts he used or reacted against. Parkinson called his disease 'shaking palsy' (*paralysis agitans*).[5] At the end of the eighteenth century, the medical meaning of 'paralysis' was very wide: Sauvages had defined it as a loss of *motion* and *sensation*[6] as had Vogel[7] and Cullen.[8] Indeed, this definition was still official teaching for medical students at the beginning of the nineteenth century.[9] By 1819, things had changed little and paralysis was still defined as 'the abolition or weakening of *sensation* and voluntary movement – or of only one of these faculties – in one part of the body.'[10] Indeed, by 1834 (long after Parkinson's death) Roche was still defining paralysis as a 'diminution or total loss of motility or *sensation*.'[11] However odd this view of paralysis might sound to modern medical ears,[12] it is the definition that Parkinson had in mind when writing on his disease.

A re-reading of Parkinson's definition

Sufficient has been published on the life of James Parkinson (1755–1824) not to need iteration here.[13] Indeed, little in his political and literary biography will help to understand his choice of words or clinical bias.[14] In a definition of 'shaking palsy' quoted *ad nauseam*, he wrote: 'Involuntary tremulous motion, with lessened muscular power, in parts not in action and even when supported; with a propensity to bend the trunk forwards, and to pass from a walking to a running pace: *the senses and intellects being uninjured*.'[15]

Two claims therein merit re-reading: ' . . . lessened muscular power' and 'the senses and intellects being uninjured'. Nineteenth century physicians interpreted 'lessened muscular power' as meaning *paresis* and this caused some debate;[16] after the 1860s, the same words were interpreted as meaning 'inability to exercise (normal) muscular power on account of rigidity.' Interestingly enough, it is likely that Parkinson actually meant *paresis*! Likewise, his second claim has been interpreted as meaning that the 'disease' was not accompanied by insanity (injured *senses*) or dementia (*intellects*).[17] Important from the psychiatric viewpoint is the question of what did Parkinson mean by 'senses'. An historical – as opposed to an anachronistic – reading of the text suggests that he meant 'sensory modalities' (i.e. functions such as vision or touch) rather than 'reason'. This would be in keeping with the logic of his medical argument, i.e. of his wanting to demonstrate that his disease was *not just another form of paralysis* (and hence involved the 'senses', as strokes often did). Parkinson believed that PD was a *different form* of paralysis characterized by tremor (*agitans*) and festination (*scelotyrbe*) but not by *sensory impairment*: 'having made the necessary inquiries respecting these two affections . . . which appear to be characteristic symptoms of the disease, it becomes necessary, in the next place, to endeavour to *distinguish this disease from others* . . .'.[18] Indeed, there was little reason (whether medical or historical) for his wanting to define a physical disease by saying: 'by the way, it is not accompanied by insanity'![19] The new reading would also tally with the fact that one of his cases, the Count of Lordat, *was in fact affected of severe mental disorder*.[20]

In regards to the word 'intellects' it is likely that Parkinson actually meant cognition, for elsewhere in his monograph he says: 'the unimpaired state of the intellects.'[21] His wanting to deny the presence of cognitive symptoms also makes sense (for the reasons giving above) for, at the time, intellectual impairment *was considered to be* part and parcel of 'paralysis'.[22] Indeed, none of the nine patients mentioned by Parkinson (mean age = 60 years) was reported as having dementia; this would make sense for a group of subjects with early onset PD and short survival (due to lack of treatment). It would also be in keeping with a suggestion that dementia only began to be reported as a complication of PD after anti-muscarinic agents were introduced as treatment during the 1850s.[23]

The right interpretation of Parkinson's claims must wait for the discovery of new evidence. It is also a pity that Parkinson never seems to have finished his monograph. Analysis of its structure suggests that it was meant to have *two parts* each dedicated to justifying one of the claims in his definition; in the event, he seems to have completed only the *first part* (i.e. Chapter 2) which dealt with tremor and festination. The *second part*, where he might have justified his claim about the 'senses and intellects', was never completed.

History of the main symptoms

Parkinson's interest in tremor and festination (to the detriment of akinesia and rigidity) poses an interesting historical problem. One obvious explanation is that his patients *did not show these signs* (indeed, of his nine cases only five seem fully to have met diagnostic criteria!); another explanation is that by the beginning of the nineteenth century, the 'conceptualization' of rigidity and akinesia had not yet been completed. This seems to be the view of Schiller, who has suggested that the separation of rigidity from 'spasms' only took place after the 1860s.[24] The same could be said of akinesia (inability to move not due to impairment of voluntary motor mechanisms) which does not seem to have been separated from paralysis until after Parkinson's monograph.[25]

On the other hand, much had been written on tremor before Parkinson's time; indeed, he used this knowledge deftly. For example, from the time of Galen it was known that there were static and dynamic tremors; during the eighteenth century, Van Swieten called the former *palpitatio* (and believed that it was a convulsive phenomenon), and the latter *tremor* (and related it to paralysis).[26] Cullen claimed that tremor was always 'symptomatic to palsy, asthenia or convulsions and therefore not be treated of by itself.'[27] Parkinson complained that 'tremor has been adopted, as a genus, by almost every nosologist; but always unmarked, in their several definitions, by such characters as would embrace this disease.'[28] He then described the natural history of tremor in his own disease: insidious onset, slight sense of weakness, fatigue, and then gradual interference with tasks such as writing and eating.[29]

Up to the middle of the nineteenth century, tremors remained in the words of Romberg: 'the bridge which conducts from the region of convulsions to the paralyses',[30] i.e. Van Swieten hypothesis was still valid. Romberg included tremors under 'neuroses of motility' and dealt with prototypical examples: mercurial tremor, tremor potatorum (alcoholic), senilis, febrilis, and paralysis agitans.[31] In 1841, Hall reintroduced the term 'paralysis agitans' and (surprisingly early) reported slight delirium and lethargy as occasional symptoms of the disease.[32] Few years later, Charcot complained that since 1817 PD had been neglected in France, and went on to demonstrate various sub-types of tremor. He also distinguished between intentional and rest tremor but acknowledged that this had been known to Galen and Van Swieten.[33] He quoted Gubler's view of tremor as being an *astasie musculaire* and attributed to Ordenstein the final separation between multiple sclerosis and PD.[34] In 1877, Jackson put forward a cerebellar hypothesis of tremor by making use of his negative–positive dichotomy, and suggested that tremor and rigidity were on a continuum.[35]

Parkinsonism and the neuroses during the nineteenth century

Until the time of Charcot and Lereboullet,[36] PD was still classified as a 'neurosis'. In practice, this meant that, as Axenfeld put it (after reviewing all available information on lesions): 'PD must provisionally remain in the class of the neuroses given that it is not characterized by an identical and constant lesion'.[37] Charcot thought likewise: 'paralysis agitans is at the moment a *névrose* in the sense that we cannot identify any characteristic lesion.'[38]

However, the notion of neuroses was changing during this period, and the specialty of neurology was being constructed out of conditions in which 'constant' focal lesions had been identified as responsible for motor and sensory symptoms. The rest of diseases with motor or sensory symptoms remained classified as 'neuroses' (see list in Axenfeld, 1883). In the event, physiology offered a partial solution by re-defining 'lesion' in 'functional' terms, i.e. giving up the idea that there always had to be structural damage. This change allowed PD (as it did epilepsy) to be incorporated into neurology *without needing to have a 'constant' anatomical lesion*.

Early neuropathology and aetiology

But research into the brain pathology of PD continued. For example, Meynert suggested that it might be associated with a disorder of the basal ganglia.[39] In 1893, Blocq and Marinesco reported a case of unilateral parkinsonism with destruction of Substantia Nigra by a tuberculoma.[40] Based on this and other pathological findings Brissaud favoured the *Locus Niger*.[41] Then, Lewy reported the first important series (60 cases) showing lesions in Striatum and Globus Pallidus and inclusion bodies which have since carried his name.[42] In 1919, Tretiakoff described three cases of encephalitis lethargica showing inflammatory lesions in the Substantia Nigra.[43] Gringer found pallidal necrosis in a subject with a combination of parkinsonian and catatonic features who had attempted suicide with carbon monoxide.[44] Following Critchley's 1929 paper, Keschner and Sloane described lesions of Substantia Nigra in association with arteriosclerotic parkinsonism.[45] The more recent history of PD is beyond the scope of this chapter.[46]

No definite views on aetiology were expressed during this earlier period, but psychological causes such as emotional shock and excessive bodily fatigue featured prominently, together with physical factors such as exposure to cold and wet, and wounds and injuries involving peripheral nerves.[47]

Psychiatry and parkinsonism

A crucial question is why did it take so long for psychiatric symptoms to be accepted as part of PD? There may be various reasons for this: one, that *ab initio* patients did not live for long enough to show them; other, that everyone followed Parkinson's injunction and refused to accept that when present, psychiatric symptoms were actually part of the disease; yet another, that there were theoretical reasons for such refusal.[48] Be that as it may, it was only during the twentieth century that it was fully accepted that PD may be accompanied by personality changes, insanity, depression, and cognitive impairment.

BENJAMIN BALL In 1881, Benjamin Ball[49] read a paper *On the relations between insanity and Paralysis agitans* before the Mental Disease Section of the International Medical Congress in London.[50] Therein, he stated: 'Few reports have been published concerning the psychological implications of Parkinson's disease and psychosis has not been one of them.'[51] He reported a case taken from the literature who had developed hallucinations following treatment with potassium bromide[52] and another two with irritability and depression.[53] He disagreed with the view that the association was coincidental: 'I think otherwise; a large number of Parkinsonian patients present psychological disorders extending from simple irritability to psychosis; far from being an exception I would say that a slight degree of cognitive impairment (*perturbation intellectuelle*) is the rule.'[54]

The ensuing debate illustrates the empirical attitude characteristic of British medicine at the time. Bucknill enjoined that only statistical evidence could substantiate the association, and Tuke that Ball's cases were just Kahlbaumian catatonias[55] accompanied by severe motor disturbance![56] Others supported Ball indirectly by reporting cases of their own; for example, Huggard described a patient with PD and recurrent mania (Ball was to include it in his paper of 1882) and Atkins another with hallucinations.[57] Mercier sided with Ball and made the important observation that the motor disorder of PD might often conceal the psychological disorder. In his summing up, Ball exhorted the audience to report new cases.

His request did not go unheeded. Parant described a case with nocturnal delusions, and another with sensory changes that induced the patient to believe that his extremities were larger than normal.[58] He considered as exaggerated Ball's claim that psychiatric disorders were the rule rather than the exception, and suggested that a causal link (mediated by the cortex) existed between the neurological and psychological manifestations of PD.[59] This view reveals that alienists dissociated themselves earlier enough from the 'spinal theory' of PD (popular at the time) in order to make plausible claims about the 'psychiatric' dimension to the disease (which most sited on the cortex).

REGIS The debate continued, and Régis identified two opposing views. According to some such as Parkinson himself, Charcot, Brissaud and others, the association between psychiatric symptoms and PD was irrelevant; according to others such as Ball, Parant, Régis, Luys, Roger, and Bechet, the symptoms were part of the disease.[60] Régis distinguished two types of psychological symptoms in PD: 'Elementary psychological disturbances and delusional or psychotic states.'[61] The former comprised mood disorder, intellectual apathy, hypersensitivity, irritability, asthenia, torpidity, lethargy, nightmares, and deterioration of mental functions; the latter 'depression with delusions of ruin, guilt, hypochondria and suicidal ideation . . . [the patients] exhibit a dissociation between their subjective experience of illness and its expression [that is] Pierret's paramimia.'[62] Occasionally, dementia, confusion, oniric states[63] and nocturnal hallucinosis could be found. Régis did not consider the possibility that some symptoms might result from intoxication with *hyoscyamus* or *atropine*, drugs prescribed for Parkinson's disease during this period.[64] Dutil supported the view that mental symptoms were important in PD, but rejected an explanation based on 'degeneration' theory on the grounds that patients improved from their delusions.[65]

Similar findings were reported elsewhere. In a review of the subject, König reported five female patients showing irritability, hypochondria, depression, and short-lived psychotic states characterized by paranoid hallucinatory and melancholic features and suicidal ruminations.[66] In a series of 282 patients, Mjönes described up to 40 per cent with 'reactive' or 'organic' psychopathology including neurotic and affective disorders, depressive illness, schizophrenia-like psychosis, and confusional states.[67]

The 'reactivity' hypothesis

Not everyone agreed with the view that mental symptoms were frequent or indeed part of the disease, and (particularly neurologists) supported a 'reactive' mechanism. Gowers, for example, wrote: 'The intellect may be unaffected throughout, except by the irritability which usually accompanies the physical restlessness, or by mental depression, which is chiefly the *natural result of the physical ailment*.'[68] Many years later, Wilson repeated this without paying any attention to the work done in the interim!: 'mental symptoms are mostly limited to depression and irritability, the *natural outcome, perhaps, of an incurable disease*, anything beyond these is to be ascribed to accompanying arteriosclerosis or some incidental condition . . . on the intellectual side there may be noted some bradyphrenia or slowness of thought yet it is probably *more apparent than real*.'[69]

Vulpian was equally simplistic: 'Intelligence remains unchanged to the very end, likewise it can be ascertained that there is no thought disorder, delusions or hallucinations.'[70] Brissaud also claimed that patients keep their intellect to the very end but made an interesting point, namely, that they become 'selfish in their approach to life, only taking but not giving' to the point that carers get eventually fed up; when this happens the patient sulks, feels abandoned, and can become paranoid (*délire de la suspicion*).'[71]

Other French neurologists, however, were more open and included mental symptoms in their description. For example, Charcot himself wrote that 'at a given moment, intellect becomes blurred and memory is lost';[72] and Marchand that: 'patients frequently present irritability, affective disorder and cognitive impairment.'[73] Claude was even more explicit, and quoted the work of Ball and Parant.[74] Thus, the 1881 London meeting seemed to have encouraged the view that psychiatric symptoms were part of PD. Further support accrued from the kaleidoscopic nature of cases with parkinsonism and mental disorder seen in the wake of the encephalitis lethargica epidemic of the late 1910s.[75]

Parkinsonism and encephalitis lethargica

The association between parkinsonian and mental symptoms observed in the post-encephalitic state led to a revision of views on both the nature of mental symptoms and of motor disorders in psychiatry. Von Economo believed that 'delusional ideas might have to be given a lesser role' in diagnosis.[76] Post-encephalitic states often showed rigidity without tremor, akinesia, compulsive behaviour, akathisia, blepharospasm, tics, torticollis, oculogyric crisis, attacks of hyper-apnoea with forced expiration, seborrhoea, sialorrhoea, distrophia adiposo genitalis, disturbance in temperature control, and psychic torpor. Some of these features had not been described before in relation to parkinsonism. Similar symptoms were later on reported in patients taking neuroleptic medication.[77]

The epidemic of encephalitis lethargica that occurred at the end of the First World War was not a new phenomenon.[78] An epidemic of *nona* had taken place in Northern Italy towards the end of the nineteenth century[79] and Von Economo believed it to be similar to the one he named in 1917. A decade after the Italian epidemic, Kleist reported cases 'with psychosis and delirium, slight fever and hyperkinesis, which in turn passed into a state of akinetic parkinsonian rigidity.'[80] It is also of interest to notice that the second case reported by Ball in 1882 was that of a 32 year-old Italian with akinesia, dysarthria, and peripheral vasomotor disturbance.[81]

It would seem, however, that the epidemic of 1917–1921 caused far more post-encephalitic cases than earlier ones.[82] Indeed, it has been suggested that the increased incidence of parkinsonism observed after the First World War resulted from subclinical infections acquired during this period.[83] This conclusion and the assumptions upon which it was based were later challenged on both statistical[84] and clinical[85] grounds. It has also been claimed that symptoms apparently pathognomonic of post-encephalitic parkinsonism can be present in the idiopathic and so-called arteriosclerotic types. This notwithstanding, the distinctive psychiatric sequelae are still used to characterize the post-encephalitic form.[86] Earlier beliefs that post-encephalitic parkinsonism was associated with lesions predominantly in Substantia Nigra whilst the idiopathic form resulted from striatal impairment have been now replaced by a unitary view.[87]

Bradyphrenia and arteriosclerotic parkinsonism

In 1929, MacDonald Critchley published a classical paper on *arteriosclerotic parkinsonism*. parkinsonism he defined as a 'symptomatic variety of paralysis agitans'.[88] Critchley claimed that there was no major clinical difference between the idiopathic and arteriosclerotic varieties, and on this he sought the support of Souques[89] and Foix and Nicolesco[90] who also believed that the important aspect of PD was not the cause but the site of the lesion. Critchley concluded that an arteriosclerotic insult to the basal ganglia would cause the same syndrome but also observed that *incomplete* forms were common such as immobility of expression, short-stepping gait, and cerebello-pallidal syndromes. Akinesia was particularly common but tremor was rare; onset was often sudden and age of onset late. There were cases associated with marked intellectual impairment. During the 1960s, when the reaction came against all 'arteriosclerotic' states, some writers called Critchley's syndrome into question.[91]

The paper also drew attention to *bradyphrenia* and *bradykinesia*, phenomena until then only studied by French neuropsychiatrists. Bradyphrenia had been described in 1922 by F. Naville to refer to a specific type of mental slowness with impaired initiative but normal praxia, memory and cognition seen in post-encephalitic states. The author suggested that bradyphrenia ought to be differentiated from dementia praecox, dementia, and brain damage.[92] Critchley himself defined bradyphrenia as 'a failure in mental elasticity' and called it 'mental viscosity.'[93] The concept of *bradykinésie*, in turn, had been proposed by Rene Cruchet in 1921[94] to refer to 'states of slowness in the starting and execution of voluntary actions without there being either paralysis or trouble with coordination',[95] also found in post-encephalitic patients. Both states have returned to fashion in current neuropsychiatry in respect to so-called sub-cortical dementia and to other clinical phenomena assumed to reflect frontal lobe involvement.

The Parkinsonian personality

During the 1920s and 1930s, psychosomatic medicine enjoyed a period of popularity, and some suggested that PD might be caused by psychological factors. For example, Jelliffe considered oculogyric crisis (then described associated with post-encephalitic parkinsonism) to be a substitutive action, i.e. a 'looking away' from a threatening reality.[96] This was challenged by Kubie[97] and a debate ensued.[98] Jelliffe also believed that post-encephalitic compulsive respiratory disorders resulted from a neurotic defect[99] and that rigidity reflected unconscious hostility.[100]

As late as the early 1940s, Sands suggested that states of chronic emotional tension might render subjects prone to PD,[101] and Schwab *et al.* stated that chronic anxiety might cause irreversible neuronal change.[102] Booth characterized PD patients as showing 'urge towards action, industriousness and motor activity, striving for independence, authority, and success within a rigid, usually moralistic behaviour pattern ... the symptoms appear when the personality attitude cannot be carried on successfully';[103] the author based his views on a sample of 66 uncontrolled PD patients (of varied aetiology) and studied by means of the Rorschach Test.

Parkinsonism and the neuroses

The study of this association was only possible after PD ceased to be considered as a 'neurosis' in the old sense of the term, and the 'five' current neuroses had been established. Mjönes reported that many of his cases showed 'psychoneurosis' and psychogenic mental depression.[104] Anxiety, depression, hypochondriacal preoccupations, and dysphoria have also been reported following surgery for PD.[105] Sensory symptoms such as formication[106] and temperature changes[107] may, however, lead to pseudo-hypochondriacal complaints.

Obsessive–compulsive symptoms featured prominently among the sequelae of encephalitis lethargica. Von Economo observed compulsive behaviour and ruminations[108] and Mayer Gross and Steiner reported similar symptoms during the acute stage.[109] Schilder suggested that the disease 'liberated motor impulses' but only one of his seven cases presented with a 'marked degree of akinesis and paralysis agitans posture.'[110] Grimshaw reported three additional encephalitic cases with obsessional features in support of an organic theory of obsessional symptoms and observed that German authors had often 'found symptoms similar to obsessions in post-encephalitic Parkinsonism.'[111]

Affective disorder and parkinsonism

Ball wrote: 'The psychiatric complication takes the form of depression. Frequently, it constitutes a real lypemania[112] accompanied by suicidal behaviour, hallucinations, and stupor.'[113] Régis iterated this view: 'Patients first show depressive features, sadness, painful resignation and intellectual apathy; then they develop melancholic psychosis with delusions of ruin, guilt, hypochondria and suicide.'[114] Five female PD patients reported by König also suffered from severe depression and showed hypochondriacal and paranoid features.[115] In a study of 201 cases of post-encephalitic parkinsonism, Neal found 17 cases with depression and 8 with hypomania.[116] Indeed, hypomania had been reported earlier[117] but was believed to be uncommon.[118]

As has been mentioned above, the early British neurological literature considered affective disorder to be an 'understandable' response to the motor disability. It is, therefore, important to know whether throughout the history of PD authors have ascertained whether the intensity of the depression was proportional to duration or severity of illness. Mjönes, for example, found that depression was out of proportion with the neurological deficit.[119] More recently, it has been suggested that depression only develops in vulnerable personalities and bears no relation to illness severity.[120] The debate has continued but its analysis would bring us perilously near to the present.

Schizophrenia and parkinsonism

Since the 1880s, insanity (characterized by delusions and hallucinations) has been considered as an occasional feature of PD. The finding that encephalitis lethargica was occasionally accompanied by a schizophrenia-like state reinforced this view. However, analysis of the early literature shows that the visual hallucinations reported by some PD cases occurred in the presence of clouding of consciousness and, therefore, might have been due to anticholinergic toxicity.[121] When symptoms actually occurred in clear consciousness, the question arises as to whether these were schizophrenia-like states.

Be that as it may, these reports are not common. Patrick and Levy found none in a series of 146 cases;[122] in 282 patients, Mjönes only found 2.1% with 'schizophrenic' symptoms;[123] and Hollister and Glazener reported 8 cases of schizoprenialike illness (some antedating the onset of Parkinson's disease) among 36 hospital cases of PD subjects collected in a period of ten years.[124] Unfortunately, some of these latter patients had been receiving maintenance neuroleptics for their chronic schizophrenia, so that the diagnosis of PD is not safe.

Most schizophrenic symptoms (from hallucinatory states to delusional, psychomotor, and personality deterioration) have been reported in post-encephalitic states.[125] For example, paranoid-hallucinatory states may be as frequent as 20%.[126] In this regard, two important reviewers have concluded: 'schizophrenia-like psychoses have long been accepted as sequelae of encephalitis lethargica, but no firm data on their actual incidence have been located; *Parkinsonism is commonly associated with the psychosis*; opinion is divided on the degree of resemblance of the psychosis to schizophrenia; and there is no good evidence of personality or genetic predisposition to schizophrenia in patients with post-encephalitis psychoses.'[127]

Doubts have also been voiced elsewhere as to the genuineness of such schizophrenic states. For example, Schilder believed that psychotic states with insight and without personality splitting did not constitute schizophrenia.[128] The diagnostic use of complex categories such as insight and splitting, however, is unwarranted in this context. In regard to this debate, Von Economo commented: 'Many psychiatrists are of the opinion that the main difference between schizophrenia and these post-encephalitic states is the fact that the disturbance of motility and psycho-motorium in the former are caused *secondarily*, i.e. they are purely psychological and based on delusions, whereas in post-encephalitic process the primary cause rests in anatomical lesion of the basal ganglia.'[129] 'The question may be asked whether after our experience with encephalitis lethargica this position should not be revised ... The old, but not antiquated, conception of Meynert, that in these forms of dementia praecox not only the cerebral cortex but also the deep grey masses of the brain-stem are affected, may have to be adopted and adapted, with the conclusion that these disturbances of motility and changes in personality and character are primarily caused by specific anatomical alterations.'[130]

At least one recent author has sided with this view and claimed that schizophrenia is an epiphenomenon of encephalitis lethargica.[131] After explaining that catatonic symptoms, 'before they made neurological sense in the wake of lethargic encephalitis, were endowed with psychological meaning and regarded as physical expression of an abnormal mental or emotional state'[132] the late Richard Hunter concluded: 'the concept of psychosis or schizophrenia is a historical accident. The abnormal mental state is not the illness, nor even its essence or determinant, but an epiphenomenon. Had the epidemic of encephalitis broken out only ten years earlier, or had its manifestations in endemic form been recognized for what they were, psychiatry would look very different today.'[133] Hunter also reported that a study of long-stay mental hospital patients labelled 'schizophrenic' confirmed that some 60–70% had motor signs corresponding to an extrapyramidal disorder.[134]

Unfortunately for his hypothesis, outbreaks of encephalitis had already occurred, as mentioned above, before 1917. This fact, however, should not obscure Hunter's central point, namely, that psychology alone is not sufficient to explain the motor disturbance of catatonia.[135] Indeed, combinations of catatonia and parkinsonism have been reported,[136] perhaps reflecting a common sub-stratum.

Witold Aubrun

Given the currency of the view that cognitive impairment is common in both early and late onset PD, the historian must ask why this complication was not observed earlier in the history of the disease. As mentioned above, one reason might have been that subjects died too early to show dementia; other that the (untreated) physical manifestations of the disease masked mental changes; another that dementia, when present, was considered to be a manifestation of senility; yet another that treatments have been a factor in the presentation of dementia; and a final reason might be that current instruments for measuring cognition are more sensitive than earlier ones.

Be that as it may, it is only during the early 1860s that Charcot reported blurring of intellect and loss of memory; this is of some interest for it historically coincides with the early usage of anti-muscarinic agents.[137] For the rest of the century, most writers, including neurologists, only refer to intellectual weakness during the *terminal stage* of the illness (and one wonders how often patients were by then already in delirium). No psychometric studies of the phenomenon seem to have been carried out until after the First World War. The reason for this was not necessarily the lack of instruments or psychometric methodology for both were available by the 1910s.[138]

Under the supervision of Piéron and Guillain (of Guillain–Barré syndrome fame), Witold Aubrun completed his doctoral thesis on the cognitive state of parkinsonians in 1937.[139] This work is interesting on two accounts: first, it is one of the earliest experimental studies of cognitive functions in PD, and secondly, it makes use of 'normed' psychometric instruments. Although by current standards the work is flawed, it was none the less pathbreaking. The first innovation was its use of entry criteria for patient selection; the second was the exclusion of elderly subjects to avoid contaminating the sample with dementias of other origin; the third was the use of a structured interview and protocol including questions on perception, state of consciousness, cognitive function, attention, remote memory, and recent memory (Ziehen's test, a form of paired learning), orientation, praxia, mood, personality, and sleep. Finally, physical examination and blood tests were also carried out.

A full psychological assessment of all 20 patients was also performed by means of Piéron's 'Psychological battery for professional orientation' which included 11 sections, and for which French norms existed. On the basis of the wealth of data obtained, the author concluded that parkinsonian patients *were cognitively impaired.* Unfortunately, he did not use inferential statistics to prove his points.[140]

Other movement disorders

In addition to the movement disorders explored above, psychiatric patients may also exhibit tics, spasmodic torticollis, blepharospasm, writer's cramp, oculogyric crisis, akathisia, restless legs, headbanging, punding, stereotypies, posturing, agitation, mannerisms, etc. In general, these signs are no longer considered as expressing a disorder in a 'unitary brain function'. For example, the tics of Tourette syndrome are considered as part of a stable cluster of signs and symptoms; spasmodic torticollis, blepharospasm, and writer's cramp are regarded as *formes frustres* of torsion dystonia.[141] Akathisia and oculo-gyric crisis are blamed on neuroleptics, although there is good historical evidence that both movement disorders were described before these drugs became available.[142] Restless legs and headbanging are now classified as primary sleep disorders although their mechanism remains mysterious. Punding is seen in chronic amphetamine abuse. Stereotypies, posturing, agitation, and mannerisms, on the other hand, still remain on the borderlines between neurology and psychiatry. This section will only deal with such 'movement' disorders as have been touched upon in the psychiatric literature.

Akathisia is a good example of this. Whilst the word and concept were created around 1900, the actual clinical phenomenon had been noticed before. Thus Trousseau reported the case of one of the chamberlains of Napoleon III who suffered from

severe restlessless of the legs and when in court (and even in the presence of the
emperor) had to walk around every few minutes.[143] On 7th November 1901, Dr
Lad Haskovec, a neuropsychiatrist from Prague, reported to the *Société de Neurologie*
of Paris two cases. One was that of a 40 year-old man who for the last three weeks
had complained of 'generalized tremor and inability to rest'. He also 'felt vertigo,
weakness, leg shaking and the fear that he might fall any time', and needed to
change position every few minutes; his neurological examination was basically
normal. The second case was a man of 54 with episodic restlessness, shaking, and
inability to stay quiet. Haskovec compared their clinical state to the motor phenomena of neurasthenia, astasia–abasia, and 'l'atrémie'. He then suggested that the
new term *akathisie* (formed by the privative α̅ and καθίζω – to be made to sit down)
was used to name what he considered to be a functional and transitory disorder
that resulted from cortical or sub-cortical over-excitation.[144]

In 1903, Haskovec returned to the topic to acknowledge that Raymond and
Janet had described the further case of Rul, a 42 year-old man with similar symptoms; the authors had not agreed with Haskovec's explanation of the syndrome but
were willing to 'adopt the term akathisia'.[145] Haskovec replied that whilst his case
was an expression of a movement disorder (*lésion motrice primaire*), that of Reymond
and Janet belonged to the class of emotional symptoms (*appartient á la sphère
emotive*).[146] In 1923, Sicard introduced the term *tasikinesia* to refer to patients who
cannot stop moving.[147] In 1923, Robert Bing, the great neurologist from Basle,
utilized the term *akathisia* to name a sign in some parkinsonian patients who
'cannot remain still ... they stretch and move their legs about restlessly'.[148] In
1968, Delay and Deniker proposed a further distinction: 'longer lasting hyperkin-
esias may consist of akathisia (inability to remain lying down) and tasikinesia
(tendency to continue moving)'.[149] In 1960, Winkelman attempted to bring
together these two contradictory aspects of akathisia.[150] The clinical and aetiological aspects of akathisia have not yet been clarified.[151]

Another important psychiatric disorder of motility concerns the so-called stereotypies which refer to 'repetitive behaviours such as verbal expression, gestures or
attitudes'[152] which seem to occur automatically and are not adaptive in relation to
the ongoing psychosocial frame. Falret coined the term in the 1860s: ' these
patients ... repeat exactly in form and expression the same idea, in other words,
their delusion is completely *stereotyped*' (my italics).[153] Ten years later, Kalhbaum
used the same word to refer to repetitive behaviours in catatonia:[154] 'Notable are
also the bizarre stereotyped movements observed in large asylums: one patient will
grasp his nose every few minutes, another rotate his arms around his head . . .'[155]
Lagriffe, then took up the term to name some of the movement disorders in
dementia praecox and suggested that 'stereotyped gestures are different from stereotyped attitudes in that they are not only seen in catatonia.'[156] In his great 1916
book (based on his doctoral thesis), Abely took the concept further by suggesting
that the term stereotypy named multiple phenomena which were not necessarily

pathological; some started life as 'intentional movements' and only become automatic later on.[157] Kraepelin used the term in a narrow sense: 'we almost always meet in the train of thought of the patients indications of stereotypy, of the persistence of single ideas. If the patient continues talking, the same ideas and expressions usually turn up again and again from time to time. Occasionally, the persistence gets the mastery of the train of thought to such an extent that the patients for weeks and months always move in the same monotonous sphere of ideas, and cannot be brought out by any means'.[158]

Kraepelin's concept of stereotypy was nearer Falret's than Kahlbaum's. Whilst in the former writers the central issue is a repetitive idea or delusion governing behaviour, Kahlbaum considers stereotypies as a motor disorder. When it developed, the psychoanalytical view was also ideational in that it emphasized the 'auto-erotic' aspects of negativism and the stereotypies.[159] By 1936, when Paul Guiraud wrote his masterly paper, there were, therefore, three theoretical approaches to the disorder.[160] According to the first, stereotypies were (like tics or tremors) only motor phenomena whose understanding did not require the presence of a voluntary act or a sematic content. The second theory, as represented by Falret, Abely and Kraepelin, proposed that stereotypies were ideational in nature, i.e. *ab initio* were the expression of a mental image, even if later on they became fully automatic; writers supporting this psychiatric view tended to reserve the term for the phenomena seen in dementia praecox. The third approach (attributed to Bleuler,[161] Minkowski[162] and Kläsi[163]), Guiraud called: 'theory of autistic thinking'; according to this view, stereotypies are phenomena which occur in a particular semantic space and have little to do with reality or the rest of the mental life. Guiraud himself concluded that there was little point in using the term for a wide variety of repetitive disorders and that to have clinical use its meaning needed to be narrowed down to refer only to phenomena with fixed course and exact repetition. The former (wide meaning) were seen in hebephrenia, chronic schizophrenia, and Pick's disease; the latter in catatonia, Alzheimer's disease, and post-encephalitic states.[164] Little has been advanced on our knowledge of stereotypies since.[165]

Summary

This chapter has mainly dealt with the history of parkinsonism and its relationship to mental symptoms. It has shown that Parkinson's purported claim that there were no mental symptoms in the disease can be interpreted in various ways. It has also shown how this misinterpretation was used by some to play down the importance of depression, personality disorders and dementia in PD. The relevance of the work of Ball, Parant, Régis and others to the development of the psychiatry of PD has been emphasized. A separate analysis has been carried out of the historical development of specific mental disorders as has of the contribution of encephalitis lethargica, arteriosclerotic parkinsonism, bradykinesia, bradyphrenia, and anti-muscarinic medication. Then a history of akathisia and stereotypies was presented.

NOTES

1 Editorial. On Parkinson's disease, 1992.
2 Duvoisin, 1987.
3 The problem with negative definitions or definitions by exclusion (of which 'idiopathic' is a good example) is that they depend on the sensitivity and power of current and future tests, i.e. the more refined the detection procedure, the smaller the 'idiopathic' group.
4 Parkinsonism may be caused by toxic, vascular, immunological, and tumoural factors and by neuroleptic drugs (see Schwab and England, 1968).
5 For an excellent discussion of Parkinson's monograph and its intellectual context, see Morris, 1989.
6 *Motus aut tactus, vel utriusque, in uno tantum artu debilitas*, p. 23, para 169, in Cullen, 1803.
7 *Sensus motusve aut utriusque defectus in singulari parte externa* p. 91, para 126, Cullen, 1803.
8 *Motus voluntarii nonnulli tantum imminuti, saepe cum sopore* p. 284, para 43, Cullen, 1803.
9 For example, the Edinburgh vade-mecum read: paralysis is 'a sudden loss of tone and vital power in a certain part of the body' . . . 'in the slighter forms of the disease, it only affects a particular muscle' 'in the higher degrees of the disease the paralytic affection is diffused over a whole limb . . . and sometimes it affects a whole side of the body, in which case it is called hemiplegia' . . . 'Sometimes there occurs a total loss of sense while motion is entire' . . .' p. 335 in Vademecum of the London Hospitals, 1803.
10 Chamberet, 1819.
11 Roche, 1834.
12 The explanation for this wide definition is that 'paralysis' was then used as a clinical (*pars per toto*) generalization of the symptoms of apoplexy and hence both loss of motor and sensory function had to be included. Evidence for this view can be found in Middleton's Dictionary: 'palsy in medicine is a disease wherein the body, or some of its members, lose their motion, and sometimes their sensation of feeling. This disease is never acute, is often tedious, and in old people, almost incurable; and the patient for the most part drags a miserable life. For the vigour of his mind, together with his memory, are lost or vastly impaired; he totters and shakes, and becomes a dismal sight; as if no longer a man, but an animal half dead' (Middleton *et al.*, 1780).
13 Critchley, 1955; Tyler and Tyler, 1986.
14 Parkinson, 1817.
15 p. 1, Parkinson, 1817.

16 Bourneville, the editor of Charcot's *Leçons*, tells (Appendix II, Vol. 1,
     p. 394 Charcot, Oeuvres, 1886) that in the lecture of 19th November
     1876, Charcot criticized the term 'paralysis' as inappropiate on the basis
     that muscle power was well preserved, and suggested *Maladie de Parkinson*
     instead. Charcot confirmed this in a letter to a Dr. Nunn dated 5th May
     1884 (Critchley, 1955). Not everyone agreed. For example, William
     Gowers believed that paralysis agitans was adequate and that there was
     no need to use an eponym
     (p. 636, Gowers, 1893).
17 p. 654, Jelliffe and White, 1929.
18 p. 27, Parkinson, 1817.
19 Parkinson had clinical experience with mental illness. For years, he was
     the visiting physician to the Hoxton madhouse and would not have
     hesitated to use the word 'insanity' (rather than the more ambiguous one
     uninjured senses); Morris, *The Madhouse Doctor*, 1989.
20 'A more *melancholy object* I never beheld. The patient, naturally a
     handsome, middle-sized, sanguine man, of cheerful disposition, an active
     mind, appeared much emaciated, stooping and *dejected*', (my italics) (p.
     40), Parkinson, 1817.
21 p. 45, Parkinson, 1817.
22 p. 251, Chamberet, 1819; Middleton *et al.*, 1780.
23 Anti-muscarinic treatment may have prolonged life, thus allowing the
     dementia to appear, or more likely to have caused itself the cognitive
     impairment (Miller *et al.*, 1987).
24 Schiller, 1986; for a general historical account of involuntary movement,
     see Barbeau, 1958.
25 Ajuriaguerra, 1975.
26 p. 61, Demange, 1887.
27 p. 338 in Vademecum of the London Hospitals, 1803; Latin definition in
     p. 286, Cullen, 1803.
28 p. 2, Parkinson, 1817.
29 pp. 3–7, Parkinson, 1817.
30 p. 230, Romberg, 1853.
31 pp. 231–235, Romberg, 1853.
32 Hall, 1841.
33 pp. 158–160, Charcot, 1886.
34 Charcot was referring here to the work of his protégée, Ordenstein, 1868.
     In a footnote, however, Charcot felt forced to accept that it had not been
     Ordenstein, after all, who had first proposed the difference between the
     two conditions: 'Cohn, nonetheless, had already noticed that in two cases
     with multiple plaques in brain and spinal cord, tremor only appeared
     when the patients wanted to carry out a movement but never during rest
     or sleep' (p. 161, Charcot, 1886).
35 '1. in health the cerebellar influx is fully antagonised; in 2. the early
     stages of paralysis agitans it is intermittently antagonised – the movement
     constituting each single tremor occurring betwixt the cerebral impulses; in
     3. the late stages it is not antagonized at all, and there is such a stream of

cerebellar impulses that rigidity occurs. We have cerebral paresis with cerebellar tremor; later, cerebral paralysis with cerebellar rigidity'; (p. 454 in Jackson, 1932).

36 Lereboullet and Bussard, 1884.

37 p. 699, Axenfeld, 1883.

38 pp. 161–162, Charcot, 1886.

39 Meynert, 1871. For a superb history of the basal ganglia, see Schiller, 1967.

40 Blocq and Marinesco, 1893.

41 Brissaud, 1899.

42 Lewy, 1913; also the charming historical account Lewy wrote when visiting Pennsylvania for the 1940 Meeting of the *Association for Research in Nervous and Mental Disease:* Lewy, 1942.

43 Tretiakoff, 1919.

44 Gringer, 1926.

45 Keschner and Sloane, 1931.

46 For this, see pp. 176–187, Rose, 1989.

47 Bristowe, 1894; Lereboullet and Bussard, 1884.

48 For example, Axenfeld felt that the lesions 'should be in the spinal cord' (p. 699, Axenfeld, 1883). Thus, insanity could not be part of a disease which did not affect the brain.

49 Benjamin Ball (1834–1893) was of British extraction, and the first incumbent to the chair of Mental Diseases (1877) at Sainte-Anne, the famous French psychiatric establishment.

50 Report. Mental Diseases Section, 1881.

51 p. 23, Ball, 1882.

52 The case had been published by Althaus in 1870 (quoted in Ball, 1882).

53 Published by Nichol in 1875 (quoted in Ball, 1882).

54 p. 24, Ball, 1882.

55 For an analysis of Kahlbaum's catatonias, see Chapter 16, this book.

56 Report, Mental Disease Section, 1881.

57 The case was published by Atkins, 1882.

58 Parant, 1883.

59 Parant, 1892.

60 Régis, 1906.

61 p. 784, Régis, 1906.

62 p. 785, Régis, 1906. *Paramimia* is defined as a lack of congruence between ideas and gestures, pp. 194–211, Dromard, 1909. Pierret led a group of French neuropsychiatrists interested in the analysis of facial expression in both neurological and psychiatric disease (for details, see pp. 116–118, Régis, 1906).

63 The 'oniric' state was an important descriptive and explanatory concept in French psychiatry. It referred to hallucinatory and other 'automatic' behaviours resulting from the breakthrough of dream activity during wakefulness (Chapter 3, this book).

64 See, for example, Marchand, 1909.

65 p. 875, Dutil, 1903.

66 König, 1912.
67 p. 73, Mjönes, 1949.
68 p. 648, Gowers, 1893.
69 pp. 933, Wilson, 1954.
70 p. 657, Vulpian, 1886.
71 p. 489, Brissaud, 1893.
72 p. 179, Charcot, 1886.
73 p. 493, Marchand, 1909.
74 p. 603, Claude, 1922.
75 Economo, 1931; also Leader, Encephalitis lethargica, 1981.
76 p. 162, Economo, 1931.
77 Delay and Deniker, 1968; Petit *et al.*, 1979.
78 Economo, 1931.
79 Editorial. La nona, 1890.
80 p. 8, Economo, 1931.
81 Ball, 1882.
82 p. 154, Brill, 1974.
83 Poskanzer and Schwab, 1963.
84 Selby, 1968; Pallis, 1971.
85 Martin *et al.*, 1973.
86 Leader, 1981.
87 Denny-Brown, 1962; Adams and Victor, 1977.
88 p. 23, Critchley, 1929.
89 Souques, 1921.
90 Foix and Nicolesco, 1925.
91 Eadie and Sutherland, 1964; Pallis, 1971.
92 Naville, 1922.
93 pp. 50–51, Critchley, 1929.
94 p. 7, Verger and Cruchet, 1925.
95 p. 19, Verger and Cruchet, 1925.
96 p. 215, Jelliffe, 1932.
97 Kubie, 1933.
98 Jelliffe, 1935.
99 Jelliffe, 1926.
100 Jelliffe, 1940.
101 Sands, 1942.
102 Schwab *et al.*, 1951.
103 Booth, 1948.
104 Mjönes, 1949.
105 Asso *et al.*, 1969.
106 Formication refers to tactile hallucinations of ants crawling under the skin (Berrios, On Tactile hallucinations, 1982.)
107 Snider *et al.*, 1976.
108 Economo, 1931.
109 Mayer-Gross, 1921.
110 Schilder, 1929.
111 p. 229, Grimshaw, 1964.

112 Lypemania was a term coined by Esquirol to refer to depression, (Chapter 12, this book).
113 p. 31, Ball, 1882.
114 p. 785, Régis, 1906.
115 König, 1912.
116 Neal, 1942.
117 Report, 1881.
118 Souques, 1921.
119 Mjönes, 1949.
120 Warburton, 1967.
121 Warnes, 1967; Johnson *et al.*, 1981.
122 Patrick and Levy, 1922.
123 Mjönes, 1949.
124 Hollister and Glazener, 1961.
125 Dimitz and Schilder, 1921; McCowan and Cook, 1928; Economo, 1931.
126 Steck, 1926, 1931; Hall, 1929.
127 pp. 131–132, Davison and Bagley, 1969.
128 Schilder, 1929.
129 p. 132, Economo, 1931.
130 It could not have been put more succinctly and foresightedly; p. 162, Economo, 1931.
131 Hunter, 1973.
132 p. 363, Hunter, 1973.
133 p. 364, Hunter, 1973.
134 Jones and Hunter, 1969.
135 Ajuriaguerra, 1975; Berrios, On Stupor revisited, 1981; Saß, 1981.
136 Bromsberg, 1930; Farran-Ridge, 1926.
137 Bourgeot, 1926.
138 See chapter 7, this book, for information on the influence of the work of Binet and Simon, Jaspers, Toulouse and others.
139 Aubrun, 1937; this author also wrote a paper on emotional reactions in PD subjects: Aubrun, 1937.
140 It must be admitted, however, that statistical analysis of Aubrun's data is not easy on account of the excessive number of variables, the small size of the sample, frequent missing data, and absence of controls. Re-analysis proved particularly difficult for the present author for Aubrun reported no raw scores or measures of dispersion.
141 Lees, 1985.
142 For a superb study of oculogyric crisis, see Jelliffe, 1932.
143 p. 139, Bing, 1925.
144 Haskovec, 1901.
145 p. 76, Vol. 2, Janet, Les obsessions. . . 1919.
146 Haskovec, 1903.
147 Sicard, 1923.
148 Bing, 1923.
149 p. 253, Delay and Deniker, 1968.
150 Winkelman, 1960.

151 Gibb and Lees, 1986; Sachdev, 1994.

152 p. 538, Postel, 1993.

153 p. 193, Falret, Des maladies mentales. . . 1864.

154 For a full discussion of Kahlbaum's diagnostic criteria and cases, see Chapter 16, this book.

155 p. 49, Kahlbaum, 1874.

156 p. 143, Lagriffe, 1913.

157 Abely, 1916.

158 p. 21, Kraepelin, 1919.

159 p. 77, Abraham, 1942.

160 Guiraud, 1936.

161 Bleuler, 1911.

162 Minkowski, 1927.

163 Kläsi, 1922.

164 pp. 268–269, Guiraud, 1936.

165 See, for example, Beckman and Zimmer, 1981; Godard, 1991; Manschreck, 1993; Liddle, 1994.

PART V

Miscellany

CHAPTER 18

Personality and its disorders

Words and concepts related to aspects of behaviour now addressed as 'personality' (or disorders of) have been known for millenia.[1] The historian must identify the moment when such descriptions appeared and the scientific and social forces that made them possible. Subordinate questions concern the conceptual pedigree of 'personality trait' as it is important to know whether it is different from that of 'symptom'. Likewise, it is important to understand why 'type' and 'trait' have taken turns as the units of clinical analysis for personality disorder. Other questions might also be answered from the historical perspective: What is the relationship between 'trait' and 'dimension'? Has the old notion of 'moral insanity' anything to do with the more recent one of 'psychopathic behaviour'? Is the latter best conceived as a disorder of personality or as a form of insanity? Should the 'neuroses' be considered as periodic forms of personality disorder? What is the relationship between psychoses and disorder of personality? When did the concept of psychopathic personality become contaminated by 'moral' nuances? Are terms currently favoured any better than older ones such as moral insanity, impulsion, impulsive insanity, lucid insanity, volitional insanity, psychopathy, monomania, non-delusional insanity, or reasoning insanity? This chapter will focus on the nineteenth century and after. Historical scholarship on this period is beginning to accumulate.[2]

The nineteenth century intellectual background

As repeatedly mentioned in this book, there were two psychological theories during the nineteenth century. Faculty psychology[3] (the oldest) conceived the mind as a set of powers, faculties or functions; the most popular being a tripartite division into intellectual (cognitive), emotional (orectic), and volitional (or conative).[4] Associationism, first propounded by Hobbes, Locke and other British philosophers,[5] included the assumption that the mind is an empty slate and that knowledge originated from simple ideas (obtained by the senses) or from combinations of simple ideas by means of rules of association.[6] By the late eighteenth century, Thomas Reid and other Scottish philosophers[7] as well as Kant[8] had expressed a preference for different versions of Faculty Psychology, their main argument for this being that experience alone could not explain all knowledge, i.e. that 'innate' structures were necessary. At the beginning of the nineteenth century both psychological theories vied for supremacy. Faculty Psychology[9] inspired phrenology, a view that gave rise to the earlier typologies of personality.[10] Associationism, in turn, was instrumental in the development of psychophysics and quantification in psychology.[11] Both theories contributed to the creation of the concepts of trait, type, and character.

Relevant nineteenth century terms

Constitution, temperament, self, character, and personality are all terms older than the nineteenth century; during this period, however, they were refurbished with new meanings.[12]

'Constitution' and 'temperament'

Since Greek times, the word 'constitution' has played an important descriptive and explanatory role in western medicine.[13] Equivalent to 'diathesis',[14] 'conformation of the body' or 'habit' (in the sense of 'pyknic' habit), constitution was used until the end of the nineteenth century to refer to 'the harmonious development and maintenance of the tissues and organs of which the body is made up.'[15] This body-centred view, however, was in contrast to the original Hippocratic usage which emphasized environmental variables, e.g. 'the climactic conditions of such a marked type as to give a distinguishing character to a period of time' or 'to denote a fixed type prevalent at any particular time.'[16] It is beyond the scope of this chapter to dwell on the process that led to this change in meaning.[17] Suffice it to say that, at the end of the nineteenth century, the concept of personality was modelled on that of constitution to mean 'harmonious' organization of psychological parts.

The word 'temperament' was equally influential; in Greek medicine it provided a 'biological' explanation for the individuality of the self and its traits.[18] One of its versions, the Hippocratic four-fold humoural view of the temperaments, lasted well into the eighteenth century, when Richerand substituted the humours by the size and predominance of certain bodily organs; this view, in turn, was challenged by Royer-Collard who claimed that there was neither physiological nor post-mortem evidence to support the claim that the size of the heart, brain or liver were in any way related to behaviour.[19] The last attempt to return to the classical notion of temperament was made in 1887 by Stewart.[20] The notion of temperament, however, remains alive in all modern attempts to seek an organic substratum for personality 'types'.[21]

'Self'

Up to the nineteenth century, the philosophical analysis of character, personality, and consciousness revolved around the concept of 'self'. Although ideas equivalent to self can be found in pre-Cartesian writings, there is agreement that this notion only achieved clarity in the work of Descartes,[22] and later in that of Locke, Leibniz, and Kant.[23] By the end of the nineteenth century, three views of self were recognized: the old Cartesian one as 'consciousness or self-awareness', and two newer ones, self as a 'core or structure' or as a 'bundle of relationships'.[24] All three were important to the development of the notions of character and personality.

Descartes conceived of the self as an enduring substance providing man with 'ontological continuity'. This view, which in his philosophy doubled up as a solution to the 'personal identity' problem,[25] was challenged by Hume[26] who questioned the existence of such a substance, and re-defined the self as a series of perceptual moments, linked up by memory episodes. During the nineteenth century, this emphasis on subjectivity continued, eventually leading to the full 'psychologisation' of the self. Humean scepticism, however, had undermined so much the ontological view[27] that the issue of personal identity also remained problematic for the psychological version of the self. This is one of the reasons why, during the last century, refurbished concepts such as character, constitution and, in the event, personality, were made to act as conceptual props for the personal identity problem.

Towards the end of the century, writers such as Royce and Baldwin offered a re-definition of the self in terms of human relationships,[28] i.e. claimed that the continuity of one's self and character and also the sense of identity were based on feedback from others. This developmental view has been the starting point for twentieth century 'interactionist' theories of personality.[29]

'Character'

Of Classical provenance, the term 'character' was revived by Kant to name the empirical and logical aspects of objects.[30] During the nineteenth century, this approach was used to explore the 'unchangeable' behavioural core that made an individual different from others.[31] Noticing its psychological potential, J.S. Mill suggested that a new book on human 'characters' needed writing, and in 1861, Alexander Bain – his one time secretary – produced his *On the study of character, including an estimate of phrenology*. Character thus became the preferred name for 'psychological type'.[32] 'Characterology' became the science of character, and soon found a niche within the new science of psychology. By the early twentieth century, the word 'character' was replaced by 'personality', which by then had acquired a wider meaning (see below).

During the early nineteenth century, however, the 'innate' view of 'character'[33] was challenged by the belief that even ingrained behaviours were shaped by the environment. Maine de Biran[34] made popular the mechanism of *habitude* (habit) to explain why certain behaviours, on account of their persistence and inflexibility, might appear to the observer as innate and / or inherited.[35] *Habitude*, itself, has a complex semantic past[36] which included references to the 'form of being' of objects, *regardless of their origin* (in the sense, for example, of 'leptosomic habitus'). Through the concept of *habitude*, however, Maine de Biran[37] and later Ravaisson[38] succeeded in drawing attention to 'learning' components in the formation of character. No wonder that, by the second half of the century, the term habitude had become incorporated into medical parlance.[39] Terms derived from the same Latin stem were later used by Kretschmer[40] and Sheldon[41] to refer to specific types of human physique.

'Personality'

'Personality' started life as a philosophical word, for example, Aquinas meant by it the 'condition or mode of appearance of a person' (*person* being the Greek word for mask). The term was 'psychologised' by Hume and Kant, and the process completed by Maine de Biran and J.S. Mill. During most of the nineteenth century, however, 'personality' was used to refer to the *subjective* aspects of the self and hence had a different meaning from the current one.[42]

This is the reason why Janet as late as 1896 pleaded that 'the study of personality, still conceived of as a metaphysical problem, should become a topic for experimental psychology.'[43] Influenced by Comte, Janet had identified two periods in the history of personality: during the metaphysical one, lasting up to the beginning of the nineteenth century, writers attempted (not always successfully) to distinguish personality from a substance or principle; the next or associationistic period was characterized by a search for the mental elements underlying the feeling of unity of the self or personality. Janet suggested that a third or scientific period should be started by studying personality in objective terms, and by applying the acquired knowledge to the mentally ill. Janet remained deeply interested in the concept and, as late as 1929, gave a magnificent series of Lectures at the *Collège de France* on the psychological evolution of personality.[44]

However, Janet's periodization is likely to have been inaccurate as perusal of Continental works on personality during this period shows that the three approaches co-existed.[45] It is true, however, that writers wanted to equate personality with self-awareness. One of them was Jeanmaire – the greatest of French historians of personality during the nineteenth century – who complained that the concept of personality was caught between the scepticism of the British empiricists and the rationalism of the French spiritualists, and recommended a purely 'psychological' analysis (as Maine de Biran had, indeed, attempted to do).[46] Likewise, after examining the use of the term 'personality' in twelve popular French books published between 1874 and 1882, Beaussire concluded that scientific psychology had not yet resolved the problem, that whilst 'personality manifests itself by means of consciousness, the latter is not sufficient to constitute the personality.'[47]

Perusal of nineteenth century books on 'disorders',[48] 'variations',[49] or 'alterations'[50] of personality shows that their authors did not conceive of personality types or disorders in the current sense; instead, they analysed the mechanisms of awareness of the self, and phenomena concerning the disintegration of consciousness such as somnambulism, hysterical anaesthesia, automatic writing, hallucinations, multiple personalities, and memory disorders. This suggests that, at the time, clinical and experimental writers shared the view that personality was tantamount to 'internal self'. During the early twentieth century, attempts were made to escape from this narrow approach by suggesting that pathological changes in awareness (as those listed above) reflected alterations in the 'perception' of the personality rather than in the personality itself.[51] These earlier beliefs might also explain why the DSM III-R category 'personality disorders' has been translated in France not as *troubles de la personnalité* but as *personnalités pathologiques*.[52]

Types, traits and their measurement

Faculty Psychology and associationism also made possible the view that mind and behaviour were divisible into recognizable parts or 'traits'; thus, for the first time, monolithic descriptions of human character[53] were broken up into their putative simple components thereby transforming 'molar' into 'molecular' descriptions. These components or 'traits' became the unit of analysis of human behaviour and soon encouraged the development of measurement scales. Finally, as theories of brain localization gained acceptance, correlation were sought between traits and brain sites.

The concept of 'type' has an interesting history.[54] *Typus*, originally meaning 'mark' or 'impression', was used by Plato to refer to model, form, scheme, or cluster of features. Galen imported *typus* into medicine to refer to the 'form' of a disease, and Juan Huarte[55] and La Bruyère[56] used the term to refer to socially recognizable patterns of behaviour. These served as models for the physiognomic[57] and phrenological.[58] 'typologies' that became popular during the first half of the nineteenth century, and in relation to which the new concept of character was developed.

The measurement of psychological data started in earnest towards the end of the nineteenth century, and in addition to sensory events, reaction times, and memory performance, efforts were also made to quantify personality traits.[59] Such impetus was helped by the work of Francis Galton (a cousin of Charles Darwin), and by the expansion of statistics and probability theory which, in the event, permeated western science.[60] The notion of 'correlation' (discovered by Galton) provided a new form of 'scientific' evidence for the view that personality traits clustered together; Galton believed that 'the fundamental and intrinsic differences of character that exist in individuals are well illustrated by those that distinguish the two sexes, and which begin to assert themselves even in the nursery . . . the subject of character deserves more statistical investigation than it has yet received.'[61] He also believed that intellectual differences had a 'hereditary' origin[62] and in his book on *Hereditary Genius*, Galton wrote: 'during the fourteen years that have elapsed since this book was published, numerous fresh instances have arisen of distinction being attained by members of the gifted families whom I quoted as instances of heredity, thus strengthening my argument.'[63] Twentieth century methods of measurement of personality and physique have been influenced by Galton's anthropometric indices.

Personality, character and psychopathic disorders

'Personality disorders' are defined by DSM III-R as clusters of 'personality traits [which] are inflexible and maladaptive and cause either significant functional impairment or subjective distress.'[64] 'Personality trait' thus remains the conceptual unit of analysis, and is defined as 'enduring pattern of perceiving, relating, and thinking about the environment and oneself exhibited in a wide range of important social and personal contexts.'[65] Clinicians are 'directed to find a single specific personality disorder that adequately describes the person's disturbed personality functioning. Frequently this can be done only with difficulty, since many people exhibit traits that are not limited to a single personality disorder.'[66] In its definition, ICD-10 even introduces an explanatory mechanism: 'conditions and patterns of behaviour [that] emerge early in the course of individual development, as a result-ant of both constitutional factors and social experience, while others are acquired later in life.'[67]

To the historian, however, both accounts of personality disorder are but palimp-sests whose European origins are barely concealed by a layer of 'empirical' varnish. To reveal the original meanings, the clinician must scratch the surface away and remind himself of the rich French and German conceptual tradition of thinking on character and personality. During the last century, as has been described above, terms such as personality, personality disorder, character, temperament, consti-tution, self, type, and trait changed and exchanged meanings. These permutations were presided over by factors scientific, ideological, and social.[68]

Nineteenth century concepts

In nineteenth century psychiatry, diagnostic categories were created for a number of reasons; some named disorders sharing clinical features in common (active naming), others named fuzzy clinical states not fitting into any category (passive naming or naming by exclusion); yet others named clinical states that seemed to have only one feature in common (e.g. *Manie sans délire*, moral insanity, and *folie lucide*); this latter variety is discussed presently.

Manie sans délire

It is not clear whether Pinel[69] intended 'mania without delusions' to be a new category. His taxonomy, based on Faculty Psychology, empirical observation, and a determination to preserve the notion of 'total insanity', included four categories: manie (*délire général*), mélancolie (*délire exclusif*), démence (*abolition de la pensée*), and idiotisme (*obliteration des facultés intellectuelles et affectives*). These definitions cut across the universe of mental disorders in ways which are opaque to current clin-icians, indeed, they would find it hard to fit their patients into any of them.

Manie, Pinel subdivided into *manie avec délire* and *manie sans délire*. The view of the historian is obscured here by the meaning of the French words *délire* and *manie*.

During this period, the former referred to disorders of either intellect, emotions, or conation, and hence cannot be fully translated as 'delusion' (which since the seventeenth century, had in English an exclusively intellectualistic meaning);[70] *manie*, in turn, referred to states of persistent furor and florid psychosis and had little to do with the current notion of mania.[71] This is the reason why Pinel needed to ask: can mania exist without a lesion of the intellect?[72] He believed that it could, and criticized John Locke for 'considering mania as inseparable from *délire*: when I started working at Bicêtre, I used to think like this author, and I was not a little surprised to see many patients who at no time showed any lesion of the intellect, and who were dominated by a sort of furor, as if their affective faculties were disordered.'[73]

As examples, Pinel reported the case of a self-indulgent young man suffering from temper tantrums during which he would kill his pet animals; after attacking a woman he was forcefully admitted into hospital. Another man, with 'a more advanced state of the same form of insanity' had periodic attacks of furor started by intense thirst, pain in his bowels, constipation, and a feeling of heat which spread to his chest, neck and face 'making them red' and his 'arterial pulses fast and visible';[74] he would then attack the first person he found; insight into this behaviour would make him contrite and suicidal.[75] The third case was that of a chronic patient, who after claiming improvement and looking normal, was released only to become agitated and aggressive after joining a political demonstration. Pinel suggested that all three patients shared a disease characterised by disordered affect (*facultés affectives léses*). But, lest the reader draws the wrong conclusions, it should be remembered that by this Pinel did not mean depression, euphoria or anxiety, but simply 'furor' and aggression.

What Pinel meant by *manie sans délire* was also obscure to his contemporaries and followers as attested by later disagreements. Some German writers accepted the new 'disease' with reservation (e.g. Hoffbauer, Reil, Heinroth), others (like Henke) rejected it, based on the principle of unity of the human mind, and on the belief that mental functions could not become diseased independently.[76] In France, Esquirol, although accepting the Faculty Psychology principle that mental functions could become ill independently, was uneasy about the notion of *manie sans délire*. Alienists from other groups (e.g. Falret) opposed it from the start. As late as 1866, in a famous debate at the *Société Médico-Psychologique*, the crucial argument was repeated by Falret junior that the only reason for entertaining a category such as *manie sans délire* was its use in court.[77] Analysis of Pinel's work suggests that he was trying to construct a new form of insanity, whose definition was no longer based on the presence of delusions but which still had forensic value.[78]

Monomania

Esquirol was unhappy with *manie sans délire*. He rarely, if ever, used the term and soon enough propounded another – *monomanie*: 'Pinel, more than other alienists, has drawn the attention of observers to this condition that is called reasoning mania (folie raisonnante) but which our illustrious master called manie sans délire. Fodéré[79] has also accepted its existence and called it fureur maniaque . . . but does this variety of mania, in which the sufferers preserve the sanity of their reason whilst abandoning themselves to the most condemnable acts, really exist? Can there be a pathological state in which men are irresistibly led to perform acts that their conscience rejects. I do not think so. I have seen many patients deploring these impulses, and all intimated that at the time of the act they felt something which they could not explain, that their brain was under pressure, and that they experienced great difficulty in the exercise of their reason.'[80] 'Thus, all the clinical cases of manie sans délire, as reported by other authors, belong into monomania or lypemania, species of insanity characterised by fixed and specific delusions.'[81]

But Esquirol's 'monomania' did not fare well either[82] and was killed in 1854 at a meeting of the Société Médico-Psychologique when it was said that it offered no advantage over Pinel's old notion.[83] Even more damning was the claim that it was tautological, i.e. that the behaviour that monomania tried to explain often was the only evidence for its existence (as in the case of 'suicidal monomania').[84]

Moral insanity

The view that this diagnostic category was a fore-runner of 'psychopathic disorder' has been discredited by a number of historians.[85] Whitlock put it neatly: 'there [is] not the remotest resemblance between their examples [Pinel's and Prichard's] and what today would be classed as psychopathic personality.'[86] But, what was, then, Prichard attempting to describe? Like Pinel, Esquirol and Georget (his only sources), Prichard[87] was influenced by the Scottish version of Faculty Psychology and from this perspective he called into question Locke's delusional definition of insanity. This had become an embarrassment to alienists appearing in court, for unless delusions were clearly elicited, judges would not countenance an insanity plea.[88] Definitions of insanity purely based on delusions also went against the view, fashionable in Prichard's time, that affective and volitional insanities were real clinical possibilities.[89]

There is little doubt that the category 'moral insanity' was created by Prichard to include both affective and volitional insanities.[90] In general, insanity was for the English writer 'a disorder of the system by which the sound and healthy exercise of the mental faculties is impeded or disturbed.'[91] This definition not only required that, on each occasion, states such as organic delirium, stupor, and apoplexy be ruled out but that a 'positive' diagnosis was made. Prichard's list of positive mental conditions included melancholia, mania, partial insanity, and incoherence (dementia) (all still conceived in their pre-nineteenth century meaning). Prichard added to it an extra category, 'moral insanity', to refer to a rag-bag of behavioural disorders whose only common feature was an absence of delusions. He criticized Pinel's poor choice of cases to illustrate his category manie sans délire, and even reported a private conversation with Esquirol in which the Frenchman admitted feeling uneasy about Pinel's view.

Pinel, Esquirol and Prichard had different reasons for wanting to create a form of insanity without delusions. Prichard's worry related to finding a niche for cases of manic-depressive illness with *no psychotic features*. Thus, he described as typical 'moral insanities' cases where 'tendency to gloom and sorrow is the predominant feature . . . the individual, though surrounded with all the comforts of existence . . . becomes sorrowful and desponding. All things present and future are to his view involved in dreary and hopeless gloom' 'a state of gloom and melancholy depression occasionally gives way after an uncertain period to an opposite condition of preter-natural excitement: in other cases this is the primary character of the disease' 'in this form of moral derangement the disordered condition of the mind displays itself in a want of self-government, in continual excitement, an unusual expression of strong feelings' 'a female modest and circumspect becomes violent and abrupt in her manners, loquacious, impetuous, talks loudly and abusively'.[92] Consistent with this interpretation is also the fact that Prichard's cases often got better[93] and that their illness had late onset (e.g. in old age).[94] Furthermore, eccentricities of behaviour alone or bad propensities were for him not sufficient to make the diagnosis.[95]

Prichard, therefore, was not talking about psychopathic personalities at all. He did for British psychiatry, however, what Pinel had done for his own: break away from the intellectualistic definition of insanity by broadening its boundaries to the point that symptoms affecting other mental functions might be sufficient to diagnose insanity. By successfully creating the moral insanity category he incorporated manic-depressive states with no delusions or hallucinations into the main stream of the insanities (psychoses). Apart from being forensically convenient, this move also encouraged the development of a more detailed descriptive psychopathology for the affective disorders.

Folie lucide

Ulysse Trélat, a French alienist and revolutionary of the first half of the nineteenth century,[96] coined the term *Folie lucide* to name an array of behavioural disorders: 'the patients I am to describe have not been studied before. Lucid madmen, in spite of their disturbed reason, answer all questions to the point, and to the superficial observer look normal.'[97] Unfortunately, Trélat only succeeded in reporting a motley collection of seventy-seven subjects which included 'idiots, satyrs and nympho-maniacs, monomaniacs, erotomaniacs, dipsomaniacs, kleptomaniacs, lucid maniacs, suicidals, adventurers and dissolutes, the jealous, the haughty, the cruel, and the inert.' He claimed that up to 56% of these cases had a family history of insanity, and that the law had not, until then, been firm enough when dealing with them.

Trélat's book had good reviews[98] in spite of the fact that it was written in a format and style already obsolete at the time, offered no clinical criteria for the classification of patients, and ignored the clinical advances made on a number of the clinical conditions he had included. It gives the impression that, because of his busy political life, Trélat had been living, as far as psychiatry was concerned, in a time warp. It is, therefore, all the more strange that Tuke thought that *folie lucide* was but a synonym of moral insanity![99]

Impulsion

During the late nineteenth century, aggressive acts committed by the insane were characterized as 'unreflective or involuntary' and dealt with under the notion of impulsion.[100] Some explained these acts as unmotivated motor explosions that occurred without warning; others as disorders of the will i.e. as irresistible feelings difficult to control.[101] The category 'impulsive insanity'[102] was created to include behavioural states, such as homicidal and suicidal monomania.[103] For example, in his book on the *Frontiers of Insanity*, Hesnard[104] classified the *déséquilibrés* into *passionnés* and *inpulsifs*. Until the end of the nineteenth century, impulsive insanity remained associated with *manie sans délire, folie avec conscience*, and other categories characterized by impulsive acts, and absence of other symptoms.

By the time of Magnan, impulsive insanity had become linked to degeneration theory, in whose association it remained until the twentieth century. Impulsion and impulsive insanity provided the kernel around which the notion of psychopathic personality was eventually to become organised.[105] By the 1930s, impulsions were seen as stereotyped actions of affective, motor, or obsessive origin.[106] However, the volitional explanation, once popular, declined after the concept of 'will' came under scrutiny.[107] After 1900, impulsions began also to be explained in psychodynamic terms although, after the epidemic of encephalitis lethargica, the organic view, once again, came to the fore. Cruchet, for example, reported that, in childhood, encephalitis gave rise to severe antisocial behaviour (the so-called *Apache* or *perverse* children syndrome).[108] In French psychiatry, interest in the study of impulsion lasted well into the second half of this century; for example, Porot and Bardenat classified impulsion as spontaneous or reflex, and constitutional or acquired, and suggested that each subtype be assessed in terms of its affective loading, degree of awareness, and inhibitory capacity.[109]

Degeneration theory and personality

Degeneration theory is the general term for a view developed by Benedict Morel,[110] a French alienist born in Austria, according to which noxae such as alcoholism[111] and masturbation might alter the human seed leading, in successive generations, to melancholia, mania, and dementia as well as to physical stigmata.[112] Morel was a Roman Catholic and his theory was permeated by the metaphor of the Fall;[113] he also assumed a sort of Lamarckian mechanism for the inheritance of acquired traits. Valentin Magnan, and later followers, played down these religious overtones whilst emphasising the neurobiological aspects of the theory.[114]

Without the framework of degeneration theory,[115] the concept of psychopathic inferiority[116] would have made little sense. Other factors were equally important such as pre-Darwinian phrenological beliefs on the criminal mind,[117] the atavistic criminology of Lombroso,[118] Darwinism itself,[119] the model of the hierarchical nervous system propounded by Spencer and Jackson,[120] and the view that some human beings are born with a higher propensity to eccentric and anti-social behaviour.[121] Degeneration theory, in turn, helped with the survival of endangered categories such as *folie raisonnante*[122] and contributed to the development of later typologies such as those by Kretschmer,[123] Schneider,[124] Kahn,[125] and Henderson.[126] (see below). Degenerational views were still detectable in the France of the 1930s, for example, in the so-called 'doctrine of the constitutions'.[127]

Psychopathic disorders

The terms psychopathic personality (and disorder) have disappeared from current classifications. ICD-10 incorporates them into 'dissocial personality disorder' (F60.2), and DSM IV into cluster B (antisocial personality disorder; 301.7). The behaviours to which these terms referred, however, remain diagnostically relevant, and hence their turbulent history needs exploration.[128] During the late nineteenth century, the adjective 'psychopathic' meant 'psychopathological' and applied to *any and all forms* of mental disorder.[129]

But a narrower meaning was to appear in the work of Koch[130] who, under 'psychopathic inferiority', grouped abnormal behavioural states resulting from 'weakness of the brain' which could not, however, be considered as 'diseases' in Kahlbaum's sense. Such states could be chronic or acute, congenital or acquired. Psychopathic inferiorities were a manifestation of degeneration, ranging from mild to severe and giving rise to anti-social behaviours. Years later, Schneider remarked that Koch's classificatory criterion had been 'moral' rather than scientific, and that, in this regard, the 'psychopathies' were 'essentially, a German problem.'[131]

Gross

Another landmark in the evolution of psychopathy is the work of Otto Gross, the Austrian alienist, well known for his hypothesis of cerebral 'secondary function'.[132] According to this view, differences in the time nervous cells took to regain electrical steady-state (after a primary discharge) modulated the character of the individual. In his book on the *Psychopathic Inferiorities*, Gross[133] differentiated between subjects with short secondary function, who responded rapidly to stimuli but were distractible, and those with longer secondary functions (or 'inferiorities') who showed slowness and 'narrowness of' consciousness. Gross influenced Jung who re-baptized Gross's types as extroverts and introverts, respectively.[134]

The impact of psychodynamic views

Current views on the personality disorders remain descriptive and their explanation biological.[135] At the turn of the century, however, psychodynamic models contributed to their analysis and are briefly mentioned here. For example, Pierre Janet[136] was a propounder of 'psychological automatism', a model of the mind based on the hierarchical levels of Hughlings Jackson,[137] and popular at the end of the nineteenth century.[138] Janet used this model to explain mental symptoms and also the 'alterations of the personality'. Mental or psychological automatism he defined as a situation in which part of the mental apparatus escaped the control of the will (and of consciousness) to function in an independent manner. There were normal and pathological forms of mental automatism, and Janet considered the latter the supreme law of human mental activity. For example, in hysterical and dissociative states there was a disconnection between the conscious and unconscious aspects of the personality.[139]

Janet also used another mechanism called 'reduction in psychological tension'. For example, *psychasthénie* was characterized by both psychological automatism and a marked reduction in energy levels.[140] Maurel has suggested that Janet's view is the culmination of a long tradition of European thinking on 'automatic' behaviour started with the mechanical models of Descartes.[141] Psychological automatism remained a popular mechanism in French psychiatry, for example, and was central to the work of de Clérambault.[142]

Freud was not particularly interested in these issues. In 1915, for example, when dealing with character types, he noted that 'when carrying out psychoanalytical treatment the physician's interest is by no means primarily directed to the patient's character' for 'he is far more desirous to know what the symptom signifies'; eventually, however, he will find that resistance may be 'justly attributed to the latter's character.'[143] There is little reference in this paper to the concept of 'character-type' itself. Nonetheless, Freud identified a group of patients who, when ask to renounce certain sources of pleasure, pleaded to be considered as 'exceptions', and another group whose main problem was that their lives had been 'wrecked by success'. Little is discussed in the way of specific mechanisms for these types.

Later psychodynamic writers, however, did show interest in the concept of personality[144] and their contribution is reflected in the development of two important and partially related concepts, namely, 'character neurosis'[145] and the 'borderline states', of which only the latter seems to remain in fashion. Character neurosis was defined as a clinical situation in which the conflict, instead of appearing in the guise of symptoms, appears as character modifications; indeed, the concept was never altogether clear. As Laplanche and Pontalis have perceptively written: 'that the notion remains so ill-defined is no doubt due to the fact that it raises not only *nosographical* problems (what are the specific attributes of character neurosis?) but also both *psychological* questions regarding the origin, basis and function of character and the *technical* question of what place ought to be given to the analysis of so-called character-defences' (*italic* in original).[146] Furthermore, there is the historical dependence of this notion on context and theory: for as long as psychoanalysis defined the 'neuroses' in terms of *symptom clusters*, there was no difficulty in differentiating them from the *character neuroses*; but, after the Second World War, so-called 'structural' models came into fashion and the neuroses were conceived of as patterns or configurations of forces, conflicts and relationships, thus making a 'phenomenological' differentiation between neuroses and character neurosis difficult indeed.

On the other hand, the notion of 'borderline' state has fared better;[147] whether conceived as a form of attenuated psychosis or as a personality disorder, this concept has been sustained by a complex psychodynamic machinery. This notwithstanding, it requires much empirical work before it can be freely used in conventional clinical practice.[148]

Schneider

Kurt Schneider published the first edition of *Psychopathic Personalities* in 1923, as part of Aschaffenburg's *Handbuch der Psychiatrie*.[149] The book was so successful that, by opting for the term 'personality', he rendered 'temperament' and 'character' obsolete. The best is perhaps the ninth edition, in which a long preface and a riposte to critics is included. This little work, like others by Schneider, assumes an 'empirical' and descriptive style which conceals much theoretical contraband. Schneider conceived of the 'psyche' as a harmonious combination of intelligence, personality, and feelings and instincts, and defined 'personality' as the stable 'composite of feelings, values, tendencies and volitions,'[150] thereby excluding cognitive functions and corporal sensations. Abnormal personality, he defined as a state of divergence from the mean, acknowledging that 'ideal' definitions of normality were also important.

Psychopathic personalities were a subclass of abnormal personalities, and referred to those 'who themselves suffer, or make society suffer, on account of their abnormality.'[151] Abnormal and psychopathic personalities were not pathological in a 'medical sense', and hence fell outside the 'disease' model; nonetheless, they had somatic bases. Schneider had little to say on abnormal personality *per se*, and concentrated on ten psychopathic groupings: hyperthymic, depressive, insecure, fanatical, lacking in self-esteem, labile in affect, explosive, wicked, aboulic, and asthenic. These categories, he conceived as 'forms of being' and not as 'diagnostic' entities,[152] and readily accepted that there was nothing new in what he was saying. They might even be, as Kahn[153] suggested, 'reactive and episodic'.[154] Schneider did not see any relationship between his types and the neuroses or psychoses[155] although he suggested that personality, whether normal or abnormal, might modulate the 'form' of the psychoses.

As Schneider himself noticed, his book enjoyed 'a wide circle of readers'; nonetheless, it was subject to much criticism. For example, Edmund Mezger, a professor of criminology at Munich, found his definition of normality 'unworkable in the courts'.[156] Unfortunately, he also believed that 'in the last analysis all psychopathy must be called degeneration'[157] and quoted in his support the now notorious book by Baur *et al.*[158] Mezger's views illustrate the way in which the notion of psychopathic personality became entangled in the eugenic atrocities committed in Germany at the time.[159]

A more determined attack on the book took place at the 105th meeting of the Swiss Society of Psychiatry, when F. Humbert and A. Repond scorned Schneider's definition of psychopathic as being 'tautological' and 'a mêlée of sociological, characterological and constitutional criteria.'[160] Humbert also accused Schneider of having 'borrowed' his clinical categories from others, and of creating artificial separations (e.g. between depressives and hyperthymics) without foundation in clinical reality. Based only on French sources, Humbert denied the existence of psychopathic disorders as a separate category and suggested that they were either attenuated forms of psychotic illness (schizothymic, cyclothymic, etc.) or acquired states, 'childhood neuroses of character'[161] which might be susceptible to psychodynamic treatment. Schneider curtly replied that it was 'self-deception to believe that there are no psychopaths, and that abnormal personalities are only developmental syndromes.'[162]

Kahn

In 1928, Eugen Kahn's published his *Psychopathischen Persönlichkeiten* as part of Bumke's *Handbuch der Geisteskrankheiten*. By 'psychopathic' he 'designated a large number of characteristics or conditions which lie in the broad zone between mental health and mental illness (psychosis).'[163] Like Schneider, Kahn believed that a 'psychopathic personality' makes 'its bearer or society suffer';[164] 'personality' he conceived as a three-legged structure finally determined by the relative contribution of impulse, temperament and character but 'not everything in the psychopathic personality was psychopathic.'[165] It is not difficult to identify the influence of William Stern[166] in Kahn's complex claim that: 'by psychopathic personality we understand those discordant personalities which on the causal side are characterized by quantitative peculiarities in the impulse, temperament, or character strata, and in their unified goal-striving activity are impaired by quantitative deviations in the ego- and foreign evaluation.'[167] Kahn classified psychopathic personalities in terms of its three components: the first group included impulsive, weak, and sexual psychopaths; the second hyper- hypo- and poikilothymic ones; and the third ego-overvaluers, undervaluers and ambitendents. The Schneiderian groups he called 'complex psychopathic states', and suggested that they should be analysed out in terms of physique, impulse-life, temperament and character.

Henderson

D.K. Henderson's book on *Psychopathic States* was an extended version of his Salmon Memorial Lectures. This simple, influential, and badly referenced work revolved around a version of the concept of 'constitution' that Adolf Meyer[168] (Henderson's teacher) had himself borrowed from Frédéric Paulhan.[169] Henderson defined constitution as 'the whole being, physical and mental, it is all partly inborn, partly environmental, and is in a state of flux varying from day to day and even from hour to hour',[170] and psychopathic state as 'the name we apply to those individuals who conform to a certain intellectual standard, sometimes high, sometimes approaching the realm of defect but yet not amounting to it, who throughout their lives, or from a comparatively early age, have exhibited disorders of conduct of an anti-social or asocial nature, usually of a recurrent or episodic nature, which, in many instances, have proved difficult to influence by methods social, penal or medical care and treatment, and for whom we have no adequate provision of a preventive or curative nature . . . [it] constitutes a true illness for which we have no explanation.'[171]

Henderson believed that the proportion of 'psychopathic states, not only amongst the prison population, but in ordinary social life, is very high indeed and that in our ordinary work we do not realise half-seriously enough that it is the psychopathic state which constitutes the rock on which our prognosis and treatment in relation to many psychoneurotic and psychotic states becomes shattered.'[172] He described three clusters of personality features: predominantly aggressive, passive, and creative; each including core and accessory behaviours: in the first group suicide, murder and assault, alcoholism and drug addiction, epilepsy, and sex variants; in the second, cycloid and schizoid states; and talent in the third. Werlinder has suggested that in this last grouping, Henderson was influenced by the French concept of *dégénéré supérieur*.[173] Craft rightly commented: 'although Henderson continued to use this term, most authors have found it difficult to use'.[174]

Later typologies

New typological classifications appeared in the early twentieth century; although conceptually similar to earlier ones, they sought to correlate personality type with bodily shape and mental disorder. In this, they differed from nineteenth century efforts which tended to conceive personality disorders as *formes frustres* of insanity. But once insanity was narrowed down into the new concept of 'psychosis' the notion of *forme frustre* lost meaning. This process set a number of disorders asunder; some, like the obsessive-compulsive states, were incorporated into the class of the new 'neuroses';[175] others formed the core of the 'character' disorders.

Typologies based on the old definition of constitution became rare during the second half of the nineteenth century. Thus, the popular treatise on *Our Temperaments* by Alexander Stewart can be considered as the last manifestation of the Hippocratic humoural and physiognomonic approaches;[176] this author claimed to have identified, amongst British people, examples of sanguine, bilious, lymphatic and nervous temperament. Earlier on, Beneke, in Germany, had suggested a bipolar typology: scrofulous-phthisical versus rachito-carcinomatous, based on three-dimensional measurements of internal organs; he believed that most people fitted into one of these body types; and that organ-size correlated with age and disease.[177] Di Giovanni was also interested in the relationship between the size of internal organs and morbidity[178] as was Galton, who attempted to identify the features and dimensions constituting the typical English face and bodily shape.[179]

But it was C.G. Jung who, at the turn of the century, rescued the concept of 'type' for the twentieth century: no longer interested in stereotyped behavioural forms or humours, he suggested that the human personality was a combination of 'dimensions'.[180] Following the neurophysiological speculations of Otto Gross,[181] Jung proposed a dimension of introversion–extroversion along which mental functions such as thinking, feeling, sensation and intuition could be graded. Gross also influenced the work of the Dutch psychologists G. Heymans and E.D. Wiersma[182] who propounded eight characters: amorphous, apathetic, nervous, sentimental, sanguine, phlegmatic, choleric, and impassioned.

Typologies based on speculative biology also developed during this period. For example, Berman believed that since 'a single gland can dominate the life history of an individual' it was possible to identify 'endocrine types' such as adrenal, pituitary, thyroid, thymo-centric, and gonado-centric.[183] In 1921, Kretschmer propounded a simpler and more influential typology.[184] Following Kraepelin's division of the psychoses, he suggested cycloid and schizoid temperaments, which he believed influenced most aspects of human behaviour. There were also four types of physique: asthenic or leptosomatic, athletic, pyknic or pyknosomatic, and dysplastic. Correlations were then postulated between manic-depressive illness and pyknic type, and between schizophrenia and leptosomatic, asthenic and (less frequently) dysplastic physique. During the 1940s, Kretschmer's work was criticized on methodological grounds, particularly in Great Britain.[185] The development of new typologies, however, continued in other places. For example, in the USA, Sheldon created a scale for measuring temperament whose items (representing a combination of behavioural traits) factorized out into three components: viscerotonia, somatotonia, and cerebrotonia.[186]

During the 1920s, the French developed a more conceptual approach to human personality which they called the doctrine of the 'constitutions'.[187] This was soon broadened into a theory of mental disorder.[188] According to Dupré[189] 'personality, whether normal or pathological, represented the sum or synthesis of all organic and functional activities' and 'mental diseases were, in effect, diseases of the personality', 'mental diseases result from anomalies of general sensibility, of alterations of organic consciousness, in a word, of vices – whether constitutional or acquired – of the nervous system.'[190] Dupré postulated eight groups: with unstable physical sensibility (i.e. hypo- and hyperesthesics, and coenesthopathics); with unstable motor function; the emotive (i.e. erethics); those with disordered appetite, instinct, and mood; the paranoid; and those with pathological imagination (i.e. mythomanics). When present in a minor degree, these types tinged the personality; when excessive, they caused mental illness. Dupré doctrine, the last important manifestation of the degeneration theory in France, was influenced by the ideas of Bouchard, Magnan, and particularly Duprat, who in 1899 published an important book on *L'Instabilité Mentale* which contained the germ of the doctrine of constitutions.[191]

Two other important French works related to the notion of constitution appeared during this period. One was the book by G. Genil-Perrin on *Les Paranoiaques* where play is made of *la constitution paranoiaque*,[192] and which follows Dupré's ideas closely. Genil-Perrin identified five dimensions in the paranoid personality: pride, mistrust, false judgment, inadaptability, and *bovarysme*, a French notion which Jules de Gaultier defined as 'the power given to man to think of himself as that which he is not.'[193] The other important book on the paranoid personality is Jacques Lacan's doctoral thesis of 1932. This work, written in a clear and powerful style, gives little indication of what was to follow! Its first chapter was a devastating critique of the traditional concept of personality: 'our work has exposed the vulgar beliefs concerning personality, its metaphysical basis, and the impossibility of drawing from this a scientific definition.'[194] Following Hesnard, Lacan suggested that, instead of talking about 'disorders of personality', one should study the 'disorders of personalisation' (*troubles de personnalisation*).[195] He also commented upon Genil-Perrin's ideas without quoting him: 'Such is the paranoid constitution, namely, the complex of pride, mistrust, false judgment, and social inadaptability; this effort, like others, tries to derive complex manifestations from a simple psychological property that might be innate, such as psychorigidity.'[196] Lacan drew three types of conclusions: 'critical, dogmatic and hypothetical', the latter of which included the view that his method of study led to identifying the life events (particularly from infancy) that determine disease, and the pre-logical conceptual structures that the psychosis generates.[197]

The aftermath

Current definitions of personality disorder, whether enshrined in DSM IV, ICD-10, or in British approaches[198] are composites of traits based on three sources of data: the direct reporting of subjective (and hopefully unedited) experiences, autobiographical accounts, and narratives by others. Their reliability (and validity) are, therefore, dependent on the degree of convergence of these sources: the higher the convergence the more stable the cluster or profile. In some cases they may be stable enough to warrant the search for a neurobiological substratum.

Historically, all three sources of information required justification. Subjective accounts were allowed only after introspection became legitimised as a method of analysis;[199] and autobiographical and biographical accounts only after mental disorders began to be conceived as longitudinal processes.[200] Likewise, the idea that stable profiles had to have a neurobiological substratum is an offshoot of the old anatomo-clinical model of disease.[201] More recently, another evidential method has emerged, to wit, statistical corroboration. Thus, anecdotal observation is no longer considered a guarantee for convergence, instead everything seems to revolve around the plausibility of certain pattern recognition techniques (like cluster and principal component analysis). This switch in scientific paradigm is perhaps the only difference that the historian can find between nineteenth and twentieth century approaches to personality or character disorders.

Summary

In general terms, this chapter has found that the concept of 'personality disorder' appeared in the psychiatric literature of the nineteenth century only after character and personality had been psychologically defined, and 'self' become a 'mental' function. The language of 'types' and 'traits' originated from the phrenological and psychometric traditions, respectively. What nowadays is called personality was last century called character, temperament, and constitution. During that period, the concept of 'disordered' character included reference to an 'organic' substratum; and that of personality disorder meant alteration of consciousness (e.g. hysterical dissociations). This would explain why, up to the First World War (and to a certain extent to the present time), the *psychiatric* and *psychological* views of 'personality' (and its disorders) have not fully converged.

During the nineteenth century, there were three causal models of personality 'disorder'. According to Faculty Psychology, they resulted from failures in the mental faculty of the 'will'; associationism postulated a loss of coherence between cognitive, emotional and volitional information; and the 'automatism' hypothesis, following a Jacksonian model, suggested that personality disorders resulted from lower forms of behaviour escaping the control of higher ones (i.e. there was a horizontal 'splitting' of consciousness). All three models made use of explanations based on degenerational (genetic) and acquired (learning) mechanisms. Hence, views on personality disorders seemed more unified than in fact they were.

Intellectual context and historical fashion, rather than empirical research, determined the successive predominance of these views. Thus, after the concept of 'will' fell out of fashion, volitional models of psychopathy rapidly disappeared. Likewise, the 'developmental' dimension was only added after the inception of Freudian ideas. Current neurobiological explanations are but a return of earlier views according to which behaviour, whether normal or pathological, is dependent upon specific neurobiological events.

NOTES

1 Theophrastus, 1967.
2 Werlinder, 1978; Blair, 1975; Craft, 1965; Ellard, 1988; Lantéri-Laura,

1979; Fullinwider, 1975; Gurvitz, 1951; Huertas, 1987; Kageyama, 1984; Lewis, 1974; Maughs, 1941; Motte-Moitreux, 1990; Pichot, 1978; Saussure, 1946; Schmiedebach, 1985; Smith, 1979; Whitlock, 1967; 1982.

3 Versions of this theory have existed since Classical times, see Blakey, 1850.

4 Berrios, On Historical background to abnormal psychology, 1988.

5 Warren, 1921.

6 Hoeldtke, 1967.

7 Brooks, 1976.

8 Hilgard, 1980.

9 Albrecht, 1970.

10 Spoerl, 1936; Hécaen and Lantéri-Laura, 1978.

11 Claparède, 1903.

12 Berrios, On Descriptive psychopathology, 1984.

13 Pinillos and López Piñero, 1966.

14 On this term, see the great work by Castan, 1867.

15 p. 381, Quain, 1894.

16 p. 141, Jones in Hippocrates, 1972.

17 Pinillos and López Piñero, 1966; Quain, 1894; Jones, in Hippocrates, 1972; Brochin, 1876.

18 Haupt, 1858; Dechambre, 1886; Staehelin, 1941; Roccatagliata, 1981; Royer-Collard, 1843.

19 Royer-Collard, 1843.

20 Stewart, 1887.

21 Bloor, 1928; Burt, 1938; Eysenck, 1951; Dublineau, 1943.

22 Frondizi, 1952; Perkins, 1969; Viney, 1969.

23 Burns, 1979; Strauss, 1991.

24 Abbagnano, 1961.

25 Penelhum, 1967.

26 Pears, 1975.

27 Hamilton, 1859.

28 Baldwin and Stout, in Baldwin, 1901; on the 'moral' aspects of the self, see Gusdorf, 1948; on its 'pathology', Cicchetti and Toth, 1994.

29 Ekehammar, 1974.

30 Ferrater Mora, 1958.

31 Roback, 1927.

32 Azam, 1885.

33 This is the sense in which Theophrastus used it: 'I shall never cease to marvel, why it has come about that, albeit the whole of Greece lies in the same clime and all Greeks have a like upbringing, we have not the same constitution of character', p. 37, Theophrastus, 1967.

34 Maine de Biran, 1929.

35 Moore, 1970.

36 Lalande, 1976.

37 Delacroix, 1924.

38 Ravaisson, 1984.

39 Dechambre, On Habitude, 1886.

40 Kretschmer, 1936.

41 Sheldon, 1942.

42 Jeanmaire, 1882.

43 p. 97, Janet, 1896.

44 Janet, 1929.

45 Paulhan, 1880; Renouvier, 1900; Martí y Juliá, 1899; Caillard, 1894;
    Galton, 1895; Beaussire, 1883.

46 Jeanmaire, 1882.

47 p. 317, Beaussire, 1883.

48 Ribot, 1912.

49 Paulhan, 1882.

50 Binet, 1892.

51 Anonymous, Personalidad, 1921; Dwelshauvers, 1934.

52 Garrabé, 1989.

53 For example, those described by Theophrastus, 1967.

54 Abbagnano, 1961.

55 Juan Huarte (1535–1592) was an Spanish physician and philosopher who
    in 1575 published an original work, *Examen de Ingenios para las Scienzias
    . . .* where he developed a typology of the human mind relating vocations
    to capacities to undertake trades and professions; he also proposed that the
    brain was composed by various independent organs each of which was in
    charge of a different mental function or ability; pp. 72–76, Ullersperger,
    1954.

56 In 1688, Jean de La Bruyère (1645–1696) produced the first modern
    French translation of Theophrastus's *The Characters* to which he added a
    series of realistic and ironic portraits of the many human types he saw
    around him whilst working as a teacher of the grandson of the Prince de
    Condé.

57 Caro-Baroja, 1988.

58 Spurzheim, 1826.

59 Boring, 1961; Zupan, 1976.

60 Hacking, 1990; Porter, 1986; Gigerenzer *et al.*, 1989.

61 pp. 39–42, Galton, 1883.

62 Buss, 1976.

63 p. 57, Galton, 1979.

64 p. 335, APA, DSM III-R, 1987.

65 p. 335, APA, DSM III-R, 1987.

66 p. 336, APA, DSM III-R, 1987.

67 WHO, ICD-10, 1992.

68 Allport, 1937; Anonymous, Personalidad, 1921; Jeanmaire, 1882; Ribot,
    1912; Tyrer and Ferguson, 1990; Werlinder, 1978.

69 Pinel, 1809.

70 For a full discussion of this issue see Chapter 5, this book.

71 Berrios, On Depressive and manic states, 1988.

72 p. 155, Pinel, 1809.

73 pp. 155–156, Pinel, 1809.

74 These attacks are redolent of acute porphyria.
75 p. 157, Pinel, 1809.
76 Motte-Moitreux, 1990; SMP, Debate on reasoning insanity, 1866; Falret, Discussion sur la folie raisonnante, 1866.
77 Falret, 1866.
78 Motte-Moitreux, 1990.
79 F.E. Fodéré (1764–1835) alienist with vitalist beliefs who specialized in forensic medicine (on 'vitalism', see Wheeler, 1939).
80 p. 95, Vol. 2, Esquirol, 1838.
81 p. 96, Esquirol, 1838.
82 Kageyama, 1984; Saussure, 1946; Goldstein, 1987; Alvarez-Uría, 1983.
83 Brierre de Boismont, 1853; SMP, Debate on monomania, 1854; Falret, De la non-existence. . ., 1864.
84 Berrios and Mohanna, 1990.
85 Whitlock, 1967; 1982; Smith, 1981; Ey, La notion de 'maladie morale' 1978.
86 p. 57, Whitlock, 1982.
87 Prichard, 1835.
88 In England, this reached its highest point after the creation of the McNaughton rules; West and Walk, 1977.
89 Based on the belief that mental functions could become diseased independently.
90 Müller, 1899.
91 p. 2, Prichard, 1835.
92 pp. 17–21, Prichard, 1835.
93 p. 26, Prichard, 1835.
94 p. 25, Prichard, 1835.
95 p. 23, Prichard, 1835.
96 Trélat, 1861.
97 p. xxx, Trélat, 1861.
98 Lunier, 1861.
99 Tuke, 1892.
100 Bourdin, 1896.
101 Ribot, 1904.
102 Dagonet, 1870.
103 Grasset, 1908; Grivois, 1990.
104 Hesnard, 1924.
105 Caroli and Olie, 1979.
106 Ey, On Impulsions, 1950.
107 Horwicz, 1876; Aveling, 1925; Daston, 1982; Kimble and Perlmuter, 1970; Keller, 1954.
108 Cruchet, 1943.
109 Porot and Bardenat, in Porot, 1975.
110 Morel, 1857.
111 Bynum, 1984.
112 Dallemagne, 1895; Ribot, 1906; Mairet and Ardin-Delteil, 1907.

113 Liégeois, 1991.
114 Saury, 1886.
115 Genil-Perrin, 1913.
116 Koch, 1891; Gross, 1909.
117 Gall, 1825.
118 Peset, 1983; Pick, 1989.
119 Hilts, 1982.
120 Berrios, On Positive and negative symptoms and Jackson, 1985.
121 Saury, 1886.
122 Saury, 1886; Sérieux and Capgras, 1909.
123 Kretschmer, 1936.
124 Schneider, 1950.
125 Kahn, 1931.
126 Henderson, 1939.
127 Charpentier, 1932; Delmas, 1943.
128 Craft, 1965; Maughs, 1941; Pichot, 1978.
129 Werlinder, 1978; Schmiedebach, 1985.
130 Koch, 1891.
131 Schneider, 1950.
132 Gross, 1904. The son of the Austrian criminologist Hans Gross (1847–1915), Otto Gross (1877–1920) led a conflictive life and died of a complication of drug addiction. After medical training he taught psychopathology at Graz but soon gravitated towards bohemian and anarchist groups. His sympathetic views on psychopathy were in stark contrast to his father's.
133 Gross, 1909.
134 Jung, 1964.
135 Cloninger, 1987.
136 Janet, 1889.
137 Balan, 1989.
138 SMP, On *L'Automatism Psychologique de Pierre Janet 100 Ans Après*, 1989; Grivois, 1992.
139 Garrabé, 1989.
140 Janet, 1919.
141 Maurel, 1989.
142 Ey, On *Une Théorie Mécaniciste*, 1952.
143 Freud, Introductory, 1963.
144 Blum, 1953.
145 On this, see superb papers by Baudry, 1983 and Liebert, 1988.
146 p. 67, Laplanche and Pontalis, 1973.
147 Kernberg, 1967; Shapiro, 1978; Kohut and Wolf, 1978; Perry and Klerman, 1978; Liebowitz, 1979; Akiskal *et al.*, 1985; Aronson, 1985.
148 Modestin, 1980.
149 Schneider, 1950.
150 p. 25, Schneider, 1950.
151 p. 27, Schneider, 1950.
152 p. 70, Schneider, 1950.

153 Kahn, 1931.

154 p. 74, Schneider, 1950.

155 p. 76, Schneider, 1950.

156 p. 60, Mezger, 1939; Mezger, 1944.

157 p. 64, Mezger, 1944.

158 Baur *et al.*, 1927.

159 Müller-Hill, 1988; Weindling, 1989.

160 p. 180 Humbert, 1947.

161 p. 194, Humbert, 1947.

162 p. 29, Schneider, 1950.

163 p. 55, Kahn, 1931.

164 pp. 56–57, Kahn, 1931.

165 p. 60, Kahn, 1931.

166 William Stern (1871–1938) sponsored a form of holistic functionalism and followed W. Dilthey's concept of understanding.

167 p. 69, Kahn, 1931.

168 Meyer, 1903.

169 Paulhan, 1894. Paulhan (1856–1931) was a disciple of Ribot and one of the great psychologist–philosophers of the late nineteenth century. He combined associationism with the holistic spiritualism that touched all French thinkers during this period.

170 p. 32, Henderson, 1939.

171 pp. 16–17, Henderson, 1939.

172 p. 37, Henderson, 1939.

173 Werlinder, 1978.

174 p. 13, Craft, 1965.

175 Berrios, On Obsessive–compulsive disorder, 1989.

176 Stewart, 1887.

177 Beneke, 1881.

178 Giovanni, 1919.

179 pp. 1–17, Galton, 1883.

180 Jung, 1964.

181 Gross, 1904.

182 Heymans, 1906.

183 p. 202, Berman, 1922.

184 Kretschmer, 1936.

185 Rees, 1961.

186 Sheldon, 1942.

187 Dupré, 1925.

188 Gayat, 1984.

189 Dupré, 1984.

190 p. 79, Dupré, 1984.

191 Duprat, 1899.

192 pp. 175–261, Genil-Perrin, 1926.

193 The term was a derivative of the name of *Madame Bovary*, the novel by Flaubert, it was introduced by Gaultier, 1902.

194 p. 35, Lacan, 1975.

195 p. 43, Lacan, 1975.
196 p. 52, Lacan, 1975.
197 p. 350, Lacan, 1975.
198 Ferguson and Tyrer, 1990.
199 Boring, 1953; Danziger, 1980; Wilson, 1991; also Lyons, 1986.
200 Pistoia del, 1971.
201 Ackerknecht, 1967.

CHAPTER 19

Self-harm

Early nineteenth century views on suicide or self-harm were but a continuation of concepts created in previous centuries.[1] The Enlightenment debate on suicide reflected a clash between religious views and the new liberalism, and this, to a certain extent, repeated itself after the 1800s. A good illustration is the work of Madame de Staël who, after writing an apology of suicide in 1796, published a rejoinder in 1812. This much neglected tract is entitled *Réflexions sur le Suicide*: 'In my work on the *Influence of Passions* I defended the act of Suicide, but I repent now of having penned those thoughtless words. I was then a proud and vivacious young woman: but what is the use of living but having the hope of improving oneself?[2] Another representative of the liberal view was Cesare Beccaria[3] who in his *Dei delitti e delle pene* wrote: 'Suicide is a crime that cannot be punished for when punishment is meted out it either falls upon the innocent or upon a corpse. In the latter case it will have no effect upon the living, in the former it is tyrannical and unfair as political rights dictate that punishment must be personal.'[4]

After the 1820s, the moral debate became 'medicalized', i.e. it was shaped by changes in the notion of mental disease and in psychological theory. As Lanteri-Laura and del Pistoia have observed: 'at the end of the eighteenth century [suicide] ceased to be condemned on the basis of religiously inspired tradition: the secularisation of the law no longer made it permissible to punish it as a revolt against God. Nevertheless, it remained a shocking act; so psychiatry was invited to take charge of it, since society still regard it as a threat to established order.'[5]

The rise of the anatomo-clinical model of disease transformed the concept of mental illness and this, in turn, led to a disintegration of the old view of 'total insanity'. The 'partial' insanities (e.g. monomania and lypemania) offered a new medical way of explaining suicide. Changes in psychological theory were equally important: the rise of Faculty Psychology made possible the clinical existence of non-intellectual insanities (i.e. insanities whose primary disorder was to be found in the emotions or volition).[6] This concept, once again, offered the medical establishment a second model for self-harm behaviour as suicidal individuals could be called 'insane' or 'alienated' without, in fact, having to show delusions or hallucinations. One way or the other, alienists became able to protect families of suicidal persons from religious and legal persecution. In fact, by the end of the eighteenth century, laws against completed suicide had ceased to be regularly enforced as they caused as much trouble to the enforcers as they did to the families of the deceased.[7]

There is no full agreement amongst scholars[8] as to the balance of arguments, during the first half of the nineteenth century, in regard to the view that all suicidal acts were the result of 'pathological' behaviour. To explore this, a definitional base-line of representative eighteenth century views is needed, and these are nowhere better expressed than in the *French Encyclopedia*. Diderot stated that the imputation of suicide should depend upon the ascertaining of *mental state* (*situation d'esprit*); subjects being unimputable when found to be suffering from a brain disorder (*cerveau derange*); depression (*tombe dans une noire melancolie*); or delirium (*phrénesie*).[9] The French doctrine, up to the 1760s, seems to have been that at least some amongst the mentally ill could not be declared *felo de se*; and although only three categories of mental disorder are mentioned, it is clear that the first – *cerveau derange* – was meant to include cases without obvious clinical features. The idea that some mental disorders could lead to suicide was not, of course, new: as J.C. Schmitt has shown, since the Medieval period states such as *accidia, tristitia, despera-tio, taedium vitae*, and *frenesia* had been regularly mentioned in this regard; the problem, for the historian is to give such states a clinical identity; indeed, some may have had no recognizable clinical boundaries.[10]

Towards the end of the eighteenth century, the abuse of the 'psychiatric' view of suicide encouraged some to put forward narrower views: for example, the French protestant Jean Dumas, in his book of 1773, attacked the defence of suicide contained in both Montesquieu's LXXVIth *Letter persane* and Holbach's *Système de la Nature*.[11] In England, E. Burton, a former Fellow of Trinity College, Cambridge, also worried about the medical excuse and stated: 'where ten destroy themselves through insanity, hundreds destroy themselves coolly and deliberately . . .'; unfortunately, 'a state of lunacy becomes a matter of purchase . . . thus it generally happens that the result of all these public inquiries into the cause of voluntary death is a state of lunacy; which implies that no one can in the full possession of his senses, resolutely and deliberately destroy himself.'[12] Bayet has made a similar commentary in regard to the French situation.[13]

Moore, also from Trinity College wrote in his magnificent two-volume book: 'that suicide implies no necessity of an absolute and permanent madness is agreed on all hands',[14] and 'suicide, then, whether deliberate or precipitate, no more 'necessarily' implies madness or lunacy than every other great crime can be said to do.'[15] And even in the case of known madness, Moore claimed, there might be imputability. In this he was only echoing Blackstone: 'if a lunatic can be proved to have committed suicide during a lucid interval he is adjudged in the eye of the law a *felo de se*.'[16]

So, the view that only a proportion of persons who committed suicide were actually mentally ill, or that mental illness may not be an explanation even when present at the time, was already well developed during the eighteenth century.[17]

The same claim was to continue into the following century, except that, as has been mentioned above, new concepts made the debate drift in other directions. It is, therefore, surprising that during the 1890s, and with the benefit of hindsight, Èmile Durkheim felt able to say that the 'psychiatric' conception of suicide was an absolute belief amongst nineteenth century alienists.

The nineteenth century debate, however, is interesting in its own right because it generated new questions – some of these still current – such as the relationship between suicide and heredity, brain localization and the value of national statistics.[18] This issue became particularly important towards the end of the century when, under the influence of degeneration theory, suicide regained a moralistic dimension by being considered as a stigma of degeneration.[19] By the 1880s, agreement developed between French, German, British, Italian, and Spanish alienists on the definition and classification of suicide, and on the role played in its pathogenesis by heredity, mental illness, and social factors. This consensus was reached through the publication of major works in the main European languages.[20] These books formulated what will here be called the 'standard view'. This view was reached by steps, and these will be here briefly described.

Esquirol: creator of the 'standard view'

Accounts of nineteenth century psychiatric views on suicide are made to start with Esquirol: 'suicide shows all the features of mental alienation of which it is but a symptom. There is no need to search for a special brain site for suicide as it can be found associated with all kinds of clinical situations being, as it is, secondary to both acute delirium and to the chronic delusional states; post-mortem studies have not thrown much light on the subject.'[21] Thus he wrote in his 1838 book (a final summary of his work); the original version of the chapter on suicide, however, had appeared as early as 1821 and is different in various ways. This is, probably, the reason why Esquirol is quoted by both camps. One the one hand, writers like Durkheim,[22] Halbwachs,[23] Achille-Delmas,[24] and Giddens[25] who see him as the champion of the 'psychiatric' thesis; on the other, by those who see him as the representative of the 'standard view',[26] namely, that only some suicides are caused by mental illness.[127]

In 1821, Esquirol defined suicide in a broad fashion: 'this phenomenon is observed in the most varied circumstances . . . and shaped by the same uncertainties that affect mental illness; doubtless, suicide is idiopathic, but it can frequently be secondary.'[28] He listed dying 'for the highest motives', 'for social delusions' (*idées fausses, mais accréditées*), impulsive emotion, organic delirium, mania (in the old fashion sense of this term), hypochondria, lypemania, and para-suicide (which Esquirol called *suicide simulé*).[29] He concluded: 'from what has been said it can be concluded that suicide is a phenomenon that follows a large number of, and has diverse, presentations; this phenomenon cannot, therefore, be considered as a disease. The general conclusions drawn from having considered suicide as a *sui generis* disease have been proven wrong by experience.'[30]

These views were tightened in their 1838 version, and Esquirol's definition became narrower. Consequently, the 'psychiatric' explanation acquired relatively more importance. But even then, these later views were not as absolute as Durkheim presented them. For example, when discussing treatment Esquirol stated: 'suicide is an act secondary to severe emotional upheaval (*délire de passion*) or insanity (*folie*)' . . . 'treatment should rest on the understanding of causes and determinant motives of suicide.'[31] It is unlikely, therefore, that for Esquirol suicide was *always* a form of monomania; indeed, it is unlikely that it was always a form of insanity. A twentieth century interpretation of Esquirol's views by Charles Blondel also gave him the benefit of the doubt by making the point that, although Esquirol might have claimed that most suicides entailed some sort of abnormal or upset state of mind, he was only too aware of the role of social factors.[32] Blondel also accused Esquirol's successors of having hardened his views, particularly by neglecting his acceptance of social factors.[33] Giddens has also suggested that Esquirol's views were more flexible than Durkheim's version of them.[34]

Interpretation of what Esquirol really said is bedevilled by the ambiguous meaning of a number of French clinical concepts: *aliénation mentale, folie, délire de passion,* and *symptomatique*. A detailed analysis of these issues is beyond the scope of this chapter. Briefly, however, the word *folie* was a generic term used to refer to various states of madness and hence to long lasting diseases.[35] Things are more complicated in relation to *délire*, which has no direct English rendition; from the beginning of the nineteenth century, much confusion has been caused by translators rendering *délire* into the English term 'delirium'; in fact, it rarely means organic brain syndrome and mostly means delusion; but it may also mean something far more complex than that.[36] Hence, the presence of *délire* does not necessarily indicate a diagnosis of *folie* or madness. Spaulding and Simpson (the English translators of Durkheim) rendered *délire* as *delirium* throughout, thereby obscuring the meaning of the term. In the case of *délire de passion*, meaning is clearer: Esquirol believed that *délire* could follow any major emotional upheaval: 'passions (i.e. emotions) can so affect our sensations, ideas, judgments and decisions that it is not surprising that violent excitement may cause *délire*: in this case it is sudden in onset and short lived; it can also be the lingering product of lasting emotions (*passion chronique*).'[37] This means that Esquirol and many of his followers used *délire de passion* to refer to any state of temporary emotional upheaval (such as that caused by a social or personal crisis); this description did not entail at all the presence of a disease (i.e. *folie*).[38]

It can be concluded, therefore, that Esquirol was saying that, during the suicidal act the individual *was always in an altered mental state* but that this might only be a *short lived emotional upheaval*, and not insanity. This interpretation is shared by Blondel: 'it is a fact that madmen kill themselves and that such suicides are pathological. It is a different fact that men said to be normal also kill themselves. But they are not normal in the moment of the act. They only do it under the effect of a strong emotion', 'this disorder of the emotions that Esquirol makes the basis of his second category of suicide can be precipitated by life events and the tendencies of individuals.'[39] This interpretation is reinforced by the view, expressed by Esquirol himself, that the treatment of suicidal behaviour must focus on the subject's 'motivations and reasons'.

Other French holders of the 'standard' view

In a popular book, Brierre de Boismont also presented a balanced view of the association between insanity and suicide.[40] For unclear reasons, Durkheim ignored Brierre de Boismont's repeated claims that 'suicide is not always evidence of mental illness'[41] and that 'the disease of spleen, when accompanied by tendency to suicide, cannot be considered as a variety of mental illness unless it is accompanied by a disorder of emotions or thinking. To make such a state yet another form of insanity is to justify the reproach, oft-times addressed at alienists, that they see their fad everywhere. Spleen has more social than personal origins.'[42]

Another important representative of the 'standard' view was G-F Étoc-Demazy[43] whose views were expressed in a book that appeared in 1844,[44] and in a paper published in 1846 as a rejoinder to Bourdin's book,[45] Étoc-Demazy intimated that he had never been able to convince himself that all suicides were the result of mental illness. He criticized the *a priori* (and, according to him, clinically weak) approach taken by Bourdin, and offered instead his notion of *aberration morbid passagère*,[46] a continuation of Esquirol's notion (discussed above) of *délire de passion*. He rejected the view that all suicides were mentally ill and concluded: 'the insistence with which some authors want to consider suicide as a form of mental alienation, stems from an exaggerated human fondness for life.'[47]

E. Lisle also defended the 'standard' view. His book on suicide, appeared the same year as Brierre's, was awarded the coveted Imperial Academy Prize of Medicine.[48] Lisle attacked Esquirol whom he interpreted (wrongly) as defending the 'psychiatric' thesis and explained this distortion as resulting from the fact that he (Esquirol) had always worked in mental hospitals and hence only seen the most severe and pathological end of the patient population. Lisle reduced *ad absurdum* the view that all suicide was a form of madness by applying the same argument to homicide. He also attacked Falret for inventing the notion of *melancolie suicide*[49] and made fun of him by claiming that, perhaps, all classical suicidal heroes were, at the time of their death, suffering from melancholia! He also dismissed Bourdin's book as insignificant, and as trying to propagate the doctrine of monomania.[50] More importantly, he criticized his method of reasoning by induction, i.e. trying to demonstrate a point of view from theoretical premises without resorting to empirical evidence. He denied the existence of the so-called 'suicidal monomania' in which suicidal behaviour was the only evidence for the existence of the disease, and concluded that, if the clinical facts were observed, the view that all suicides are 'pathological' would soon be dispelled.

But not all defenders of the 'standard' view necessarily argued from a medical perspective; Bertrand, for example, wrote from a deeply religious viewpoint, and his award wining book received the imprimatur of Gousset, then Archbishop of Reims.[51] Predictably, Bertrand started by saying that suicide is an act against God, family and fatherland. He believed that moral freedom must be preserved at all costs, and this led him to accuse Bourdin of believing that man was like a clock, and paradoxically, to deny the view that all suicides must be the result of madness. He concluded that 'to put forward the view that all suicides are the result of mental alienation, and hence not imputable, is a dangerous and serious mistake which can give rise to undesirable moral consequences.'[52] He differentiated between acute and chronic suicide (the terminology was Esquirol's)[53] and included in the latter alcoholism (this about 100 years before Menninger's identical claim in *Man against himself*).

Non-French holders of the 'standard' view

The standard view was held by renowned alienists outside France. For example, Prichard wrote: 'the prevalent opinion is that insanity is not always the cause of suicide, though the verdict of lunacy is generally brought by juries, owing to the extreme barbarity of the law on this subject. M Fodéré[54] has expressed long ago the opinion that suicide is always the result of madness. Though every one would wish to be of the same sentiment, it seems difficult to maintain it when we consider the frequent and almost ordinary occurrence of suicide in some countries' 'like the impulse to homicide, this propensity to suicide is simply a moral perversion,[55] and therefore neither of these affections fall within the restricted definition of insanity.'[56] Griesinger was equally balanced in his views: 'the pathological and aetiological history of suicide does not belong entirely to psychiatry; in fact, whatever some writers have said, we cannot conclude that suicide is always a symptom or a result of insanity.' [57]Bucknill and Tuke wrote: 'We have had occasion to remark that the act of self-destruction may originate in different, and even opposite conditions of mind. Hence, it is quite clear that the suicide act cannot always be properly referred to disorder of the same group of feelings' 'and here it may be observed, in regard to suicide in general, that the question so often asked *is suicide the result of cerebro-mental disease* [italics in original] must be answered both affirmatively and negatively. That the act may be committed in a perfectly healthy state of mind cannot, for a moment, be disputed.'[58]

Defenders of the 'psychiatric thesis'

During the first half of the nineteenth century there were, however, some whose views approached the caricature drawn by Durkheim; one such was Cazauvieilh when writing on 'rural' suicide.[59] This French alienist put forward the extreme view that there were three types of suicide and *all were psychiatric disorders*. In the purest Faculty Psychology tradition, he listed suicides resulting from disorders of thought, affection and volition (*délire de intelligence*, affections, and *actions*). 'Real' suicides, he defined as acts accompanied by willingness and clear consciousness. He considered as 'accidental' all deaths in the insane when there was no formed *intent* to die. Loyal to Esquirol, he defended a concept of monomania that, at the time, had already been called into question.[60] He considered suicide and homicide as related acts and reported sixteen post-mortem studies searching for the *siège de l'organe dont les souffrances portent au meurtre de soi-même*.[61]

The aftermath

By the 1880s, the psychiatric debate on whether suicide was *always* due to mental illness (the 'psychiatric' thesis) had been decided in favour of the view that it was not (the 'standard' view). Most alienists entertained a broad definition of suicide, and consequently all manner of 'social' events were accepted as potential causes.[62] Of this view many non-medical men – except perhaps, Durkheim – were aware: for example, Westcott[63] listed amongst the supporters of the standard view Blandford, Leuret, Gray, Bucknill and Tuke, Des Ètangs,[64] and Littré.[65] Morselli, whom no one could accuse of softness,[66] expressed a similar sentiment: 'just as madness may go on without any attempt at suicide, so the suicidal determination is formed in the healthiest of minds, which then carry it out with the coolness inspired by the most perfect logic.'[67] Brouc discussed suicide as a 'social event',[68] and Legoyt went as far as discussing the very social variables that played such an important role in Durkheim's argument.[69] The 'standard view' was carried without difficulty into the twentieth century.

In his assessment of the controversy between the psychiatric and standard views, Viallon restated that Ètoc-Demazy, Cerise, Belhomme, Chereau, Palmer and Gray 'had reacted with force against' the 'psychiatric thesis';[70] Pilcz agreed with Kraepelin that only thirty per cent of suicides seem to be related to diagnosable mental illness;[71] and Serin concluded, after a detailed survey, that 'a third [of suicides] were conceived and executed in the absence of psychopathology'.[72]

Things should have been allowed to rest there. With hindsight, it seems clear that much of the nineteenth century debate (including Durkheim's contribution), had been conceptual rather than empirical, i.e. resulted from confusion in regard to the definition of suicide; but after Durkheim's book, disagreement also resulted from the way in which 'social' was to be defined. It is beyond dispute that most nineteenth century alienists managed to include 'social' facts as causes of suicide. However, by the time of Durkheim, and probably as a result of his contribution, 'social fact' acquired a wider and more abstract meaning.[73] Analysis of this shift, which has to do with the gradual development of sociology during the nineteenth century, is beyond the scope of this chapter.

However, it seems as if, by the very end of the century, 'the social' had became accepted as a higher, irreducible, and omnipresent level of explanation.[74] This was good for sociology and for the professionalization of her practitioners, but created explanatory splits in a number of regions of reality, one of which was mental illness and suicide. Durkheim was, in a way, unfair to accuse early nineteenth century psychiatrists of not fully accepting the social explanation of suicide for, during that period, such concepts were not yet part of the intellectual *armamentarium* of alienists. For example, for Esquirol 'social' meant environmental in relation to specific individuals; he had little thought for general social laws. For Durkheim, on the other hand, it meant general, the result of objective laws equally applicable to all people. Whilst for Esquirol the 'dependent' variable for social explanations was the behaviour (e.g. suicide) of a given individual, for Durkheim it became the social facts themselves, as expressed in large group statistics.

And these differences became more obvious by the time the controversy flared up again in France in the 1930s. It started in 1926, with the publication by Maurice de Fleury[75] of an update of the 'psychiatric thesis' whose only new feature was the incorporation of the 'neuroses'. It must be remembered that up to the 1880s, 'mental disorder' basically referred to the 'insanities' (organic states, melancholia, etc.). Between this time and the 1930s, however, and thanks to the work of Janet, Freud and others, the neuroses[76] and the personality disorders were included under the rubric 'mental disorder'. When Fleury and Achille-Delmas[77] claimed that all suicides resulted from mental disorder, they meant by this both the old insanities and the new neurotic conditions, particularly the anxiety states. This is why, few years later, Deshaies felt able to claim that about one-third of the psychiatric causes of suicide fell into this latter category.[78]

Maurice Halbwachs replied in 1930 in a classical book that went further than Durkheim's in its re-affirmation of the 'social thesis' of suicide.[79] By Halbwachs's time, the 'social' explanation had become fully consolidated, and he had no difficulty in making the claim that all suicides were socially originated, including those in which alienists might show clear mental illness for, after all, *mental illness* was also social in origin. This claim, albeit legitimate from a conceptual point of view, did upset alienists then as much as it might upset some now; the reason for this being that psychiatrists always deal with individual cases, and grand social causes seems to be beyond their perception and remedial manipulation. Consequently, they deny or neglect their existence or try to re-define them in simpler and tangible ways. This is the explanation for Achille-Delmas' ill-tempered argument.[80] On occasions, his 1932 book is naive and conceptually uncouth but it only conveys the perplexity of a generation of alienists *vis á vis* the sociological explanation of suicide.

But one obvious thing to do, when faced with multiple levels of explanation, is blend them. This is precisely what Blondel, a man who since the 1910s had shown great sensitivity for the 'sociological'[81] did in his book of 1933.[82] He chastised

Achille-Demas for 'inventing a phrenology without organology'[83] and accused Halbwachs of resuscitating a needless conflict (*En cette querelle les partis extrêmes semblend tous deux dans leur tort*).[84] He wrote: 'in regard to suicide, it would be dangerous to reject the sociological explanation; but it would be equally dangerous not to acknowledge the role of the pathological which although it may have social causes and lead to social effects, *may not be social at all*.'[85] Whether or not Blondel was successful in his eclecticism remains to be seen. To many current clinicians, old issues such as the definition of suicide, the informational value of suicide statistics, and the ways in which these should be collected and interpreted[86] have not yet been solved; as has not the crucial question of whether they are susceptible to empirical solution.

ACKNOWLEDGEMENT To Dr M. Mohanna, Consultant Psychiatrist, Lincolnshire, for his invaluable help with the writing of sections of this chapter.

NOTES

1 See excellent chapter on suicide by professor John McManners, 1985; also MacDonald and Murphy, 1990; Rosen, 1971; Crocker, 1952; Doughty, 1926; Bartel, 1960; pp. 204–246, Fedden, 1938.
2 p. 296 in Mme la Baronne de Staël, 1820. This volume includes her *Réflexions sur le Suicide*. In 1821, Esquirol also commented about her change of mind: 'In the enthusiasm of youth, Madame de Staël seemed to have approved of suicide, later she recanted.' p. 241, Esquirol, 1821.
3 Cesare Bonesana, Marquis de Beccaria (1733–1781) was educated by the Jesuits and decided on a philosophical career after reading Montesquieu's *Lettres Persans*. He wrote *Dei delitti* when he was 25, and at the instigation of his friends who used to find him boring and sluggish. At the time he had read widely, and was influenced by Diderot, Helvetius, Voltaire, D'Alambert, Buffon, and Hume.
4 p. 89, Beccaria, 1868.
5 pp. 324–325, Lantéri-Laura Del Pistoia, 1970.
6 Berrios, On Historical aspects of the psychosis, 1987; Berrios, On Historical background to abnormal psychology, 1988.
7 McManners, 1985.
8 Blondel, 1933; Ey, On *Le suicide pathologique*, 1950.
9 Diderot and D'Alembert, Vol 14, 1765.
10 Schmitt, 1976.
11 Although of French origin, Dumas worked in Leipzig where he died in 1799. He also published literary criticism and poetry. His main work was: *Traité du Suicide ou du Meurtre Volontaire de soi-même*, 1773.
12 pp. 15–16 in Burton, 1790.
13 Bayet, 1922.
14 p. 326, Moore, 1790.
15 p. 329, Moore, 1790.

16 p. 326, Blackstone, 1775–1779.

17 Rosen, 1971.

18 Voisin, 1882; Krugelstein, 1841.

19 pp. 8–9, Saury, 1886.

20 These include Winslow, 1840; Lisle, 1856; Brierre de Boismont, 1856;
    Morselli, 1881.

21 p. 639, Esquirol, 1838.

22 Durkheim, 1897.

23 Halbwachs, 1930.

24 Achille-Delmas, 1932.

25 Giddens, 1978.

26 Berrios and Mohanna, 1990.

27 One of the earliest to recognize this was Griesinger, 1861. He first quoted
    Esquirol's well-known lines: 'I believe that I have proved that an
    individual will only put an end to his life when he is deluded, and that
    suicides are mentally diseased' (p. 183, Esquirol, 1838). Then he
    commented: 'Esquirol expresses himself *less absolutely* in other parts of the
    book' (my italics) (p. 256, Griesinger, 1861).

28 p. 269 Esquirol, 1821.

29 p. 214, Esquirol, 1821.

30 p. 214, Esquirol, 1821.

31 p. 655, Esquirol, 1838.

32 pp. 33-56, Blondel, 1933.

33 p. 55, Blondel, 1933.

34 Footnote 26, in Giddens, 1965: 'Esquirol himself did *allow that social factors*
    play a certain role in the aetiology of mental disorder and, consequently,
    suicide' (my italics). It is arguable whether this is the case.
        The issue here is, however, whether Esquirol felt that all individuals
    who had committed suicide were mentally disordered. I do not think he
    did, although he often stated that, during the act, suicidal persons are in
    an 'upset state of mind'; unfortunately, – like all alienists during his
    period – to refer to such disturbance of mind (however temporary) he used
    terms such as delusion, passion, or transient insanity; this gives the
    impression that he is talking about real madness.

35 See Cotard, 1878.

36 For this, see Esquirol: Délire, 1814.

37 p. 255, Esquirol, 1814.

38 On the role of the passions in the aetiology of mental disease, see Berrios,
    On The psychopathology of affectivity, 1985.

39 pp 42–43, Blondel, 1933.

40 Alexandre Jacques François Brierre de Boismont (1797–1881) was a
    prolific writer who published work on homicidal monomania, and
    hallucinations. In 1840, on account of his political views he lost the
    opportunity to replace Esquirol at the Charenton.

41 p. 135, Brierre de Boismont, 1856.

42 p. 181, Brierre de Boismont, 1856.

43 Gustave François Ètoc-Demazy (1806–1893) trained under Ferrus and

Pariset and wrote on stupor (see Chapter 16, this book), monomania, and medico-legal topics.

44 Ètoc-Demazy, 1844.

45 Bourdin, 1845. Bourdin was a rabid defender of the view that suicide was always a form of mental disease, and fits well into Durkheim's stereotypy. However, he was not an alienist, although he also wrote on catalepsy and alcoholism. He claimed that suicide was always a monomania: 'frequently, suicide was the earliest manifestation of monomania' (p. 8); thus the view that suicide was not pathological was based on 'incomplete observations' (p. 7). He also complained that 'it was legislators and philosophers who had criminalized the act of suicide' (p. 20): 'If I showed that suicide constitutes a real disease, that all its aspects, when considered in themselves and in their relationship and origins, are no different from the array of ordinary symptoms [of mental illness], I would have freed suicidal individuals from all culpability . . .' (p. 21). Bourdin's book is rambling, sententious, and obsolete in terms of clinical argument.

46 p. 347, Étoc-Demazy, 1846.

47 p. 362, Étoc-Demazy, 1846.

48 Lisle, 1856.

49 Falret, 1822.

50 Monomania was a diagnosis invented by Esquirol which achieved certain popularity, particularly in forensic psychiatry. It was never fully accepted by those not belonging to Esquirol's school and after severe attack during the 1950s, it gradually disappeared (Kageyama, 1984; Debate on Monomanie. SMP, 1854; Falret, De la non-existence de la monomanie, 1864; Linas, 1871).

51 Bertrand, 1857. Bertrand was well known in the USA (Kushner, 1986).

52 p. 56, Bertrand, 1857.

53 p. 219, Esquirol, 1838.

54 Emmanuel Françoise Fodéré (1764–1835) was a physician in the eighteenth century mould: he held vitalist principles and his views on insanity were an offshoot from his medico-legal preoccupations. He defined délire as a 'disease in which freedom had been lost'.

55 When used by alienists, 'moral' meant 'psychological', had little moralistic overtones, and carry no implication in regards to duration.

56 pp. 400–401, Prichard, 1835.

57 pp. 256–257, Griesinger, 1861.

58 pp. 201–203, Bucknill and Tuke, 1858.

59 Cazauvieilh, 1840. A disciple of Esquirol, and organicist au outrance, Cazauvieilh wrote a classical paper on epilepsy (see Berrios, Epilepsy and insanity during the 19th century, 1984). After leaving La Salpêtrière, he worked in various provincial hospitals until he settled in the asylum of Liancourt-Oise. He reported in his book suicide cases from four regions: Gironde, Landes, Seine and Oise.

60 p. v, Cazauvieilh, 1840.

61 p. 175, Cazauvieilh, 1840.

62 See, for example, masterly summaries by Morselli, 1881; Legoyt, 1884;

Ritti, 1884; also a Discussion on suicide and its psychiatric aspects. Various, 1898 and Strahan, 1893.

63 Westcott, 1885.
64 Des Ètangs, 1857.
65 Littré, 1881.
66 Guarnieri, 1988.
67 p. 272, Morselli, 1881.
68 Brouc, 1836.
69 Legoyt, 1884.
70 Viallon, 1901–1902.
71 Pilcz, 1908.
72 p. 358, Serin, 1926.
73 pp. 466 and ff, Durkheim, 1894.
74 Parain-Vial, 1966; pp. 1–38, Duverger, 1961.
75 Fleury, 1926.
76 For an account of the process of incorporation of the neurosis, see López Piñero and Morales Meseguer, 1970; also Oppenheim, 1991.
77 Achille-Delmas, 1932.
78 Deshaies, 1947.
79 Halbwachs, 1930. This author (1877–1945) died in a Nazi concentration camp.
80 Achille-Delmas, 1932.
81 Blondel, 1914; 1964. The second of these books shows Blondel's awareness of the work of Comte, Durkheim, Tarde, and Halbwachs. He had trained both under Lévy-Bruhl and Deny (the latter one of the great French alienists of the early twentieth century).
82 Blondel, 1933.
83 p. 132, Blondel, 1933.
84 p. 3, Blondel, 1933.
85 p. 4, Blondel, 1933.
86 See, for example, the old paper by Selvin, 1958; also Lester, 1994.

References

Aaron R.I. *John Locke*, London, Oxford University Press, 1965.

Aarsleff H. *The Study of Language in England 1780–1860*. Minneapolis, University of Minnesota Press, 1983.

Abbagnano N. *Dizionario di Filosofia*, Turin, Unione Tipografico Torinese, 1961.

Abeles M. and Schilder P. Psychogenic loss of personal identity. *Archives of Neurology and Psychiatry*, 1935, 34: 587–604.

Abely X. *Les Stéréotypies*. Thèse de Médecine, Université de Toulouse, 1916.

Abraham K. *Selected Papers*. Translated by D. Bryan and A. Strachey, London, Hogarth Press, 1942, pp. 64–79 (paper originally published in 1908).

Abrams R., Taylor M.A. and Stolurow K.A.C. Catatonia and mania, patterns of cerebral dysfunction. *Biological Psychiatry*, 1979, 14: 111–17.

Achille-Delmas F. *Psychologie Pathologique du Suicide*. Paris, Alcan, 1932.

Ackerknecht E. *Kurze Geschichte der Psychiatrie*, Stuttgart, Enke, 1957.

Ackerknecht E. Preface. In Griesinger W. *Mental Pathology and Therapeutics*, New York, Hafner Publishing Company, 1965.

Ackerknecht E. *Medicine at the Paris Hospital 1794–1848*, Baltimore, Johns Hopkins Press, 1967.

Adams R.D. and Victor M. *Principles of Neurology*, New York, McGraw-Hill, 1977.

Agassi J. *Toward an Historiography of Science. History and Theory*. Studies in the Philosophy of History. Beiheft 2, Wesleyan University Press, 1963.

Aguirre J.M. and Guimón J. (eds.) *Vida y Obra de Julián de Ajurriaguerra*. Madrid, Aran, 1992.

Ahlheid, A. Considerazione sull'esperienza nihilistica e sulla sindrome di Cotard nelle psicosi organiche e sintomatiche. *Il Lavoro Neuropsichiatrico*, 1968, 43: 927–45.

Ajuriaguerra J. de. The concept of akinesia. *Psychological Medicine*, 1975, 5: 129–37.

Ajuriaguerra J. de and Garrone G. Désafferentation partialle et psychopathologie. In *Désafferentation Expérimentale et Clinique* (Symposium Bel Air II) Geneva, Georg, pp. 91–157, 1965.

Ajuriaguerra J. de, Hécaen H., Lagani E. and Sadoni R. Maladie de Schilder-Fox, Étude anatomoclinique d'un cas. *Presse Médicale*, 1953, 61: 1756–9.

Akhtar S. and Brenner I. Differential diagnosis of fugue-like states. *Journal of Clinical Psychiatry*, 1979, 40: 381–5.

Akiskal H.S. Dysthmic disorders. *American Journal of Psychiatry*, 1983, 140: 11–20.

Akiskal H.S. and Weise R.W. The clinical spectrum of so-called 'minor' depressions. *American Journal of Psychotherapy*, 1992, 46: 9–22.

Akiskal H.S. and McKinney W. Depressive disorders: toward an unified hypothesis. *Science* 1972, 182: 20–9.

Akiskal H.S., Yerevanian B.I., Davis G.C., King D. and Lemmi H. The nosologic status of borderline personality: clinical and polysomnographic study. *American Journal of Psychiatry*, 1985, 142: 192–8.

Albarracín Teulón A. *La Teoria Celular. Historia de un Paradigma*. Madrid, Alianza Editorial, 1983.

Albert M.L. Subcortical dementia. In Katzman R., Terry R.D. and Bick K.L. (eds.) *Alzheimer's Disease*, New York, Raven Press, pp. 173–180, 1978.

Albrecht F.M. A re-appraisal of faculty psychology. *Journal of the History of Behavioral Science*, l970, 6: 36–40.

Albrecht T. Manischdepressives Irresein und Arteriosklerose. *Allgemeine Zeitschrift für Psychiatrie*, 1906, 63: 402–47.

Albury W.R. Experiment and explanation in the physiology of Bichat and Magendie. *Studies in the History of Biology*, 1977, 1: 47–131.

Alexander F.G. and Selesnick S.T. *The History of Psychiatry*. New York, Harper and Row, 1966.

Alexander M. D. *The Administration of Madness and Attitudes Towards the Insane in Nineteenth Century Paris*. Doctoral Dissertation, Johns Hopkins Press, Baltimore, 1976.

Allier R. *Les Défaillances de la Volonté au Temp Present*, Paris, Alcan, 1891.

Allier R. *The Mind of the Savage*, London, Bell, 1929.

Allport G.W. *Personality*, New York, Henry Holt, 1937.

Alonso Fernández F. *Fundamentos de la Psiquiatría Actual*, 2 vols (3rd edn.) Madrid, Editorial Paz Montalvo, 1977.

Alston W.P. Pleasure, in Edwards P. (ed.) *The Encyclopaedia of Philosophy* (Vol. 6). New York, Macmillan, 1967.

Altschule M.D. *The Development of Traditional Psychopathology*, New York, Wiley, 1976.

Alvarez A. and del Rio P. Prólogo a la edición en lengua castellana. in Vygotski L.S. *Obras Escogidas*. Vol. 1, Madrid, Centro de Publicaciones del M.E.C., 1991.

Alvarez-Uría F. *Miserables y Locos*. Barcelona, Tusquets, 1983.

Alzheimer A. Über eine eigenartige Erkrankung der Hirnrinde. *Allgemeine Zeitschrift für Psychiatrie und Psychisch-Gerichtlich Medizine*, 1907, 64: 146–8.

Alzheimer A. Über eigenartige Krankheitsfälle des späteren Alters. *Zeitschrift für die gesamte Neurologie und Psychiatrie*, 1911, 4: 356–85.

American Psychiatric Association. *Diagnostic and Statistical Manual of Mental Disorders* (third edn.). Washington DC, APA, 1980.

American Psychiatric Association. *Diagnostic and Statistical Manual of Mental Disorders*. Third Edition, Revised. Washington. DC. American Psychiatric Association, 1987.

American Psychiatric Association: *Diagnostic and Statistical Manual of Mental Disorders*. Fourth Edition. Washington. DC. American Psychiatric Association, 1994.

Anderson E.W., Threthowan W.H. and Kenna J.C. An experimental investigation of simulation and pseudodementia. *Acta Psychiatrica et Neurologica Scandinavica*, 1959, 34 (Supplement 132): 5–42.

Andral (no initial). Amnesie *Dictionnaire de Médicine*, Paris, Gabon, pp. 166–169, 1829.

Andreasen N.C. Should the term 'thought disorder' be revised? *Comprehensive Psychiatry*, 1982, 23: 291–9.

Angell J.R. Pleasure, in Baldwin J.M. (ed.): *Dictionary of Philosophy and Psychology*. London, Macmillan, 1901.

Anonymous. An exposure of the unphilosophical and unchristian expedients adopted by antiphrenologists, for the purpose of obstructing the moral tendencies of phrenology. A review of John Wayte's Book. *The Phrenological Journal and Miscellany*, 1832, 7: 615–22.

Anonymous. Nervousness. *Journal of Psychological Medicine and Mental Pathology*, 1860, 13: 218–33.

Anonymous. Luigi Luciani. *Rivista de Patologia Nerviosa e Mentale*, 1919, 24: 256.

Anonymous. Augusto Tamburini. *Rivista de Patologia Nerviosa e Mentale*, 1919, 24: 255–6.

Anonymous. Catalepsia. *Enciclopedia Universal Illustrada Europeo-Americana*, Vol. 12, Bilbao, Espasa-Calpe, 1921.

Anonymous. Confusión. *Enciclopedia Universal Illustrada Europeo-Americana*, Vol. 14, Madrid, Espasa-Calpe, pp. 1198–2000, 1921.

Anonymous. Fatiga. *Enciclopedia Universal Ilustrada Europeo-Americana*, Vol. 23, pp. 376–380, Bilbao, Espasa-Calpe, 1921.

Anonymous. Personalidad. *Enciclopedia Universal Illustrada* Europeo-Americana, Vol. 43, Bilbao, Espasa-Calpe, pp. 1173–1184, 1921.

Anonymous. Mosso A. *Enciclopedia Universal Illustrada Europeo-Americana*, Vol. 36, Barcelona, Hijos de Espasa, pp. 1317–1318, 1923.

Anonymous. Visión Beatífica y Visionario. *Enciclopedia Universal Illustrada Europeo-Americana*, Vol. 69, Bilbao, Espasa-Calpe, pp. 435–443, 1930.

Anonymous. Editorial. Epidemic myalgic encephalomyelitis. *British Medical Journal*, 1978, i: 1436–7

Anonymous. On the influence of Unzer on Crichton. *Journal of Psychological Medicine and Mental Pathology* 1854, 7: 519.

Apel K.-O. Dilthey's distinction between 'explanation' and 'understanding' and the possibility of its 'mediation'. *Journal of the History of Philosophy*, 1987, 25: 131–49.

Arbousse-Bastide P. Auguste Comte et la Folie. In Bastide R. (ed.) *Les Sciences de la Folie*, Paris, Mouton, pp. 47–72, 1972.

Arieti S. Discussion of Rado's theory and therapy: the theory of schizotypal organization and its application to the treatment of decompensated schizotypal behaviour. In Scher S.C. and Davis H.R. (eds.): *The Outpatient Treatment of Schizophrenia*. New York, Grune and Straton, 1960.

Arieti S. *The Interpretation of Schizophrenia*. New York, Basic Books, 1974.

Aristotle. *De Anima*, Books II and III (translated by D.W. Hamlyn) Oxford, Clarendon Press, 1968.

Aristotle. Nicomachean ethics. In Barnes J. (ed.), *The Complete Works of Aristotle*. Princeton, Princeton University Press, 1984.

Aristotle. *Parva Naturalia* (translated by W.S. Hett) Loeb Classical Library, London, Heinemann, 1986.

Arkes H.R. and Garske J.P. *Psychological Theories of Motivation*, California, Brooks, 1977.

Armstrong D.M. *Bodily Sensations*, London, Routledge and Kegan Paul, 1962.

Arnaud. F.L. Sur le délire des negations. *Annales Médico-Psychologiques*, 1892, 50:387–403.

Arnaud M. Un cas d'illusion de 'déjà vu' ou de 'fausse mémoire'. *Annales Médico-Psychologiques*, 1896, 54: 455–71.

Arnaud S. La Senescenza Precoce nei Melancolici. *Rivista di Patologia Nervosa e Mentale*, 1899, 4: 362–7.

Arndt E. Über die Geschichte der Katatonie. *Centralblatt für Nervenheilkunde und Psychiatrie*, 1902, 25: 81–121.

Arnold T. *Observations on the Nature, Kinds, Causes, and Preventions of Insanity, Lunacy, or Madness*, Vol. 1, Leicester, G. Ireland, 1782.

Arnold T. *Observations on the Nature, Kinds, Causes and Prevention, of Insanity*, 2nd edn., London, Phillips, 1806.

Duran, pp. 785–789, 1754.

Arondel A. *Sur les Hallucinations des Moignons*, Paris, Doin, 1898.

Aronson T.A. Historical perspectives on the borderline concept: a review and critique. *Psychiatry*, 1985, 48: 209–22.

Asso D., Crown S., Russell J.A. and Logue V. Psychological aspects of the stereotactic treatment of Parkinsonism. *British Journal of Psychiatry*, 1969, 115: 541–3.

Astruc P. Les Sciences Médicales et leurs representants dans *L'Encyclopédie*. *Revue d'Histoire des Sciences*, 1950, 3: 359–68.

Atkins R. A case of paralysis agitans in which insanity occurred. *Journal of Mental Science*, 1882, 28: 534–6.

Atlas S. Salomon Maimon. In Edwards P. (ed.) *The Encyclopedia of Philosophy*, Vol. 5, New York, McMillan, 1967.

Aubanel H. *Essai sur les Hallucinations*, Thèse de la Faculté de Médecine de Paris N° 343, submitted on 21st August 1839.

Aubrun W.P.A.J. *L'État Mental des Parkinsoniens. Contribution a son Étude Expérimentale*, Paris, Baillière, 1937.

Aubrun W.P.A.J. Résponses aux emotions-chocs chez les Parkinsoniens. *Année Psychologique*, 1937, 37: 140–71.

Augustine. *Confessions and Enchiridion.* (translated and edited by A.C. Outler) Library of Christian Classics, Vol. VII, London, Westminster Press, 1955.

Austin J.L. *How to do Things with Words*, Oxford, Clarendon Press, 1962.

Aveling F. The psychology of conation and volition. *British Journal of Psychology*, 1925, 16: 339–53.

Axenfeld A. *Traité des Névroses*, 2nd edn., Paris, Baillière, 1883.

Azam E. Amnésie périodique. *Annales Médico-Psychologiques*, 1876, 34: 5–35.

Azam E. Le caractére dans les maladies. *Annales Médico-Psychologiques*, 1885, 43: 386–406.

Azouvi F. Des sensations internes aux hallucinations corporelles: de Cabanis a Lélut. *Revue Internationale d'Histoire de la Psychiatrie*, 1984, 2: 5–19.

Baars B.J. *A Cognitive Theory of Consciousness*. Cambridge, Cambridge University Press, 1988.

Babinski J. Définition de l'hystérie. *Société de Neurologie de Paris*, Séance of 7th November 1901. *Ouvres Scientifiques* Paris, Masson, pp. 457–464, 1934.

Bachelard G. *La formation de l'esprit scientifique*. Paris, Vrin, 1938.

Bacon C.E. Visual pseudo-hallucinations: psychotherapy case study of a long-standing perceptual disorder. *Psychopathology* 1991, 24: 361–4.

Bacon, F. *The Physical and Metaphysical Works*. London, Bohn, 1858.

Bagenoff T. La cyclothymie. In Marie A. (ed.) *Traité International de Psychologie Pathologique-* Vol. 2, Paris, Alcan, pp. 709–722, 1911.

Baguenier-Desormeaux A. Étude sur le traitement moral et ses origines philosophiques. *Mémoire pour le C.E.S. de Psychiatrie*, Ronéot, Angers, 1983.

Baillarger J. De l'ètat désigné chez les aliénés sous le nom de stupidité. *Annales Médico-Psychologiques*, 1843, 1: 76, 256.

Baillarger J. Des hallucinations. *Mémoires de l'Académie Royale de Médecine*, 1846, 12: 273–475.

Baillarger J. Doit-on dans la classification des maladies mentales assigner une place á part aux pseudo-paralysies générales? *Annales Médico-Psychologiques*, 1889, 41: 521–5.

Baillarger J. De la mélancolie avec stupeur. *Annales Médico-Psychologiques*, 1853, 5: 251–76.

Baillarger J. De la folie á double-forme. *Annales Médico-Psychologiques*, 1854, 6: 367–91.

Baillarger J. La théorie de l'automatisme étudiée dans le manuscrit d'un monomaniaque. *Annales Médico-Psychologiques*, 1856, 2: 54–63.

Baillarger J. Note sur le délire hypochondriaque considerée comme symptome et comme signe précurseur de la paralysie générale. *Annales Médico-Psychologiques*, 1860, 6: 509–14.

Baillarger J. Sur la théorie de la paralysie générale. *Annales Médico-Psychologiques*, 1883, 35: 18–52; 191–218.

Baillarger J. Physiologie des hallucinations: les deux theories. *Annales Médico-Psychologiques*, 1886, 4: 19–39.

Bain A. *The Emotions and the Will*, London, Longmans, Green and Co., 1859.

Bain A. *The Senses and the Intellect*, second edition, London, Longman, Green, Longman, Roberts, and Green, 1864.

Bain A. The feelings and the will viewed physiologically. *Fortnightly Review*, 1866, 3: 375–88.

Bain A. *Mind and Body: The Theories of their Relationship*, London, Henry S. King, 1874.

Bain A. *The Emotions and the Will*, second edition, London, Longmans, Green and Co., 1875.

Bain A. *Dissertations on Leading Philosophical Topics*. London, Longmans, Green and Co., 1903.

Balan B. Sur le role de l'imaginaire dans la pratique psychiatrique au XIX Siècle. *Revue d'Histoire des Sciences et de Leurs Applications*, l972, 25: 171–90.

Balan B. Les fondements psychologiques de la notion d'automatism mental chez John Hughlings Jackson. *L'Information Psychiatrique*, 1989, 69: 610–19.

Baldwin J.M. *Dictionary of Philosophy and Psychology* New York, MacMillan, 1901.

Ball B. De la torpeur cérébrale. *L'Encéphâle*, 1881, 1: 369–78.

Ball B. De l'insanité dans la paralysie agitante. *L'Encéphâle*, 1882, 2: 22–32.

Ball B. *Leçons sur les Maladies Mentales*. Second Edition, Paris, Asselin et Houzeau, 1890 (first edition 1880).

Ball B. Des obsessions en pathologie mentale *Annales de Psychiatrie et d'Hypnologie*, 1892, 2: 1–15.

Ball B. and Chambard E. Délire aigu. In Dechambre A. and Lereboullet L. (eds.) *Dictionnaire Encyclopédique des Sciences Médicales*. Vol. 26, Paris, Masson, pp. 408–434, 1881.

Ball B. and Chambard E. Démence. In Dechambre A. and Lereboullet L. (eds.) *Dictionnaire Encyclopédique des Sciences Médicales*, Vol. 26, Paris, Masson, pp. 559–635, 1881.

Ball B. and Ritti E. Délire. In Dechambre A. and Lereboullet L. (eds.) *Dictionnaire Encyclopédique des Sciences Médicales*, Vol. 26, Paris, Masson, pp. 315–434, 1881.

Ballet G. Contribution a l'étude de l'état mental des héréditaires dégénérés. *Archives Générales de Médecine*, 1881, 21: 257–75; 427–41.

Ballet G. *Le Langage Intérieur et les Diverses Forms de L'Aphasie*. Paris, Alcan, 1886.

Banister H. and Zangwill O.L. John Thompson McCurdy (1886–1947). *British Journal of Psychology*, 1949, 40: 1–4.

Bannour W. *Jean-Martin Charcot et l'Hystérie*, Paris, Métailié, 1992.

Barbé, A. Idées de négation dans la senilité. *L'Encéphale*, 1912, 7: 557–8.

Barbeau A. The understanding of involuntary movements: an historical approach. *Journal of Nervous and Mental Disease*, 1958, 127: 469–89.

Barnes B. *Scientific Knowledge and Sociological Theory*. London, Routledge and Kegan Paul, 1972.

Barnett S.A. The 'Expression of the Emotions'. In Barnett S.A. (ed.): *A Century of Darwin*, London, Mercury Books, pp. 206–230, l962.

Barr M.W. *Mental Defectives, their History, Treatment and Training*. Philadelphia, Blackiston's Son and Co., 1904.

Barrett A.M. Presenile, arteriosclerotic and senile disorders of the brain and cord. In White W.A. and Jellife S.A. (eds.): *The Modern Treatment of Nervous and Mental Diseases*, London, Kimpton, pp. 675–709, 1913.

Barrough P. *The Methods of Physicke*, London, Vautrollier, 1583.

Barrucand D. *Histoire de L'Hypnose en France*, Paris, Presses Universitaires de France, 1967.

Bartel R. Suicide in 18th century England. *Huntington Library Quarterly*, 1960, 23: 145–58.

Bartels I. Über Wortneubildung bei Geisteskranken. *Allgemeine Zeitschrift für Psychiatrie*, 1888, 45: 598–661.

Bartenwerfer H.G. *Beiträge zum Problem der psychischen Beanspruchung*, Cologne, Opladen, 1960.

Barthes R. Sémiologie et Médicine, in Bastide R. (ed.) *Les Sciences de la Folie*, Paris, Mouton, pp. 37–46, 1972.

Bartley S.H. and Chute E. *Fatigue and Impairment in Man*, New York, McGraw Hill, 1947.

Baruk H. Automatisme et troubles des mécanismes de la pensée intérieure dans la psychiatrie française et dans la psychologie interprétative de Freud. In Bastide R. (ed.) *Les Sciences de la Folie*, Paris, Mouton, 1972.

Baruk H. *La Psychiatrie Française de Pinel á nos Jours*, Paris, Presses Universitaires de France, 1967.

Baruk H., Launay J. and Berges K. Experimental catatonia and psychopathology of neuroleptics. *Journal of Clinical and Experimental Psychopathology*, 1958, 19: 277–91.

Bash K.W. *Lehrbuch der allgemeinen Psychopathologie. Grundbegriffe und Klinik*, Stuttgart, George Thième, 1955.

Bastian Ch. On the neural processes underlying attention and volition. *Brain*, 1892, 15: 1–34.

Bastian H.C. Consciousness. *Journal of Mental Science*, 1870, 15: 501–23.

Bateman Sir F. *The Idiot: his Place in Creation and his Claims on Society*, 2nd edn., London, Jarrold and Sons, 1902.

Battie W.A. *Treatise on Madness*, London, J. Whiston and B. White, 1758.

Baudry F.D. The evolution of the concept of character in Freud's writings. *Journal of the American Psychoanalytic Association*, 1983, 31: 3–31.

Baur E., Fischer E. and Lenz F. *Menschliche Erblichkeitslehre und Rasenhygiene*, Munich, Springer, 1927.

Bayet A. *Le Suicide et la Morale*, Paris, Alcan, 1922.

Bayfield R. *A Treatise de Morborum Capitis Essentiis et Prognosticis*, London, Tomlins, 1663.

Bayle A.L.J. *Recherches sur les Maladies Mentales*, Paris, Thèse de Médecine, 1822.

Bayle A.L.J. *Traité des Maladies du Cerveau*. Paris, Gabon et Compagnie, 1826.

Beaugrand E. Alienation. In Dechambre A. and Lereboullet L. (eds.) *Dictionnaire Encyclopédique des Sciences Médicales*. Vol. 3, Paris, Masson, pp. 11–50, 1865.

Beauroy R. Rêve et délire: une révision. *L'Evolution Psychiatrique*, 1973, 38: 693–722.

Beaussire E. La personnalité humaine d'après les théories récents. *Revue de Deux Mondes*, 1883, 55: 316–61.

Beccaria C. *De los Delitos y de las Penas* (translated by Juan Antonio de las Casas) Madrid, Alianza, 1868 (first published, 1764).

Bech P. Quality of life in psychosomatic research. A psychometric model. *Psychopathology*, 1987, 20: 169–79.

Beck A.T. *Depression: Clinical, Experimental and Theorical Aspects*. New York, Hoeber, 1967.

Beck A.T. The development of depression: a cognitive model, in Friedman R, Katz M. (eds.) *The Psychology of Depression: Contemporary Theory of Research*. Silver Spring Md, Winston and Sons, 1974.

Beckmann H. and Zimmer R. Durch Außenreiz induzierte Stereotypie in ethologischer Sich. *Archiv für Psychiatrie und Nervenkrankheiten*, 1981, 230: 81–9.

Bédard P., Larochelle L., Poirier L.J. and Sourkes T.L. Reversible effects of L-dopa on tremor and catatonia Induced by α-methyl-*p*-tyrosine. *Canadian Journal of Physiology and Pharmacology*, 1970, 48: 82–6.

Bedford E. Emotions. In Gustafson D.F. (ed.) *Essays in Philosophical Psychology*, London, McMillan, pp. 77–98, 1964.

Beebe-Center J.G. Feeling and emotion. In Helson H. (ed.) *Theoretical Foundations of Psychology*, New York, Nostrand, pp. 142–175, 1951.

Bcech H.R. (cd.) *Obsessional States*, London, Methuen, 1974.

Behan P.O., Behan W.M.H. and Bell E.J. The post-viral fatigue syndrome. *Journal of Infections*, 1985, 10: 211–22.

Behr F., Croq L. and Vauterin C. Sémiologie des conduites de fugue. *Encyclopédie Médico-Chirurgicale* (Paris) Psychiatrie, 37113 A10, 2, 1985.

Beljahow S. Pathological changes in the brain in dementia senilis. *Journal of Mental Science*, 1889, 35: 261–62.

Bell Sir C. *The Anatomy and Philosophy of Expression, as connected with the Fine Arts*. 3rd edn., London, John Murray, 1844 (1st edn., 1806).

Bell Sir C. *The Nervous System of the Human Body*, London, Longman, 1830.

Benedikt M. Über Platzschwindel. *Allgemeine Wiener Medizinische Zeitung*, 1870, 15: 488–90.

Benedikt M. *Aus meinem Leben. Erinnerungen und Errterungen*, Wien, Konegen, 1906.

Beneke F.W. *Konstitution und Konstitutionelles kranksein des Menschen*, Marbourg, Elwert, 1881.

Benon R. Les ictus amnésiques. *Annales Médico-Psychologiques*, 1909, 67: 207–19.

Benon R. *La Mélancolie*, Paris, Marcel Vigné, 1937.

Benon R. and Froissart P. Fugue et vagabondage. Définition et étude clinique. *Annales Médico-Psychologiques*, 1908, 66: 305–12.

Benon R. and Froissart P. Les fugues en pathologie mentale. *Journal de Psychologie Normale et Pathologique*, 1909, 6: 293–330.

Benrubi J. *Les Sources et les Courants de la Philosophie Contemporaine en France*, Paris, Alcan, 1933.

Benson D.F. Psychiatric aspects of aphasia. *British Journal of Psychiatry*, 1973, 123: 555–66.

Bentall R.P., Kaney S. and Dewey M.E. Paranoia and social reasoning: an attribution theory analysis. *British Journal of Clinical Psychology*, 1991, 30: 13–23.

Benton A.L., Allen M.W. van and Fogel M.L. Temporal orientation in cerebral disease. *Journal Nervous Mental Disease*, 1964, 139: 110–19.

Bercherie P. *Les fondements de la clinique. Histoire et structure du savoir psychiatrique*. La Bibliotheque d'Ornicar, Paris, 1980.

Bercherie P. *Genèse des Concepts Freudians*, Paris, Navarin, 1983.

Bercherie P. *Géographie du Champ Psychanalytique*, Paris, Navarin, 1988.

Berger K. Über die Psychosen des Klimakteriums. *Monatschrift für Psychiatrie und Neurologie*, 1907, 22: 13–52.

Bergeron M. Fugues. In *Encyclopédie Médico-Chirurgicale*. Psychiatrie, 37140 E10, 1956.

Bergmann J. Der Begriff des Deseins und das Ich-Bewusstseins. *Archiv für systematische Philosophie* 1896, 2: 145–73; 289–316.

Berliner Medicinisch-psychologische Gesellschaft *Berliner klinische Wochenschrift*, 1877, 14: 706–708; 720–22.

Berman L. *The Glands Regulating the Personality*, New York, McMillan, 1922.

Bernard P. and Trouvé, S. *Sémiologie Psychiatrique*, Paris, Masson, 1977.

Bernard-Leroy E. *L'Illusion de Fausse Reconnaissance. Contribution a l'étude des conditions psychologiques de la reconnaissance des souvenirs*. Paris, Alcan, 1898.

Bernard-Leroy E. Sur l'illusion dite 'dépersonnalisation'. *Revue Philosophique*, 1898, 46: 157–62.

Berner P. and Naske R. Wahn. In Müller Ch. (ed.), *Lexicon der Psychiatrie*. Heidelberg, Springer, 1973.

Bernheim H. *Automatisme et Suggestion*, Paris, Alcan, 1917.

Bernt-Larsson H. Über das Déjà vu und andere Täuschungen des Bekanntheitsgefühls. *Zeitschrift für der gesamte Neurologie und Psychiatrie*, 1931, 133: 521–39.

Bernutz. (no initial) Amnesie *Noveau Dictionnaire de Médicine*, Vol. 2, Paris Baillière, pp. 52–56, 1865.

Berrington W.P., Liddell D.W. and Foulds G.A. A re-evaluation of the fugue. *Journal of Mental Science*, 1956, 102: 280–6.

Berrios G.E. Delirium and confusion in the 19th century: a conceptual history. *British Journal of Psychiatry*, 1981, 139: 439–49.

Berrios G.E. Stupor revisited. *Comprehensive Psychiatry*, 1981, 22: 466–78.

Berrios G.E. The two manias. *British Journal of Psychiatry*, 1981, 139: 258–9.

Berrios G.E. Stupor: a conceptual history. *Psychological Medicine*, 1981, 11: 677–88.

Berrios G.E. Tactile hallucinations: conceptual and historical aspects. *Journal of Neurology, Neurosurgery and Psychiatry*, 1982, 45: 285–93.

Berrios G.E. Orientation failures in medicine and psychiatry. *Journal of the Royal Society of Medicine*, 1983, 76, 249–56.

Berrios G.E. Descriptive psychopathology: conceptual and historical aspects. *Psychological Medicine*, 1984, 14: 303–13.

Berrios G.E. Epilepsy and insanity during the 19th century. A conceptual history. *Archives of Neurology*, 1984, 41: 978–81.

Berrios G.E. Delusional parasitosis and physical disease. *Comprehensive Psychiatry*, 1985, 26: 395–403.

Berrios G.E. 'Depressive pseudodementia' or 'melancholic dementia': a 19th century view. *Journal of Neurology, Neurosurgery and Psychiatry*, 1985, 48: 393–400.

Berrios G.E. Hallucinosis. In Frederiks J.A.M. (ed.), *Handbook of Clinical Neurology, Vol. 46, Neurobehavioural Disorders*, Amsterdam, Elsevier, pp. 561–572, 1985.

Berrios G.E. Obsessional disorders during the nineteenth century. In Bynum W.F., Porter R. and Shepherd M. (eds.) *The Anatomy of Madness*, Vol. 1, London, Tavistock, pp. 166–187, 1985.

Berrios G.E. Positive and negative symptoms and Jackson. *Archives of General Psychiatry*, 1985, 42: 95–7.

Berrios G.E. Presbyophrenia: clinical aspects. *British Journal of Psychiatry*, 1985, 147: 76–9.

Berrios G.E. Presbyophrenia: the rise and fall of a concept. *Psychological Medicine*, 1986, 16: 267–75.

Berrios G.E. The psychopathology of affectivity. conceptual and historical aspects. *Psychological Medicine* 1985, 15: 745–58

Berrios G.E. Dementia during the seventeenth and eighteenth centuries: a conceptual history. *Psychological Medicine*, 1987, 17: 829–37.

Berrios G.E. Historical aspects of the psychoses: 19th century issues. *British Medical Bulletin*, 1987, 43: 484–98.

Berrios G.E. Introduction to Eugen Bleuler. In Thompson C. (ed.) *The Origins of Modern Psychiatry*, New York, Wiley, pp. 200–209, 1987.

Berrios G.E. Depressive and manic states during the nineteenth century. In Georgotas A. and Cancro R. (eds.) *Depression and Mania*, New York, Elsevier, pp. 13–25, 1988.

Berrios G.E. and Hauser R. The early development of Kraepelin's ideas on classification: a conceptual history. *Psychological Medicine*, 1988, 18: 813–21.

Berrios G.E. Historical background to abnormal psychology. In Miller E. and Cooper J. (eds.) *Adult Abnormal Psychology*, Edinburgh, Churchill Livingstone, pp. 26–51, 1988.

Berrios G.E. Melancholia and depression during the 19th century. *British Journal of Psychiatry*, 1988, 153: 298–304.

Berrios G.E. Non-cognitive symptoms and the diagnosis of dementia. Historical and clinical aspects. *British Journal of Psychiatry*, 1989, 154 (suppl. 4): 11–16.

Berrios G.E. Obsessive–compulsive disorder: its conceptual history in France during the 19th Century. *Comprehensive Psychiatry*, 1989, 30: 283–95.

Berrios G.E. Alzheimer's disease: a conceptual history. *International Journal of Geriatric Psychiatry*, 1990; 5: 355–65.

Berrios G.E. Feelings of fatigue and psychopathology. *Comprehensive Psychiatry*, 1990, 31: 140–51.

Berrios G.E. Melancholic stupor: a conceptual history. In Stephanis C.N., Soldatos C.R. and Rabavilas T. (eds.) *Psychiatry: A World Perspective*, Vol. 4, Amsterdam, Excerpta Medica, pp. 918–27, 1990.

Berrios G.E. Memory and the cognitive paradigm of dementia during the 19th century: a conceptual history. In Murray R.M. and Turner T.H. (eds.) *Lectures on the History of Psychiatry*, London, Gaskell, pp. 194–211, 1990.

Berrios G.E. A theory of hallucinations. *History of Psychiatry* 1990, 1: 145–50.

Berrios G.E. Affective disorders in old age: a conceptual history. *International Journal of Geriatric Psychiatry*, 1991, 6: 337–46.

Berrios G.E. British psychopathology since the early 20th century. In Berrios G.E. and Freeman H. (eds.): *150 years of British Psychiatry 1841–1991*, London, Gaskell, pp. 232–44, 1991.

Berrios G.E. Delusions as 'wrong beliefs': a conceptual history. *British Journal of Psychiatry*, 1991, 159 (Suppl. 14): 6–13.

Berrios G.E. Positive and negative signals: a conceptual history. In Marneros A., Andreasen N.C. and Tsuang M.T. (eds.), *Negatives versus Positive Schizophrenia*, Berlin, Springer, pp. 8–27, 1992.

Berrios G.E. Phenomenology, psychopathology and Jaspers: a conceptual history. *History of Psychiatry*, 1992, 3: 303–27.

Berrios G.E. and Chen E. Recognising psychiatric symptoms: relevance to the diagnostic process. *British Journal of Psychiatry*, 1993, 163: 308–14.

Berrios G.E European views on personality disorders: a conceptual history. *Comprehensive Psychiatry*,1993, 34: 14–30.

Berrios G.E. A conceptual history in the nineteenth century. In Copeland J., Abou-Saleh M. and Blazer D. (eds.), *Principles and Practice of Geriatric Psychiatry*, Chichester, Wiley, pp. 11–16, 1994.

Berrios G.E. History of Parkinson's disease. In Berrios G.E. and Porter R. (eds.) *A History of Clinical Psychiatry*, London, Athlone Press, pp. 95–112, 1995.

Berrios G.E. and Luque R. Cotard's delusion or syndrome? A conceptual history. *Comprehensive Psychiatry* 1995, 36:218–223.

Berrios G.E. and Beer D. The notion of unitary psychosis: a conceptual history. *History of Psychiatry*, 1994, 5: 13–36.

Berrios G.E. and Freeman H. (eds.) *Alzheimer and the Dementias*, London, Royal Society of Medicine, 1991.

Berrios G.E., Henri Ey, Jackson et les idées obsédantes. *L'Evolution Psychiatrique*, 1977, 62: 685–99.

Berrios G.E. and Morley S. Koro-like symptoms in non-Chinese subjects. *British Journal of Psychiatry*, 1984, 145: 331–4.

Berrios G.E. and Quemada, J.I. Andre Ombredane and the psychiatry of multiple sclerosis: a conceptual and statistical history. *Comprehensive Psychiatry*, 1990, 31: 438–48.

Berrios G.E. and Mohanna M. Durkheim and French views on suicide during the 19th century. *British Journal of Psychiatry*, 1990, 156: 1–9.

Berrios G.E. Hallucinations: selected historical and clinical aspects. In Critchley E.M.R. (ed.) *The Neurological Boundaries of Reality*. London, Farrand Press, pp. 229–50, 1994.

Berrios G.E. Historiography of mental symptoms and diseases. *History of Psychiatry* 1994, 5: 175–90.

Berrios G.E., Marková I.S. and Olivares J.M. Retorno a los sítomas meutales: hacia una nueva metateoría *Psiquiatría Biologica*, 1995, 2:13–24.

Berrios G.E. and Porter R. (eds.) *The History of Clinical Psychiatry*. London, Athlone Press, 1995.

Berrios G.E., Gairin, I. and Fuentenebro F. Statistical Analysis of Janet's 234 cases of Psychasthenia, 1996 (in press).

Berrios G.E. and Luque R. Cotard's syndrome: analysis of 100 cases. *Acta Psychiatrica Scandinavica*.

Berthier M. Note. *Annales Médico-Psychologiques*, 1869, 27: 58.

Bertolini M.M. *Il Pensiero e la Memoria. Filosofia e Psicologia nella 'Revue Philosophique' de Théodule Ribot (1876–1916)*, Parma, Angeli, 1991.

Bertrand A. *La Psychologie de l'Effort et Les Doctrines Contemporaines*, Paris, Alcan, 1889.

Bertrand L. *Traité du Suicide Considéré dans ses Rapports avec la Philosophie, la Théologie, la Médicine, et la Jurisprudence*, Paris, Baillière, 1857.

Berze J. *Die Primäre Insuffizienz der psychischen Aktivität*, Leipzig, Deuticke, 1914.

Bessière R. La presbyophrénie. *L'Encéphale*, 1948, 37: 313–42.

Bessière T. Les stéréotypies démentielles. *Annales Médico-Psychologiques*, 1906, 64: 206–13.

Bevan-Lewis. *Textbook of Mental Diseases*. London, Charles Griffin and Co, 1899.

Bianchi L.A. *Textbook of Psychiatry*, London, Baillière, Tindall and Cox, 1906.

Bick P.A. The syndrome of intermetamorphosis. In Christodoulou G.N. (ed.) *The Misin-dentification Syndromes*, Basel, Karger, pp. 131–135, 1986.

Biervliet J.J. van Observations et documents sur les paramnésies. *Revue Philosophique*, 1894, 38: 47–9.

Billod E. Maladies de la volonté. *Annales Médico-Psychologiques*, 1847, 10: 15–35; 170–202; 317–47.

Billod E. Des Diverses formes de lypémanie. *Annales Médico-Psychologiques*, 1856, 2: 308–38.

Billod E. De la lésion de l'association des idées. *Annales Médico-Psychologiques*, 1855, 18: 540–52.

Binet A. *Les Altérations de la Personnalité*, Paris, Alcan, 1892.

Binet A. Review of: la psychologie des sentiments. *Psychological Review* 1896, 3: 673–7.

Binet A. and Simon Th. Sur la nécessité d'établir un diagnostic scientifique des états inférieurs de l'intelligence. *L'Année Psychologique*, 1905, 11: 163–90.

Binet A. and Simon Th. Définition des principaux états mentaux de l'aliénation. *L'Année Psychologique*, 1910, 16: 61–371.

Binet A. and Simon Th. L'arriération. *L'Année Psychologique*, 1910, 16: 349–60.

Binet A. and Simon Th. La confusion mentale. *L'Année Psychologique*, 1911, 17: 278–300.

Bing R. Über einige bemerkenswerte Begleitersscheinungen der extrapyramidalen Rigidität (Akathisie, Mikrographie, Kinesia Paradoxa). *Schweitzer medizinische Wochenschrift*, 1923, 53: 167–71.

Bing R. *Tratado de las enfermedades nerviosas*. 3rd edn. Translated into Spanish by M. Montaner and M. Montaner-Toutain. Barcelona, Usón, 1925.

Biographie Universelle Ancienne et Moderne, ou Dictionnaire de tous les Hommes, Vol. 13, Bruxelles, H Ode, 1843–1847.

Black S.E. Pseudopods and synapses: the amoeboid theories of neuronal mobility and the early formulation of the synapse concept. *Bulletin of the History of Medicine*, 1981, 55: 34–58.

Blackstone W. *Commentaries on the Laws of England*, London, 1775–1779 (quotation taken from the 15th Edition).

Blair D. The medicolegal implications of the terms 'psychopath', 'psychopathic personality' and 'psychopathic disorder'. *Medicine, Science and Law*, 1975, 15: 51–61; 110–23.

Blakey R. *History of the Philosophy of the Human Mind*, 4 vols., London, Longman, Brown, Green and Longmans, 1850.

Blankenburg W. Anankastische Psychopathie. In Müller Ch. (ed.) *Lexicon der Psychiatrie*, Berlin, Springer, pp. 406–7, 1973.

Blankenburg W. (ed.) *Wahn und Perspectivität*, Stuttgart, Enke, 1991.

Blanc C. Conscience et inconscient dans la pensée neurobiologique actuelle. In Ey H. (ed.) *L'Inconscient*. Paris, Desclée de Brouwer, pp. 181–253, 1966.

Blancard S. *The Physical Dictionary wherein the terms of Anatomy, the Names and Causes of Diseases, Chirurgical Instruments, and their Use, are Accurately Described*, London, John and Benjamin Sprint, 1726.

Blashfield R.K. Feighner *et al*. Invisible colleges and the Matthew effect. *Schizophrenia Bulletin* 1982, 8: 1–6.

Blasius D. *Der vervaltete Wahnsinn. Eine Sozialgeschichte des Irrenhauses*. Fischer Taschenbuck, Frankfurt, 1980.

Bleuler E. *Affectivität, Suggestibilität, Paranoia* Halle, Carl Marhold, 1906.

Bleuler E. *Dementia Praecox oder Gruppe der Schizophrenien*, Leipzig, Deuticke, 1911.

Bleuler E. *Textbook of Psychiatry*, New York, McMillan, 1924.

Bleuler E. *Dementia Praecox or the Group of the Schizophrenias* (translated by J. Zinkin), New York, International Universities Press, 1950.

Bleuler E. *Afectividad, Sugestibilidad, Paranoia* (translated by B. Llopis), Madrid, Morata, 1969.

Bleuler M., Willi J. and Bühler H.R. *Akute Psychische Begleiterscheinungen Körperlicher Krankheiten*, Stuttgart, Thième, 1966.

Blocq P. and Marinesco G. Sur un cas de tremblement parkinsonian hemiplegique symptomatique d'une tumeur du péduncule cérébrale. *Comptes Rendus Société Biologique de Paris*, 1893, 45: 105.

Blondel, Ch. Délire systématisé de transformation et de négation chez une intermittente. *L'Encéphale*, 1912, 7:74–5.

Blondel, Ch. Mélancolie avec délire des négations. *L'Encéphale* 1912, 7: 552–7.

Blondel Ch. *La Conscience Morbide. Essai de Psycho-Pathologie Générale*, Paris, Alcan, 1914.

Blondel Ch. *Le Suicide*. Strassbourg, Librairie Universitaire D'Alsace, 1933.

Blondel Ch. *Introduction á la Psychologie Collective*, Paris, Colin, 1964 (first publication, 1928).

Bloom F., Segal D.S., Ling N. and Guillemin R. Endorphins: profound behavioural effects in rats suggest new aetiological factors in mental illness. *Science*, 1976, 194: 630–2.

Bloor C. *Temperament. A Survey of Psychological Theories*, London, Methuen, 1928.

Bloor D. *Knowledge and social imagery*. 2nd edn, University of Chicago Press, Chicago, 1991.

Blount J.H. On the terms delusion, illusion, and hallucination. *Asylum Journal of Mental Science* 1856, 2: 494–505; 3: 508–16.

Blum G.S. *Psychoanalytic Theories of Personality*. New York, McGraw-Hill, 1953.

Blumer G. The coming of psychasthenia. *Journal of Nervous and Mental Disease*, 1906, 33: 336–53.

Boas G. Introduction. In Maine de Biran's *The Influence of Habit on the Faculty of Thinking* (translation by M.D. Boehm) London, Baillière, 1929.

Bobes M.M. *La Semiótica como Teoría Lingüística*, Madrid, Gredos, 1973.

Bobon J. *Introduction Historique á l'ètude des Néologismes er des Glossolalies in Psychopathologie*, Paris, Masson, 1952.

Bock G.R. and Marsh J. (eds.) *Experimental and Theoretical Studies of Consciousness*. Ciba Foundation Symposium 174, Chichester, Wiley, 1993.

Boisseau F.G. *Nosografía Orgánica*. In 8 volumes, Valencia, Mompié, 1830.

Bollote G. Moreau de Tours 1804–1884. *Confrontations Psychiatriques*, 1973, 11: 9–26.

Bolton J.S. Maniacal-depressive insanity. *Brain*, 1908, 31: 301–18.

Bolton J.S. The histological basis of amentia and dementia. *Archives of Neurology*, 1903, 2: 424–612.

Bolton L.C. Amentia and dementia: a clinico-pathological study. *Journal of Mental Science*, 1906, 52: 427–90.

Bondy M. Psychiatric antecedents of psychological testing (before Binet). *Journal of the History of the Behavioral Sciences*, 1974, 10: 180–94.

Bonhoeffer K. *Die symptomatischen Psychosen*. Im Gefolge von akuten Infektionen und inneren Erkrankungen, Leipzig, Deuticke, 1910.

Bonhoeffer K. Die exogenen Reaktionstypen. *Archiv für Psychiatrie und Nervenkrankheiten*, 1917, 58: 58–70.

Bonin W.F. *Lexicon der Parapsychologie und ihrer Grenzgebiete*, Bern, Schweiz, 1976.

Bonnet Ch. *Essai Analytique sur les Facultés de l'áme*, 2nd edn., Vol. 14, Neuchatel, Fauche, 1769.

Bonnet Ch. *Essay de Psychologie*. Neuchatel, Fauche, 1783.

Booth G. Psychodynamics in Parkinsonism. *Psychosomatic Medicine*, 1948, 10: 1–12.

Borgese G.A. Romanticism. *Encyclopaedia of the Social Sciences* Vol. 13. New York, Charles Scribner and Sons, 1934; pp. 287–314.

Boring E.G. *Sensation and Perception in the History of Experimental Psychology*, New York, Appleton-Century-Crofts, 1942.

Boring E.G. *A History of Experimental Psychology*. New York, Appleton-Century-Crofts, 1950.

Boring E.G. A history of introspection. *Psychological Bulletin*, 1953, 50: 169–89.

Boring E.G. The beginning and growth of measurement in psychology. *Isis*, 1961, 52: 238–57.

Bostroem A. Über Presbyophrenie. *Archiv für Psychiatrie und Nervenkrankheiten*, 1933, 99: 339–54.

Boswell J. *The Life of Dr Johnson*, 2 Vols, London, Dent, 1791.

Bouchard R. *Sur l'Evaluation du Temps dans Certains Troubles Mentaux*, Thèse de Paris, Vigot frères Editeurs, 1926.

Boucher L. Note sur une forme particulière d'obsession chez une héréditaire. *Normandie Médicale*, 1890, 5: 285–286, 309–10.

Bouchut E. *De l'état Aigu et Chronique du Névrosisme appelé Névropathie aiguë Cérébro-Pneumo-Gastrique*, Paris, 1860.

Bouillaud J. Amnésie. In Andral, Bégin, Blandin (eds.) Vol. 2, *Dictionnaire de Médicine et de Chirurgie Pratiques*, Paris, Gabon, 1829.

Boulenger J.P. and Uhde T.W. Crises Aigües d'angoisse et phobies. Aspects historiques et manifestations cliniques du syndrome d'agoraphobie. *Annales Médico-Psychologiques*, 1987, 145: 113–31.

Bourdin C.E. *Du Suicide Considéré Comme Maladie*. Paris, Batignolles, Hennuyer et Turpin, 1845.

Bourdin V. De L'Impulsion. Sa définition, ses formes et sa valeur psychologique. *Annales Médico-Psychologiques*, 1896, 54: 317–39.

Bourgeois M. Le syndrome de Cotard aujourd'hui. *Annales Médico-Psychologiques*, 1969, 127: 534–44.

Bourgeois M. Jules Cotard et son syndrome. Cent ans après. *Annales Médico-Psychologiques*, 1980, 138: 1165–80.

Bourgeois M. and Geraud M. Eugène Azam (1822–1899). *Annales Médico-Psychologiques*, 1990, 148: 709–17.

Bourgeot H. *Contribution a l'ètude de la Belladona et en Particulier de ses Alcaloïdes Totaux dans les etats Parkinsoniens*. Thèse a la Faculté de Médecine et de Pharmacie de Lyon, Lyon, Bosc, 1926.

Bourneville D.M. and Regnard P. *Iconographie Photographique de la Salpêtrère*, 3 Vols, Paris, Delahaye, 1873–1880.

Boutonier J. *L'Angoisse*, Paris, Presses Universitaires de France, 1945.

Boutroux É. De l'Influence de la philosophie ècossaise sur la philosophie Française. In *Ètudes d'Histoire de la Philosophie*, Paris, Alcan, pp. 413–443, 1908.

Boutroux É. La Philosophie in France depuis 1867. In *Nouvelles Études d'Histoire de la Philosophie*. Paris, Alcan, pp. 139–93, 1927.

Bowman I.A. *William Cullen (1710–90) and the Primacy of the Nervous System*, Indiana University PhD Thesis, History of Science, Xerox University Microfilms, Michigan, Ann Harbor, 1975.

Boyer L. Histoire de la médicine. In Dechambre A. and Lereboullet L (eds.) *Dictionnaire Encyclopédique des Sciences Médicales*, Vol. 6, Paris, Masson, pp. 1–209, 1873.

Boyer P. *Les Troubles du Langage en Psychiatrie*, Paris, Presses Universitaires de France, 1981.

Boyle M. Is schizophrenia what it was? A re-analysis of Kraepelin's and Bleuler's population. *Journal of the History of the Behavioural Sciences*, 1990, 26: 323–33.

Boza R.A. and Liggett S.B. Pseudohallucinations: radio reception through shrapnel fragments. *American Journal of Psychiatry*, 1981, 138: 1263–4.

Braceland F.J. Foreword. In Mora G. and Brand J.L. (eds.) *Psychiatry and Its History*. Springfield, C.C. Thomas, 1970, pp. vii–x.

Bradley F.H. The definition of the will. *Mind* 1902, New Series, N° 44, 437–69.

Bramwell J.M. On imperative ideas. *Brain*, 1894, 17: 331–51.

Braudel F. *La Historia y las Ciencias*. Alianza Editorial, Madrid, 1980.

Bräutigam W. Zwang. In Müller Ch. (ed.) *Lexicon der Psychiatrie*, Berlin, Springer, pp. 586–7, 1973.

Brazier M.A.B. *A History of Neurophysiology in the 17th and 18th Centuries. From Concept to Experiment*, New York, Raven Press, 1984.

Brentano F. *Psychology from an Empirical Standpoint* (translated by A.C. Rancurello, D.B. Terrell and L.L. McAlister) London, Routledge and Kegan Paul, 1973 (First Edition, 1874).

Brett G.S. *History of Psychology* (edited and abridged by R.S. Peters) London, Allen and Unwin, 1953.

Bricke J. Hume's Associationistic psychology. *Journal of the History of the Behavioral Sciences*, 1974, 10: 397–409.

Brierre de Boismont A. Du Délire aigu *Memoires de l'Académie de Médecine*, 1845, 11: 477–595.

Brierre de Boismont A. De l'état des facultés dans les délires partiels ou monomanies. *Annales Medico-Psychologiques*, 1853, 5: 567–91.

Brierre de Boismont A. *Du Suicide et de la Folie Suicide*. Paris, Baillière, 1856.

Brierre de Boismont A. *Des Hallucinations*. third edition, Paris, Baillière, 1862.

Brill H. Post-encephalitic states or conditions. In Arieti S. (ed.) *American Handbook of Psychiatry*, New York, Basic Books, pp. 152–165, 1974.

Brissaud É. De L'Anxiété Paroxystique. *Semaine Médicale*, 1890 (no vol) pp. 410–411.

Brissaud É. *Leçons sur les Maladies du Système Nerveux* (First Edition) Paris, Masson, 1893.

Brissaud É. *Leçons sur les Maladies Nervouses*, Vol. 2, Second Edition, Paris, Masson, 1899.

Brissaud É. Compte Rendu du XIIe Congrès des Médecins Aliénists et Neurologistes. *Revue Neurologique*, 1902, 2: 762–3.

Bristowe J.S. 'Paralysis agitans' in *Quain's Dictionary of Medicine*, Vol. 2, London, Longman, Green and Co., 1894.

British Journal of Psychology, 1910.

Broca P. Perte de la parole, ramollissement chronique et destruction partielle du lobe anterieur gauche du cerveau. *Bulletin de la Société d'Anthropologie*, Paris, 1861, 2: 235–8.

Brochin M. Constitutions Médicales. Constitutions èpidémiques. In Dechambre A. and Lereboullet L. (eds.) *Dictionnaire Encyclopédique des Sciences Médicales*, Vol. 19, Paris, Masson, pp. 751–806; 1876.

Brocq L. Quelques aperçus sur les dermatoses prurigineuses. *Annales de Dermatologie et Syphiligraphie*, 1892, 3: 1100.

Bromsberg W. Mental symptoms in chronic encephalitis. *Psychiatric Quarterly*, 1930, 4: 537–66.

Bronisch T. Dysthyme Störungen. *Nervenarzt*, 1990, 61: 133–9.

Brooks G.P. The faculty psychology of Thomas Reid. *Journal of the History of the Behavioral Sciences*, 1976, 12: 65–77.

Brouc M. Considerations sur le suicide de notre époque. *Annales d'Hygiène Publique et the Médecine Légale*, 1836, 6: 223–62.

Broussais F.J.U. *De l'Irritation et de la Folie*, Paris, Delaunay, 1828.

Brown J. *Elementos de Medicina del Doctor Juan Brown* (translated from the Latin by Joaquín Serrano Manzano) Vol. 2, Madrid, Imprenta Real, 1800.

Brown P. Pierre Janet: alienist reintegrated. *Current Opinion in Psychiatry*, 1991, 4: 389–95.

Brown T. *Lectures on the Philosophy of the Human Mind*, Edinburgh, William Tait, 1828.

Brown-Séquard C.E. Inhibition. In Dechambre A. and Lereboullet L. (eds.) *Dictionnaire Encyclopédique des Sciences Médicales*, Vol. 52, Paris, Masson, pp. 1–19, 1889.

Browne J. Darwin and the face of madness. In Bynum W.F., Porter R. and Shepherd M. (eds.) *The Anatomy of Madness*, Vol. 1, London, Tavistock, pp. 151–65, 1985.

Browne, J. Darwin and the expression of the emotions. In Kohn D. (ed.) *The Darwinian Heritage*, Princeton, Princeton University Press, pp. 307–26, 1985.

Browne J.C. Clinical Lectures on Mental and Cerebral Diseases. *British Medical Journal*, 1874, i: 601–5.

Bruce L.C. Physical symptoms of acute confusional insanity. *Lancet*, 1935, i: 550–1.

Bruchon-Schweitzer M. *Une Psychologie du Corps*. Paris, Presses Universitaires de France, 1990.

Brunschvicg L. *Le Progrès de la Conscience dans la Philosophie Occidentale*, 2 Vols, Paris, Alcan, 1927.

Brush E.N. An analysis of one hundred cases of acute melancholia. *British Medical Journal*, 1897, ii: 777–9.

Buccola G. L'idee fisse. In Tamburini A. (ed.) *Memorie della Clinica Psichiatrica della R. Universita di Modena* Serie IIᵃ, Reggio-Emilia, Calderini, pp. 1–29, 1880.

Buchan J. Concerning volition. In *The Philosophy of Human Nature*, London, Richmond, pp. 298–319, 1812.

Buchanan A. Delusional memories: first rank symptoms? *British Journal of Psychiatry*, 1991, 159: 472–4.

Büchner E.F. A study of Kant psychology. *Psychological Review* (Monograph Supplement), 1897, 4: 1–87.

Bucknill J. and Tuke D.H. *A Manual of Psychological Medicine*, London, John Churchill, 1858.

Buffon M. le Comte Histoire naturelle de l'homme, de la vieillese et de la mort, Vol. 4, *Histoire Naturelle de l'Homme*, Paris, De L'Imprimerie Royale, 1774.

Bugard P. *La Fatigue. Physiologie – Psychologie – et Médecine Sociale*, Paris, Masson, 1960.

Bühler K. *Ausdruckstheorie. Das System an der Geschichte aufgezeigt*, Stuttgart, Gustav Fischer, 1968.

Bulbena A and Berrios G.E. Pseudodementia: facts and figures. *British Journal of Psychiatry*, 1986, 148: 87–94.

Bullen F.S. Olfactory hallucinations of the insane. *Journal of Mental Science*, 1899, 45: 513–33.

Burckard E. Les conceptions psychiatriques de Wernicke. *Travaux de la Clinique Psychiatrique de Strasbourg*, 1931, 9: 45–141.

Burger-Prinz H. and Jacob H. Anatomische und klinische Studien zur senilen Demenz. *Zeitschrift für die gesamte Neurologie und Psychiatrie*, 1938, 161: 538–43.

Burgermeister J.J. Tissot R. and Ajuriaguerra J. de. Les hallucinations visuelles des ophthalmopathies. *Neuropsychologie*, 1964, 3: 9–38.

Burnham W.H. Memory, historically and experimentally considered. *American Journal of Psychology*, 1888–89, 2: 39–90; 225–70; 431–64; 568–622.

Burns R.B. *The Self, Theory, Measurement, Development and Behaviour*, London, Longman, 1979.

Burt C. The analysis of temperament. *British Journal Medical Psychology*, 1938, 17: 158–80.

Burt C. The concept of consciousness. *British Journal of Psychology*, 1962, 53: 229–42.

Burton E. *Suicide, a Dissertation*, London, Vint, 1790.

Burton R. *The Anatomy of Melancholy*, London, Chatto and Windus, 1883 (First Edition, 1620).

Bury M.R. Social constructionism and the development of medical sociology. *Sociology of Health and Illness*, 1986, 8: 137–69.

Bury M.R. Social constructionism and medical sociology: a rejoinder to Nicolson and McLaughlin. *Sociology of Health and Illness*, 1987, 9: 439–41.

Buss A.R. Galton and the birth of differential psychology and eugenics: social, political and economic forces. *Journal of the History of the Behavioral Sciences*, 1976, 12: 47–58.

Butterfield H. *The Whig Interpretation of History*. Charles Scribner's Sons, New York, 1931.

Buvat J. and Buvat-Herbaut M. Dysperception de l'image corporelle et dysmorphophobies dans l'anorexie mentale. A propos de 115 cas des deux sexes. I, II, III. *Annales Médico-Psychologique*, 1978, 136: 547–61; 563–80; 581–92.

Buzzard Sir E.F. Discussion on the diagnosis and treatment of the milder forms of the manic-depressive psychosis. *Proceedings of the Royal Society of Medicine*, 1930, 23: 881–95.

Bynum W.F. Alcoholism and degeneration in 19th century European medicine and psychiatry. *British Journal of Addiction* 1984, 79: 59–70.

Bynum W.F. Rationales for therapy in British psychiatry 1780–1835. *Medical History*, 1964, 18: 317–34.

Bynum W.F. *Science and the Practice of Medicine in the Nineteenth century.* Cambridge, Cambridge University Press, 1994.

Cabaleiro Goas M. *Temas psiquiátricos.* Madrid, Montalvo, 1966.

Cabanis P.J.G. *On the Relations between the Physical and Moral Aspects of Man.* 2 Vols., Mora G (ed.) Baltimore, The Johns Hopkins University Press, 1981.

Caillard E.M. Personality as the outcome of evolution. *Contemporary Review* 1894, 65: 713–21.

Cairns H., Oldfield F., Pennybacker J. and Whitteridge D. Akinetic mutism with an epidermoid cyst of the third ventricle. *Brain*, 1941, 64: 273–90.

Calmeil L.F. Démence. In *Dictionaire de Médicine on Repertoire General des Sciences Médicales*, Second Edition, Paris, Bechet, pp. 70–85, 1835.

Calmeil L.F. *Traité des Maladies Inflammatoires du Cerveau*, 2 Vols, Paris, Baillière, 1859.

Calmeil L.F. Lypémanie. In Dechambre A, Lereboullet L (eds) *Dictionnaire Encyclopédique des Sciences Médicales*, Vol. 55. Paris, Masson, 1869.

Campbell, S., Volow, M.R. and Cavenar, J.O. Cotard's syndrome and the psychiatric manifestations of thyphoid fever. *American Journal of Psychiatry*, 1981, 138: 1377–8.

Camuset L. Le Congrés de médicine mentale á Blois. *Annales Médico-Psychologiques* 1892, 50: 177–83.

Camuset L. Review of Chaslin's 'La confusion mentale primitive'. *Annales Médico-Psychologiques*, 1897, 5: 317.

Canguilhem G. *Le Normal et le Pathologique*, Paris, Presses Universitaires de France, 1966.

Cantor G.N. The Edinburgh phrenology debate: 1803–1828. *Annals of Science*, 1975, 32: 195–218.

Caparrós A. H. *Ebbinghaus. Un Funcionalista Investigador Tipo Dominio*, Barcelona, Publicacions Universitat de Barcelona, pp. 177–205, 1986.

Capgras J.M.J. Contribution a l'étude de la névrose d'angoisse. *Annales Médico-Psychologiques* 1936, 61: 397–404.

Capgras, J.M.J. and Daumezón, G. Syndrome de Cotard atypique. *Annales Médico-Psychologiques*, 1936, 94: 806–12.

Carlson E.T. The nerve weakness of the 19th century. *International Journal of Psychiatry*, 1970, 9: 50–4.

Carlson E.T. and Dain N. The psychotherapy that was moral treatment. *American Journal of Psychiatry*, 1960, 117: 519–24.

Carlson E.T. and Simpson M.M. Models of the nervous system in eighteenth century psychiatry. *Bulletin of the History of Medicine*, 1969, 43: 101–15.

Carlsson A., Lindqvist M. and Magnusson T. 3,4-Dihydroxyphenylalanine and 5-hydroxytryptophan as reserpine antagonists. *Nature* (London), 1957, 180: 1200–1.

Caro Baroja J. *Historia de la Fisiognomica.* Madrid, Istmo, 1988.

Caroli F. and Olie J.P. *Nouvelles Formes de Déséquilibre Mental*, Paris, Masson, 1979.

Caron M. *Étude Clinique de la Maladie de Pick*, Paris, Vigot Fréres, 1934.

Carpenter P.K. Descriptions of schizophrenia in the psychiatry of Georgian Britain: John Haslam and James Tilly Matthews. *Comprehensive Psychiatry*, 1989, 30: 332–8.

Carpenter P.K. Thomas Arnold: a provincial psychiatrist in Georgian England. *Medical History*, 1989, 33: 199–216.

Carpenter W.B. *Principles of Mental Physiology*, London, C. Kegan Paul and Co., 1879.

Carpenter W.B. and Power H. *Principles of Human Physiology* (8th edn.) London, J. and A. Churchill, 1876.

Carroll J.B. (ed.) *Language, Thought and Reality: Selected writings of Benjamin Lee Whorf*. Cambridge, Mass., MIT Press, 1956.

Cash T.F. and Pruzinsky T. (eds.) *Body Images. Development, Deviance, and Change*. New York, The Guilford Press, 1990.

Castan L. *Traité Élémentaire des Diathèses*, Paris, Delahaye, 1867.

Castel R., Castel F. and Lovell A. *La Société Psychiatrique Avancé*. Grasset et Fasquelle, Paris, 1979.

Castel R. *L'Ordre Psychiatrique. L'Age d'Or de l'Alienisme*. Minuit, Paris, 1977.

Cattell J.McK. Mental tests and measurements. *Mind*, 1890, 15: 373–81.

Castilla del Pino C. *Teoría de la Alucinación*, Madrid, Alianza, 1984.

Cautela J.R and Kastelbaum R. A reinforcement survey schedule for use in therapy, training and research. *Psychological Reports*, 1967, 20: 1115–30.

Cauwenbergh L. J. Chr. A. Heinroth (1773–1843): psychiatrist of the German Romantic era. *History of Psychiatry*, 1991, 2: 365–83.

Cazauvieilh J.B. *Du Suicide et l'Aliénation Mentale et des Crimes contra les Personnes, Comparés dans leurs Rapports Reciproques. Recherches sur ce Premier Penchant chez les Habitants des Campagnes*, Paris, Baillière, 1840.

Cenac M. *De Certains Langages créés par les aliénés: Contribution á l'étude des 'Glossolalies'*, Thèsis de Médicine, Paris, 1925.

Cerise L. Du Délire de Sensation par M. Michéa. *Annales Médico-Psychologiques*, 1848, 11: 132–9.

Chaika E. Thought disorder or speech disorder in schizophrenia. *Schizophrenia Bulletin* 1982, 8: 587–91.

Chambard E. Idiotie. In Dechambre A. and Lereboullet L. (eds.) *Dictionnaire Encyclopédique des Sciences Médicales*. Vol. 51, Paris, Masson, pp. 507–27, 1888.

Chamberet (no initial): Paralysis in *Dictionnaire des Sciences Médicales*, Vol. 39, Paris, Panckouke, 1819.

Chan T. and Berrios G.E. Intuition: a neglected concept in psychiatry. *History of Psychiatry* (in press), 1996.

Chapman L.J, Chapman J.P, Raulin M.L: Scales for physical and social anhedonia. *Journal of Abnormal Psychology* 1976, 85: 374–82.

Charbonnier-Debatty M. *Maladies de Mystiques*. Brussels, Manceaux, 1875.

Charcot J.M. *Clinical Lectures on Senile and Chronic Diseases* (translated by William S. Tuke) London, The New Sydenham Society, 1881.

Charcot J.M. *Oeuvres Complètes*, Paris, Delahaye, 1886.

Charcot J.M. *L'Hystérie* (Textes Choisis et Présentés par E. Trillat) Paris, Privat, 1971.

Charcot J.M. *The Tuesday Lessons* (translated and commented by C.G. Goetz), New York, Raven Press, 1987.

Charcot J.M. and Magnan V. De l'onomatomanie. *Archives de Neurologie*, 1885, 10: 157–168.

Charlton W. *Weakness of the Will*, Oxford, Blackwell, 1988.

Charpentier R. De L'ideé de dégénérescence dans la doctrine des constitutions. *Journal Neurologie Psychiatrie*, 1932, 32: 137–69.

Charpentier, T. Le Congrés de médicine mentale á Blois. *Annales Médico-Psychologiques*, 1892, 50: 177–83.

Chaslin P. La confusion mentale primitive. *Annales Médico-Psychologiques* (seventh series), 1892, 16: 225–73.

Chaslin Ph. *La Confusion Mentale Primitive*. Paris, Asselin et Houzeau, 1895.

Chaslin Ph. *Eléments de Sémiologie et de Clinique Mentale*, Paris, Asselin et Houzeau, 1912.

Chaslin Ph. Contribution a l'ètude des rapports du délire avec les hallucinations. *Annales Médico-Psychologiques*, 1890, 12: 45–70.

Chaslin Ph. La 'psychiatrie' est-elle une langue bien faite? *Revue Neurologique*, 1914, 26: 16–23. (English translation in *History of Psychiatry*, 1995)

Chaslin Ph. Review of *Allegmeine Psychopathologie* by K. Jaspers. *Annales Médico-Psychologiques*, 1914, 72: 621–62.

Chaslin Ph. La confusion mentale. *Annales Médico-Psychologiques*, 1915, 6: 276–89; 413–43.

Chaslin Ph. Quelques mots sur la confusion mentale. *Annales Médico-Psychologiques*, 1920, 6: 356–66.

Chatel J.C. and Peel R. The concept of neurasthenia. *International Journal of Psychiatry*, 1971, 9: 36–49.

Chereau A. Rostan. In Dechambre A. and Lereboullet L. (eds.) *Dictionnaire Encyclopédique des Sciences Médicales*, Vol. 84, Paris, Masson, pp. 238–240, 1877.

Cheyne G. The *English Malady or a Treatise of Nervous Diseases of all Kinds*. London, Strahan, 1733.

Chiarugi V. *On Insanity and its Classification*, Translation of G. Mora, Canton, Watson, p. 230, 1987 (1st edn. 1793).

Christian J. Hallucination. In Dechambre D.A. and Lereboullet A. (eds.) *Dictionnaire Encyclopédique des Sciences Médicales*, Vol. 48, Paris, Masson, pp. 77–120, 1886.

Christodoulou G.N. Delusional Hyperidentification of the Frégoli Type. *Acta Psychiatrica Scandinavica*, 1976, 54: 305–14.

Christodoulou G.N. (ed.) *The Delusional Misidentification Syndromes*, Basel, Karger, 1986.

Chronique: Le XXXIIIe Congrès des Médecins Aliénists et Neurologistes de France et des Pays de Langue Française, Le Puy, 1913. *Annales Médico-Psychologiques*, 1913, 71: 129–53.

Cicchetti D. and Toth S.L. (eds.) *Disorders and dysfunctions of the self. New York, University of Rochester Press*, 1994.

Cicero. De Senectute, De Amicitia, De Divinatione (translated by W.A. Falconer) London, Loeb, 1923.

Claparède É. *L'Association des Idées*, Paris, Doin, 1903.

Claparède É. Feelings and emotions. In Reymert M.L. (ed.) *Feelings and Emotions*, New York, Clark University Press, pp. 124–138, 1928.

Claparède H. *La Psychologie Animale de Charles Bonnet* (Mémoire Publié á l'Occasion du Jubilé de l'Université, 1559–1909) Geneva, Georg, 1909.

Clark M.J. 'Morbid introspection' unsoundness of mind, and British psychological medicine, *c.*1830-*c.*1900. In Bynum W.F., Porter R. and Shepherd M. (eds.) *The Anatomy of Madness*, Vol. 3, London, Tavistock, 71–101, 1985.

Clarke B. *Mental Disorders in Earlier Britain: Exploratory Studies*. University of Wales Press, Cardiff, 1975.

Clarke E. (ed.) *Modern Methods in the History of Medicine*. Athlone Press, London, 1971.

Clarke E. and Jacyna L.S. *Nineeenth-Century Origins of Neuroscientific Concepts*. Berkeley, University of California Press, 1987.

Claude H. *Précis de Pathologie Interne. Maladies du Système Nerveux*, 2 Vols., Paris, Baillière, 1922.

Claude H. and Ey H. Hallucinations, pseudo-hallucinations et obsessions. *Annales Médico-Psychologiques*, 1932, 90: 273–316.

Claude H. and Lévy-Valensi J. *Les Ètats Anxieux*, Paris, Maloine, 1938.

Clervoy P., Lassagne M. and Juglard G. Les Hallucinations dans l'oeuvre de Henri Ey. *L'Information Psychiatrique*, 1993, 69: 899–911.

Cloninger C.R. A systematic method for clinical description and classification of personality variants. *Archives of General Psychiatry*, 1987, 44: 573–88.

Clouston T.S. *Clinical Lectures on Mental Disease*. 2nd edn., London, Churchill, 1887.

Cobb I.G. *A Manual of Neurasthenia (Nervous Exhaustion)*. London, Baillière, Tindall and Cox, 1920.

Code Napoléon. Edition Originale et Seule Officielle, Paris, de l'Imprimerie Impériale, 1808.

Cohen A. Descartes, consciousness, and depersonalisation: viewing the history of philosophy from a Straussian perspective. *The Journal of Medicine and Philosophy*, 1984, 9: 7–27.

Cohen G.D. Historical views and evolution of concepts. In Reisberg B. (ed.) *Alzheimer's Disease*, New York, The Free Press, pp. 29–34, 1983.

Cohen R. Das Anhedonie-Konzept in der Schizophrenie-Forschung. *Nervenarzt* 1989 60: 313–17.

Cohn (no initial). Ein Beiträg zur Lehre der Paralysis Agitans. *Wiener Medizinischen Wochenschrift*, 1860, pp. 321–327.

Coleman W. Health and hygiene in the *Encyclopédie*. *Journal of the History of Medicine*, 1974, 29: 399–421.

Colloque International De Bruxelles, *Folie et Déraison á la Renaissance*, Brussels, Editions de l'Université de Bruxelles, 1976.

Colodrón A. Bartolome Llopis (1906–1966). *History of Psychiatry*, 1991, 2: 219–24.

Colonna d'Istra F. L'influence du moral sur la physique d'après Cabanis et Maine de Biran. *Revue de Métaphysique et de Morale*, 1913, 21: 451–61.

Combe G. *Elements of Phrenology*, Tenth Edition, Edinburgh, MacLachlan and Stewart, 1873.

Combet, C.L. In Berbiguier A.V.C. *Les Farfadets*, Paris, Jérôme Millon, 1990.

Comelles J.M. *La razón y la sinrazón*. Barcelona, PPU, 1988.

Condillac Étienne Bonnot de. *Oeuvres Philosophiques de Condillac*, edited by G. Le Roy, Paris, Presses Universitaires de France, 1947 (first edition, 1754).

Conrad K. *Die beginnende Schizophrenie*, Stuttgart, Thième, 1958.

Conrad K. Die symptomatischen Psychosen. In Grühle H.W. and Mayer-Gross W. (eds.) *Psychiatrie der Gegenwart*, Vol. 2, Berlin, Springer, 1960.

Conry Y. Thomas Willis ou le premier discours rationaliste en pathologie mentale. *L'information Psychiatrique*, 1982, 58: 313–23.

Constantinidis J., Richard J. and Ajuariaguerra J. de. Dementias with senile plaques and neurofibrillary changes. In Isaacs A.D. and Post F. (eds.) *Studies in Geriatric Psychiatry*, Chichester, Wiley and Sons, pp. 119–152, 1978.

Conway M.A., Rubin D.C., Spinnler H. and Wagenaar W.A. (eds.) *Theoretical Aspects on Autobiographical Memory*. Dordrecht, Kluwer Academic Publishers, 1992.

Cooter R. *The Cultural Meaning of Popular Science. Phrenology and the Organization of Consent in Nineteenth Century Britain*. Cambridge, Cambridge University Press, 1984.

Cooter R. Phrenology and British alienists, c.1825–1845. *Medical History*, 1979, 20: 1–21; 135–51.

Copland J. *Dictionary of Practical Medicine*, Vol. 1, London, Longmans, pp. 290–293, 1858.

Corbin A. *The Foul and the Fragrant: Odor and the French Imagination*, Cambridge MA, Harvard University Press, 1986.

Cordeiro J.C. États délirants du troisième age. *L'Encéphale*, 1973, 62: 20–55.

Cordes E. Die Platzangst (Agoraphobie), Symptom einer Erschöpfungsparese. *Archiv für Psychiatrie und Nervenkrankheiten*, 1872, 3: 521–74.

Costello. Depression: loss of reinforcers or loss of reinforcer effectiveness? *Behavioural Therapy* 1972, 3: 240–7.

Cotard, J. Du délire hypocondriaque dans una forme grave de melancolie anxieuse. *Annales Médico-Psychologiques*, 1880, 4:168–74.

Cotard J. Folie. In Dechambre A. and Lereboullet L. (eds.) *Dictionnaire Encyclopédique des Sciences Médicales*, Paris, Masson, Vol. 39, pp. 271–306, 1878.

Cotard J. Du délire des negations. *Archives de Neurologie*, 1882, 4: 152–70; 282–96.

Cotard J. De l'aboulie et de l'inhibition en pathologie mentale. In *Études sur les Maladies Cérébrales et Mentales*, Paris, Baillière, pp. 358–65, 1891.

Cotard J. De l'origine psycho-motrice du délire. In *Études sur les Maladies Cérébrales et Mentales*, Paris, Baillière, pp. 416–29, 1891.

Cotard J. De l'Origine Psycho-Sensorielle ou Psycho-Motrice du Délire. In *Études sur les Maladies Cérébrales et Mentales*, Paris, Baillière, pp. 366–73, 1891.

Cotard J. *Études sur les Maladies Cérébrales et Mentales*. Paris, Baillière, 1891.

Cotard, J. and Prévost, J.L. ètudes physiologiques et pathologiques sur le ramollissement cérébral. In *Études sur les Maladies Cérébrales et Mentales* Paris, J.B. Baillière, 1891 (originally published in 1865).

Cotard, J. Étude sur l'atrophie partielle du cerveau. In *Études sur les Maladies Cérébrales et Mentales* Paris: J.B. Baillière, 1891 (originally published in 1868).

Cotard, J. Perte de la vision mentale dans la melancolie anxieuse. In *Études sur les Maladies Cérébrales et Mentales* Paris J.B. Baillière, 1891.

Cottereau M.J. Les Nevroses I. Historique des nevroses. *La Revue de Medicine*, 1975, 13: 903–10.

Coupland W.C. Philosophy of mind. In Tuke D.H. (ed.) *A Dictionary of Psychological Medicine*, Vol. 1, pp. 27–49. London, J. and A. Churchill, 1892.

Courbon P. De la dualité ètiologique de la manie et de la mélancolie. *L'Encephale*, 1923, 18: 27–31.

Cousin V. *Elements of Psychology* (translated by Caleb Henry) London, Trübner, 1856.

Cousin V. *Fragmens Philosophiques*, Paris, A. Sautelet et Compagnie, 1826.

Cowles E. The mental symptoms of fatigue. *New York Medical Journal* 1893, i: 345–52.

Craft M. *Ten Studies into Psychopathic Personality*. Bristol, Wright, 1965.

Cranfield P.F. A seventeenth century view of mental deficiency and schizophrenia: Thomas Willis on 'stupidity and foolishness'. *Bulletin of the History of Medicine*, 1961, 35: 291–316.

Creutzfeldt H.G. Über eine eigenartige herdförmige Erkrankungen des Zentralnervensystem. *Zeitschrift für die gesamte Neurologie und Psychiatrie*, 1920, 57: 1–18.

Crichton A. *An Inquiry into the Nature and Origin of Mental Derangement. Comprehending a Concise System of the Physiology and Pathology of the Human Mind and a History of the Passions and their Effects*, 2 Vols. London, T. Cadwell and W. Davies, 1798.

Crichton-Browne J. Senile dementia. *British Medical Journal*, 1874, i: 601–3; 640–3.

Cristiani, A. *Delirio di Negazione*. Rome, Nuova Rivista, 1892.

Critchley E.M.R. The neurology of familiarity. *Behavioural Neurology*, 1989, 2: 195–200.

Critchley M. Arteriosclerotic Parkinsonism. *Brain*, 1929, 52: 23–83.

Critchley M. Pre-senile psychoses. *Proceedings of the Royal Society of Medicine*, 1938, 31: 1447–53.

Critchley M. (ed.) *James Parkinson 1755–1824*, London, MacMillan, 1955.

Critchley M. The neurology of psychotic speech. *British Journal of Psychiatry*, 1964, 110: 353–64.

Crocker L.G. The discussion of suicide in the 18th century. *Journal of the History of Ideas*, 1952, 13: 47–52.

Cruchet R. *Nuevos Conceptos de Patología Nerviosa*. Buenos Aires, Editorial Médico-Quirúrgica, 1943.

Cudworth R. *The Intellectual System of the Universe*, London, 1837 (First Edition, 1678).

Culbetian C. *Hallucinations de Moignon*, Paris, Alcan, 1902.

Cullen W. *Institutions de Médicine pratique*. 2 Vols, French Translation of Ph. Pinel, Paris, Duplain, 1785.

Cullen W. *Synopsis Nosologiæ Methodicæ*, 6th edn., Edinburgh, W. Creech, 1803.

Cullen W. *The Works of William Cullen*. Edited by John Thomson. 2 Vols, Edinburgh, William Blackwood, 1827.

D'Assigny M. *The Art of Memory*, London, Bell, 1706.

d'Aumont Arnulphe. Délire. In Diderot and D'Alambert (eds.) *Encyclopédie ou Dictionnaire Raisonné des Sciences, des Arts, et de Métières*. Vol. 4, Paris, Briasson, David, Le Breton,

d'Istria F.C. La psychologie de Bichat. *Revue de Metaphysique et de Morale*, 1926, 23:1–38.

Dagonet M.H. Des impulsions dans la folie et de la folie impulsive. *Annales Médico-Psychologiques*, 1870, 4: 5–32; 215–59.

Dagonet M.H. De la stupeur. *Annales Médico-Psychologiques*, (fifth series), 1872, 7: 161–359.

Dagonet M.H. *Noveau Traité Élémentaire et Pratique des Maladies Mentales*, Paris, Baillière, 1876.

Dagonet M.H. Conscience et Aliénation Mentale. *Annales Médico-Psychologiques*, 1881, 5: 368–97; 6: 19–32.

Dagonet M.H. *Traité des Maladies Mentales*, Paris, Baillière, 1894.

Dallemagne J. *Dégénérés et Déséquilibrés*, Paris, Alcan, 1895.

Damirón Ph. *Essai sur l'Histoire de la Philosophie en France*, 2 Vols, Paris, Schubart et Heideloff Libraires, 1828.

Dana C.L. A discussion on the Classification of the melancholias. *Medical Record*, 1904, 66: 1033–5.

Danion J.M., Keppi J. and Singer L. Un approche historique de la doctrine des dégénérescences et des constitutions psychopathiques. *Annales Médico-Psychologiques*, 1985, 144: 271–80.

Danziger K. The history of introspection reconsidered. *Journal of the History of the Behavioral Sciences*, 1980, 16: 241–62.

Danziger K. *Constructing the Subject. Historical Origins of Psychological Research*, Cambridge, Cambridge University Press, 1990.

Darwin C. *The Descent of Man*, London, Murray, 1883 (1st edn., 1871).

Darwin C. *The Expression of the Emotions in Man and Animals*, London, Murray, 1904 (First Edition, 1872).

Darwin E. *Zoonomia*, 2 Vols, London, U. Johnson, 1794–1796.

Daston L.J. The theories of will versus the sciences of mind. In Woodward W.R. and Ash M.G. (eds.) *The Problematic Science. Psychology in the 19th Century*, New York, Praeger, pp. 88–115, 1982.

Dastre A. *La Vie et la Mort*, Paris, Flammarion (no year).

Daumezón G. Legitimité de l'intérêt pour l'histoire de la psychiatrie. *L'Information Psychiatrique* 1980, 65: 647–53.

Daumezón G. Ph. Chaslin. *Confrontations Psychiatriques*, 1973, 11: 27–39.

Dauzat A. *La Philosophie du Langage*. Paris, Flammarion, 1912.

Davaine C. Monstres. Monstruosité. In Dechambre A. and Lereboullet L. (eds.) *Dictionnaire Encyclopédique des Sciences Médicales*, Vol. 61, Paris, Masson, pp 201–64, 1874.

Davies W.G. Consciousness and 'unconscious cerebration'. *Journal of Mental Science*, 1873, 19: 202–17.

Davison K. and Bagley C.R. Schizophrenia-like psychoses associated with organic disorders of the central nervous system: a review of the literature. In Herrington R.N. (ed.) Current Problems in Neuropsychiatry, *British Journal of Psychiatry*, Special Publication N° 4, Kent, Headley Brothers, 1969.

De Clérambault G. *OEuvre Psychiatrique*. Vol. 2, Paris, Presses Universitaires de France, 1942.

De Cool, E. *Contribution a l'étude du délire des négations*. Thése de Paris, 1893.

De Garmo C. *Herbart and the Herbartians*, New York, Scribner's, 1896.

De Martis, D. Un caso di sindrome di Cotard. *Rivista Sperimentale di Freniatria*, 1956, 80:491–514.

De Sanctis, S. Negativismo vesanico e allucinazione antagonistiche. *Bolletino della Societa Lancisiana degli Ospedale di Roma* 1896, 16: 1–13.

Dechambre A. Songe. In Dechambre A. and Lereboullet L. (eds.) *Dictionnaire Encyclopédique des Sciences Médicales*, Vol. 95. Paris, Masson, pp. 408–33, 1881.

Dechambre A. Habitude. In Dechambre A. and Lereboullet L. (eds.) *Dictionnaire Encyclopédique des Sciences Médicales*, Vol. 48, Paris, Masson, pp. 8–15, 1886.

Dechambre A. Tempérament. In Dechambre A. and Lereboullet L. (eds.) *Dictionnaire Encyclopédique des Sciences Médicales*, Vol. 95, Paris, Masson, pp. 312–25, 1886.

Dechambre A. Maurice Krishaber. In Dechambre A. and Lereboullet L. (eds.) *Dictionnaire Encyclopédique des Sciences Médicales*, Vol. 52, Paris, Masson, p. 777, 1889.

Deerborn G.U.N. The concept of psychogenesis. *Journal of Abnormal Social Psychology*, 1937, 32: 207–17.

DeFelipe J. and Jones E.G. (eds.) *Cajal on the Cerebral Cortex. An Annotated Translation of the Complete Writings*, Oxford, Oxford University Press, 1988.

Dejerine J. and Gauckler E. *Les Manifestations Fonctionnelles des Psychonévroses. Leur Traitement par la Psychotherapie*, Paris, Masson, 1911.

Del Greco, F. Delirio e forme paranoiche in rapporto ad altri delirii e condizioni patogeniche. *Manicomio Moderno*, 1896, 12: 22–7.

Delacroix M.H. Maine de Biran et L'Ècole médico-psychologique. *Bulletin de la Société Française de Philosophie*, 1924, 24: 51–63.

Delasiauve L.J.F. Du diagnostic differentiel de la lypémanie. *Annales Médico-Psychologiques*, 1851, 3: 380–442.

Delasiauve L.J.F. Psychologie, de la sensibilité: sentiments, etc. *Journal de Médicine Mentale*, 1861, 1: 230–6.

Delasiauve L.J.F. Des diverses formes mentales. *Journal de Médicine Mentale*, 1861, 1: 5–14.

Delasiauve L.J.F. De la monomanie. *Journal de Medicine Mentale*, 1861, 1: 348–64.

Delay J. Le Jacksonisme et l'oeuvre de Ribot. In *Études de Psychologie Médicale*, Paris, Presses Universitaires de France, 1953.

Delay J. Jacksonism and the work of Ribot. *Archives of Neurology and Psychiatry*, 1957, 78: 505–15.

Delay J. and Deniker P. Drug-induced extrapyramidal syndromes. In Vinken P.J. and Bruyn G.W. (eds.) *Handbook of Clinical Neurology*, Vol. 6, *Diseases of the Basal Ganglia*, North-Holland, Amsterdam, pp. 248–66, 1968.

Delboeuf J. *Le Sommeil et les Rêves*. Paris, Alcan, 1885.

Deleule D. *La Psychologie. Mythe Scientifique*, Paris, Robert Laffont, 1969.

Delkeskamp C. Philosophical reflections in the 19th century Medico-Legal Discussions. In Engelhardt H.T. Jr. and Spicker S.F. (eds.) *Mental Health: Philosophical Perspective*, Dordrecht, Reidel, pp. 125–137, 1977.

Delmas F.A. Les constitutions psychopatiques. Le rôle et la signification des constitutions en psychiatrie. *Annales Médico-Psychologiques*, 1943, 101: 119–232.

Demange E. *Étude Clinique et Anatomo-Pathologique de la Vieillesse*, Paris, Ducost, 1886.

Demange E. Tremblement. In Dechambre A. and Lereboullet L. (eds.) *Dictionnaire Encyclopédique des Sciences Médicales*, Paris, Masson, Vol. 97, pp. 59–77, 1887.

Dendy W.C. *On the Phenomena of Dreams and other Transient Illusions*. London, Whittaker, Treacher and Co., 1832.

Dening T. and Berrios G.E. Autoscopic phenomena. *British Journal of Psychiatry*, 1994, 165: 808–817.

Dening T. and Berrios G.E. The Enigma of Pseudohallucinations Psychopathology (in press) 1995.

Dennett D.C. *Consciousness Explained*. London, Penguin Book, 1993 (1st edn. 1991).

Denny-Brown D. *The Basal Ganglia and their Relation to Disorders of Movement*, London, Oxford University Press, 1962.

Deny G. La Cyclothymie. *La Semaine Médicale*, 1908, No 15: 169–71.

Deny G. Représentation schématique et nomenclature des différentes formes de la psychose maniaque-dépressive. *L'Encéphale*, 1909, 4: 363–6.

Deny, G. and Camus, P. Étude nosologique et pathogenique du délire des négations. *Annales Médico-Psychologiques*, 1906, 64: 423–43.

Deny G. and Camus P. *La Psychose Maniaque-Dépressive*, Paris, Baillière, 1907.

Deny G. and Roy P. *La Démence Précoce*, Paris, Baillière, 1903.

Derombies M. *L'illusion de sosies*, Paris, Thèse de Médicine, 1935.

Des Étangs. Du suicide en France. Études sur la mort volontaire depuis 1798 jusqu'a nos jours. *Annales Médico-Psychologique*, 1857, 3: 1–27.

Descartes. *Oeuvres Choisies*, Paris, Garnier, 1919.

Descartes. The passions of the soul. In *The Philosophical Works of Descartes* (translated by E.S. Haldane and G.R.T. Rose) Cambridge, Cambridge University Press, pp. 331–427, 1967.

Deschamps A. *Les Maladies de l'esprit et les Asthénies*, Paris, Alcan, 1919.

Deshaies G. *Psychologie du Suicide*, Paris, Presses Universitaires de France, 1947.

Deshaies G. *Psychopathologie Générale*. Paris, Presses Universitaires de France, 1967.

Despine P. *De la Folie au point de vue Philosophique ou plus spécialement psychologique* Paris, Savy, 1875.

Despine P. Du rôle de la psychologie dans la question de la folie. *Annales Médico-Psychologiques*, 1876, 34: 161–75.

Deusen E.H. van Observations on a form of nervous prostration neurasthenia. *American Journal of Insanity*, 1869, 25: 44–7.

Devaux and Logre (no initials) *Les Anxious. Étude Clinique*, Paris, Masson, 1917.

Devereux G. Normal and abnormal. In *Basic Problems in Ethnopsychiatry*. The University of Chicago Press, Chicago, 1980, pp. 3–71.

Dewhurst K. *Hughlings Jackson on Psychiatry*, Oxford, Sandford Publications, 1982.

Di Mascio P. Comment naissent les théories? Le cas de la neurasthénie. *L'Evolution Psychiatrique*, 1986, 51: 625–38.

Dictionnaire Universal des Synonymes de la Langue Française, 3 Vols, Paris, edited by Benoît Morin, 1792.

Diderot and D'Alembert (eds.) *Encyclopédie ou Dictionnaire Raisonné des Sciences, des Artes, et des Métiers, par una Société de Gens de Lettres*, Paris, Briasson, David, Le Breton, Durand, 1753–1765.

Diem O. Die einfach demente Form der Dementia praecox. *Archiv für Psychiatrie und Nervenkrankheiten*, 1903, 37: 111–87.

Diethelm O. and Heffernan T. F. Felix Platter and Psychiatry. *Journal for the History of the Behavioral Sciences*, 1965, 1: 10–23.

Digby A. *Madness, Morality and Medicine*. Cambridge, Cambridge University Press, 1985.

Dihle A. *The Theory of Will in Classical Antiquity*, Berkeley, University of California Press, 1982.

Dijksterhius E.J. *The Mechanization of the World Picture*, Oxford, Oxford University Press, 1961.

Diller T. Obsessions; fixed ideas, indecisions, imperative conceptions, abulias, phobias. *The Medical News*, 1902, 81: 961–8.

Dilthey W. *Einleitung in die Geisteswissenschaften*. First Vol. Duncker und Humboldt, Leipzig, 1883.

Dilthey W. *Selected Writings*, Cambridge, Cambridge University Press, pp. 87–97, 1976.

Dimitz L. and Schilder P. Über die psychischen Störungen bei der Encephalitis Epidemica des Jahres 1920. *Zeitschrift für Neurologie und Psychiatrie*, 1921, 68: 298–340.

Discussion sur L'Hystérie. *Société de Neurologie de Paris*. Séances of 9th April and 14th May 1908. *Revue Neurologique*, 1908, 16: 375–404; 494–519.

Dodds E.R. *The Greeks and the Irrational*, California, California Press, 1951.

Domarus Von E. Zur Theories des schizophrenen Denkens. *Zeitschrift für Neurologie und Psychiatrie*, 1927, 108: 703–14.

Donath J. Zur Kenntniss des Anancasmus (psychische Zwangszustände), *Archiv für Psychiatrie und Nervenkrankeiten*, 1897, 29: 211–24.

Donegan A. Wittgenstein on Sensation. In Pritcher G. (ed.) *Wittgenstein*, London, McMillan, pp. 324–51, 1968.

Dörner K. *Bürger und Irre. Zur Sozialgeschichte und Wissenschaftsoziologie der Psychiatrie*. Europäische Verlagsanstalt, Frankfurt, 1969.

Doughty O. The English malady of the 18th century. *Review of English Studies*, 1926, 2: 257–69.

Dowbiggin I. Degeneration and hereditarianism in French mental medicine. In Bynum W.F.,

Porter R. and Shepherd M. (eds.) *The Anatomy of Madness*, Vol. 1, London, Tavistock, pp. 188–232, 1985.

Dowbiggin I. French Psychiatry and the search for a professional identity: the Société Médico-Psychologique. *Bulletin of the History of Medicine*, 1989, 63: 331–55.

Dowbiggin I. Alfred Maury and the politics of the unconscious in nineteenth-century France. *History of Psychiatry*, 1990, 1: 255–88.

Dowbiggin I. *Inheriting Madness*. Berkeley, University of California Press, 1991.

Down J.L. Observations on an ethnic classification of idiots. *London Hospital Reports*, 1866, 3: 259–62.

Doyen E. Quelques considerations sur les terreurs morbides et la délire emotif en général. *L'Encéphale*, 1885, 4: 418–38.

Drabkin I.E. Remarks on ancient psychopathology. *Isis*, 1955, 46: 223–34.

Drevet A. *Maine de Biran*, Paris, Presses Universitaires de France, 1968.

Dreyfus G.L. *Die Melancholie. Ein Zustandsbild des manisch-depressiven Irreseins*, Jena, Gustav Fischer, 1907.

Drinka G.F. *The Birth of Neurosis*. New York, Simon and Schuster, 1984.

Dromard G. *La Mimique chez les Aliénés*, Paris, Alcan, 1909.

Dromard G. Mémoire et délire; éclipses mnésiques comme sources et comme conséquences de'idées délirantes. *Journal de Psychologie Normale et Pathologiques*, 1911, 8: 252–60.

Dublineau J. La psychiatrie et le problème des tempéraments. *Annales Médico-Psychologiques*, 1943, 101: 200–18.

Dubois P. *Les Psychonévroses et leur Traitement Moral*. Paris, Masson, 1905.

Duché D.-J. *Histoire de la Psychiatrie de l'enfant*. Paris, Presses Universitaires de France, 1990.

Ducost M. De l'involution présénile dans la folie maniaque-dépressive. *Annales Médico-Psychologiques*, 1907, 65: 299–303.

Ducost M. Hallucinations dans la paralysie générale. *L'Encéphale*, 1907, 2: 158–79.

Duensing F. Das Elektroenzephalogramm bei Störungen der Bewusstseinslage. *Archives für Psychiatrie und Nervenkrankheiten*, 1949, 183: 71–115.

Dugas L. L'impression de 'l'entièrement nouveau' et cela de 'déjà vu'. *Revue Philosophique*, 1894, 38: 40–6.

Dugas L. Observations sur la Fausse mémoire. *Revue Philosophique*, 1894, 37: 34–45.

Dugas L. *Timidité*, Paris, Alcan, 1898.

Dugas L. Un cas de dépersonnalisation. *Revue Philosophique* 1898, 45: 500–7.

Dugas L: Un nouveau cas de depersonnalisation. *Journal de Psychologie Normale et Pathologique*, 1912, 9: 38–47.

Dugas L. and Moutier F. La depersonnalisation et la perception extérieure. *Journal de Psychologie Normale et Pathologique*, 1910, 7: 481–98.

Dugas L. and Moutier F. *La Depersonnalisation*, Paris, Alcan, 1911.

Dugas M., Halfon, O., Badoual A.M. *et al.* Le syndrome de Cotard chez l'adolescent. *Neuropsychiatrie Enfance Adolescence*, 1985, 33: 493–8.

Dumas (no initial). *Traité du Suicide ou du Meurtre Volontaire de soi-même*, Leipzig, 1773.

Dumas G. *Les États Intellectuels dans la Mélancolie*, Paris, Alcan, 1894.

Dumas G. L'État mental d'Auguste Comte. *Revue Philosophique*, 1898, 45: 30–60; 151–80; 387–414.

Dumas G. *Traité de Psychologie* 2 Vols. Paris, Alcan, 1923.

Duprat G.L. *L'Instabilité Mentale. Essai sur les données de la psychopathologie*. Paris, Alcan, 1899.

Dupré E. Les cénestopathies. *Mouvement Médical*, 1913, 23: 3–22.

Dupré E. Préface. In Devaux and Logre. *Les Anxieux. Étude Clinique*, Paris, Masson, 1917.

Dupré E. *Les Déséquilibres Constitutionnels du Système Nerveux*, Paris, Baillière, 1919.

Dupré E. *Pathologie de l'Imagination et de l'Émotivite*, Paris, Payot, 1925.

Dupré E. Les déséquilibres constitutionnels du système nerveux. *Revue Internationale de Histoire de la Psychiatrie*, 1984, 2: 77–91.

Dupuytren Baron de. On Nervous Delirium. *Lancet*, 1834, i: 919–23.

Durand V.J. Hallucinations Olfactives et Gustatives. *Annales Médico-Psychologiques*, 1955, 113: 777–813; and pp. 249–64.

Dureau A. Sömmerring S.T. In Dechambre A and Lereboullet L. (eds.) *Dictionnaire Encyclopédique des Sciences Médicales*, Vol. 88, Paris, Masson, 1881, pp. 319–21.

Durkheim E. Les règles de la méthode sociologique. *Revue Philosophique*, 1894, 37: 465–98.

Durkheim E. *Le Suicide*, Paris, Alcan, 1897 (translated by J.A. Spaulding and G. Simpson as *Suicide. A Study in Sociology*) London, Routledge and Kegan Paul, 1952.

Dutil A. Troubles psychiques dans la maladie de Parkinson. In Ballet G. (ed.) *Traité de Pathologie Mentale*, Paris, Doin, pp. 872–5, 1903.

Duverger M. *Méthodes des Sciences Sociales*, Paris, Presses Universitaires de France, 1961.

Duvoisin R. History of Parkinsonism. *Pharmacological Therapy*, 1987, 32: 1–17.

Dwelshauvers G. *La Psychologie Française Contemporaine*, Paris, Alcan, 1920.

Dwelshauvers G. *Traité de Psychologie*, Paris, Payot, 1934.

E.M.C. Encyclopédie Médico-Chirurgicale. *Psychiatrie*. 6 Vols, Paris, Editions Techniques, 1987.

Eadie M.J. and Sutherland J.M. Arteriosclerosis in Parkinsonism. *Journal of Neurology, Neurosurgery and Psychiatry*, 1964, 27: 237–40.

Ebbinghaus H. *Über das Gedächnis*, Leipzig, Duncker und Humbolt, 1885.

Ebbinghaus H. *Memory. A contribution to Experimental Psychology* (translated by H.A. Ruger, C.E. Bussenius and E.R. Hilgard), New York, Dover, 1964 (1st edn. 1885).

Economo C. von. *Encephalitis Lethargica*, Oxford, Oxford Medical Publications, 1931.

Edel A. Happiness and pleasure. In Wiener P.P. (ed.) *Dictionary of the History of Ideas*. Vol. 3, New York, Charles Scribner's Sons, pp. 374–87, 1973.

Edgell B. *Theories of Memory*, Clarendon Press, Oxford, 1924.

Editorial. La nona, the so-called new disease. *British Medical Journal*, 1890, i: p. 748.

Editorial. Mental Obsessions. *British Medical Journal*, 1901, ii: 100.

Editorial. Parkinson's disease: One illness or many syndromes. *Lancet*, 1992, 339: 1263–4.

Editors, 'Intelligence and its measurement'. *Journal of Educational Psychology*, 1921, Vol. 12.

Edwards W. and Tversky A. (eds.) *Decision-Making*. London, Penguin, 1967.

Eeden V. Les Obsessions. *Revue de l'Hypnotisme*, 1892, 6: 5–14.

Ehrenwald H. Anosognosie und depersonalisation. *Der Nervenarzt*, 1931, 4: 681–8.

Eigen J.P. Delusions in the Courtroom: the role of partial insanity in early forensic testimony. *Medical History*, 199, 35: 25–49.

Eisler (ed.) *Wörterbuch der Philosophischen Begriffe*, Vol. 2, Berlin, Mitler und Sohn, 1904.

Ekehammar B. Interactionism in personality from a historical perspective. *Psychological Bulletin*, 1974, 81: 1026–948.

Ellard J. Did schizophrenia exist before the eighteenth century. *Australian and New Zealand Journal of Psychiatry*, 1987, 21: 306–14.

Ellard J. The history and present status of moral insanity. *Australia and New Zealand Journal of Psychiatry*, 1988, 22: 383–9.

Ellenberger H. *The Discovery of the Unconscious*, London, Allen Lane, 1970.

Engel-Janosi F. *The growth of German historicism*. Studies in History and Political Science, Series 62, N° 2, Johns Hopkins University, 1944.

Engstrom E.J. Emil Kraepelin. *Leben und Werk des Psychiaters im Spannungsfeld zwischen positivischer Wissenschaft und Irrationalität*. Dissertation presented to the Ludwig-Maximilians-Universität, Munich, 1990.

Enoch, D. and Trethowan, W. *Uncommon Psychiatric Syndromes* 3rd edn. Oxford: Butterworth and Heinemann, 1991.

Erdmann B. Vorstellung. *Viertel-jarsch für wissenschaftliche Philosophie*, 1886, 10: 307–15.

Errera P. Some historical aspects of the concept phobia. *Psychiatric Quarterly*, 1962, 36: 325–36.

Erwin E. *Behaviour Therapy Scientific, Philosophical and Moral Foundations*. Cambridge, Cambridge University Press, 1978.

Esquirol E. *Des Passions considérées comme Cause, Symptomes et Moyens Curatifs de l'Aliénation Mentale*, Paris, Librairie des Deux-Mondes, 1980 (First Published, 1805).

Esquirol E. Démence. In *Dictionnaire des Sciences Médicales, par une Societé de Médicins et de Chirurgiens*, Paris, Panckoke, Vol. 8, pp. 280–93, 1814.

Esquirol E. Délire. In Adelon, Alard, Alibert et al. (eds.) *Dictionnaire des Sciences Médicales*, Paris, Panckoucke, pp. 251–9, 1814.

Esquirol, E. Démonomanie. In *Dictionnaire des Sciences Médicales*, Paris, Panckouke, pp. 294–318, 1814.

Esquirol E. Hallucinations *Dictionaire des Sciences Médicales*, Paris, Panckouke, 1817.

Esquirol E. Mélancolie. In *Dictionnaire des Sciences Médicales*, Paris, Panckoucke, 1820.

Esquirol E. Suicide. In Adelon, Alard, Alibert et al. (eds.) *Dictionnaire des Sciences Médicales*, Paris, Panckoucke, pp. 213–83, 1821.

Esquirol E. *Des Maladies Mentales Considérées sous les Rapports Médical, Hygienique et Médico-Legal*, 2 Vols, Paris, Baillière, 1838.

Esquirol E. *De la Lypémanie ou Mélancholie*, Fedida P. and Postel J. (eds.) Paris, Sandoz Editions, 1976.

Étoc-Demazy G.F. *De la Stupidité Considerée ches les Aliénés. Recherches Faites á Bicêtre et á la Salpêtrière*, Paris, Didot le Jeune, 1833.

Étoc-Demazy G.F. *Recherches Statistiques sur le Suicide, Appliquées á l'Hygiène Publique et á la Médicine Legal*, Paris, Baillière, 1844.

Étoc-Demazy G.F. Sur la folie dans la production du suicide. *Annales Médico-Psychologiques*, 1846, 7: 338–62.

Evans B. *The Psychiatry of Robert Burton*, New York, Columbia University Press, l944.

Evans C.O. *The Subject of Consciousness*, London, Allen and Unwin, 1970.

Evans P. Henri Ey's Concepts of the organization of consciousness and its disorganization: an extension of Jacksonian theory. *Brain*, 1972, 95: 413–40.

Ey H. Confusion et délire confuso-onirique. ètude N° 24. In *Études Psychiatriques*, Vol. III, Paris, Desclée De Brouwer, pp. 325–428, 1954.

Ey H. Les Psychoses Périodiques maniaco-depressives. Étude N° 25. In *Études Psychiatriques*, Vol. 3, Paris, Desclée de Brouwer, pp. 429–518, 1954.

Ey H. La Discussion de 1855 à la Société Médico-Psychologique surl l'hallucination et l'état actuel du problème de l'activité hallucinatoire. *Annales Médico-Psychologique*, 1935, 93: 584–613.

Ey H. Esquirol et le problème des hallucinations. *L'Evolution Psychiatrique*, 1939, 1: 21–44.

Ey H. Impulsions. Étude N° 11 In *Études Psychiatriques*, Vol. 2, Paris, Desclée de Brouwer, pp. 163–212, 1950.

Ey H. Le Suicide Pathologique. Étude N° 14 In *Études Psychiatriques. Aspects Séméiologiques*, Vol. 2, Paris, Desclée de Brouwer, pp. 341–78, 1950.

Ey H. Anxiété Morbide. Étude N° 15. In *Études Psychiatriques Aspects Sémiologiques*, Paris, Desclée de Brouwer, pp. 379–426, 1950.

Ey, H. Délire de negations. Étude N° 16. In *Études Psychiatriques*, Vol. 2, Paris: Desclée de Brower, pp 427–52, 1950.

Ey H. Hypocondrie. Étude N° 17. In *Études Psychiatriques*, Vol. 2, Paris, Desclée de Brouwer, 1950.

Ey H. *Estudios sobre los Delirios*, Madrid, Paz Montalvo, 1950.

Ey H. Une théorie mécaniciste. Étude N° 5. In *Ètudes Psychiatriques*, Vol. 1, Paris, Desclée de Brouwer, pp. 83–102, 1952.

Ey H. Le développement 'mechaniciste' de la psychiatrie. Étude N° 3 In *Études Psychiatriques*, Vol. 1, Paris, Desclée de Brouwer, p. 56, 1952.

Ey H. Le rêve, 'fait primordial' de la psychopathologie. Étude N°8. In *Études Psychiatriques*. 2nd edn., Vol. 1, Paris, Desclée de Brouwer, pp. 187–283, 1952.

Ey H. Structure et déstructuration de la conscience. Étude N° 27, In *Études Psychiatriques*, Vol. 3, Paris, Descle de Bouwer, pp. 653–760, 1954.

Ey H. *La Conscience*, Paris, Presses Universitaires de France, 1963.

Ey H. Les Hallucinoses, *L'Encéphale*, 1957, 46: 564–73.

Ey H. *Traité des Hallucinations* 2 Vols, Paris, Masson, 1973.

Ey H. *Des Idées de Jackson a un Modèle Organo-Dynamique en Psychiatrie*, Paris, Privat, 1975.

Ey H. La notion de 'maladie morale' et de 'traitement moral' dans la psychiatrie Française et Allemande du debut du XIXme Siècle. *Perspectives Psychiatriques*, 1978, 1: 12–35.

Ey H. and Mignot H. La Psychologie de J. Moreau de Tours. *Annales Médico-Psychologiques*, 1947, 2: 225–41.

Ey H., Marty P. and Dublineau J. *Psychopathologie Générale. Comptes Rendus Des Séances. Premier Congrés Mondial De Psychiatrie*, Vol. 1, pp. 98–104, Paris, Hermann, 1952.

Ey H., Bernard P. and Brisset Ch. *Manuel de Psychiatrie*, Fourth Edition, Paris, Masson, 1974.

Ey H., Bernard P, Brisset Ch, *Manuel de Psychiatrie* (5th edn.). Paris, Masson, 1978.

Eysenck H.J. Cyclothymia and schizothymia as dimensions of personality. I. historical review. *Journal of Personality*, 1951, 19: 123–52.

Fabre Dr. (ed.) *Dictionnaire des Dictionnaires de Medicine Français et Etrangers*, Paris, Béthune et Plon, 1840.

Fabre Dr. (ed.) *Bibliothéque du Médicin-Practicien*, Paris, J.B. Baillière, 1849.

Facon E., Steriade M. and Wertheim N. Hypersomnie prolongée engendrée par des lesions bilatérales du système activateur médial et le syndrome thrombotique de la bifurcation du tronc basilar. *Revue Neurologique*, 1958, 98: 117–33.

Falret J.P. *De l'Hypocondrie et du Suicide. Considérations sur les Causes, sur le Siége et le Traitement de ces Maladies, sur Moyens d'en Arrêter les Progrès et d'en Prévenir le Développement.* Paris, Croullebois, 1822.

Falret J.P. De la non-existence de la monomanie. In *Des Maladies Mentales et des Asiles d'Aliénés*, Paris, Baillière, pp. 425–48, 1864.

Falret J.P. Délire. In *Des Maladies Mentales et des Asiles d'Aliénes* Paris, Asselin, 1864.

Falret J.P. *Des Maladies Mentales et des Asiles d'Aliénés, Leçons Cliniques and Considérations Générales*, Paris, Baillière, 1864.

Falret J.P. *Leçons Cliniques de Médecine Mentale faites a la Salpêtrière. 1re Partie: Symptomatologie Générale des Maladies Mentales*, Vol. 1, Paris, Baillière, 1854.

Falret J.P. Mémoire sur la folie circulaire. *Bulletin de l'Académie de Médicine*, 1854, 19: 382–415.

Falret J.P. Obsessions intellectuelles et emotives. *Archives de Neurologie*, 1889, 2: 274–93.

Falret Jules. Note. *Gazette des Hôpitaux*, 14th January, 1851.

Falret Jules. De la catalepsie. *Archives Générales de Médicine*, 1857, 10: 206–21; 455–66.

Falret Jules. Amnésie. In Dechambre A. and Lereboullet L.(eds.) *Dictionnaire Encyclopédique des Sciences Médicales*, Vol. 3, Paris, Asselin and Masson, pp. 725–42, 1865.

Falret Jules. Aphasie, Aphémie, Alalie. In Dechambre A. and Lereboullet L. (eds.) *Dictionnaire Encyclopédique des Sciences Médicales*, Vol. 5, Paris, Masson, pp. 605–44, 1866.

Falret Jules. Discussion sur la folie raisonnante. *Annales Médico-Psychologiques*, 1866, 24: 382–426.

Falret, Jules. Nécrologie. *Annales Médico-Psychologiques* 1889, 47: 319–24.

Falret, Jules. Le Congrés de médicine mentale à Blois. *Annales Médico-Psychologiques* 1892, 50:177–83.

Fancher R.E. Brentano's psychology from an empirical standpoint and Freud's early metapsychology. *Journal of the History of the Behavioral Sciences*, 1977, 13; 207–27.

Farran-Ridge C. Some symptoms referable to the basal ganglia occurring in dementia praecox and epidemic encephalitis. *Journal of Mental Science*, 1926, 72: 513–23.

Farrell B.A. The progress of psychology. *British Journal of Psychology*, 1978, 69: 1–8.

Faure H. *Hallucinations et Réalité Perceptive* Paris, Presses Universitaires de France, 1965.

Fava G.A. Morselli's legacy: dysmorphophobia. *Psychotherapy and Psychosomatics*, 1992, 58: 117–18.

Fawcett J, Clark C, Scheftner WA *et al.* Assessing anhedonia in psychiatric patients. *Archives General Psychiatry*, 1983, 40: 79–84.

Fearn J. *An Essay on Consciousness or a Series of Evidences of a Distinct Mind*, 2nd edn., London, Longman, 1812.

Fechner G.T. *Elements of Psychophysics*, Vol. 1, New York, Holt, Rinehart and Winston, 1966.

Fedden H.R. *Suicide*, London, Peter Davies, 1938.

Fellner von Feldegg F. *Beiträge zur philosophie des Gefühls; gesammelte kritisch-dogmatische Aufsätze über zwei Grundproblemen*, Leipzig, Barth, 1900.

Fenichel O. *The Psychoanalytical Theory of Neurosis*, London, Kegan, Paul, Trench, Trubner, 1945.

Féré Ch. Un spasme de cou coïncidant avec des hallucinations visuelles unilatérales. *Comptes Rendus de la Société de Biologie*, 1896, 3: 269–71.

Féré Ch. *The Pathology of Emotions* (rendered into English by R. Park) London, The University Press, 1899.

Féré Ch. *Sensación y Movimiento* (translation of the 1887 French Edition by Ricardo Rubio) Madrid, Fernando Fé, 1903.

Ferguson B. and Tyrer P. Classifying personality disorder. In Tyrer P. (ed.) *Personality Disorders*, London, Wright, pp. 12–32, 1990.

Ferraro A.L.L. Luigi Luciani (1840–1919) In Haymaker W. and Schiller F. (eds.) *The Founders of Neurology*, Springfield, Charles Thomas, pp. 233–237, 1970.

Ferrater Mora J. *Diccionario de Filosofia*. Buenos Aires, Editorial Sudamericana, 1958.

Ferriar J. *An Essay Towards a Theory of Apparitions*, London, 1813.

Ferster C. Animal behavior and mental illness. *Psychological Record*, 16: 345–56, 1966.

Feuchtersleben von E. *Lehrbuch der ärztlichen Seelenkunde*. Wien, Carl Gerold, 1845.

Feuchtersleben von E. *On the Dietetics of the Soul*, London, Churchill, 1852 (First German Edition, 1838).

Feuchtersleben von E. *The Principles of Medical Psychology. Translated by H.E. Lloyd and B.G. Babington*. London, Sydenham Society, 1847 (First German Edition, 1845).

Fields W.S. and Lamak N.A. *A History of Stroke*, New York, Oxford University Press, 1989.

Finzi, J. Sul Sintoma Disorientamiento. *Rivista di Patologia Nervosa e Mentale*, 1899, 4: 347–62.

Fischer O. Miliare Nekrosen mit drusigen Wucherungen der Neurofibrillen, eine regelmaessege Verandaerung der Hirnrinde bei seniler Demenz. *Monatsschrift für Psychiatrie und Neurologie*, 1907, 22: 361–72.

Fischer O. Ein weiterer Beitrag zur Klinik und Pathologie der presbyophrenen Demenz. *Zeitschrift für die gesamte Neurologie und Psychiatrie*, 1912, 12: 99–135.

Fischer-Homberger E. On the medical history of the doctrine of imagination. *Psychological Medicine*, 1979, 9: 619–28.

Fischhoff B. and Beyth-Marom R. Hypothesis evaluation from a Bayesian perspective. *Psychological Review*, 1983, 90: 239–60.

Fish F. The Varieties of Delusion. *International Journal of Psychiatry*, 1968, 6: 38–40.

Fishbein I.L. Involutional Melancholia and Convulsive Therapy. *American Journal of Psychiatry*, 1949, 106: 128–35.

Fishgold H. and Mathis P. Obnubilations, Comas at Stupeurs. Études Electroencephaliques. *Electroencephalography and Neurophysiology*, 1959, (Suppl. 2).

Flanagan O. *Consciousness Reconsidered*. Cambridge, Mass, MIT Press, 1992.

Flashar H. *Melancholie und Melancholiker in den medinischen Theorien der Antike*, Berlin, W.D. Gruyter, 1966.

Fleck L. *Genesis and Development of a Scientific Fact*. University of Chicago Press, Chicago, 1979.

Fleck U. Über die Bewußtseinstrübung bei den exogenen Reaktionsformen (Bonhoeffer). *Nervenarzt*, 1956, 27: 433–40.

Flemming C.F. *Pathologie und Therapie der Psychosen*, Berlin, August Hirschwald, 1859.

Fleury M. *Les Grands Symptômes Neurasthéniques*, Paris, Alcan, 1901.

Fleury M. *De L'Angoisse Humaine*, Paris, Les Editions de France, 1926.

Flournoy H. Hallucinations liliputiennes atypiques chez un vieillard opéré de la cataracte. *L'Encéphale*, 1923, 18: 566–79.

Flournoy Th. Le cas de Charles Bonnet. Hallucinations visuelles chez un vieillard opéré de la cataracte. *Archives de Psychologie*, 1902 (Geneva) 1: 1–23.

Floyd W.F. and Welford A.T. (Eds) *Symposium on Fatigue* London, Lewis, 1953.

Fodor J.A. *Psychological Explanation*, New York, Randon House, 1968.

Fodor J.A. *The Modularity of the Mind*, Cambridge, MIT Press, 1983.

Foix Ch. and Nicolesco J. *Les Noyaux Gris Centraux*. Paris, Masson, 1925.

Follin S and Azoulay J. Les altérations de la conscience de soi. *Encyclopédie Médico-Chirurgicale*, 37125A10, 1978.

Follin S. and Azoulay J. La dépersonnalisation. *Encyclopédie Médico-Chirurgicale*, 37125A30, 1979.

Fonseca da A.F. Affective equivalents. *British Journal of Psychiatry*, 1963, 109: 464–9.

Förstl H. Angermeyer M. and Howard R. Karl Philipp Moritz' Journal of Empirical Psychology (1783–1793): an analysis of 124 case reports. *Psychological Medicine*, 1991, 21: 299–304.

Förstl, H. and Beats, B. Charles Bonnet's description of Cotard's delusion and reduplicative paramnesia. *British Journal of Psychiatry*, 1992, 160: 416–18.

Förstl H. and Rattay-Förstl B. Karl Philipp Moritz and the Journal of Empirical Psychology: an introductory note and a series of case reports. *History of Psychiatry*, 1992, 3:95–116.

Förstl H. and Sahakian B.A. Psychiatric presentation of abulia – three cases of left frontal lobe ischaemia and atrophy. *Journal of the Royal Society of Medicine*, 1991, 84: 89–91.

Fortenbaugh W.W. *Aristotle on Emotion*, London, Academic Books, 1975.

Foucault M. *Maladie Mentale et Psychologie*, Paris, Presses Universitaires de France, 1954.

Foucault M. *Histoire de la Folie a l'Age Classique*, Gallimard, Paris, 1972.

Fouks L., Potiron G. and Moukalou R. L'Angoisse et l'Anxiété dans la Psychopathologie de Pierre Janet. *Annales Médico-Psychologiques*, 1986, 144: 461–71.

Foulquié P. *La Volonté* Paris, Presses Universitaires de France, 1972.

Fournier A. *Syphilis du Cerveau*, Paris, Baillière, 1875.

Foville A. Fils Idiotie, imbécillité. In Anger B. *et al.* (ed.) *Noveau Dictionnaire de Médicine et de Chirurgie pratiques*. Vol. 18, Paris, Baillière, pp. 363–75, 1874.

Foville A. Les aliénés voyageurs ou migrateurs. Étude clinique sur certains cas de lypémanie. *Annales Médico-Psychologiques*, 1875, 14: 5–45.

Foville A. Folie á double forme. *Brain*, 1882, 5: 288–323.

Franck A.D. Apathie. In Franck A.D. (ed.) *Dictionnaire des Sciences Philosophiques*. Paris Hachette, p. 78, 1875.

Franck A.D. Signes. In Franck A.D. (ed.) *Dictionnaire des Sciences Philosophiques*, Paris, Hachette, pp. 1608–16, 1875.

Franck A.D. Système. In Franck A.D. (ed.) *Dictionnaire des Sciences Philosophiques*, Paris, Hachette, pp. 1703–4, 1875.

Fraser A.C. in Locke J. *An Essay Concerning Human Understanding* (Vol 1). New York, Dover, 1959.

Freeman W. Eduard Brissaud (1852–1909) In Haymaker W. and Schiller F. (eds.) *The Founders of Neurology*, Springfield, Thomas, pp. 417–20, 1970.

Freud S. A reply to criticisms on the anxiety neurosis. In *Collected Papers*, Vol. 1, London, The Hogarth Press, pp. 107–27, 1953 (First published, 1895).

Freud S. The justification for detaching from neurasthenia a particular syndrome: the anxiety neurosis. In *Collected Papers*, Vol. 1, London, The Hogarth Press, pp. 76–106, 1953 (First published, 1894).

Freud S. *On Aphasia*. Translated by E. Stengel. London, Imago, 1953 (First published, 1891).

Freud S. Trauer und Melancholie. *Gesammelte Werke*, Vol. 10, Frankfurt, Fischer, 1963 (first published, 1917).

Freud S. Introductory lectures in psychoanalysis, in Strachey J (trans-ed.): *The Standard Edition of the Complete Works of Sigmund Freud* (Vol. 16). London, Hogarth Press and the Institute for Psychoanalysis, 1963 (First published, 1917).

Freud S. Notes on a case of paranoia. *The Standard Edition of the Complete Works of Sigmund Freud* (Vol. 12). London, Hogarth Press and the Institute for Psychoanalysis, 1963 (First Published, 1911).

Friedrich G. *Die Krankheiten des Willens vom Standpunkte der Psychologie ans betrachtet, im Anschlusse au die Untersuchung des Normalen (gesunde) Willens, in Bezug auf Entwicklungensstufen, Ziele und Merkmale*. München, S. Friedriech, 1885.

Fritsch J. Die Verwirrheit. *Jahrbücher für Psychiatrie*, 1879, 2: 27–89.

Fritzsch T. *Juan Federico Herbart*, Barcelona, Labor, 1932.

Frondizi R. *Substancia y Función en el Problema del Yo*, Buenos Aires, Editorial Losada, 1952.

Fuchs T. and Lauter H. Charles Bonnet Syndrome and Musical Hallucinations in the Elderly. In Katona C. and Levy R. (eds.) *Delusions and Hallucinations in Old Age*, London, Gaskell, pp. 187–200, 1992.

Fuentenebro F. Delirio. Un enfogue pragmático de la dialogiciad delirante *Revista de Psiquiatría de la Facultad de medicina de Barcelona*, 1995 22: 42–47.

Fulcher J.R. Puritans and the passions: the faculty psychology in American puritanism. *Journal of the History of Behavioural Science*, l973, 9: 123–39.

Fuller S.C. A study of the neurofibrils in dementia paralytica, dementia senilis, chronic alcoholism, cerebral lues and microcephalic idiocy. *American Journal of Insanity*, 1907, 63: 415–68.

Fuller S.C. Alzheimer's Disease (Senium Praecox): The report of a case and review of published cases. *Journal of Nervous and Mental Disease*, 1912, 39: 440–55; 536–57.

Fullinwider S.P. Insanity as the loss of self: the moral insanity controversy revisited. *Bulletin History of Medicine*, 1975, 49: 87–101.

Fullinwider S.P. Sigmund Freud, John Hughlings Jackson, and speech. *Journal of the History of Ideas* 1983, 44: 151–8.

Furukawa T. Charles Bell's Description of the phantom limb phenomenon in 1830. *Neurology*, 1990, 40: 1830.

Gajdusek D.C. and Zigas V. Degenerative disease of the central nervous system in New Guinea. The endemic occurrence of 'Kuru' in the native population. *New England Journal of Medicine*, 1957, 257: 974–8.

Gall F.J. *Fonction du Cerveau*, Paris, Baillière, 1825.

Gallup G.G. and Maser J.D. Tonic Immobility: evolutionary underpinnings of human catalepsy and catatonia. In Maser J.D. and Seligman M.E.P. (eds.) *Psychopathology: Experimental Models*, San Francisco, W.H. Freeman, pp. 334–57, 1977.

Galtier-Boissière (ed.) *Larousse Médical Illustré*, Paris, Larousse, 1929.

Galton F. *Hereditary Genius*, London, Friedmann, 1979 (1st edn., 1869).

Galton F. *Inquiries into Human Faculty*, London, Dent, no date; 1st edn., McMillan, 1883.

Galton F. Personality. *Nature*, 1895, 62: 517–18.

Gangler-Mundwiller D. Mélancolie et Désespérance. Médicine et Morale au Quinzième Siècle. In *La Mélancolie dans la Relation de l'âme et du Corps*, L.M.S. No. 1, Université de Nantes, 1979.

Gardair J. *Philosophie de St. Thomas: les passions et la volonté*, Paris, Lethielleux, 1892.

Gardiner H.M. Metcalf R.C. and Beebe-Center J. G. *Feeling and Emotion. A History of Theories*, New York, American Book Company, 1937.

Gardiner H.M. The definition of feeling. *Journal of Philosophy, Psychology and Scientific Method*, 1906, 3: 57–62.

Garety P.A. and Hemsley D.J. Characteristics of delusional experience. *European Archives of Psychiatry and Neurology*, 1987, 236, 294–8.

Garmany G. Acute anxiety and hysteria. *British Medical Journal*, 1955, ii: 115–17.

Garnier A. *Traité des Facultés de L'Ame*, 3 Vols, Paris, Hachette, 1852.

Garnier, P. Le Congrés de médicine mentale à Blois. *Annales Médico-Psychologiques*, 1892, 50: 177–83.

Garrabé J. *Dictionnaire Taxinomique de Psychiatrie*, Paris, Masson, 1989.

Garrabé J. Dissociation et refoulement. *Annales Médico-Psychologiques*, 1989, 147: 1011–16.

Garrabé J. (ed.) Philippe Pinel. Paris, Les Empêcheurs de Penser en Rond, 1994.

Garth T.R. *Mental Fatigue*. Ph Thesis, Columbia Univ., 1918.

Gasser J. La notion de mémoire organique dans l'oeuvre de Th. Ribot. *History and Philosophy of the Life Sciences*, 1988, 10: 293–313.

Gauchet M and Swain G. *La Pratique de l'Esprit Humain*. Gallimard, Paris, 1980.

Gauld A. *The Founders of Psychical Research*. London, Routledge and Kegan Paul, 1968.

Gaultier J. *Le Bovarysme*, Paris, Mercure de France, 1902.

Gaupp R. Die Depressionszustände des höheren Lebensalters. *Münchener Medizinische Wochenschrift*, 1905, N° 22: 1531–7.

Gautheret F. Historique et position actuelle de la notion de scheme corporel. *Bulletin de Psychologie* 1961, 11: 41–9.

Gayat G. Introduction à la Lecture de la Leçon Inaugurale d'Ernest Dupré. *Revue Internationale Histoire de la Psychiatrie*, 1984, 2: 67–76.

Gelder M.G. Is cognitive therapy effective? Discussion paper. *Journal of the Royal Society of Medicine*, 1983, 76: 938–42.

Gelenberg A.J. and Mandel M.R. Catatonic reactions to high-potency neuroleptic drugs. *Archives of General Psychiatry*, 1977, 34: 947–50.

Genil-Perrin G.P.H. *Histoire des Origines et de l'Évolution de l'Idée de Dégénérescence en Médicine mentale*. Paris, A Leclerc, 1913.

Genil-Perrin G.P.H. *Les Paranoiaques*, Paris, Maloine, 1926.

Georget E. J. Catalepsie. In Adelon M. (ed.) *Dictionnaire de Médicine*, Vol. 6, Paris, Béchet, pp. 479–489, 1834.

Georget E.J. *De la Folie. Considérations sur Cette Maladie*, Paris, Crevot, 1820.

Georget E.J. Délire. In *Dictionnaire de Médicine ou Répertoire Général des Sciences Médicales Considérées sous les Rapports Théorique et Pratique*, Vol. 10, Second Edition, Paris, Béchet, 1835.

Georgin B. Remarques sur le discours nosologique en psychiatrie. *L'Evolution Psychiatrique*, 1980, 45: 5–17.

Giannelli, A. Sul delirio sistematizzato di negazione. *Rivista di Psicologia, Psichiatria e Neurologia* 1897, 6: 231.

Gibb W.R.G. and Lees A.J. The clinical phenomenon of akathisia. *Journal of Neurology, Neurosurgery and Psychiatry*, 1986, 49: 861–6.

Gibbs C.J., Gajdusek D.C., Asher D.M. *et al.*. Creutzfeldt-Jakob Disease: transmission to the chimpanzee. *Science*, 1968, 161: 388–9.

Gibson E.T. A clinical summary of 106 cases of mental disorder of unknown etiology arising in the fifth and sixth decades. *American Journal of Insanity*, 1918, 75: 221–49.

Giddens A. The suicide problem in French sociology. *British Journal of Sociology*, 1965, 16: 3–18.

Giddens A. Introduction to the translation by Goldblatt H. of Halbwachs M. *The Causes of Suicide*, London: Routledge and Kegan Paul, 1978.

Gigerenzer G., Swijtink Z., Porter T., Daston L., Beatty J. and Kruger L. *The Empire of Chance*, Cambridge, Cambridge University Press, 1989.

Gillespie R.D. Hypochondria. *Guy's Hospital Reports*, 1928, 78: 408–60.

Gillespie R.D. The clinical differentiation of types of depression. *Guy's Hospital Reports*, 1929, 79: 306–44.

Gillespie R.D. Amnesia. *Archives of Neurology and Psychiatry*, 1937, 37: 748–64.

Gilman S.L. *Seeing the Insane*, New York, John Wiley, 1982.

Giné y Partagás D. *Tratado Teórico-práctico de Frenopatología*. Madrid, Moya y Plaza, 1876.

Gineste T. Naissance de la psychiatrie infantile (destins de l'idiote, origine des psychoses). In Postel J. and Quetel C. (eds.) *Nouvelle Histoire de la Psychiatrie*. Paris, Privat, pp. 499–516, 1983.

Giovanni A. di. *Clinical Commentaries Deduced from the Morphology of the Human Body*, London, Eyre, 1919.

Glatzel J. Zum Problem der sogenannten Pseudohalluzination. *Fortschritte der Neurologie, Psychiatrie und ihrer Grenzgebiete* 1970, 38: 348–64.

Glauber I.P. Observations on a primary form of anhedonia. *Psychoanalytic Quarterly*, 1949, 18: 67–78.

Globus G.G. The Problem of consciousness. In Goldberger L. and Rosen V.H. (eds.) *Psychoanalysis and Contemporary Science*, Vol. 3, New York, International University Press, pp. 40–69, 1975.

Globus G.G., Maxwell G. and Savodnik I. (eds.) *Consciousness and the Brain*, New York, Plenum Press, 1976.

Gloor P., Olivier A. and Quesney L.F. The role of the limbic system in experiential phenomena of temporal lobe epilepsy. *Annales of Neurology*, 1982, 12: 129–44.

Godard D. Éthologie clinique: Étude des stéréotypies. *Annales Médico-Psychologiques* 1991, 149: 615–30.

Goddard H.H. Feeblemindedness: a question of definition. *Journal of Psycho-Asthenics* 1928, 33: 219–27.

Goldstein J. *Console and Classify. The French Psychiatric Profession in the Nineteenth Century*, Cambridge, Cambridge University Press, 1987.

Goldstein K. Methodological approach to the study of schizophrenic thought disorder. In Kasanin J.S. and Lewis N.D.C. (eds.) *Language and Thought in Schizophrenia*. New York, Norton, pp. 17–40, 1944.

Gombault N. La démence terminale dans les psychoses. *Annales Médico-Psychologiques*, 1900, 58: 213–49.

Gómez J. Hysterical Stupor (letter). *British Journal of Psychiatry*, 1980, 136: 105.

Gomulicki B.R. The development and present status of the trace theory of memory. *British Journal of Psychology* (Monograph Suppl. 29), Cambridge, At The University Press, 1953.

Gontard A. The development of child psychiatry in 19th century Britain. *Journal of Child Psychology and Psychiatry*, 1988, 29: 569–88.

Gordon B. de: *Lilio de Medicina*, Sevilla, Ungut and S. Polonio, 1495.

Gosling F.G. *Before Freud: Neurasthenia and the American Medical Community 1870–1910*, Urbana, University of Illinois Press, 1987.

Got J.A. *Contribution á l'etude du syndrome de Cotard, sa valeur pronostique*. Bordeaux: Thèse N° 9, 1912.

Gowers W.B. *A Manual of Diseases of the Nervous System*, 2nd edn., 2 Vols, London, Churchill, 1893.

Gowers W.B. Abiotrophy. *Lancet*, 1902, i, 1003–7.

Grant R.L. Concepts of aging: an historical review. *Perspectives in Biology and Medicine*, 1963, 6: 443–78.

Grasset J. *Les Maladies de l'Orientation et de l'Équilibre*, Paris, Alcan, 1901.

Grasset J. *Semi-Locos y Semi-Responsables.* (Translation by G. Gonzáles) Madrid, Saenz de Jubera, 1908.

Gratiolet L.P. *Mémoires Sur Les Plis Cérébraux De L'homme Et Des Primates*, Paris, Bertrand, 1854.

Gratiolet L.P. Communication, *Bulletin de La Société de Anthropologie*, 1861, 2: 66, 238, 421.

Grave S.A. *The Scottish Philosophy of Common Sense*, Oxford, Clarendon Press, 1960.

Grave S.A. Thomas Brown. In Edwards P. (ed.) *The Encyclopedia of Philosophy*, Vol. 1, New York, McMillan, pp. 401–403, 1967.

Grayson D.A. Limitations on the use of scales in psychiatric research. *Australian and New Zealand Journal of Psychiatry*, 1988, 22: 99–108.

Green A. Conceptions of affect. *International Journal of Psychoanalysis*, 1973, 58: 129–56.

Green J.C. Biology and social theory in the 19th century: Auguste Comte and Herbert Spencer. In Clagett M. (ed.) *Critical Problems in the History of Science*, Madison, University of Wisconsin Press, pp. 419–446, 1952.

Greenberg, D.B., Hochberg, F.H. and Murray, G.B. The theme of death in complex partial seizures. *American Journal of Psychiatry*, 1984, 141: 1587–9.

Greenway A.P. The incorporation of action into associationism: the psychology of Alexander Bain. *Journal of the History of the Behavioral Sciences*, 1973, 9: 42–52.

Griesinger W. *Mental Pathology and Therapeutics* (translated by C.L. Robertson and J. Rutherford), London, The New Sydenham Society, 1867.

Griesinger W. Einen wenig bekannten psychopathischen Zustand. *Archiv für Psychiatrie und Nervenkrankheiten*, 1868, 1: 626–35.

Griesinger W. *Die Pathologie und Therapie der psychischen Krankheiten*, 2nd edn, Stuttgart, Krabbe, 1861.

Grimm J. and Grimm W. *Deutsches Wörterbuch*, Vol. 12, Leipzig, S. Hirzel, 1956.

Grimshaw L. Obsessional disorders and neurological illness. *Journal of Neurology, Neurosurgery and Psychiatry*, 1964, 27: 229–31.

Gringer R.R. Parkinsonism following carbon monoxide poisoning. *Journal of Nervous Mental Diseases*, 1926, 64: 18–28.

Grivois H. (ed.) *Les Monomanies Instinctives*, Paris, Masson, 1990.

Grivois H. (ed.) *Autonomie et Automatisme dans la Psychose*, Paris, Masson, 1992.

Grmek M.D. *On Ageing and Old Age*, Den Haag, W. Junk, 1958.

Gros M. Contribution a l'Étude de l'agoraphobie (peur des espaces). *Annales Médico-Psychologiques*, 1885, 43: 394–407.

Gross O. Dementia sejunctiva. *Neurologisches Centralblatt*, 1904, 23: 1144–6.

Gross O. *Zerebrale Sekundärfunktion*, Leipzig, Vogel, 1904.

Gross O. *Über psychopathische Minderwertigkeiten*. Wien und Leipzig. Wilhelm Braumüller, 1909.

Gruber H.E *Darwin on Man*, Chicago, University of Chicago Press, 1981.

Gruman G.J. A history of idea about the prolongation of life. *Transactions of the American Philosophical Society*, 1966, 56: 1–97.

Grünbaum A.A. Pseudovorstellung und Pseudohalluzination. *Zeitschrift für die gesammte Neurologie und Psychiatrie* 1917, 37: 100–9.

Guarnieri P. Between soma and psyche: Morselli and psychiatry in late nineteenth century Italy. In Bynum W.F., Porter R. and Shepherd M. (eds.) *The Anatomy of Madness*, Tavistock, London, Vol. 3, pp. 102–24, 1988.

Gubser A. Fatigue. In Eysenck H.J., Arnold W. and Meili R (eds.) *Encyclopedia of Psychology*, Vol. 1, London, Search, pp. 369–71.

Gueniot M. D'une hallucination du toucher (ou hétérotopie subjective des extrémiteé) particulière a certains amputés. *Journal de Physiologie de l'Homme et des Animaux (Brown-Séquard)*, 1861, 4: 416–30.

Guillain G.J.M. *Charcot 1825–1893. His Life and Work*, London, Pitman, 1959.

Guiraud P. Analyse du symptome stéréotypie. *L'Encéphale*, 1936, 31: 229–69.

Guislain J. *Leçons Orales sur les Phrénopathies ou Traité Théorique et Pratique des Maladies Mentales*, 3 Vols, Gand, Hebbelynck, 1852.

Gull W.W. *A Collection of the Published Writings of W.W. Gull* (edited by T. Acland), 2 Vols, London, New Sydenham Society, 1894.

Gurney E. Hallucinations. *Mind*, 1885, 10: 161–99.

Gurney E., Myers F.W.H. and Podmore E. *Phantasms of the Living*, 2 Vols, London, 1886.

Gurvitz M. Developments in the concept of psychopathic personality (1900–1950). *British Journal of Delinquency*, 1951, 2: 88–102.

Gurwitsch A. *Théorie du champ de la Conscience*, Paris, Desclée de Brouwer, 1957.

Gusdorf G. *La Découverte de Soi*. Paris, Presses Universitaires de France, 1948.

Haas F.J. *Essai sur les Avantages Cliniques de la Doctrine de Montpellier*. Baillière, Paris, pp. 115–154, 1864.

Hacking I. Imre Lakatos's philosophy of science. *British Journal for the Philosophy of Science* 1979, 30: 381–410.

Hacking I (ed.) *Scientific Revolutions*. Oxford, Oxford University Press, 1981.

Hacking I. *The Taming of Chance*, Cambridge, Cambridge University Press, 1990.

Hadlow W.J. Scrapie and Kuru. *Lancet*, 1959, ii: 289–90.

Haenel T. *Zur Geschichte der Psychiatrie. Gedanken zur allgemeinen und Basler Psychiatriegeschichte*. Basel, Birkhäuser, 1982.

Häfner H. The concept of disease in psychiatry. *Psychological Medicine*, 1987, 17: 11–14.

Hagen F.W. *Studien auf dem Gebiete der ärztlichen Seelenheilkunde*. Erlangen, Besold, 1861.

Hagen F.W. Zur Theorie der Hallucination. *Allgemeine Zeitschrift für Psychiatrie* 1868, 25: 1–107.

Hahn L. Panizza. In Dechambre A. and Lereboullet L. (eds.) *Dictionnaire Encyclopédique des Sciences Médicales*, Vol. 72, Paris, Masson, 1884.

Haigh E. Xavier Bichat and the medical theory of the eighteenth century. *Medical History*, Supl. N° 4, London, Wellcome Institute for the History of Medicine, 1984.

Hakkébousch B.M. and Geier T.A. De la Maladie d'Alzheimer. *Annales Médico-Psychologiques*, 1913, 71: 358.

Halbwachs M. *Les Causes du Suicide*, Paris, Alcan, 1930.

Halgren E, Walter R.D., Cherlow D.G. and Crandall P.H. Mental phenomena evoked by electrical stimulation of the human hippocampal formation and amygdala. *Brain*, 1978, 101: 83–117.

Hall M. *On the Diseases and Derangements of the Nervous System* London, Baillière, 1841.

Hall S.B. Mental Aspects of Epidemic Encephalitis. *British Medical Journal*, 1929, i: 444–6.

Hall T.S. *Ideas Of Life And Matter*, Vol. 2, Chicago, University of Chicago Press, 1969.

Hall V.M.D. The contribution of the physiologist William Benjamin Carpenter (1813–1885) to the development of the principles of the correlation of forces and the conservation of energy. *Medical History*, 1979, 23: 129–55.

Haltenhof L. Vertige paralysant. *Bulletin de L'Academie de Médicine*, 1887, 51: 334–51.

Hamilton E. and Cairns E. (eds.) *Collected Dialogues of Plato* Bollinger Series, New Jersey, Princeton University Press, 1973.

Hamilton M. (ed.) *Fish's Clinical Psychopathology*, Bristol, Wright, 1974.

Hamilton Sir W. *Lectures on Metaphysics and Logic, edited by H.L Mansel and J. Veitch*, 4 Vols, Edinburgh, William Blackwood and Sons, 1859.

Hammond W.A. Unilateral hallucinations. *Medical News (New York)*, 1885, 47: 681–9.

Hankoff L.D.S. Ancient descriptions of organic brain syndrome: the 'Kordiakos' of the Talmud. *American Journal of Psychiatry*, 1972, 129: 233–6.

Hanson N R. *Patterns of Discovery*, Cambridge, Cambridge University Press, 1958.

Hare E. The origin and spread of dementia paralytica. *Journal of Mental Science*, 1959, 105: 594–626.

Hare E. Schizophrenia as a different disease. *British Journal of Psychiatry*, 1988a, 153: 521–31.

Hare E. Schizophrenia before 1800? The case of the Revd George Trosse. *Psychological Medicine*, 1988, 18: 279–85.

Hare E. The history of 'nervous disorders' from 1600 to 1840, and a 'comparison' with modern views. *British Journal of Psychiatry*, 1991, 159: 37–45.

Hare E. A Short note on pseudo-hallucinations. *British Journal of Psychiatry*, 1973, 122: 469–76.

Hare E. The changing content of psychiatric illness. *Journal of Psychosomatic Research* 1974, 18: 283–9.

Harrow M., Grinker R.R., Holzman P.S. and Kayton L. Anhedonia and schizophrenia. *American Journal of Psychiatry*, 1977, 134: 794–7.

Harrow M. and Quinlan D. Is disordered thinking unique to schizophrenia? *Archives of General Psychiatry*, 1977, 34: 15–21.

Hart B. *The Psychology of Insanity*. Cambridge, Cambridge University Press, 1916.

Hartenberg P. Le névrose d'angoisse. *Revue de Médicine*, 1901a, 21: 464–84; 612–21; 678–99.

Hartenberg P. *Les Timides et la Timidité*, Paris, Alcan, 1901b.

Hartenberg P. and Valentin P. The role de l'émotion dans la pathogénie et la thérapeutique des aboulies. *Revue de Psychologie Clinique and Thérapeutique* 1897, 1: 15–20; 45–8.

Hartley D. *Observations on Man, his Frame, his Duty and his Expectations*, Sixth Edition, London, Thomas Tegg and Son, 1834 (First Edition, 1749).

Hartmann H. and Schilder P. Zur Klinik der Amentia. *Zeitschrift für die gesamte Neurologie*, 1924, 92: 531–96.

Hartmann R. and Witter H. Le concept d'*Antrieb* en psychiatrie allemande. *L'Evolution Psychiatrique*, 1966, 31: 25–31.

Harvey P. and Heseltine J.E. *The Oxford Companion to French Literature*, Oxford, Clarendon Press, 1959.

Haskovec L. L'Akathisie. *Revue Neurologique* 1901, 9: 1107–9. (Translation in *History of Psychiatry*, 1995, 6: 245–248.)

Haskovec L. Nouvelles remarques sur l'akathisie. *Nouvelle Iconographie de la Salpêtrière*, 1903, 16: 287–96. (Translation in *History of Psychiatry* 1995, 6: 248–251.)

Haslam J. *Observations on Madness and Melancholy: Including Practical Remarks on those Diseases; together with cases: and an account of the Morbid Appearances on Dissection*, London, J. Callow, 1809.

Hassler R. Striatal control of locomotion, intentional actions and integrating and perceptive activity. *Journal of Neurological Science*, 1978, 36: 187–224.

Haupt T von. *Die Temperamente des Menschen im gesunden und kranken Zustande* Würzburg, Stahel, 1858.

Hausser-Hauw C. and Bancaud J. Gustatory hallucinations in epileptic seizures. *Brain*, 1987, 110: 339–59.

Hearnshaw L.S. *A Short History of British Psychology 1840–1940*, London, Methuen, 1964.

Hearnshaw L S. *The Shaping Of Modern Psychology*. London, Routledge, 1987.

Hécaen H. and Ajuriaguerra J. de: *Méconnaisances et hallucinations corporelles*. Paris, Masson, 1952.

Hécaen H. and Albert M.L. *Human Neuropsychology*, New York, John Wiley, 1978.

Hécaen H. and Dubois J. *La Naissance de la Neuropsychologie du Langage (1825–1865)* Paris, Flammarion, 1969.

Hécaen H. and Lantéri-Laura G. *Evolution des Connaissances et des Doctrines sur les Localisations Centrales*, Paris, Desclée de Brouwer, 1978.

Heckel F. *La Névrose d'Angoisse. et les États d'Émotivité Anxieuse*, Paris, Masson, 1917.

Hecker E. Die Hebephrenie. *Archiv für pathologische Anatomie und Physiologie und für klinische Medizin*, 1871, 52: 394–429.

Heiberg J.L. Geisteskrankheiten im klassischen Altertum. *Allegemeine Zeitschrift für Psychiatrie*, 1927, 86: 1–44.

Heidenhein R. *Hypnotism and Animal Magnetism*. London, Kegan Paul, 1899.

Heinroth J.C. *Textbook of Disturbances of Mental Life. Or Disturbances of the Soul and their Treatment*. (translated by J. Schmorak), Baltimore, Johns Hopkins University Press, 1975 (1st German edn., 1818).

Heins T., Gray A. and Tennant M. Persisting hallucinations following childhood sexual abuse. *Australian and New Zealand Journal of Psychiatry*, 1990, 24: 561–5.

Helmer O. and Rescher N. On the epistemology of the inexact sciences. *Management Science*, 1959, 8: 25–52.

Hemsley D.R. and Garety P.A. The formation and maintenance of delusions: a Bayesian analysis. *British Journal of Psychiatry*, 1986, 149: 51–6.

Henderson D.K. *Psychopathic States*, New York, Norton, 1939.

Henderson D.K. Robert Dick Gillespie. *American Journal of Psychiatry*, 1945, 102: 572–3.

Henderson V.H. Paul Broca's less heralded contributions to aphasia research. Historical perspective and contemporary relevance. *Archives of Neurology*, 1986, 43: 609–12.

Herbart J.F. *A Text-book in Psychology* (trans M. Smith). New York, Appleton, 1895 (first published, 1834).

Hering E. Über das Gedächtniss als eine allgemeine Funktion der organisierten Materie. *Vortrag gehalten in der feierlichen Sitzung der Kaiserlichen Akademie der Wissenschaften in Wien am XXX*, Wien, 1870.

Hering E. *Memory. Lectures on the specific energies of the nervous system*. Chicago, The Open Court Publishing Company, 1913.

Herman M., Harpham D. and Rosenblum M. Non-schizophrenic catatonic states. *New York State Journal of Medicine*, 1942, 43: 643–7.

Hermie L. Die Degenerationslehre in der Psychiatrie. *Fortschritte Neurologie Psychiatrie*, 1986, 54: 69–79.

Herodotus. *Histories*. Loeb's Classical Library. Book VI. London, W. Heinemann, 1971.

Herrmann D.J. and Chaffin R. *Memory in Historical Perspective*, Berlin, Springer, 1988.

Herzen A. *Fisiologia de la Voluntad*, Second Edition, Madrid, Iravedra, 1880 (first edition, 1873).

Hesnard A. and Laforgue R. Aperçu historique des mouvement psychanalytique en France. *L'Evolution Psychiatrique*, 1925, 1: 11–26.

Hesnard A. *Les Psychoses et les Frontières de la Folie*, Paris, Flammarion, 1924.

Hesnard A. *De Freud á Lacan*, Paris, Les Editions ESF, 1971.

Hesse M B. *Models and Analogies in Science*. University of Notre Dame Press, Notre Dame, Indiana, 1966.

Hesse M B. Reasons and evaluations in the history of science. In Teich M. and Young R. (eds.) *Changing Perspectives in the History of Science. Essays in Honour of Joseph Needham*, London, Heinemann, pp 127–147, 1973.

Hett W.S. Introduction. In *Aristotle*. Vol. 8, Loeb Edition, London, Heinemann, 1986.

Heymans G. and Wiersma E. Beiträge zur speziellen Psychologie auf grund einer Massenunterschung. *Zeitschrift für Psychologie*, 1906, 42: 81–127; 253–301.

Higier H. Über unilaterale Hallucinationen. *Wiener Klinik*, 1894, 20: 139–70.

Hilgard E.R. The trilogy of mind: cognition, affection and conation. *Journal of the History of the Behavioral Sciences*: 1980, 16: 107–17.

Hilts V.L. *Statist and Statistician: Three Studies in the History of Nineteenth Century English Statistical Thought*, PhD Dissertation, Harvard University, 1967 (published by Arno Press, 1981).

Hilts V.L. Obeying the laws of hereditary descent: phrenological views on inheritance and eugenics. *Journal of the History of the Behavioral Science*, 1982, 18: 62–77.

Hinde R.A. Energy models of motivation. *Symposia of the Society for Experimental Psychology*. Vol. 14, Cambridge, Cambridge University Press, pp. 199–213, 1960.

Hippocrates: *Works*, (with and English translation by W.H.S. Jones) Loeb Classical Library, London, William Heinemann, 1972.

Hobbes T. *English Works* (edited by Sir William Molesworth), London, John Bohn, 1839–1845.

Hobbes T. *Leviathan* (version edited by C.B. Macpherson), London, Penguin Books, 1968 (first published in 1651).

Hobbes T. Quoted in 'Stupor' entry of *Oxford English Dictionary*, second edition.

Hoch A. *Benign Stupors*, Cambridge, Cambridge University Press, 1921.

Hodges H.A. *The Philosophy of Wilhelm Dilthey*. Connecticut, Greenwood, 1952.

Hodges J.R. *Transient Amnesia*, London, Saunders, 1991.

Hodges J.R. and Ward C.D. Observations during Transient Global Amnesia. *Brain*, 1989, 112: 595–620.

Hoeldtke R. The history of associationism and British medical psychology. *Medical History*, 1967, 11: 46–64.

Hoenig J. The clinical usefulness of the phenomenology of delusions. *International Journal of Psychiatry*, 1968, 6: 41–5.

Hoenig J. The concept of schizophrenia: Kraepelin–Bleuler–Schneider. *British Journal of Psychiatry*, 1983, 142: 547–56.

Hoenig J., Tiakley J.G. and Meyer A. The diagnosis of stupor. *Psychiatrie et Neurologie*, 1959, 137: 128–44.

Hoeres W. Der Wille als reine Vollkommenheit nach Duns Scotus *Salzburger Studien Z., Phil.*, 1; Munich, Salzburg Press, 1962.

Hoff P. Zum Krankheitsbegriff bei Emil Kraepelin. *Nervenarzt*, 1985, 56: 510–13.

Hoffbauer J.C. *Médicine légale relative aux aliénés et aux sourds-muets ou les lois appliquées aux désordres de l'intelligence* (translated by A.M. Chambeyron with notes by Esquirol and Itard) Paris, Baillière, 1827 (first German edition 1808).

Höffding H. *Outlines of Psychology* (translated by M.E. Lowndes), London, McMillan, pp. 221–307, 1892.

Holland H. *Chapters on Mental Physiology*. London, Longman, Brown, Green, and Longman, 1852.

Hollander B. The cerebral localization of melancholia. *Journal of Mental Science*, 1901, 47: 458–85.

Hollander B. *The Mental Functions of the Brain. An Investigation into their Localization and their Manifestation in Health and Disease*, London, Grant Richards, 1901.

Hollander B. *The First Signs of Insanity*, London, Stanley Paul, 1912.

Hollander B. *Brain, Mind and the External Signs of Intelligence*, London, George Allen and Unwin, 1931.

Hollander E., Leabowitz M.R., Winchel R. *et al.* Treatment of body-dysmorphic disorder with serotonic re-uptake inhibitors. *American Journal of Psychiatry*, 1989, 146: 768–70.

Hollister L.E. and Glazener F.S. Concurrent paralysis agitans and schizophrenia. *Diseases of the Nervous System*, 1961, 22: 187–9.

Holton G. *Thematic Origins of Scientific Thought*. Harvard University Press, Cambridge, Massachusetts, 1973.

Hopewell-Ash E.L. *Melancholia in Everyday Practice*, London, Bale, 1934.

Horwicz A. Histoire du développement de la volunté. *Revue Philosophique*, 1876, 1: 488–502.

Houzeau J.C. *Études sur les Facultés Mentales des Animaux Comparées a Celles de l'Homme*, Paris, Hachette, 1872.

Howells J.G. Dementia in Shakespeare's King Lear. In Berrios G.E. and Freeman, H.L. (eds.) *Alzheimer and the Dementias*, London, Royal Society of Medicine, pp. 101–109, 1991.

Huber G. and Gross G. *Wahn*, Stuttgart, Enke, 1977.

Huber J-P. and Gourin P. Le vieillard dément dans l'antiquité classique. *Psychiatrie Française*, 1987, 13: 12–18.

Huertas R. *Locura y Degeneración: Psiquiatría y Sociedad en el Positivismo Francés*. Madrid, Consejo Superior de Investigaciones Científicas, 1987 (English translation has appeared in *History of Psychiatry*, 1992–3).

Humbert F. Les états dits psychopathiques constitutionnels; terms, notions et Limites. *Schweizer Archives Neurologie Psychiatrie*, 1947, 59: 179–95.

Hume D. *A Treatise of Human Nature*, Selby-Bigge edn., Oxford, Clarendon Press, 1888.

Humbolt W. von *On Language* (Transl. by Peter Health) Cambridge, Cambridge University Press, 1988 (first German edition 1836).

Hunter K.M. *Doctor's Stories. The Narrative Structure of Medical Knowledge*, Princeton, Princeton University Press, 1991.

Hunter R. Psychiatry and neurology. Psychosyndrome or brain disease. *Proceedings of the Royal Society of Medicine*, 1973, 66: 359–64.

Hunter R. and McAlpine I. In Battie W.A. *Treatise on Madness*, London, Dawson of Pall Mall, 1962.

Hunter R. and McAlpine I. *Three Hundred Years of Psychiatry 1535–1860*, New York, Oxford University Press, 1963.

Hutton P.H. The art of memory reconceived: from rhetoric to psychoanalysis. *Journal of the History of Ideas*, 1987, 48: 371–92.

ICD-9: *Glossary and Guide to their Classification in accordance with the Ninth Revision of the International Classification of Diseases*, Geneva, World Health Organization, 1978.

ICD-10 *Classification of Mental and Behavioural Disorders*, Geneva, World Health Organization, 1992.

Ingram W.R., Barris R.W. and Ranson S.W. Catalepsy. *Archives of Neurology and Psychiatry*, 1936, 35: 1175–97.

Ioteyko J. *La Fatigue*, Paris, Flammarion, 1920.

Ireland W.W. On hallucinations, especially of sight and hearing. In *The Blot upon the Brain*, 2nd edn., Edinburgh, Bell and Bradfute, pp. 1–55, 1893.

Ireland W.W. On fixed ideas. In *The Blot upon the Brain*, Edinburgh, pp. 189–205, Bell and Bradfute, 1893.

Irwin F.W. The concept of volition in experimental psychology. In Clarke F.P. and Nahm M.C. (eds.) *Philosophical Essays in Honor of E.A. Singer Jr.* Philadelphia, University of Pensylvania Press, 1942.

Iversen G.R. *Bayesian Statistical Inference*, London, Sage, 1984.

Jackson J.H. A lecture on softening of the brain. *Lancet*, 1875, ii: 335–9.

Jackson J.H. On the comparative study of diseases of the nervous system, *British Medical Journal*, 1889, ii, 355–64.

Jackson J.H. The factors of insanities. *Medical Press and Circular*, 1894, ii: 615–26.

Jackson J.H. On imperative ideas. *Brain*, 1895, 18: 318–22.

Jackson J.H. *Selected Writings of John Hughlings Jackson*, 2 Vols, London, Hodder and Stoughton, 1932.

Jackson S.W. Force and kindred notions in eighteenth century neurophysiology and medical psychology. *Bulletin of the History of Medicine*, 1970, 64: 397–410; 539–54.

Jackson S.W. Unusual mental states in mediaeval Europe: I: Medical syndromes of mental disorders 400–1100 AD. *Journal of History of Medicine and Allied Science*, 1972, 27: 262–97.

Jackson S.W. Two sufferers' perspectives on melancholia: 1690s to 1790s. In Wallace IV E.R. and Pressley L.C. (eds.) *Essays in the History of Psychiatry*, W.M.S. Hall Psychiatric Institute of the South Carolina, Department of Mental Health, pp. 559–71, l980.

Jackson S.W. Melancholia and partial insanity. *Journal of the History of Behavioural Science*, 1983, 19: 173–84.

Jackson S.W. Melancholia and mechanical explanation in eighteenth century medicine. *Journal of History of Medicine and Allied Sciences*, 1983, 38: 298–319.

Jackson S.W. *Melancholia and Depression*, New Haven, Yale University Press, 1986.

Jacobs W.G. Bewuβtsein. In Krings H., Baumgartner H.M. and Wild Ch. *Handbuch Philosophischer Grundbegriffe*, Vol. 1, München, Kösel, pp. 232–46, 1973.

Jacques A. Faculties de l'Ame. In Franck A. (ed.) *Dictionnaire des Sciences Philosophiques* (Second Edition), Paris, Hachette, pp. 511–16, 1875.

Jacyna L.S. Somatic theories of mind and the interests of medicine in Britain. *Medical History*, 1982, 26: 233–58.

Jakob A. Über eine multiplen Sklerose klinisch nahestehende Erkrankung des Zentralnervensystem (spastiche Pseudosklerose) mit bemerkenswertem anatomischem Befunde. Mitteilung eines vierten Falles. *Medizinischen Klinik*, 1921, 17: 372–6.

Jalley M. Lefebvre J.P and Feline A. Essai sur les maladies de la tête par E. Kant. *L'Evolution Psychiatrique*, 1977, 42: 203–30.

James A.R.W. L'hallucination simple? *Revue D'Histoire Litteraire de la France*, 1986, 6: 1024–37.

James F.E. Some observations on the writings of Felix Platter (1539–1614) in relation to mental handicap. *History of Psychiatry*, 1990, 2:103–8.

James W. *The Principles of Psychology*, Vol. 2, London, McMillan, 1891.

James W. *The Varieties of Religious Experience*. London, Longmans, Green and Co., 1903.

Janet P. *L'Automatisme Psychologique*, Paris, Alcan, 1889.

Janet P. Résumé historique des études sur le sentiment de la personnalité. *Revue Scientifique*, 1896, 5: 98–103.

Janet P. *Névroses et Idées Fixes*, 2 Vols, Paris, Alcan, 1898.

Janet P. *Les Névroses*, Paris, Flammarion, 1909.

Janet P. L'oeuvre psychologique de Th Ribot. *Journal de Psychologie Normal et Pathologique*, 1916, 12: 268–82.

Janet P. *Les Obsessions et la Psychasthénie*, Third Edition, Paris, Alcan, 1919 (First Edition, 1903).

Janet P. *Les Médications Psychologiques*, 3 Vols, Paris, Alcan, 1919.

Janet P. *De L'Angoisse a L'Extase*, 2 vols, Paris, Alcan, 1926.

Janet P. *L'Evolution Psychologique de la Personnalité*, Paris, Chahine, 1929.

Janet P. Nécrologie. Eugène-Bernard Leroy. *Journal de Psychologie Normale et Pathologique*, 1933, 30: 664–72.

Janet P. and Séailles G. *A History of the Problems of Philosophy*, Vol. 1, Psychology, London, McMillan, 1902.

Janzarik W (ed.) *Psychopathologie als Grundlagenwissenschaft*, Enke, Stuttgart, 1979.

Jardine N. *The Fortunes of Inquiry*, Clarendon Press, Oxford, 1986.

Jardine N. *The Scenes of Inquiry*, Clarendon Press, Oxford, 1991.

Jaspers K. Die Methoden der Intelligenzprüfung und der Begriff der Demenz. *Zeitschrift für die gesamte Neurologie and Psychiatrie*, 1910, 1: 402–52.

Jaspers K. Einfersuchtswahn. Ein Beitrag zur Frage: 'Entwicklung einer Persönlichkeit oder Prozess'. *Zeitschrift für the gesamte Neurology und Psychiatrie*, 1910, 1: 567–637.

Jaspers K. Zur Analyse der Trugwahrnemungen (Leibhaftigkeit und Realitätsurteil). *Zeitschrift für die gesamte Neurologie und Psychiatrie*, 1911, 6: 460–534.

Jaspers K. Die Trugwahrnemungen. *Zeitschrift für die gesamte Neurologie und Psychiatrie, (Referate und Ergebnisse)*, 1912, 4: 289–354.

Jaspers K. Über Leibhaftige Bewusstheiten (Bewusstheitsstäuschungen). Ein psychopathologischen Elementarsymptom. *Zeitschrift für Patho-Psychologie*, 1913, 2: 151–61.

Jaspers K. *Allgemeine Psychopathologie*, Fifth Edition, Berlin, Springer, 1948.

Jaspers K. *General Psychopathology* A translation of the Seventh German Edition by J. Hoenig and M.W. Hamilton, Manchester, Manchester University Press, 1963.

Jastrow J. Obsession. In Baldwin J.M. (ed.) *Dictionary of Philosophy and Psychology*, Vol. 2, London, MacMillan, 1901.

Jeanmaire Ch. *L'Idée de la Personnalité dans la Psychologie Moderne*, Toulouse, Douladoure-Privat, 1882.

Jeannerod M. *Le Cerveau-Machine. Physiologie de la Volunté*, Paris, Fayard, 1983.

Jefferson G. The nature of concussion. *British Medical Journal*, 1944, i: 1–5.

Jelliffe S.E. Cyclothemia. The mild forms of manic-depressive psychosis and the manic-depressive constitution. *American Journal of Insanity*, 1911, 67: 661–75.

Jelliffe S.E. and White W.A. *Diseases of the Nervous System*, 5th edn., London, Lewis, 1929.

Jelliffe S.E. Post encephalitic respiratory disorders. Psychopathological considerations. *Journal of Nervous and Mental Disease*, 1926, 64: 503–27.

Jelliffe S.E. Psychopathology of forced movements in oculogyric crises. New York, *Nervous and Mental Disease Monograph*, 1932, Series N° 55.

Jelliffe S.E. The psychopathology of the oculogyric crises and its funeral by Dr Lawrence S. Kubie, *Psychoanalytic Quarterly*, 1935, 4: 360–6.

Jelliffe S.E. The Parkinsonian body posture: some considerations on unconscious hostility. *Psychoanalytic Review*, 1940, 27: 467–79.

Jellinger K., Gerstenbrand F. and Pateisky K. Die Protrahierte Form der posttraumatischen Enzephalopathie. *Nervenarzt*, 1963, 34: 145–63.

Jennett W.B. and Plum F. The persistent vegetative state: a syndrome in search of a name. *Lancet*, 1972, i: 734–7.

Jeste D.V., del Carmen R., Lohr J.B. and Wyatt R.J. Did schizophrenia exist before the eighteenth century? *Comprehensive Psychiatry*, 1985, 26: 493–503.

Jobe T.H. Medical theories of melancholia in the 17th and early 18th centuries. *Clio-Medica*, 1976, 11: 217–29.

Joffroy A. Las hallucinations unilatérales. *Archives de Neurologie*, 1896, 4: 97–112.

Johnson A.L., Hollister L.E. and Berger P.A. The anticholinergic intoxication syndrome: diagnosis and treatment. *Journal of Clinical Psychiatry*, 1981, 42: 313–7.

Johnson S. *A Dictionary of the English Language*, London, J. and P., Knopton, T. Longman, 1755.

Johnston D. *The Rethoric of Leviathan*, Princeton, Princeton University Press, 1986.

Johnstone E., Crow T.J. and Frith C.D. The dementia of dementia praecox. *Acta Psychiatrica Scandinavica*, 1978, 57: 305–24.

Jolivet R. *Introducción a Kierkegaard*, Madrid, Gredos, 1950.

Jones K. *A History of the Mental Health Services*. Routledge and Kegan Paul, London, 1972.

Jones M. and Hunter R. Abnormal movements in patients with chronic psychiatric illness. In Crane G.E. and Gardner P. (eds.) *Psychothropic Drugs and Dysfunctions of the Basal Ganglia: A Multi-Disciplinary Workshop*, US Public Health Service Publication N° 1938, Washington, Government Printing Office, pp. 53–64, 1969.

Jong H. de Experimental catatonia in animals and induced catatonic stupor in man. *Diseases of the Nervous System*, 1956, 17: 137–9.

Joseph, A.B. Cotard's syndrome in a patient with co-existent Capgras' syndrome, syndrome of subjective doubles, and palinopsia. *Journal of Clinical Psychiatry*, 1986, 47: 605–6.

Joseph, A.B. and O'Leary, D.H. Brain atrophy and inter-hemispheric fissure in Cotard's syndrome. *Journal Clinical Psychiatry*, 1986, 47: 518–20.

Jouard G. Recension du traité médico-philosophique sur l'aliénation Mentale ou la manie par Phillipe Pinel, *Bibliothèque Française*, ouvrage périodique, pp. 105–117, N° VIII, Frimaire, An X, Décember 1880.

Jourdan (no initial). Confusion. In *Dictionaire des Sciences Médicales*, Paris, Panckouke, 1813.

Juliard P. *Philosophies of Language in Eighteenth Century France*, The Hague, Mouton, 1970.

Jung C.G. The psychology of dementia praecox. In *The Collected Works*, Vol. 3, London, Routledge and Kegan Paul, pp. 1–151, 1972 (First Edition, 1907).

Jung C.G. *Über die Psychologie der Dementia praecox: Ein Versuch*, Falle, Carl Marhold, 1907.

Jung C.G. *Tipos Psicológicos* (translation by Ramón de la Serna), Buenos Aires, Editorial Sudamericana, 1964.

Kaan H. *Der neurasthenische Angsteffekt bei Zwangsvorstellungen und der primordiale Grübelzwang*. Leipzig, Deutike, 1892.

Kageyama J. Sur l'histoire de la monomanie. *L'Evolution Psychiatrique*, 1984, 49: 155–62.

Kahlbaum K. *Die Gruppirung der psychischen Krankheiten und die Eintheilung der Seelenstörungen*, Danzig, A.W. Kafemann, 1863.

Kahlbaum K.L. Die Sinnesdelirien. *Allgemeine Zeitschrift für Psychiatrie*, 1866, 23: 1–86.

Kahlbaum K.L. Über Spannunsirresein. *Archiv für Psychiatrie und Nervenkrankheiten*, 1870, 2: 502.

Kahlbaum K.L. *Die Katatonie, oder das Spannungsirresein*, Berlin, Kirschwald, 1874.

Kahlbaum K.L. *Catatonia*, Baltimore, Johns Hopkins University, 1973.

Kahn E. Die anankastische Psychopathen. In Bumke O. (ed.) *Handbuch der Geisteskrankheiten*, Vol. 5, Part 1, Berlin, Springer, 1928.

Kahn E. *Psychopathic Personalities*, New Haven, Yale University Press, 1931.

Kandinsky V. Zur Lehre von den Hallucinationen. *Archiv für Psychiatrie und Nervenkrankheiten*, 1881, 11: 453–64.

Kandinsky V. *Kritische und Klinische Betrachtungen im gebiete der Sinnestäuschungen*. Berlin, Verlag von Friedländer and Sohn, 1885.

Kanner L. *A History of the Care and Study of the Mentally Retarded*. Charles C Thomas, Springfield, Illinois, 1964.

Kant E. *Anthropologie in pragmatischer Hinsicht abgefaßt*. 2nd Edition, Königsberg, Friedrich Nicolovius, 1800.

Kant E. *Anthropologie* (translated by J. Tissot), Paris, Ladrange, 1863.

Kant E. A Sömmerring. De l'organ de l'ame. In *Anthropologie*, translated by J. Tissot, Paris, Ladrange, pp. 441–446, 1863.

Kant E. *Critique of Practical Reason* (translation by T.K. Abbott), London, Longman, 1909.

Kant E. *Critique of Judgement (translated by J.H. Bernard)*, London, Longman, 1914 (First Edition 1790).

Kant E. *Antropología*. (translated by José Gaos), Madrid, Revista de Occidente, 1935.

Kant E. *Anthropology from a Pragmatic Point of View (translated with an introduction and notes by Mary J. Gregor)* The Hague, Martinus Nijhoff, 1974 (First Edition, 1798).

Kasanin J. and Haufmann E. Disturbances in concept formation in schizophrenia. *Archives of Neurology and Psychiatry*, 1938, 40: 1276–82.

Kasanin J.S. and Lewis N.D.C. (eds.) *Language and Thought in Schizophrenia*, New York, Norton, 1944.

Kastenbaum R. and Ross B. Historical perspectives on care. In Howells J. (ed.) *Modern Perspectives in the Psychiatry of Old Age*, Edinburgh, Churchill Livingstone, pp. 421–49, 1975.

Katona C. and Levy R. (eds.) *Delusions and Hallucinations in Old Age*, London, Gaskell, 1992.

Katz D. *El Mundo de las Sensaciones Tactiles*, Madrid, Revista de Occidente, 1930 (translation of Der Aufbau der Tastwelt. *Zeitschrift für Psychologie und Physiologie den Sinnesorgane*, 1925, suppl. II).

Katz J. Psychophysiological contributions to phantom limbs. *Canadian Journal of Psychiatry*, 1992, 37: 282–98.

Katzenstein R. *Karl Ludwig Kahlbaum. Und sein Beitrag zur Entwicklung der Psychiatrie*, Zürich, Juris, 1963.

Kazdin A.E. Evaluation of the pleasure scale in the assessment of anhedonia in children. *Journal of the American Academy of Childhood and Adolescent Psychiatry*, 1989, 28: 364–72.

Kearns A. Cotard's syndrome in a mentally handicapped man. *British Journal of Psychiatry*, 1987, 150: 112–14.

Keller W. *Psychologie und Philosophie des Wollens*, Basel, Reinhardt, 1954.

Kemperman C.J.F. and Hutter J.M. Pseudohallucinations in diabetic eye-disease: a natural Rorschach test? *Netherlands Journal of Medicine*, 1989, 35: 201–3.

Kendell R.E. *The Classification of Depressive Illnesses*, London, Oxford University Press, 1968.

Kendler K.S., Glazer W.M. and Morgenstern H. Dimensions of delusional experience. *American Journal of Psychiatry* 1983, 140: 466–9.

Kenny A. *Action, Emotion and Will*. London, Routledge, Kegan and Paul, 1963.

Kenny A. Descartes. *A Study of his Philosophy*. New York, Random House, 1968.

Kenny A. *Aristotle's Theory of the Will*. London, Duckworth, 1979.

Kenny A. *Aquinas*, Oxford, Oxford University Press, 1980.

Kensies F. *Arbeitshygiene der Schule auf Grund von Ermüdungsmessen*, Berlin, Reuther und Reichard, 1898.

Kenyon F.K. Hypochondriasis: a survey of some historical, clinical and social aspects. *British Journal Medical Psychology*, 1965, 38: 117–33.

Kernberg O. Borderline personality organization. *Journal American Psychoanalytic Association*, 1967, 15: 641–85.

Keschner M. and Sloane P. Encephalitic, idiopathic and arteriosclerotic parkinsonism. *Archives of Neurology and Psychiatry*, 1931, 25: 1011–14.

Ketal R. Affect, mood, emotion and feeling. Semantic consideration. *American Journal of Psychiatry*, 1975, 132: 1215–17.

Keup W. (ed.) *Origin and Mechanisms of Hallucinations*, New York, Plenum Press, 1970.

Kevles D. *In the Name of Eugenics: Genetics and the Uses of Human Heredity*, New York, Wiley, 1985.

Kiloh L.G. Pseudo-dementia. *Acta Psychiatrica Scandinavica*, 1961, 37: 336–51.

Kim J. *Supervenience and Mind*, Cambridge, Cambridge University Press, 1993.

Kimble G.A. and Perlmuter L.C. The problem of volition. *Psychological Review*, 1970, 77: 361–84.

Kinderman P. Attentional bias, persecutory delusions and the self-concept. *British Journal of Clinical Psychology*.1994, 67: 53–66.

King L.S. Signs and symptoms. *Journal of the American Medical Association*, l968, 206: 1063–5.

King L.S. *Medical Thinking*. Princeton, Princeton University Press, pp. 131–83, 1982.

Kirkegaard S. *El Concepto de la Angustia*, Madrid, Espasa Calpe, 1959.

Klaf F.S. and Hamilton J.G. Schizophrenia – a hundred years ago and today. *Journal of Mental Science*, 1961, 128: 819–27.

Kläsi J. *Über die Bedeutung und Entstehung der Stereotypien*. Berlin, Karger Verlag, 1922.

Klein E. *A Comprehensive Etymological Dictionary of the English Language*, Vol. 2, Amsterdam, Elsevier, 1967.

Klein D B. *A History of Scientific Psychology*, London, Routledge and Kegan Paul, 1970.

Klein D.B. The Scottish school and its 'faculties'. In *A History of Scientific Psychology*, London, Routledge, Kegan and Paul, pp. 638–698, l970.

Klein D.F. Endogenomorphic depression: a conceptual and terminological revision. *Archives in General Psychiatry* 31: 447–54, 1974.

Klein D.F, Gittelman R. and Quitkin F. *et al. Diagnosis and Drug Treatment of Psychiatric Disorder: Adults and Children.* Baltimore, Williams and Wilkins, 1980.

Klein D.F. Depression and anhedonia, in Clark D.C, Fawcett J. (eds.) *Anhedonia and Affect Deficit States.* New York, PMA Publishing Corp., 1987.

Kleinman A. *Social Origins Of Distress And Disease: Depression, Neurasthenia, and Pain in Modern China,* New Haven, Yale University Press, 1986.

Kleist K. Zur hirnpathologischen Auffassung der schizophrenen Grundstörungen. Die alogische Denkstörung. *Schweizer Archiv für Neurologie und Psychiatrie,* 1930, 26: 99–102.

Klosterkötter J. Schizophrenia simplex. Gibt es das? *Nervenarzt,* 1983, 54: 340–6.

Knapp T.J. and Schumacher M.T. *Westphal's Die Agoraphobie,* Lanham, University Press of America, 1988.

Knoll E. The science of language and the evolution of mind: Max Müller's quarrel with Darwinism. *Journal of the History of the Behavioral Sciences,* 1986, 22: 3–22.

Koch J.A. *Die psychopathischen Minderwertigkeiten.* Ravensburg, Maier, 1891.

Koehler K. Delusional perception and delusional notion linked to a perception. *Psychiatria Clinica,* 1976, 9: 45–58.

Koffka K. *The Growth of the Mind,* Second Edition, London, Kegan Paul, 1928.

Kogan A.A. *Cuerpo y Persona.* México, Fondo de Cultura Económica, 1981.

Koh S.E., Grinker R.R., Marusartz N.T. and Forman P. Affective memory and schizophrenic anhedonia. *Schizophrenia Bulletin,* 1981, 7: 292–307.

Kohut H. and Wolf E.S. The disorders of the self and their treatment: an outline. *International Journal of Psycho-Analysis,* 1978; 59: 413–25.

Kolle K. Carl Friedrich Flemming. In Kolle K. (ed.) *Grosse Nervenärzte,* Vol. 3, Stuttgart, George Thième, pp. 61–68, 1963.

König H. Zur Psychopathologie der Paralysis Agitans. *Archiv für Psychiatrie und Nervenkrankheiten,* 1912, 50: 285–305.

Koninck de C. Introduction á l'ètude de l'âme. *Lavel Théologique et Philosophique,* 1947, 3: 9–65.

Korkina M.V. and Morozov P.V. Dysmorphophobic disorders. *Zh. Neuropath. Psikhiat. Korsakov,* 1979, 79: 111.

Koupernick C. La Psychose de laideur ou dysmorphophobie. *Entretiens de Bichat (Médecine),* 1962, 321–6.

Koupernik C., Loo H., Zarifian E. *Précis de Psychiatrie.* Paris, Flammarion, 1982.

Kraepelin E. Über Erinnerungsfälschungen. *Archiv für Psychiatrie und Nervenkrankheiten,* 1886–1887, 17: 830–43; 18: 199–239, 395–436.

Kraepelin E. Der psychologische Versuch in der Psychiatrie. *Psychologische Arbeiten,* 1896, 1: 1–91.

Kraepelin E. *Zur Überbürdungsfrage,* Jena, Fischer, 1898.

Kraepelin E. Die Arbeitskurve. *Wundts Philosophischen Studien,* 1902, 19: 459–507.

Kraepelin E. *Lectures on Clinical Psychiatry* (translated and edited by Thomas Johnstone) London, Tindall and Cox, 1904.

Kraepelin E. *Lectures on Clinical Psychiatry* (revised and edited by Thomas Johnstone) Second Edition, London, Baillière, Tindall and Cox, 1906.

Kraepelin E. *Psychiatrie. Ein Lehrbuch für Studierende und Ärzte,* Klinische Psychiatrie. Leipzig, Barth, 1910–1915.

Kraepelin E. *Dementia Praecox and Paraphrenia* (BM Barclay trans). Edinburgh, E. and S. Livingstone, 1919 (first published, 1913).

Kraepelin E. Die Erscheinungsformen des Irreseins. *Zeitschrift für die gesamte Neurologie und Psychiatrie,* 1920, 62: 1–29.

Kraepelin E. *Manic Depressive Insanity and Paranoia,* Edinburgh, E. and S. Livingstone, 1921.

Kraepelin E. *Lebenserinnerungen*, Berlin, Springer, 1983.

Krafft-Ebing R. Über Geistestörung durch Zwangsvorstellungen. *Allgemeine Zeitschrift für Psychiatrie*, 1879, 35: 303–28.

Krafft-Ebing. R. De la démence senile. *Annales Médico-Psychologiques*, 1876, 34: 306–7.

Krafft-Ebing. R. *Lehrbuch der Psychiatrie*, Fifth Edition, Stuttgart, Enke, 1893.

Kraft I. Edouard Séguin and 19th century moral treatment of idiots. *Bulletin of the History of Medicine*, 1961, 35: 393–418.

Krestchmer E. *A Textbook of Medical Psychology*, Oxford, Oxford University Press, 1934.

Kretschmer E. *Physique and Character* (translated by W.J.H. Sprott), London, Kegal Paul, Trench, Trubner and Co, 1936.

Kretschmer E. Das apallische Syndrom. *Zeitschrift für Neurologie und Psychiatrie*, 1940, 169: 576–9.

Krishaber M. Cérébro-cardiaque (névropathie). In Dechambre A. and Lereboullet L. (eds.) *Dictionnaire Encyclopédique des Sciences Médicales*, Vol. 14, Paris, Masson, pp. 100–142, 1873.

Kroll J. A Reappraisal of Psychiatry in the Middle Ages. *Archives of General Psychiatry*, 1973, 29: 276–83.

Kronecker H. Über die Ermüdung und Erholung der quergestreiften Muskeln. *Beritche der Verhandlungen d.k. saechsisch Gesell. der Wiss zu Leipzig*, 1871, 5: 710–36.

Krueger F. Das Wesen der Gefühle. Entwurf einer systematischen Theorie. *Archiv für die Gesamte Psychologie*, 1928, 65: 91–128.

Krugelstein J. Mémoire sur le suicide. *Annales d'Hygiène Publique et the Médecine Légale*, 1841, 25: 151–82.

Kubie L.S. On the psychopathology of forced movements and the oculogyric crises of lethargic encephalitis. *Psychoanalytic Quarterly*, 1933, 2: 622–6.

Kuch K. and Swinson R.P. Agoraphobia: what Westphal really said. *Canadian Journal of Psychiatry*, 1992, 37: 133–6.

Kuhn T. *The Structure of Scientific Revolutions*. Chicago University, Press, 1962.

Kühne G.E., Hempel H.D. and Koselowski G. Toward the development of operational criteria of differentiated mental states. *Psychopathology*, 1985, 18: 98–105.

Kushner H.I. American psychiatry and the cause of suicide 1844–1917. *Bulletin History of Medicine*, 1986, 60: 36–57.

Lacan J. *De la psychose paranoïque dans ses rapports avec la personnalité suivie de premiers écrits sur la paranoïa*. Paris, Éditions du Seuil, 1975 (first published in 1932).

Ladame P.L. La folie du doute et le délire du toucher. *Annales Médico-Psychologiques*, 1890, 12: 368–86.

Ladee G.A. *Hypochondriacal Syndromes*, Amsterdam, Elsevier, 1966.

Lafond, A.M. *Du délire chronique des négations comme survivance asilaire*. Paris: Thèse n° 112, 1973.

Lafora G.R. Foreword to Spanish Edition. in Mauz F. *El Pronóstico de las psicosis endógenas* (translated by L. Valenciano), Madrid, Morata, 1931 (German edition 1930).

Lafora G.R. Sobre la Presbiofrenia sin Confabulaciones. *Archivos de Neurobiologia*, 1935, 15: 179–211.

Lagache D. *Oeuvres II (1947–1952)*, Paris, Presses Universitaires de France, 1979.

Lagneau G. Cagots. In Dechambre A. and Lereboullet L. (eds.) *Dictionnaire Encyclopédique des Sciences Médicales*, Vol. 11, Paris, Masson, pp 534–557, 1869.

Lagneau L.V. *Tratado Práctico de las Enfermedades Sifilíticas*. 2 Volumes, Madrid, Imprenta de Villaamil, 1834 (translation of the 6th French edition; first French edition, 1801).

Lagriffe L. Les troubles du mouvement dans la démence précoce. *Annales Médico-Psychologiques* 1913, 71: 136–53.

Laignel-Lavastine M., Barbé A, and Delmas A. *La Pratique Psychiatrique*. Paris, Baillière et fils, 1929.

Laín-Entralgo P. *La Historia Clínica. Historia y Teoría del Relato Patográfico*, Barcelona, Salvat, 1961.

Laín-Entralgo P. *La Relación Médico-Enfermo*, Madrid, Revista de Occidente, 1964.

Laín-Entralgo P. *Historia de la Medicina*, Barcelona, Salvat, 1978.

Laín-Entralgo P. *El Diagnóstico Médico*, Barcelona, Salvat, 1982.

Laín-Entralgo, P. *El Cuerpo Humano. Oriente y Grecia Antigua*. Madrid, Espasa, 1987.

Lakatos I. and Musgrave A. (eds.) *Criticism and the Growth of Knowledge*. Cambridge, Cambridge University Press, 1970.

Lalande A. Des paramnésies. *Revue Philosophique*, 1893, 36: 485–7.

Lalande A. *Vocabulaire Technique et Critique de la Philosophie*. Paris, Presses Universitaires de France, 1976.

Lalanne (no initial). Des ètats anxieux dans les maladies mentales. *Revue Neurologique*, 1902, 2: 755–62.

Lambert C.I. The clinical and anatomical features of Alzheimer's disease. *Journal of Mental and Nervous Disease*, 1916, 44: 169–70.

Lambie J. The misuse of Kuhn in psychology. The psychologist: *Bulletin of the British Psychological Society*, 1991, 1: 6–11.

Lamy H. Hémianopsie avec hallucinations dans la partie abolie du champ de la vision. *Revue de Neurologie*, 1895, 3: 129–35.

Lanczik M. *Der Breslauer Psychiater Carl Wernicke*, Sigmaringen, Thorbecke, 1988.

Landman M. *Philosophische Anthropologie*, Berlin, Gruyter, 1958.

Landré-Beauvais A.J. *Séméiotique ou Traité des Signes des Maladies*, Second Edition, Paris, Brosson, 1813.

Lane H. *The Wild Boy of Aveyron*. London, George Allen and Unwin, 1977.

Lang J.L. Situation de l'infance handicapée. *Esprit*, 1965, 33: 588–99.

Lange J. Die Endogenen und Reaktiven Gemütserkrankungen. In Vol. 2, Bumke O. (ed.) *Handbuch der Geisteskrankheiten*, Berlin, Springer, 1928.

Lange J. *Psiquiatría*. Translated by R. Sarró. Madrid, Miguel Servet, 1942. (translation of the 4th German edition).

Lange K. *Apperception*. Boston, Heath and Company, 1900.

Langle M. *De l'action d'Arrêt ou Inhibition dans les Phénomènes Psychiques*, Paris, Thèse, 1886.

Lantéri-Laura G. *Les Apports de la Linguistique a la Psychiatrie Contemporaine*, Paris, Masson, 1966.

Lantéri-Laura G. *Histoire de la Phrénologie*, Paris, Presses Universitaires de France, 1970.

Lantéri-Laura G. La chronicité dans la psychiatrie moderne Française. *Annales*, 1972, 3: 548–68.

Lantéri-Laura G. *Lecture des Perversions. Histoire de leur Appropriation Médicale*, Paris, Masson, 1979.

Lantéri-Laura G. Conditions théoriques et conditions institutionnelles de la connaissance des perversions au XIX siècle. *L'Evolution Psychiatrique*, 1979, 45: 633–62.

Lantéri-Laura G. La Semiologie de J.P. Falret. *Perspectives Psychiatriques*, 1984, 22: 104–10.

Lantéri-Laura G. Les localisations imaginaires. *L'Evolution Psychiatrique*, 1984, 49: 379–402.

Lantéri Laura G. Acuité et pathologie mentale, *L'Evolution Psychiatrique*, 1986, 51: 403–18.

Lantéri-Laura G. L'unicité de la notion de délire dans la psychiatrie Française moderne. In Grivois H. *Psychose Naissante, Psychose Unique?* Paris, Masson, pp. 5–21, 1991.

Lantéri-Laura G. *Les Hallucinations*, Paris, Masson, 1991.

Lantéri-Laura G. and Del Pistoia L. Structural analysis of suicidal behaviour. *Social Research*, 1970, 37: 324–47.

Lantéri-Laura G. and Del Pistoia L. Diversité clinique et unité physio-psychopathologique des altérations du langage. *L'Evolution Psychiatrique*, 1980, 45: 225–52.

Lantéri-Laura G and Gros M. *La Discordance*, Paris, Unicet, 1984.

Lantéri-Laura G. and Gros M. *Essai sur la Discordance Dans la Psychiatrie Contemporaine*, Paris, Epel, 1992.

Lapassade G. *Les États Modifiés de Conscience*, Paris, Presses Universitaires de France, 1897.

Lapie P. Note sur la paramnésie. *Revue Philosophique*, 1894, 37: 351–2.

Lapie P. *Logique de la Volonté*, Paris, Alcan, 1902.

Laplanche J. and Pontalis J.B. *The Language of Psychoanalysis*, London, the Hogarth Press, 1973.

Larson J.L. *Reason and Experience. The Representation of Natural Order in the work of Carl Von Linné*, Berkeley, University of California Press, 1971.

Lasègue C. Du délire de persécution. *Archives Générales de Médicine*, 1852, 28: 129–50.

Lasègue C. Alcoolisme Subaigu, Fugue. *Archives Générales de Médicine*, 1868, ii: 159.

Lasègue C. Le délire alcoolique n'est pas un délire, mais in rêve. *Archives Générales de Médicine*, 1881, 2: 573–9.

Lasègue C. Du délire de persécution. In *Ètudes Médicales*, Vol. 1, pp. 545–566, Paris: Asselin, 1884.

Lasègue C. *Écrits Psychiatriques*. Textes Choisis et Présentés par J. Corraze, Paris, Privat, 1971.

Lashley K.S. *Brain Mechanisms and Intelligence*, New York, Dover, 1963 (first edition, 1929).

Laudan L. *Progress and its Problems: Towards a Theory of Scientific Growth*. University of California Press, Berkeley, 1977.

Lavater J.C. *Essays on Physiognomy*, London, Ward, Lock and Co., 1891.

Laycock T. *A Treatise on the Nervous Diseases of Women*, London, Longman, Orme, Brown, Green and Longman, 1840.

Laycock T. On the reflex function of the brain. *British and Foreign Medico-Chirurgical Review* Vol. 19, 1845.

Laycock T. *Mind and Brain or the Correlations of Consciousness and Organization*, Vol. 1, Edinburgh, Sutherland and Knox, 1860.

Lazarus A.P. Learning theory and the treatment of depression. *Behavioral Research and Therapy*, 6: 83–9, 1968.

Le Goc-Diaz I. Le dépersonnalisation. *Encyclopédie Médico-Chirurgicale* (Paris), 37125A[10], 6, 1988.

Le Lorrain J. A propos de la paramnésie. *Revue Philosophique*, 1894, 37: 208–10.

Le Roy, G. *La Psychologie de Condillac*, Paris, Boivin and Cie., 1937.

Leader. Acute delirium in 1845 and 1860. *American Journal of Insanity*, 1864, 21: 181–200.

Leader. Obsessions and morbid impulses. *Lancet*, 1904, i: 1441.

Leader. Encephalitis lethargica, *Lancet*, 1981, ii: 1396–7.

Leary D.E. The philosophical developments of the conception of psychology in Germany 1780–1850. *Journal of the History of Behavioural Science*, 1978, 14: 113–21.

Leary D.E. (ed.) *Metaphors in the History of Psychology*. Cambridge, Cambridge University Press, 1990.

Lechner J. *A.V.C. Berbiguier de Terre-Neuve du Thym, 'L'Homme aux Farfadets'*, Thèse de Médecine, Strasbourg, Louis Pasteur, 1983.

Lecours A.R., Cronk C. and Sébahoun-Balsamo M. From Pierre Marie to Norman Geschwind. In Lecours A.R., LHermitte F. and Bryans B. (eds.) *Aphasiology*, London, Baillière, pp. 20–29, 1983.

Lecourt D. *Marxism and Epistemology Part I; Gaston Bachelard's Historical Epistemology*, London, NLB, 1975.

Lee C. and Lance J.W. Migraine stupor. *Headache*, 1977, 17: 32–8.

Leeper R.W. A motivational theory of emotion to replace emotion as disorganized response. *Psychological Review*, 1948, 55: 5–21.

Lees A.J. *Tics and Related Disorder*. Edinburgh, Churchill and Livingstone, 1985.

Lefevre P. De L'Aphémie a l'Aphasie. Les Tribulations d'une Dénomination. *L'Information Psychiatrique*, 1988, 64: 945–54.

Leff A. Thomas Laycock and the cerebral reflex: a function arising from and pointing to the unity of nature. *History of Psychiatry*, 1991, 2: 385–408.

Legoyt A. Suicide. In Dechambre A (ed.) *Dictionnaire Encyclopédique de Sciences Médicales*, Vol. 92, Paris, Asselin, pp. 242–296, 1884.

Legrain M. Obsession and impulse. In Tuke D.H. (ed.) *Dictionary of Psychological Medicine*, Vol. 1, London, J. and A. Churchill, pp. 866–868, 1892.

Legrand du Saulle H.: *La Folie devant les Tribunaux*. Paris, Savy, 1864.

Legrand du Saulle H. *La Folie du Doute (avec délire du toucher)* Paris, Delahaye, 1875.

Legrand du Saulle H. De la Peur des Espaces (agoraphobie des Allemands). *Annales Médico-Psychologiques*, 1876, 34: 405–33.

Legrand M.A. *La Longévité á Travers les Âges*, Paris, Flammarion, 1911.

Leguil F. La phobie avant Freud, *Ornicar?*, 1979, 17: 88–105.

Leibbrand W. and Wettley A. *Der Wahnsinn, Geschichte der Abendländischen Psychopathologie* Freiburg, Karl Alber, 1961.

Leigh D. *The Historical Development of Psychiatry. Vol. 1, 18th and 19th Centuries*, Oxford, Pergamon Press, 1961.

Lemoine A. *Le Cerveau et la Pensée*. Paris, Baillière, 1875.

Lemperiere T, Feline A, Guttman A *et al. Psychiatrie de l'Adulte*. Paris, Masson, 1983.

Leon J., Antelo E. and Simpson G. Delusion of parasitosis or chronic tactile hallucinosis: hypothesis about their brain physiopathology. *Comprehensive Psychiatry*, 1992, 33: 25–33.

Leonhard K. *The Classification of the Endogenous Psychoses*, New York, John Wiley and Sons, 1979.

Lereboullet L. and Bussard T. Paralysie Agitante. In Dechambre A. and Lereboullet L. (eds.) *Dictionnaire Encyclopédique des Sciences Médicales*, Vol. 72, Paris, Masson, pp. 614–654, 1884.

Leroux (no initial). Vertige. In Dechambre A. and Lereboullet L. (eds.) *Dictionnaire Encyclopédique des Sciences Médicales*, Vol. 100, Paris, Masson, pp. 146–188, 1889.

Leroy E.B. Préoccupations hypocondriaques avec hallucinations obsédantes de l'ouïe et de l'odorat. *Comptes Rendus du Congrès de Médicines Aliénistes*, Paris, Masson, 1905.

Leroy O. *La Raison Primitive. Essai de Réfutation de la Théorie du Prélogisme*, Paris, Alcan, 1927.

Leroy R. The syndrome of Lilliputian hallucinations. *Journal of Nervous and Mental Disease*, 1922, 56: 325–33.

Lesky E. Structure and function in Gall. *Bulletin of the History of Medicine*, 1970, 44: 297–314.

Lesser I.M. and Lesser B.Z. Alexithymia: examining the development of a psychological concept. *American Journal of Psychiatry*, 1983, 140: 1305–8.

Lester D. (ed.): *Emile Durkheim Le Suicide 100 years later*. Philadelphia, The Charles Press, 1994.

Leubuscher. *Zeitschrift für Psychiatrie*, 1847, 4: 562 (quoted in Griesinger, 1861).

Leuret, F. *Fragments Psychologiques sur la Folie*, Paris, Crochard, 1834.

Levêque de Pouilly J.S. *Éloge de Charles Bonnet*, Lausanne, Henbach, 1794.

Levi A. *French Moralists. The Theory of the Passions 1585–1649*, Oxford, Clarendon Press, 1964.

Levin H.S., Peters B.H. and Hulkonen D.A. Early concepts of anterograde and retrograde amnesia. *Cortex*, 1983, 19: 427–40.

Levin K. *Freud's Early Psychology of the Neuroses. A Historical Perspective*, Sussex, The Harvester Press, 1978.

Levy M. *Traité d'Hygiène Publique et Privée*, Paris, Baillière, 1850.

Levy P.E. *Neurasthénie et Névroses. Leur Guérison Définitive en Cure Libre*, Paris, Alcan, 1917.

Lévy-Bruhl L. *Les Fonctiones Mentales dans les Sociétes Inférieures*, Paris, Alcan, 1928 (First Edition, 1910).

Lévy-Friesacher Ch. *Meynert-Freud: L'Amentia'*, Paris, Presses Universitaires de France, 1983.

Lévy-Valensi J. Mentalité primitive et psychopathologie. *Annales Médico-Psychologiques*, 1934, 92: 676–701.

Lewes G.H. *Comte's Philosophy of the Sciences*, London, George Bell and Sons, London, 1878.

Lewinsohn P. A behavioral approach to depression, in Friedman R, Katz M (eds.) *The Psychology of Depression: Contemporary Theory of Research*. Silver Spring Md, Winston and Sons, 1974.

Lewis A. Melancholia: a clinical survey of depressive states. *Journal of Mental Science*, 1934, 80: 277–378.

Lewis A. States of depression. *British Medical Journal*, 1938, ii: 875–8.

Lewis A. The study of defect. *American Journal of Psychiatry*, 1961, 117: 289–305.

Lewis A. Problems presented by the ambiguous word 'anxiety' as used in psychopathology. *The Israel Annals of Psychiatry and Related Disciplines*, 1967, 5: 105–21.

Lewis A. Paranoia and paranoid: a historical perspective. *Psychological Medicine*, 1970, 1: 2–12.

Lewis A. 'Psychogenic': a word and its mutations. *Psychological Medicine*, 1972, 2: 209–15.

Lewis A. Psychopathic personality: a most elusive category. *Psychological Medicine*, 1974, 4: 133–40.

Lewis C.T. and Short C. *A Latin Dictionary*, Oxford, Clarendon Press, 1879.

Lewis E.O. Types of mental deficiency and their social significance. *Journal of Mental Science*, 1933, 79: 298–304.

Lewis N.D.C. *Research in Dementia Praecox*, New York, Published by Supreme Council of Sovereign Grand Inspectors-General of the Thirty-third and Last Degree of the Ancient Accepted Scottish Rite of Freemasonry, New York, 1936.

Lewy F.H. Historical Introduction: The basal ganglia and their diseases. In *The Diseases of the Basal Ganglia*, Baltimore, Williams and Wilkins, pp. 1–20, 1942.

Lewy F.H. Zur pathologischen Anatomie der Paralysis Agitans. *Deutsches Zeitschrift für Nervenheilkunden*, 1913, 50: 50–87.

L'Hermitte J. Syndome de la calotte du pédoncule cérébral. Les troubles psychosensoriels dans les lésions du mésocéphale. *Revue Neurologique*, 1922, 29: 1363–4.

L'Hermitte J. L'Hallucinose pédonculaire. *L'Encéphale*, 1932, 27: 422–35.

L'Hermitte J. *Les Rêves*. Paris, Presses Universitaires de France, 1963.

Liddle P.F. Volition and schizophrenia. In David A.S. and Cutting J.C. (eds.) *The Neuropsychology of Schizophrenia*, Hove, Lawrence Erlbaum, pp. 39–49, 1994.

Liebert R.S. The concept of character: A historical review. In Glick R.A. and Meyers D.I. (eds.) *Masochism: Current Psychoanalytical Perspectives*. Hillsdale, N.J., Analytic Press, pp. 27–42, 1988.

Liebowitz M.R. Is borderline a distinct entity? *Schizophrenia Bulletin*, 1979, 5: 23–38.

Liebowitz M.R. and Klein D.F. Hysterical dysphoria. *Psychiatric Clinics of North America*, 1979, 2: 555–75.

Liebowitz M.R., Gorman J.M., Fier A.J. and Kein D. Social phobia. *Archives of General Psychiatry*, 1985, 42: 729–36.

Liégeois A. Hidden philosophy and theology in Morel's theory of degeneration and nosology. *History of Psychiatry*, 1991, 2: 419–28.

Linas A. Catalepsie. In Dechambre A. and Lereboullet L. *Dictionnaire Encyclopédique des Sciences Médicales*, Vol 13, Paris, Masson, pp. 59–90, 1877.

Linas A. Monomanie. In Dechambre A. and Lereboullet L. (eds.) *Dictionnaire Encyclopédique des Sciences Médicales*, Vol. 61, Paris, Mason, pp. 146–95, 1871.

Lipowski Z. *Delirium. Acute Brain Failure in Man*, Springfield, Illinois, Charles C. Thomas, 1980.

Lishman W.A. *Organic Psychiatry. The Psychological Consequence of Cerebral Disorder*, Oxford, Blackwell, 1978.

Lisle E. *Du Suicide. Statistique, Médecine, Histoire et Legislation*, Paris, Baillière, 1856.

Littré È. *Auguste Comte et la Philosophie Positive*, Paris, Hachette, 1864.

Littré E. *Dictionnaire de la Langue Française*, Supplément, Paris, Hachette, 1877–81.

Littré E. and Robin Ch. (eds.) *Dictionnaire de Médicine de P.H. Nysten* Paris, Baillière, 1858.

Llopis B. *La Psicosis Pelagrosa*, Barcelona, Editorial Científico-Médica, 1946.

Llopis B. La Psicosis Unica. *Archivos de Neurobiología*, 1954, 17: 1–39.

Llopis B. Note. *Archivos de Neurobiología*, 1954, 17: 1–34.

Llopis B. Sobre la Delusion y la Paranoia. In Bleuler E. (ed.) *Afectividad, Sugestibilidad, Paranoia* (translated by B. Llopis) Madrid, Morata, 1969.

Lloyd G.E.R. *Aristotle: The Growth and Structure of his Thought*, Cambridge, Cambridge University Press, 1968.

Lloyd G.E.R. *Demystifying Mentalities*, Cambridge, Cambridge University Press, 1990.

Loas G. and Pierson A. L'Anhédonie en Psychiatrie: revue. *Annales Médico-Psychologiques*, 147: 705–17, 1989.

Lobstein J.G. *Traité de Anatomie Pathologique*, Vol. 2, Paris, Baillière, 1838.

Locke J. *An Essay Concerning Human Understanding*, 2 Vols, New York, Dover, 1959 (First Edition, 1690).

Long E.R. The development of our knowledge of arteriosclerosis. In Cowdry E.V. (ed.) *Arteriosclerosis. A survey of the problem.* New York, MacMillan Company, 1933, pp. 19–52.

López A. '*Comprensión*' e '*interpretación*' en las ciencias del espíritu, Universidad de Murcia, Murcia, 1990.

López Ibor J.J. *La Angustia Vital*, Madrid, Paz Montalvo, 1950.

López Ibor J.J. and López-Ibor J.J. *El cuerpo y la corporalidad*. Madrid. Gredos, 1974.

López Moreno, A. *Comprensión e interpretación en las ciencias del espíritu*: Dilhey. Murcia, El Taller, 1990.

López Piñero J.M. *Orígenes históricos del concepto de neurosis*. Instituto de Historia de la Medicina, Valencia, 1963.

López Piñero, J.M. and Morales Meseguer J.M. *Neurosis y psicoterapia. Un estudio histórico*. Espasa-Calpe, Madrid, 1970.

López Piñero J.M. *John Hughlings Jackson (1835–1911)*, Madrid, Moneda, 1973.

López Piñero J.M. *Historical Origins of the Concept of Neurosis* (translated by D. Berrios), Cambridge, Cambridge University Press, 1983.

Lorenz K. The comparative method in studying innate behaviour patterns. *Symposia of the Society for Experimental Biology*, 1950, 4: 221–68.

Losserand J. Les rapports du physique et du moral de l'homme de Cabanis á Auguste Comte. *L'Evolution Psychiatrique*, 1967, 32: 573–601.

Loudet, O. and Martinez Dalke, L. Sobre la psicogénesis y el valor pronóstico del síndrome de Cotard. *Archivos Argentinos de Neurología*, 1933, 1:1–12.

Louyer-Villermay. Maladies de la mémoire. In *Dictionnaire des Sciences Médicales*, Vol. 32, Paris, Panckouke, 1819.

Lovejoy A.O. *The Great Chain of Being.* Harvard University Press, 1936.

Lowenfeld L. *Psychische Zwangserscheinungen*. Wiesbaden, Bergmann, 1904.

Lowry R. *The evolution of psychological theory*, Chicago, Aldine, 1971.

Lugaro E. La psichiatria tedesca nella storia e nell'attualita. *Rivista di Patologia Nervosa e Mentale*, 1916, 21: 337–86.

Lugaro E. Sulle pseudo-allucinazioni (allucinazione psichiche di Baillarger). Contributo a lla psicologia della demenza paranoide. *Rivista di Patologia nervosa e mentale*, 1903, 8: 1–87.

Lugaro E. Sulle allucinazioni unilaterali dell'udito. *Rivista di Patologia Nervosa e Mentale*, 1904, 9: 228–37.

Lunier (no initial). Review of Trélat's Folie Lucide. *Annales Médico-Psychologiques*, 1861, 7: 658–664.

Luque R. and Berrios G.E. Cotard's syndrome in the elderly. Historical and clinical aspects. *International Journal of Geriatric Psychiatry*, 1994, 9: 957–64.

Luyendijk-Elshout A. Of masks and mills: The enlightened doctor and his frightened patient. In Rousseau G.S. (ed.) *The Languages of Psyche. Mind and Body in Enlightenment Thought*, Berkeley, University of California Press, pp. 186–230, 1990.

Luys J. *Le Cerveau*, Paris, Baillière, 1876.

Luys J. Obnubilation Passagère de la Conscience des Choses du Monde Extérieur, ayant duré Plusieurs jours, chez un Homme Adulte, Continuant á Vivre de la Vie Commune. *L'Encéphale*, 1881, 1: 251–6.

Luys J. Des Obsessions pathologiques dans leur rapports avec l'activité automatique des elements nerveux. *L'Encéphale*, 1883, 3: 20–61.

Luys J. *Tratado de las Enfermedades Mentales*, Madrid, Teodoro, 1891 (First French Edition, 1881).

Lyons W. *The Disappearance of Introspection*. Cambridge, Mass., MIT, 1986.

Macario, M. Sur la démonomanie. *Annales Médico-Psychologiques* 1842, 1: 440–85.

McCarthy T. The operation called verstehen: towards a redefinition of the problem. In Schaffner K.F. and Cohen R.S. (eds.) *Boston Studies in the Philosophy of Science, Vol. XX, Proceedings of the 1972 Philosophy of Science Section*. Dordrecht, Reidel, pp. 167–193, 1972.

MacCarthy V.A. 'Psychological Fragments': Kirkegaard's Religious Psychology. In Smith J.H. (ed.) *Kirkegaard's Truth: the Disclosure of the Self*, New York, Yale University Press, pp. 235–265, 1981.

M'Cosh J. in Stewart D. *Outlines of Moral Philosophy*, London, William Allan, 1866.

McCowan P.K. and Cook L.C. The mental aspects of chronic epidemic encephalitis. *Lancet*, 1928, i: 1316–20.

MacCurdy J.T. *The Psychology of Emotion. Morbid and abnormal*, London, Kegan Paul, Trench, Trubner and Co, 1925.

MacDonald M. *Mystical Bedlam, Madness, Anxiety and Healing in Seventeenth Century England*, Cambridge, Cambridge University Press, 1981.

MacDonald M. and Murphy T. *Sleepless Souls: Suicide in Modern England*. Oxford, Clarendon Press, 1990.

MacDougall R. Fatigue. *Psychological Review*, 1899, 6: 203–8.

McFie J. Psychological testing in clinical neurology. *Journal Nervous Mental Disease*, 1960, 131: 383–93.

McGinn C. *The Problem of Consciousness*, Oxford, Blackwell, 1991.

McLeod R. Changing perspectives in the history of science. In *Science, Technology and Society: A Cross Disciplinarian Perspective*. Spiegel-Rosing I. and Price D.S. (eds.), Sage Publications, London, 1977, pp. 149–196.

McMahon C.E. The role of imagination in the disease process: pre-Cartesian history. *Psychological Medicine*, 1976, 6: 179–84.

McManners J. *Death and the Enlightenment*, Oxford, Oxford University Press, 1985.

MacPherson J. On the dissolution of the functions of the nervous system in insanity, with a suggestion for a new basis of classification. *American Journal of Insanity*, 1889, 45: 387–94.

MacPhillamy D.J., Lewinsohn P.M. Depression as a function of levels of desired and obtained pleasure. *J. Abnorm. Psychol.*, 1974, 83: 651–7.

Mackenzie B. Darwinism and positivism as methodological influences on the development of psychology. *Journal of the History of Behavioural Science*, 1976, 12: 330–7.

Mackenzie T.B., Rosenberg S.D. and Berger B.L. The manipulative patient: an interaction approach. *Psychiatry*, 1978, 41: 264–71.

MacKinnon F.I. The meaning of 'emergent' in Lloyd Morgan's 'Emergent evolution'. *Mind*, 1924, 33: 311–15.

Madden J.J., Luhan J.A.and Kaplan L.A. Non-dementing psychoses in older persons. *Journal of the American Medical Association*, 1952, 150: 1567–70.

Magazin zur Erfahrungsseelenkunde Vol. 9, Berlin, August Melius, 1792.

Magnan V. Considérations générales sur la folie (des héréditaires ou dégénérés). *Le Progrés Médical*, 1886–7, 14: 1089–90; 1108–12; 15: 187–90; 209–13.

Magnan V. and Saury M. Trois cas de cocainisme chronique. *Comptes Rendus, Séances et Memoire de la Société de Biologie*, 1889 (no volume): 60–3.

Magnan V. and Sérieux P. *Le Délire Chronique á èvolution Systématique*, Paris, Masson, 1892.

Magnan V. and Sérieux P. Délire chronique. In Marie A. (ed.) *Traité International de Psychologie Pathologique*, Vol. 2, Paris, Alcan, pp. 605–639, 1911.

Magrinat G, Danziger J.A., Lorenzo I.C. and Flemenbaum A. A Reassessment of Catatonia. *Comprehensive Psychiatry*, 1983, 24: 218–28.

Mahendra B. Subnormality revisited in early 19th century France. *Journal of Mental Deficiency*, 1985, 29: 391–401.

Maier H.W. *La Cocaine*, Paris, Payot, 1928.

Maimon S. Ueber den Plan des Magazins zur Erfahrungsseelentunde. *Magazin zur Erfahrungs-seelenkunde*, Vol. 1, 1792.

Maine de Biran. *The Influence of Habit on the Faculty of Thinking* (translation by M.D. Boehm) London, Baillière, 1929.

Mairet A. *De la Démence Mélancolique*, Paris, Masson, 1883.

Mairet A. and Ardin-Delteil P. *Hérédité et Prédisposition*. Montpellier, Coulet, 1907.

Maisonneuve J. and Bruchon-Schweitzer M. *Modèlos du corps et psychologie esthétique*. Paris, Presses Universitaires de France, 1981.

Makkreel R.A. *Dilthey*. Princeton, Princeton University Press, 1975.

Malcolm N. *Dreaming*. London, Routledge and Kegan Paul, 1959.

Maleval J.C. *Folies Hysteriques et Psychoses Dissociatives*, Paris, Payot, 1981.

Malson L. *Les enfants sauvages*. Paris, Union Générale d'Èditions, 1964.

Manschreck T.C. Psychomotor abnormalities. In Costello C.G. (ed.) *Symptoms of Schizophrenia*. New York, Wiley, pp. 261–290, 1993.

Mansvelt J. *Pick's Disease*, Enchede, Van der Loeff, 1954.

Mantegazza P. *Physiognomy and Expression*, London, Walter Scott, 1878.

Mapother E. Discussion on Manic-Depressive Psychosis. *British Medical Journal*, 1926, ii: 872–879.

Marandon de Montyel E. Les formes de la démence précoce. *Annales Médico-Psychologiques*, 1905, 2: 246–65.

Marc C.C.H. *De la Folie, Considérée dans ses Rapports avec les Questions Médico-Judiciaires*, 2 Vols, Paris, Baillière, 1840.

Marcé L V. Recherches cliniques et anatomo-pathologiques sur la démence senile et sur les différences qui la separent de la paralysie générale. *Gazette Médicale de Paris*, 1863, 34: 433–5; 467–9; 497–502; 631–2; 761–4; 797–8; 831–3; 855–8.

Marcé L.V. *Traité Pratique des Maladies Mentales*, Paris, Baillière, 1862.

Marcel A.J. and Bisiach E. (eds) *Consciousness in Contemporary science*, Oxford, Clarendon, 1988.

Marchand L. *Manuel de Neurologie* Paris, Doin, 1909.

Marchais P. La méthode systèmale en psychiatrie. *Annales Médico-Psychologiques*, 1977, 135: 677–95.

Marchais P. *Les Mouvances Psychopathologiques: Essai de Psychiatrie Dynamique*. Eres, Paris, 1983.

Marcil-Lacoste L. *Claude Buffier and Thomas Reid: Two Common Sense Philosophers*, Kingston, McGill-Queen's University Press, 1982.

Marco-Merenciano F. *Esquizofrenias paranoides*. Madrid, Miguel Servet, 1942.

Marek T., Noworol C. and Karwowski W. Mental fatigue at work and pain perception. *Work and Stress*, 1988, 2: 133–7.

Marie A. *Étude sur Quelques Symptoms des Délires Systématisés, et sur leur Valeur*, Paris, Doin, 1892.

Marie A. *La Démence*, Paris, Doin, 1906.

Marie A. *Mysticisme et Folie* Paris, V. Giard and E. Briére, 1907.

Marie P. Éloge de Charcot. *Bulletin de L'Académie de Médecine*, 1925, 93: 576–93.

Marillier L. Statistique des hallucinations, *Congrès Internationale de Psychologie*, Paris, 1890.

Marková I. The development of self-consciousness: Part I - Baldwin, Mead and Vygotsky. *History and Philosophy of Psychology*, 1988, BPS Newsletter N° 7 (November).

Marková I.S. and Berrios G.E. The meaning of Insight in clinical psychiatry. *British Journal of Psychiatry*, 1992, 160: 850–60.

Marková I.S. and Berrios G.E. Delusional misidentifications: facts and fancies. *Psychopathology*, 1994, 27: 136–143.

Marková I.S. and Berrios G.E. Mental symptoms: are they similar phenomena? The problem of symptom-heterogeneity. *Psychopathology* 1995, 28: 147–157.

Marková I.S. and Berrios G.E. Insight: a new model. *Journal of nervous and mental disease* (in press), 1995.

Markowitsch H.J. Transient psychogenic amnesic states. In *Transient Global Amnesia*, Berlin, Springer, pp. 181–190, 1990.

Marks I.M. *Fears and Phobias*, London, Heinemann, 1969.

Marsden C.D., Tarsy D. and Baldessarini R.J. Spontaneous and drug-induced movement disorders in psychotic patients. In Benson D.F. and Blumer D. (eds.) *Psychiatric Aspects of Neurological Disease*, New York, Grune and Stratton, pp. 219–266, 1975.

Marshall H.R. Consciousness, self-consciousness, and the self. *Mind*, 1901, 10: 98–113.

Marshall J.C. Multiple perspectives on modularity. *Cognition*, 1984, 17: 209–42.

Marshall M.E. Physics, metaphysics and Fechner's psychophysics. In Woodward W.R. and Ash M. (eds.) *The Problematic Science: Psychology in 19th Century Thought*, New York, Praeger, pp. 65–87, 1982.

Martí y Juliá D. Concepto de la Personalidad. *Revista de Ciencias Médicas de Barcelona*, 1899, 25: 281–92.

Martin J. *Une biographie française (1812–1850) d'Onésime Èdouard Séguin, premier thérapeute des enfants arriérés, d'après ses écrits et les documents historiques*. Thèse de Médecine, Saint Antoine, Paris, 1981.

Martin W.E., Young W.I. and Anderson V.E. Parkinson's disease: a genetic study. *Brain*, 1973, 96: 495–506.

Martin-Santos L. *Dilthey, Jaspers y la Comprensión del Enfermo Mental*, Madrid, Paz Montalvo, 1955.

Martini, E. *De la Folie*. Paris, Migneret, 1824.

Marx O.M. What is the history of psychiatry? *American Journal of Orthopsychiatry* 1970, 40: 593–605.

Marx O.M. History of psychology: a review of the last decade. *Journal of the History of the Behavioral Sciences* 1977, 13: 41–77.

Marx O.M. The case of the chronic patient seen in a historical perspective. In Wallace E.R. and Pressley L.C. (eds.) *Essays in the History of Psychiatry*, Columbia, W.M.S. Hall Psychiatric Institute, pp. 22–7, 1980.

Marx O.M. What is the history of psychiatry II. *History of Psychiatry* 1992, 3: 293–301.

Masselon R. *Psychologie des Déments Précoces*, Paris, Boyer, 1902.

Masselon R. Délire systématisé a base d'obsessions. *Annales Médico-Psychologiques*, 1913, 71: 513–27.

Masshoff W. Allgemeine und spezielle Pathologie der Vita Reducta. *Verhandlungen der Deutschen Gesellschaft für innere Medizin*, 1963, 69: 59–64.

Masterman M. The nature of a paradigm. In Lakatos I. and Musgrave A. (eds.) *Criticism and the Growth of Knowledge*. Cambridge, Cambridge University Press, 1970, pp. 59–89.

Masters F.W. and Greaves D.C. The quasimodo complex. *British Journal of Plastic Surgery*, 1987, 20: 204–10.

Matthey A. *Nouvelles Recherches sur les Maladies de l'Esprit Précédées de Considérations sur les Difficultés de l'Art de Guérir*. Paris, J.J. Paschoud, 1816.

Maudsley H. Certain varieties of insanity which are frequently confounded. *Lancet*, 1866, i: 363–4.

Maudsley H. *Body and Will, Being an Essay Concerning Will in its Metaphysical, Physiological and Pathological Aspects* London, Kegan Paul, 1883.

Maudsley H. *Responsibility in Mental Disease*. London, Kegan Paul & Trench, 1885.

Maudsley H. *The Pathology of Mind*. London, MacMillan and Co., 1895.

Maughs S. The concept of psychopathy and psychopathic personality: its evolution and historical development. *Journal of Criminology and Psychopathology*, 1941, 2: 329–356.

Maulitz R.C. *Morbid Appearances. The Anatomy of Pathology in the early Nineteenth Century*, Cambridge, Cambridge University Press, 1987.

Maurel H. Approche historique de la notion d'automatisme en psychiatrie. *Annales Médico-Psychologiques* 1989, 147: 946–950.

Maury L.F.A. Des hallucinations hypnagogiques. *Annales Médico-Psychologiques* 1848, 11: 26–40.

Maury L.F.A. *Le Sommeil et les Rêves. Études Psychologiques sur ces Phénomènes et les divers états qui s'y rattachent*, 4th edn., Paris, Didier, 1878.

Mauz F. *El Pronóstico de las psicosis endógenas* (translated by L. Valenciano), Madrid, Morata, 1931 (German edn. 1930).

Mavrojannis M. L'action cataleptique de la morphine chez les rats. Contribution á la théorie toxique de la catalepsie. *Comptes Rendus de la Société de Biologie*, 1903, 55: 1092–4.

May R. Fundamentos Históricos de las Modernas Teorías de la Ansiedad. In May R. (ed.) *La Angustia Normal y Patológica*, Paidós, Buenos Aires, pp. 7–24, 1968.

Mayer-Gross W. On depersonalization. *British Journal of Medical Psychology* 1935, 15: 103–26.

Mayer-Gross W. Arteriosclerotic, senile and presenile psychoses. In Fleming G.W.T.H. (ed.) Recent Progress in Psychiatry, Vol. 1, *The Journal of Mental Science*, London, Churchill, pp. 316–327, 1944.

Mayer-Gross W. and Steiner G. Encephalitis Lethargica in der Selbsbeobachtung. *Zeitschrift für Neurologie und Psychiatrie*, 1921, 73: 422–75.

Mayne R.G. *An Expository Lexicon of the terms, Ancient and Modern, in Medical and General Sciences*. London, John Churchill, 1860.

Mayr E. *The Growth of Biological Thought*, Cambridge, Mass, The Belknap Press of Harvard University Press 1982.

Meduna L.J. *Oneirophrenia*, Urbana, University of Illinois Press, 1950.

Meehl P.E. Genes and the unchangeable core. *Voices*, 10: 1974, 25–35.

Meehl P.E. Anger, anhedonia and the borderline syndrome. *American Journal of Psychoanalysis* 1975, 35: 157–61.

Meehl P.E. Hedonic capacity ten years later: some classifications, in Clark D.C., Fawcett J. (eds.) *Anhedonia and Affect Deficit States*. New York, PMA Publishing Corp, 1987.

Meehl P.E. Schizotaxia, schizotypia, schizophrenia. *American Psychologist*, 17: 827–38, 1962.

Meige H. Le Juif-errant à la Salpêtrière. *Nouvelle Iconographie de la Salpêtrière* 1893, 6: 1–118.

Meige H. and Feindel E. *Les Tics et leur Traitement*, Paris, Masson, 1902.

Meige H. and Feindel E. *Tics and their Treatment*, London, Sidney Appleton, 1907.

Meister R. *Hypochondria*, New York, Tapingler, 1980.

Mendel E. *Textbook of Psychiatry* (translated by W.C. Krauss), Philadelphia, Davis, 1907.

Menninger K. *Man Against Himself.* New York, Harcourt, Brace and World, 1938.

Mercier Ch. On imperative ideas. *Brain,* 1895, 18: 328–30.

Metzger W. *Psychologie,* Second Edition, Darmstadt, Steinkopff, pp. 140–2, 1954.

Meyer A. The frontal lobe syndrome, the aphasias and related conditions. A contribution to the history of cortical localization. *Brain,* 1974, 97: 565–600.

Meyer Ad. Melancholia. In Baldwin J.M. (ed.) *Dictionary of Philosophy and Psychology,* Vol. 2, London, McMillan, pp. 61–62, 1901.

Meyer Ad. An attempt at analysis of the neurotic constitution. *American Journal of Psychology,* 1903, 14: 90–4.

Meyer Ad. The relation of emotional and intellectual functions in paranoia and in obsessions. *Psychological Bulletin,* 1906, 3: 255–74.

Meyer E. Beitrag zur Kenntniss der akut enstandenen Psychosen und der katatonen Zustände. *Archiv für Psychiatrie und Nervenkrankheiten,* 1899, 32: 780–902.

Meyer M. *Découverte et Justification en Science.* Paris, Klincksieck, 1979.

Meyering T. *Historical Roots of Cognitive Science,* Dordrecht, Kluwer, 1989.

Meynert T. Beiträge zur differentiel Diagnose des paralytischen Irreseins. *Wiener medizinische Praktizieren,* 1871, 12: 645–7.

Meynert T. Die akuten (halluzinatorischen) Formen des Wahnsinns und ihr Verlauf. *Jahrbücher für Psychiatrie,* 1881, 2: 181–6.

Meynert T. *Psychiatry. A Clinical Treatise on Diseases of the Fore-brain* (translated by B. Sachs), New York, Putnam, 1885.

Meynert T. Amentia. In *Klinische Vorlesungen über Psychiatrie auf Wissenschaftlichen Grundlagen, für Studierende und Ärzte, Juristen und Psychologen,* Vienna, Braumüller, 1890.

Meynert, T. Amentia, die Verwirrtheit. *Jahrbücher für Psychiatrie und Neurologie,* 1890, 9: 1–112.

Mezger E. Zum Begriff der Psychopathen. *Monatschrift für Kriminologie,* 1939, 30: 190–213.

Mezger E. *Kriminalpolitik auf kriminologischer Auflage,* Third Edition, Stuttgart, Enke, 1944.

Micale M. and Porter R. (eds) *Discovering the History of Psychiatry.* New York, Oxford University Press, 1994.

Michéa C.F. Du siége, de la nature intime, des symptomes et du diagnostic de l'hypocondrie. *Mémoires de l'Académie Royale de Médecine,* 1843, 2: 573–654.

Michéa C.F. Des hallucinations, de leurs causes, et des maladies qu'elles caractérisent. *Mémoires de L'Académie Royale de Médecine,* 1846, 12: 241–71.

Michéa C.F. *Du Délire des Sensations,* Paris, Labé, 1846.

Mickle J. Mental besetments. *Journal of Mental Science,* 1896, 42: 691–719.

Mickle W.J. Katatonia: in relation to dementia praecox. *Journal of Mental Science,* 1909, 55: 22–36.

Middleton E. Turnbull W. Ellis T. and Davison J. (eds.) *The New Complete Dictionary of Arts and Sciences,* London, Alex Hogg, 1780.

Mignard M. *L'Unité Psychique et les Troubles Mentaux,* Paris, Lacan, 1928.

Mill J. *Analysis of the Phenomena of the Human Mind,* London, Longman, Green, Reader and Dyer, 1869. (First Edition 1829).

Mill J.S. *A System of Logic,* London, Longman, 1898 (First Edition, 1845).

Miller E., Berrios G.E. and Politynska B.E. The adverse effect of benzhexol on memory in Parkinson's disease. *Acta Neurologica Scandinavica,* 1987, 76: 278–82.

Millet J. Des Vertiges chez les Aliénés. *Annales Médico-Psychologiques,* 1884, 42: 38–51; 204–19.

Milner A.D. and Rugg M.D. (eds.) *The Neuropsychology of Consciousness,* London, Academic Press, 1992.

Minkowski E. Bergson's conceptions as applied to psychopathology. *Journal Nervous Mental Disease,* 1926, 63: 553–61.

Minkowski E. *La Schizophrénie. Psychopathologie des Schizoïdes et des Schizophrenes*, Paris, Payst, 1927.

Minkowski E. *Traité de Psychopathologie*, Paris, Presses Universitaires de France, 1966.

Minois G. *Histoire de la Vieillesse. De l'Antiquité á la Renaissance*, Paris, Fayard, 1987.

Mischel T. Affective concepts in the psychology of J.F. Herbart. *Journal of the History of Behavioral Science*, 1973, 9: 262–268.

Mishlove M. and Chapman L.J. Social anhedonia in the prediction of psychosis proneness. *Journal of Abnormal Psychology* 94: 384–96, 1985.

Mitchell S.W. Phantom limb. *The Lippincott Magazine*, 1871, 8: 563–9.

Mitchell S.W. An analysis of 3000 cases of melancholia. *Transactions of the Association of American Physicians*, 1897, 12: 480–7.

Mjönes H. Paralysis agitans, clinical and genetic study. *Acta Psychiatrica Scandinavica*, 1949, (Suppl) 54: 1–95.

Modestin J. Borderline: a concept analysis. *Acta Psychiatrica Scandinavica*, 1980, 61: 103–10.

Mollaret P. and Goullon M. Le coma dépaseé. *Revue Neurologique*, 1959, 101: 3–15.

Monahan W.B. *The Psychology of St Thomas Aquinas*. London, Trinity Press (undated).

Monakow C. and Mourgue R. *Introduction Biologique a l'ètude de la Neurologie et de la Psychopathologie*, Paris, Alcan, 1928.

Mondolfo R. *Un Psicologo Associazionista: E.B. de Condillac Bolonia*, Cappelli, 1924.

Monod G. *Les Formes Frustres de la Démence Précoce*, Paris, Rousset, 1905.

Monro H. On the nomenclature of the various forms of insanity. *Asylum Journal*, 1856, 2: 286–305.

Monserrat-Esteve S., Costa J.M. and Ballús C. (eds.) *Patología Obsesiva*, Málaga, Graficasa, 1971.

Montassut M. *La Dépression Constitutionnelle*, Paris, Masson, 1938.

Moore C. *Suicide: A Full Inquiry into the Subject*, 2 Vols, London, J.F.C. Rivington, 1790.

Moore F.C.T. *The Psychology of Maine de Biran*, Oxford, Clarendon Press, 1970.

Mora G. The scrupulosity syndrome. *International Journal of Clinical Psychology*, 1969, 5: 163–74.

Mora G. *Introduction to the English Translation of Catatonia* (K.L. Kahlbaum) Baltimore, Johns Hopkins University Press, 1973.

Mora G. Heinroth's Contribution to Psychiatry. In Heinroth J.C. *Textbook of Disturbances of Mental Life (translated by J. Schmorak)*, 2 Vols, Baltimore, Johns Hopkins University Press, pp. ix-lxxv, 1975.

Mora G. and Brand J.L. (eds.) *Psychiatry and its History. Methodological Problems in Research.* Charles Thomas, Springfield, Illinois, 1970.

Mora G. Cabanis, Neurology and Psychiatry. In Mora G. (ed.) *On the Relations Between the Physical and Moral Aspects of Man* by P.J.G. Cabanis, Vol. 1, Baltimore, Johns Hopkins Press, pp. 45–90, 1981.

Moravia S. The capture of the invisible: for a (pre)history of psychology in eighteenth century France. *Journal of the History of the Behavioral Sciences*, 1983, 19: 370–8.

Mordret A.E. *De la Folie a Double Forme. Circulaire - Alterne*. Paris, Baillière, 1883.

Moreau de Tours J.J. *Du Hachisch et de l'Aliénation Mentale*, Paris, Fortin, Masson et Cie, 1845.

Moreau de Tours J.J. *La Psychologie Morbide dans ses Rapports avec la Philosophie de l'Histoire ou de l'Influence des Névropathies sur le Dynamisme Intellectuel*, Paris, Masson, 1859.

Morel B.A. Du délire èmotif névrose du système nerveux ganglionaire visceral. *Archives Generales de Médecine* (Sixth Series) 1866, 385–402, 530–51, 700–7.

Morel B.A. *Ètudes Cliniques Traité Théorique et Pratique des Maladies Mentales*, 2 Vols, Paris, Masson, 1851–1853.

Morel B.A. *Traité des Dégénérescences Physiques Intellectuelles et Morales de l'Espèce Humaine*, Paris, Baillière, 1857.

Morel B.A. *Traité de Maladies Mentales*, Paris, Masson, 1860.

Morel F. (ed.) *Psychopathologie Des Délires*, Paris, Hermann, 1950.

Morel P.B.A. Morel (1809–1873). In Postel J. and Quétel C. (eds.) *Nouvelle Histoire de la Psychiatrie*, Paris, Privat, 1983.

Morenon M. and Morenon J. L'hallucination appartient au système de la langue. *L'Information Psychiatrique*, 1991, 67: 633–42.

Morgagni J.B. *The Seats and Causes of Diseases* (translated by B. Alexander). London, A. Millar and T. Cadell, 1769.

Morgan C.L. *An Introduction to Comparative Psychology*, Second Edition, London, Walter Scott, 1903 (first edition, 1894).

Morris A.D. A discussion of Parkinson's essay on the shaking palsy. In Rose C. (ed.) *James Parkinson. His life and Times*, Boston, Birkhäuser, pp. 131–148, 1989.

Morris A.D. The madhouse doctor. In Rose C. (ed.) *James Parkinson. His life and Times*, Boston, Birkhäuser, pp. 96–113, 1989.

Morrison J.R. Karl Kahlbaum and catatonia. *Comprehensive Psychiatry*, 1974, 15: 315–16.

Morselli E. *Suicide. An Essay on Comparative Moral Statistics*, London, Kegan Paul, 1881.

Morselli E. Sulla dismorfofobia et sulla tafefobia due forme non per anco descritte di Pazzia con idee fisse. *Bollettino della R. Accademia Medica*, 1891, 6: 110–19.

Morselli E. Confusion. In Baldwin J.M. (ed.) *Dictionary of Philosophy and Psychology*, London, McMillan, p. 212, 1901.

Morsier G. de Les automatismes visuels. *Schweizer medizinische Wochenschrift*, 1936, 66: 700–8.

Morsier G. de Les hallucinations. *Revue D'oto-neuro-ophtalmologie*, 1938, 16: 242–352.

Morsier G. de Le syndrome de Charles Bonnet. Hallucinations visuelles des vieillards sans déficience mentale. *Annales Médico-Psychologiques*, 1967, 125: 677–702.

Morsier G. de Ètudes sur les hallucinations, histoire, doctrines, problèmes. *Journal de Psychologie Normale et Pathologique*, 1969, 66: 281–317.

Morton P. *The Vital Sciences: Biology and the Literary Imagination 1860–1900*, London, Allen and Unwin, 1988.

Mosso A. *La Fatigue: Intellectuel et Physique*, Paris, Alcan, 1903.

Motet (no initial). Fugues de quatre et dix jours consécutives á une chute grave. *Annales Médico-Psychologiques*, 1886, 40: 128–9.

Mott F.W. Arterial degenerations and diseases. In Allbutt T.C. (ed.) *A System of Medicine*, Vol. IV, London, McMillan, pp. 294–344, 1899.

Motte-Moitreux J.F. Philippe Pinel et la manie sans délire. *L'Information Psychiatrique*, 1990, 66: 1016–21.

Mouren M.C. Rajaona F.R. Thiébaux M. and Tatossian A. Le vagabondage: aspects psychologiques et psychopathologiques. *Annales Médico-Psychologiques*, 1978, 135: 415–47.

Mourgue R. *Neurobiologie de L'Hallucination*, Bruxelles, Lamertin, 1932.

Moutier F. *L'Aphasie de Broca*, Paris, Steinheil, 1908.

Moya C.J. *The Philosophy of Action* Cambridge, Polity Press, 1990.

Mucha H. Der Katalepsie-Begriff von Kahlbaum bis zur Gegenwart. *Psychiatria Clinica*, 1972, 5: 330–49.

Müller Ch. (ed.): *Lexicon der Psychiatrie*, Heidelberg, Springer, 1973.

Müller E. Über 'moral insanity'. *Archiv für Psychiatrie und Nervenkrankheiten*, 1899, 31: 325–77.

Müller M. *Lectures on the Science of Language*, Vol. 1, London, Longmans, Green, 1882.

Müller-Freienfels R. *The Evolution of Modern Psychology* (translated by W.B. Wolfe), New Haven, Yale University Press, 1935.

Müller-Hill B. *Murderous Science. Elimination by Scientific Selection of Jews, Gypsies and others in Germany 1933–1945*, Oxford, Oxford University Press, 1988.

Mundt Ch. and Saß H. (eds.) *Für und wider die Einheitspsychose* Stuttgart, Thieme, 1992.

Munro A. and Stewart M. Body dysmorphic disorder and the DSM IV: the demise of dysmorphophobia. *Canadian Journal of Psychiatry*, 1991, 36: 91–6.

Münsterberg, H. The psychology of will. *Psychological Review*, 1898, 5: 639–45.

Murphy G. *An Introduction to Modern Psychology*, London, Routledge and Kegan Paul, 1949.

Murphy T.D. Medical knowledge and statistical methods in early nineteenth-century France. *Medical History*, 1981, 25: 301–19.

Murray D.J. Research on human memory in the nineteenth century. *Canadian Journal of Psychology*, 1976, 30: 201–20.

Musalek M., Bach M., Passweg. V and Jaeger S. The position of delusional parasitosis in psychiatric nosology and classification. *Psychopathology* 1990, 23: 115–24.

Muscio B. Is a fatigue test possible? *British Journal of Psychology*, 1921, 12: 31–46.

Myerson A. *The Nervous Housewife*. Boston, Brown and Little, 1920.

Myerson A. Anhedonia. *American Journal Psychiatry*, 1923, 2: 87–103.

Myerson A. Constitutional anhedonia and the social neurosis. *Journal of Nervous Mental Diseases*, 1944, 99: 309–12.

Myerson A. The constitutional anhedonic personality. *American Journal of Psychiatry*, 1946, 102: 774–9.

Nagera H. *Obsessional Neuroses*, New York, Jason Aronson, 1976.

Naville F. Études sur les Complications et les Séquelles Mentales de l'Encéphalite èpidémique. *L'Encéphale*, 1922, 17: 369–75.

Neal J.B. *Encephalitis: A Clinical Study*, New York, Grune and Stratton, 1942.

Nelson J.C., Charney D.S. and Quinlan D.M. Characteristics of autonomous depression. *Journal of Nervous and Mental Disease*, 1980, 168: 637–43.

Neppe V.M. Carbamazepine for withdrawal hallucinations. *American Journal of Psychiatry*, 1988, 145: 1605–6.

Nesse R.M., Carli T, Curtis G.C. and Kleinman P.D. Pseudohallucinations in cancer chemotherapy patients. *American Journal of Psychiatry*, 1983, 140: 483–5.

Netchine G. Idiotas, débiles y sabios en el siglo XIX. In Zazzo R (ed.) *Los débiles mentales*, Fontanella, Barcelona, pp 77–117, 1973.

Neuburger M. *The Historical Development of Experimental Brain and Spinal Cord Physiology before Flourens* (translated and edited, with additional material, by E. Clarke), Baltimore, The Johns Hopkins University Press, pp. 113–168, 1981.

Neugebauer R. Mediaeval and early modern theories of mental illness. *Archives of General Psychiatry*, 1979, 36: 477–83.

Neugebauer R. A doctor's dilemma: the case of William Harvey's mentally retarded nephew. *Psychological Medicine*, 1989, 19: 569–72.

Neumann E. *The Origins and History of Consciousness*, New York, Bollingen, 1964 (First Edition in German, 1949).

Neumarker K.J. *Karl Bonhoeffer*, Berlin, Springer, 1990.

Neustatter W.L. A case of hysterical stupor recovering after cardiazol treatment. *Journal of Mental Science*, 1942, 88: 440–3.

Newcombe N. and Lerner J.C. Britain between the wars: the historical context of Bowlby's theory of attachment. *Psychiatry*, 1981, 44: 1–12.

Newington H.H. Some observations on different forms of stupor and on its occurrence after acute mania in females. *Journal of Mental Science*, 1874, 20: 312–86.

Nicolson M. and McLaughlin C. Social constructionism and medical psychology: a reply to M.R. Bury. *Sociology of Health and Illness* 1987, 9:107–26.

Niery D., Snowden J.S., Northen B. and Goulding P. Dementia of frontal lobe type. *Journal of Neurology, Neurosurgery and Psychiatry*, 1988, 51: 353–61.

Nisbett R.E., Krantz D.H., Jepson C. and Kunda Z. The use of statistical heuristics in everyday inductive reasoning. *Psychological Review*, 1983, 90: 339–63.

Noël G. *Philippe Chaslin*. Thèse de Médecine N° 168. Faculté de Médecine Xavier-Buchat, 1984.

Noel P.S. and Carlson E.T. The faculty psychology of Benjamin Rush. *Journal of the History of Behavioral Science*, 1973, 9: 369–77.

Noetzli J. Über Dementia Senilis. Reported by Meyer A. *Psychological Review*, 1896, 3: 224–6.

Norman C. Acute confusional insanity. *Dublin Journal of Medical Science*, 1890, 89: 506–18.

North H.M. and Bostock F. Arteriosclerosis and mental disease. *Journal of Mental Science*, 1925, 71: 600–1.

O'Shaughnessy B. *The Will. A Dual Aspect Theory*, Vol. 1, Cambridge, Cambridge University Press, 1980.

Obarrio, J.M., Sagreras, P.O. and Petre, A.J. Melancolía delirante de fisonomía crónica. Síndrome de Cotard, curado. *La Semana Médica* 1932, 39: 1851–4.

Oberg B.B. David Hartley and the association of ideas. *Journal of the History of Ideas*, 1976, 37: 441–54.

Obici, G. Sul cosí detto 'delirio di negazione'. *Rivista Sperimentale di Freniatria*, 1900, 26: 1–29; 291–323.

Obituary. Luciani L. *British Medical Journal*, 1919, ii: 400.

Obituary. Luciani L. *Rivista di Patologia Nervosa e Mentale*, 1919, 24: 256.

Obituary. Tamburini. *Rivista di Patologia Nervosa e Mentale*, 1919, 24: 255–6.

Obituary. Tamburini. *British Medical Journal*, 1919, ii: 400.

Ochoa E. and Berrios G.E. Unilateral hallucinations: a conceptual history submitted for publication.

Oepen G., Harrington A., Spitzer M. and Fünfgeld M. 'Feelings' of conviction: On the relation of affect and thought disorder. In Spitzer M., Uehlein F.A. and Oepen G. (eds.) *Psychopathology and Philosophy*, Berlin, Springer, pp. 43–55, 1988.

Olah G. Was kann man heute unter Arteriosklerotischen Psychosen verstehen? *Psychiatrie Neurologie Wochenschrift*, 1910, 52: 532–3.

Olivares J.M. and Berrios G.E. Anhedonia: clinical aspects submitted for publication.

Oltmanns T.F. and Maher B. (eds.): *Delusional Beliefs*, New York, Wiley, 1988.

Oppenheim J. *Shattered Nerves*, Oxford, Oxford University Press, 1991.

Ordenstein L. *Sur la Paralysie Agitante et la Sclérose en Plaques Généralisées*, Thèse de Paris, Paris, Mortimer, 1868.

Osterlind S.J. *Test Item Bias*. Beverly Hills, Sage Publications, 1983.

Owen A.R.G. *Hysteria, Hypnosis and Healing. The Work of J.M. Charcot*, London, Dobson, 1971.

Owens H. and Maxmen J.S. Mood and affect: a semantic confusion. *American Journal of Psychiatry*, 1979, 136: 97–9.

Oxford English Dictionary (2nd edn): New York, Oxford University Press, 1993.

Packard F. The feeling of unreality. *Journal of Abnormal Psychology*, 1906, 1: 69–82.

Pallis C.A. Parkinsonism: natural history and clinical features. *British Medical Journal*, 1971, 3: 683–90.

Pandit G.L. *The structure and growth of scientific knowledge*, Reidel, Dordrecht, 1983.

Panizza B. Osservazioni sul Nervo Ottico, *Giornale dell'Istituto Lombardo*, Vol. 5, 1855.

Pappenheim, E. On Meynert's amentia. *International Journal of Neurology*, 1975, 9: 310–26.

Parain-Vial J. *La Nature du Fait dans les Sciences Humaines*, Paris, Presses Universitaires de France, 1966.

Parant V. La paralysie agitante examinée comme cause de folie. *Annales Médico-Psychologiques*, 1883, 10: 45–66.

Parant V. *La Raison dans La Folie*. Paris, Doin, 1888.

Parant V. 'Paralysis Agitans'. In Tuke D.H. (ed). *Dictionary of Psychological Medicine*, London, Churchill, 1892.

Parant V. Prétendue entité morbide dite démence précoce. *Annales Médico-Psychologiques*, 1905, 1: 229–41.

Parchappe J.B.M. Symptomatologie de la folie. *Annales Médico-Psychologiques*, 1850–1, 2: 1–20; 332–50; 3: 40–82; 236–49.

Parchappe J.B.M. Rapport sur la statistique de l'alienation mentale. *Annales Médico-Psychologiques*, 1856, 2: 1–6.

Parfitt D.N. and Gall C. Psychogenic amnesia: the refusal to remember. *The Journal of Mental Science*, 1944, 90: 511–31.

Pargeter W. *Observations on Maniacal Disorders*, London, Murray, 1792.

Parish E. *Hallucinations and Illusions*, London, Walter Scott, 1897 (translation of improved version of Parish E. Über die Trugwahrnehmung. *Schriften der Gessellschaft für psychologischen Forschung*, 1894: 1–246).

Parkinson J. *An Essay on the Shaking Palsy*, London, Sherwood, Neely, and Jones, 1817.

Parot F. and Richelle M. *Psychologues de la Langue Française*, Paris, Presses Universitaires de France, 1992.

Parrot J. Cerveau. VIII Ramollissement. In Dechambre A. and Lereboullet L. (eds.) *Dictionnaire Encyclopédique des Sciences Médicales*, Vol. 14, Paris, Mason and Asselin, pp. 400–431, 1873.

Parsons J. Human physiognomy explained. Croonian lectures on muscular motion for the year 1746. *Transactions Royal Society*, pp. 60–2, 1747.

Passingham R. *The Frontal Lobes and Voluntary Action*. Oxford, Oxford University Press, 1993.

Passmore J.J. *Ralph Cudworth*. Cambridge, Cambridge University Press, 1951.

Patrick H.T. and Levy D.M. Parkinson's disease. A clinical study of 146 cases. *Archives of Neurology and Psychiatry*, 1922, 7: 711–20.

Pauleikhoff B. Die Katatonie (1848–1968). *Fortschritte der Neurologie Psychiatrie und ihrer Grenzgebiete*, 1969, 37: 461–96.

Paulhan F. La Personnalité. *Revue Philosophique*. 1880, 5: 49–67.

Paulhan F. Les variations de la personnalité a l'ètat normal. *Revue Philosophique*, 1882, 13: 639–53.

Paulhan F. *L'Activité Mentale et les èléments de l'Esprit*, Paris, Alcan, 1889.

Paulhan F. *Les Caractères*, Paris, Alcan, 1894.

Paulhan F. *La Volonté*, Paris, Doin, 1903.

Paulus, J. *Le Problème de l'Hallucination et l'Évolution de la Psychologie d'Esquirol á Pierre Janet*. Paris, Les Belles Letters, 1941.

Pauw K.W. Frégoli syndrome after cerebral infarction. *Journal Nervous and Mental Disease*, 1987, 175: 433–8.

Payne R.W. Mattussek P. and George E.I. An experimental study of schizophrenic thought disorder. *The Journal of Mental Science*, 1959, 105: 627–52.

Payot L. *L'Éducation de la Volonté*, Paris, Alcan, 1931 (first edition, 1893).

Paz M. Alfred Maury, Member del'Institute, Chroniqueur de Napoléon III et du Second Empire. *Revue des Travaux de l'Academie des Sciences Morales et Politiques*, 1964, 117: 248–64.

Pears D. Hume's account of personal identity. In *Questions in the Philosophy of Mind*, London, Duckwork, pp. 208–23, 1975.

Pearson E.S. (ed.) *The History of Statistics in the 17th and 18th Centuries*, London, Griffin, 1978.

Penelhum T. Personal Identity. In Edwards P. (ed.) *The Encyclopedia of Philosophy*, Vol. 6, New York, McMillan, pp. 95–107, 1967.

Penfield W. and Porot P. The brain's record of auditory and visual experiences. *Brain*, 1963, 86: 595–696.

Perkins J.A. *The Concept of Self in the French Enlightenment*, Genève, Droz, 1969.

Perrin L. Des névrodermies parasitophobiques. *Annales de Dermatologie et Syphiligraphie*, 1896, 7: 129–38.

Perris, C. Sul delirio cronico di negazione (Sindrome di Cotard). *Neuropsichiatria* 1955, 11: 175–201.

Perrot J.C. and Woolf S.J. *State and Statistics in France 1789–1815*, London, Harwood, 1984.

Perry J.C. and Klerman G.L. The borderline patient. *Archives of General Psychiatry* 1978, 35: 141–50.

Perry R.B. *The Thought and Character of William James* (vol. 1). London, Oxford University Press, 1936.

Perusini G. Sul valore nosografico di alcuni reperti istopatologici caratteristiche per la senilitá. *Rivista Italiana di Neuropatologia, Psichiatria ed Elettroterapia*, 1911, 4: 193–213.

Peset J.L. *Ciencia y Marginación*, Barcelona, Grijalbo, 1983.

Peterman B. *The Gestalt Theory and the Problem of Configuration*, London, Kogan Paul, 1932.

Peters R. *Hobbes*, London, Peregrin Books, 1967.

Peters V.H. Psychopathology of the apallic syndrome. In Dalle Ore G. (ed.) *The Apallic Syndrome*, Berlin, Springer, pp. 59–68, 1977.

Petersen P. *Guillermo Wundt*. Madrid, Revista de Occidente, 1932.

Peterson C.A. and Knudson R.M. Anhedonia: a construct validation approach. *Journal of Personality Assesment*, 47: 539–51, 1983.

Peterson J. *Early Conceptions and Tests of Intelligence*, London, Harrap, 1925.

Petetin J.H.D. *Mémoire sur la Découverte des Phénomènes que Présentent la Catalepsie et le Somnambulisme*, Paris, Labé, 1787.

Petho B. Hundert Jahre Hebephrenie. *Psychiatrie, Neurologie und medizinische Psychologie*, 1972, 24: 305–17.

Petit G. *Essai sur une variété de pseudo-hallucinations: les auto-représentations aperceptives*, Bordeaux, Broch, 1913.

Petit M. Lepine J.P. and Lesieur Ph. Chronologie des effets extrapyramidaux des neuroleptiques et système dopaminergique nigrostriatal. *L'Encéphale*, 1979, 5: 297–316.

Petrie A. Edward Mapother. *Journal of Mental Science*, 1940, 106: 747–9.

Philippopoulos G.S. The analysis of a case of dysmorfophobia. *Canadian Journal of Psychiatry*, 1979, 24: 397–401.

Phillips J. Psychoses associated with senility and arteriosclerosis. In Mott F. W. (ed.) *Early Mental Disease*. The Lancet Extranumbers N° 2, London, Wakley and Son, pp. 146–148, 1912.

Phillips J. Involutional conditions. In Mott F.W. (ed.) *Early Mental Disease*, The Lancet Extranumbers N° 2, London, Wakley and Son, pp. 90–92, 1912.

Pic A. *Précis des Maladies des Vieillards*, Paris, Doin, 1912.

Pichot P. French pioneers in the field of mental deficiency. *American Journal of Mental Deficiency*, 1948, 53: 128–37.

Pichot P. Recent developments in French psychiatry. *British Journal of Psychiatry* 1967, 113: 11–18.

Pichot P. Psychopathic behaviour. A historical overview. In Hare R.D. and Schalling D. (eds.) *Psychopathic Behaviour: Approaches to Research*, New York, Wiley, pp. 55–70, 1978.

Pichot P. The diagnosis and classification of mental disorders in French-speaking countries: background, current views and comparison with other countries. *Psychological Medicine*, 1982, 12: 475–92.

Pichot P. The birth of the bipolar disorder. *European Psychiatry*, 1995, 10: 1–10.

Pick A. Senile Hirnatrophie als Grundlage von Herderscheinungen. *Wiener klinische Wochenschrift*, 1901, 14: 403–4. (Translation by D.M. Girling and I.S. Marková, *History of Psychiatry*, Dec. 1995.

Pick A. Über die Beziehungen der senilen Hirnatrophie zur Aphasie. *Prager medicinische Wochenschrift*, 1892, 17: 165–7 (translation by D.M. Girling and G.E. Berrios in *History of Psychiatry*, 1994, 5, 542–574).

Pick A. Zur Pathologie des Ich. *Archiv für Psychiatrie und Nervenkrankheiten*, 1904, 33: 22–33.

Pick A. Über einen weiterer Symptomenkomplex im Rahmen der Dementia senilis, bedingt durch umschriebene sträkere Hirnatrophie (gemische Apraxie). *Monatschrift für Psychiatrie und Neurologie*, 1906, 19: 97–108.

Pick D. *Faces of Degeneration: A European Disorder, c1848–1918*. Cambridge, Cambridge University Press, 1989.

Piéron H. *Thought and the Brain*, London, Kegan Paul, Trench, Trubner and Co, 1927.

Piéron H. *Vocabulaire de la Psychologie*, Paris, Presses Universitaires de France, 1968.

Pigeaud J.M. Le rôle des passions dans la pensée médicale de Pinel à Moreau de Tours. *History and Philosophy of the Life Sciences*, 1980, 2: 123–40.

Pigeaud J.M. *La Maladie de l'âme. Étude sur la Relation de l'âme et du Corps dans la Tradition Médico-Psychologique Antique*, Paris: Les Belles Lettres, 1981.

Pigeaud J.M. La Génie et la Folie: Étude sur la Psychologie Morbide de J. Moreau de Tours. *L'Evolution Psychiatrique*, 1986, 51: 587–608.

Pilcz A. Contribution a l'ètude du suicide. *Annales Médico-Psychologiques*, 1908, 7: 193–205.

Pilkington G.W. and Glasgow W.D. Towards a Rehabilitation of Introspection as a method in psychology. *Journal of Existentialism*, 1967, 7: 329–50.

Pinard G. and Lecours A.R. The language of psychotics and neurotics. In Lecours A.R., L'Hermitte F. and Bryans B. (eds.) *Aphasiology*, London, Baillière, pp. 313–335, 1983.

Pinel Ph. *Traité Médico-Philosophique sur L'Aliénation Mentale ou la Manie*, Paris, Richard, Caille et Ravier, year IX, 1801.

Pinel Ph. *A Treatise of Insanity.* (translated by D.D. Davis), Sheffield, W. Todd, 1806.

Pinel Ph. *Traité Médico-Philosophique de la Aliénation Mentale*, 2nd edn., Paris, Brosson, 1809.

Pinel Ph. *Nosographie Philosophique ou la Méthode de l'Analyse Appliquée a la Médicine*. Paris, Vol. 1, 6th edn., J.A. Brosson, 1818 (First Edition, 1798).

Pinillos J.L. López Piñero J.M. and Ballester L.G. *Constitución y Personalidad. Historia y Teoría de un Problema*, Valencia, Guerris, 1966.

Piro S. *Il Linguaggio Schizofrenico*. Milan, Giangiacomo Feltrinelli, 1967.

Pistoia del L. Le problème de la temporalité dans le psychiatrie Française Classique. *L'Évolution Psychiatrique*, 1971, 36: 445–74.

Pitman R.K. Pierre Janet on obsessive compulsive disorder. *Archives of General Psychiatry*, 1987, 44: 226–32.

Pitres A. and Régis E. Les impulsions. *Revue de Psychiatrie*, 1902, 9: 208–17.

Pitres A. and Régis E. *Les Obsessions et les Impulsions*, Paris, Doin, 1902.

Place J.L. L'hypocondrie: Éloge de Dubois d'Amiens. *L'Evolution Psychiatrique*, 1986, 51: 567–86.

Plato. *The Collected Dialogues of Plato*. Edited by E. Hamilton and H. Cairns. Bollingen Series. Princeton, Princeton University Press, 1961.

Platt A.M. and Diamond B.L. The origins and development of the 'Wild Beast' concept of mental illness and its relation to theories of criminal responsibility. *Journal of the History of the Behavioral Sciences*, 1965, 1: 355–67.

Platter F. *Praxeos seu de cognoscendis, . . .* 2 vols, Basileae, C Waldkirchius, 1602–3.

Plum F. and Posner J.B. *Diagnosis of Stupor and Coma* (Second Edition) Philadelphia, F.A. Davies, 1972.

Podoll K., Osterheider M. and Noth J. Das Charles Bonnet-Syndrom. *Fortschritte Neurologie und Psychiatrie*, 1989, 57: 43–60.

Politzer G. *Critique des Fondements de la Psychologie*. Presses Universitaires de France, 1967 (first published in 1927).

Pollit J. Moodiness: a heavenly problem? *Journal of the Royal Society of Medicine*, 1982, 75: 7–16.

Poore G. On Fatigue. *Lancet*, 1895, ii: 163–4.

Popper K. *The Logic of Scientific Discovery*, London, Hutchinson, 1968.

Porot A. *Manual Alphabétique de Psychiatrie*, Paris, Presses Universitaires de France, 1975.

Porot M. Approche d'une classification française des délires. *Annales Médico-Psychologiques* 1989, 147: 374–81.

Porter N. *The Human Intellect*, Fourth Edition, New York, Scribner's, 1868.

Porter R. *Mind-forg'd Manacles*, Athlone Press, London, 1987.

Porter T.M. *The Rise of Statistical Thinking: 1820–1900*, Princeton, Princeton University Press, 1986.

Poskanzer D.C. and Schwab R.S. Cohort analysis of Parkinson's syndrome: Evidence for a single aetiology related to a subclinical infection about 1920. *Journal of Chronic Diseases*, 1963, 16: 961–74.

Post F. *The Clinical Psychiatry of Late Life*. Oxford, Pergamon Press, 1965.

Postel J. Introduction. In Georget E. *De la Folie*, Paris, Privat, pp. 7–21, 1972.

Postel J. Naissance et decadence du traitement moral pendant la première moitie du XIX siècle. *L'Evolution Psychiatrique*, 1979, 44: 585–616.

Postel J. *Genèse de la Psychiatrie. Les Premiers ècrits de Philippe Pinel*, Paris, Le Sycomore, 1981.

Postel J. Review. *L'Evolution Psychiatrique*, 1984, 49: 697–8.

Postel J. Images de la folie au XVIIIe siècle: quelques différénces de sa représentation dans les littératures Française et Britannique au siècle des lumières. *L'Evolution Psychiatrique*, 1984, 49: 707–18.

Postel J. *Dictionnaire de Psychiatrie*. Paris, Larousse, 1993.

Postel J. and Quetel C. (eds.) *Nouvelle Histoire de la Psychiatrie*. Privat, Paris, 1983.

Postman L. Herman Ebbinghaus. *American Psychologist*, 1968, 23: 149–57.

Potain C. Cerveau (Pathologie). In Dechambre A. and Lereboullet L. (eds.) *Dictionnaire Encyclo-pédique des Sciences Médicales*, Vol. 14, Paris, Masson, pp. 214–345, 1873.

Power H. and Sedwick L.W. *The New Sydenham Society's Lexicon of Medicine and the Allied Sciences*, London, New Sydenham Society, 1892.

Pratt R. Psychogenic loss of memory. In Whitty C.M.W. and Zangwill O.L. (eds.) *Amnesia*, Second Edition, London, Butterworths, pp. 224–32, 1977.

Prevost C.M. *Janet, Freud et la Psychologie Clinique*. Paris, Payot, 1973a.

Prevost C.M. *La psycho-philosophie de Pierre Janet*. Paris, Payot, 1973b.

Price H.H. Some considerations about belief. *Proceedings of the Aristotelian Society*, 1931, 35: 229–52.

Prichard J.C. *A Treatise on Insanity and other Disorders Affecting the Mind*, London, Sherwood, Gilbert, and Piper, 1835.

Pujol R. and Savy A. *Le Devenir de L'Obsédé*, 2 Vols. Paris, Masson, 1968.

Quain R. *A Dictionary of Medicine*. 2 Vol, London, Longman, Green, and Co, 1894.

Quercy P. *Études sur L'Hallucination*, Paris, Alcan, 1930.

Quercy P. Les fondateurs de la doctrine Française de l'aphasie. *Annales Médico-Psychologiques*, 1943, 101: 161–88.

Quétel C. *History of Syphilis*. Cambridge, Polity Press, 1990 (First French edition 1986).

Quincy J. *Lexicon Physico-Medicum: or, a New Physical Dictionary*, London, Taylor, Taylor and Osborne, 1719.

Quinton A. Knowledge and belief. In Edwards P. (ed.) *The Encyclopedia of Philosophy*, Vol. 3, pp. 345–52, New York, MacMillan, 1967.

Rachlin H.L. A follow up study of Hoch's 'benign supor' cases. *American Journal of Psychiatry*, 1935, 92: 531–58.

Rachman S.J. and Hodgson R.J. *Obsessions and Compulsions*, New Jersey, Prentice-Hall, 1980.

Rack P. *Race, Culture and Mental Disorder*. Tavistock Publications, London, 1982.

Radicke (no initial). *On the Application of Statistics to Medical Enquiries (translated by F.T. Bond)*, London, The New Sydenham Society, 1861 (First appeared in Wunderlich's Archiv für physiologische Heilkunde, Vol. 2, 1858).

Rado S. and Daniels G. *Changing Concepts of Psychoanalytic Medicine*. New York, Grune and Stratton, 1956.

Rado S. *Psychoanalysis of Behaviour: Collected Papers* (2 Vols.). New York, Grune and Stratton, 1956.

Rado S. Obsessive Behaviour. In Arieti S. (ed.) *American Handbook of Psychiatry*, New York, Basic Books, 1959.

Rado S. Theory and Therapy: The theory of schizotypal organization and its application to the treatment of descompensated schizotypal behaviour, in Scher S.C. and Davis H.R. (eds.). *The Outpatient Treatment of Schizophrenia*. New York, Grune and Straton, 1960.

Ramul K. The problem of measurement in the psychology of the eighteenth century. *American Psychologist*, 1960, 15: 256–65.

Rancurello A.C. *A Study of Franz Brentano*, New York, Academic Press, 1968.

Rand B. *The Classical Psychologists*, London, Constable, 1912.

Raskin D.E. and Frank S.W. Herpes encephalitis with catatonic stupor. *Archives of General Psychiatry*, 1974, 31: 544–6.

Rath G. Neural Pathology. A pathogenetic concept of the 18th and 19th centuries. *Bulletin of the History of Medicine*, 1959; 33: 526–30.

Ratner S.T. Comparative aspects of hypnosis. In Gordon J. (ed.) *Handbook of Clinical and Experimental Hypnosis*, New York, Macmillan, 1967.

Rauzier G. *Traité des Maladies des Vieillards*, Paris, Baillière, 1909.

Ravaisson J.G.F. *La Philosophie en France au XIXe Siècle*, Second Edition, Paris, Hachette, 1885.

Ravaisson J.G.F. *De L'Habitude*, Paris, Fayard (First Edition, 1838), 1984.

Raymond F. and Janet P. *Les obsessions et la Psychasthénie*. Vol. 2. Second Edition, Paris, Alcan, 1911 (first edition, 1903).

Raymond F. Névroses et Psycho-Névroses. In Marie A. (ed.) *Traité International de Psychologie Pathologique*, Vol. 2, Paris, Alcan, pp. 1–77, 1911.

Recueil Périodique de Littérature Médicale ètrangère published by the Société de Médicine de Paris (series).

Redlich E. Die Psychosen bei Gehirnerkrankungen. In Aschaffenburg G. *Handbuch der Psychiatrie*, Leipzig, Deuticke, 1912.

Reed J.L. Schizophrenic thought disorder: a review and hypothesis. *Comprehensive Psychiatry*, 1970, 11: 403–32.

Rees L. Constitutional factors and abnormal behaviour. In Eysenck H. (ed.) *Handbook of Abnormal Psychology*, London, Pitman, pp. 344–392, 1961.

Régis E. Des hallucinations unilatérales. *L'Encéphale*, 1881, 1: 43–74.

Régis E. *Manuel Pratique de Médecine Mentale*, Paris, Doin, 1885.

Régis, E. Note historique et clinique sur le délire des négations. *Gazette Médicale de Paris*, 1893, 2: 61–4.

Régis E. *Précis de Psychiatrie*, Paris, Doin, 1906.

Régis E. and Hesnard A. Les confusions mentales. In Marie A. (ed.) *Traité International de Psychopathologie*, Vol. 2, Paris, Félix Alcan, 1911.

Reich J. The interface of plastic surgery and psychiatry. *Clinics in Plastic Surgery*, 1982: 367–77.

Reid, T. *The Works of Thomas Reid D.D*, collected by Sir William Hamilton. Fourth Edition, Edinburgh, Maclachan and Stewart, 1854.

Reil J.C. *Rhapsodieen über die Anwendung der psychischen Curmethode auf Geisteszerrüttungen*. Halle, Unveraenderten Nackdruck der Ausgabe, 1803.

Reilly T.M. and Beard A.W. Monosymptomatic hypochondriasis (letter). *British Journal of Psychiatry*, 1976, 129: 191.

Renaudin L.F.E. Observations médico-legales sur la monomanie. *Annales Médico-Psychologiques*, 1854, 6: 236–49.

Renaudin L.F.E. Observations sur les recherches statistiques relatives a l'aliénation mentale. *Annales Médico-Psychologiques*, 1856, 2: 339–360.

Rennert H. Wilhelm Griesinger und die Einheitspsychose. *Wissenschaftliche Zeitschrift der Humboldt-Universität*, 1968, 17: 15–16.

Renouvier Ch. La Personnalité. *L'Anne Psychologique* 1900, 10: 1–38.

Report. Mental Diseases Section (International Medical Congress, London) *Journal of Mental Science*, 1881, 27: 457–60.

Rescher N. *Cognitive Systematization*, Oxford, Blackwell, 1979.

Revault d'Allonnes G. *L'Affaiblissement intelectuel chez les déments. ètude clinique par la méthode d'observation expérimentale*. Thèse de Medicine, Paris, 1912.

Revault d'Allonnes, J. Une forme eclipsé du délire des négations. *Annales Médico-Psychologiques*, 1923, 83: 138–56.

Reveillé-Parise J.H. *Traité de la Vieillesse*, Paris, Baillière, 1853.

Ribot Th. Les désordres généraux de la mémoire. *Revue Philosophique*, 1880, 10: 181–214; 485–516.

Ribot Th. *Diseases of Memory*, London, Kegan Paul, Trench and Co, 1882 (1st French edn., 1881).

Ribot Th. *Les Maladies de la Personnalité*, Paris, Alcan, 1884.

Ribot Th. *La Psychologie Allemande Contemporaine*, Second Edition, Paris, Alcan, 1885.

Ribot Th. *Psychologie de l'Attention*, Paris, Alcan, 1889.

Ribot Th. Sur les diverses formes du caractère. *Revue Philosophique* 1892, 17: 480–500.

Ribot Th. Les caractéres anormaux et morbides *L'Année Psychologique*, 1896, 2: 1–17.

Ribot Th. *La Psychologie Anglaise Contemporaine. (École Expérimentale)* Third Edition, Paris, Alcan, 1896.

Ribot Th: *The Psychology of Emotions*. London, W. Scott, 1897.

Ribot Th. *Les Maladies de la Volonté*, Eighteenth Edition, Paris, Alcan, 1904 (First Edition, 1883).

Ribot Th. *L'Hérédité Psychologique*, Paris, Alcan, 1906.

Ribot Th. *Las Enfermedades de la Personalidad* (translation of R. Rubio), Madrid, Jorro, 1912.

Ribot Th. Les tendences. *Journal de Psychologie Normale et Pathologique*, 1915, 12: 284–99.

Ribot Th. *Essai sur les Passions*. 5th Edition, Paris, Alcan, 1923.

Ribstein M. Hypnagogic hallucinations. In Guilleminault C., Dement W.C., and Passouant P. (eds.) *Narcolepsy*. New York, Spectrum Publications, pp. 145–60, 1976.

Richards R.J. Lloyd Morgan's theory of instinct: from Darwinism to neo-Darwinism. *Journal of the History of Behavioral Science*, 1977, 13: 12–32.

Richardson E.P. Introduction. In Rottenberg D.A. and Hochberg F.H. (eds.) *Neurological Classics in Modern Translation*, New York, Hafner Press, pp. 95–6, 1977.

Richet Ch. *Traité de Métapsychique*. Paris, Alcan, 1922.

Richfield J. An analysis of the concept of insight. *Psychoanalytical Quarterly*, 1954, 23: 390–408.

Rieder R.O. The origins of our confusion about schizophrenia. *Psychiatry*, 1974, 37: 197–208.

Riese W. Hughlings Jackson's doctrine of consciousness. Sources, versions and elaborations. *Journal of Nervous and Mental Disease*, 1954, 120: 330–7.

Riese W. Hughlings Jackson's doctrine of aphasia and its significance today. *Journal of Nervous and Mental Disease*, 1955, 122: 1–13.

Riese W. The impact of nineteenth-century thought on psychiatry. *International Record of Medicine*, 1960, 173: 7–19.

Riese W. The sources of Hughlings Jackson's view on aphasia. *Brain*, 1965, 88: 811–22.

Riese W. *La Théorie des Passions á la Lumière de la Pensée Médicale du XVII Siècle*, New York, Bale, 1965.

Riese W. La méthode analytique de Condillac et ses rapports avec l'oeuvre de Phillipe Pinel. *Revue Philosophique*, 1968, 158: 312–36.

Riese W. *The Legacy of Philippe Pinel*, New York, Springer, 1969.

Riether A.M. and Stoudmire A. Psychogenic fugue states: a review. *Southern Medical Journal* 1988, 81: 568–71.

Rignano E. *Psicología del Razonamiento*, Madrid, Calpe, 1922 (first Italian edition, 1920).

Riklin T. Beitrag zur Psychologie der kataleptischen Zustände bei Katatonie. *Psychiatrie und Neurologie Wochenschrift*, N° 32, 1906.

Risse G.B. The Brownian system of medicine. *Clio Medica*, 1970, 5: 45–51.

Ritti A. Folie á double forme. In Dechambre A. and Lereboullet A. (eds.) *Dictionnaire Encyclopédique des Sciences Médicales*, Vol. 39, Paris, Masson, 1876.

Ritti A. Folie de doute avec délire de toucher. In Dechambre A. and Lereboullet A. (eds.) *Dictionnaire Encyclopédique des Sciences Médicales*, Vol. 39, Paris, Masson, pp. 339–48, 1876.

Ritti A. Folie avec conscience. In Dechambre A. and Lereboullet A. (eds.) *Dictionnaire Encyclopédique des Sciences Médicales*, Vol. 39, Paris, Masson, pp. 307–20, 1876.

Ritti A. *Traité Clinique de la Folie a Double Forme*. Paris, Doin, 1883.

Ritti A. Stupeur, Stupidité. In Dechambre A. and Lereboullet A. (ed.) *Dictionnaire Encyclopédique des Sciences Medicales*, Paris, Asselin, pp. 454–69, 1883.

Ritti A. Suicide. In Dechambre A. (ed.) *Dictionnaire Encyclopédique de Sciences Médicales*, Vol. 92, Paris, Asselin, pp. 296–347, 1884.

Ritti A. Éloge de J. Baillarger. *Annales Médico-Psychologiques*, 1892, 16: 5–58.

Ritti A. Éloge de Billod. *Annales Médico-Psychologiques*, 1900, 58: 11–41.

Ritti A. Review. *Annales Médico-Psychologiques*, 1913, 71: 284–9.

Roback A.A. *The Psychology of Character. With a Survey of Temperament*, London, Kegan Paul, Trench, Trubner and Co, 1927.

Roberts G. The origins of delusion. *British Journal of Psychiatry*, 1992, 161: 298–308.

Robertson A. On unilateral hallucinations and their relation to cerebral localisation. In McCormac W. *Transactions of the International Medical Congress*, Vol. III, London, Kolckman, pp. 632–3, 1881.

Robertson A. Unilateral hallucinations: their relative frequency, associations, and pathology. *Journal of Mental Science*, 1901, 47: 277–93.

Robertson G.M. Melancholia, from the physiological and evolutionary points of view. *Journal of Mental Science*, 1890, 36: 53–67.

Roccatagliata G. *Storia de la Psichiatria Antica*, Milan, Ulrico Hoepli, 1973.

Roccatagliata G. *Storia della psichiatria biologica*. Nuova Guaraldi, Florence, 1981.

Roccatagliata G. *Le Origini de la Psychoanalisi nella Culture Classica*, Rome, II Pensiero Scientifico, 1981.

Roccatagliata G. *Isteria*, Roma, Il Pensiero Scientifico, 1990.

Rocha D. La psychose maniaque-dépressive. *Annales Médico-Psychologiques*, 1906, 64: 250–62.

Roche L.Ch. Paralysie In *Dictionnaire de Médicine et de Chirurgie Pratiques*, Vol. 12, Paris, Baillière, p. 364, 1834.

Rochoux M. Psychologie. In *Dictionnaire de Médicine* (second edition) Vol. 26, Paris, Labé, pp. 280–317, 1842.

Roelens R. Une recherche psychologique méconnue, le courant 'dramatique' de G. Politzer á aujourd'hui. *La Pensée* N°103, 76–101, 1962.

Rogers D. The motor disorder of severe psychiatric illness: a conflict of paradigms. *British Journal of Psychiatry*, 1985, 147: 221–32.

Rogues de Fursac and Capgras, J. Délire mélancolique de négation et d'immortalité disparú au bout de deux ans et demi. *L'Encéphale*, 1912, 7:68–74.

Rogues de Fursac J. *Manual de Psiquiatría* (translation of Fifth French edition by J. Peset), Valencia, Editorial Publ, 1921.

Rokhline L.L. Les conceptions psychopathologiques de Kandinsky. *L'Evolution Psychiatrique*, 1971, 36: 475–88.

Romanes G.J. *Mental Evolution of Man. Origin of Human Faculty*, London, Kegan Paul, Trench and Co, 1888.

Romberg M.H. *A Manual of the Nervous Diseases of Man* (translated by E.H. Sieveking) Vol. 2, London, Sydenham Society, 1853.

Rose C. (ed.) *James Parkinson. His life and Times*, Boston, Birkhäuser, 1989.

Rosen G. The philosophy of ideology and the emergence of modern medicine in France. *Bulletin of the History of Medicine*, 1964, 20: 328–39.

Rosen G. Irrationality and madness in seventeenth and eighteenth century Europe. In Rosen G. (ed.) *Madness in Society*, Chicago, University of Chicago Press, pp. 151–71, 1968.

Rosen G. History in the study of suicide. *Psychological Medicine*, 1971, 4: 267–85.

Rosen G. Nostalgia: a 'forgotten' psychological disorder. *Psychological Medicine*, 1975, 5: 340–54.

Rosenberg C.E. Body and mind in nineteenth century medicine: some clinical origins of the neurosis construct. *Bulletin of the History of Medicine*, 1989, 63: 185–97.

Rosenthal D.M. Two concepts of consciousness. *Philosophical Studies*, 1986, 3: 329–59.

Rosmini Serbati A. *Psychology*, Vol. 3, London, Kegan Paul Trench and Co., 1888.

Ross B.M. *Remembering the Personal Past*. New York, Oxford University Press, 1991.

Ross E.D. and Mesulam M.M. Dominant language functions of the right hemisphere? Prosody and emotional gesturing. *Archives of Neurology*, 1979, 36: 144–8.

Ross T.A. *The Common Neurosis*, London, Arnold, 1923.

Rostan L.L. *Recherches sur le Ramollissement du Cerveau*, Paris, Bechet, 1819 and 1823.

Rostan L.L. *Jusqu'á quel point l'Anatomie Pathologique peut-elle éclairer la Thérapeutique des Maladies*. Thèse de concours, Paris, 1833.

Rostan, L.L. *Curso de Medicina Clínica*. In 3 Volumes. Cádiz, Imprenta de Féros, 1839 (First French edition 1830).

Rothschuh K.E. *History of Physiology* (translated by G.B. Risse) New York, Krieger, 1973.

Rouart J. Janet and Jackson. *L'Evolution Psychiatrique*, 1950, 25: 485–501.

Rouart J. *Psychose Maniaque Dépressive et Folies Discordantes*, Paris, Doin, 1936.

Roubinovitch J. *Des Variétés Cliniques de la Folie en France et en Allemagne*, Paris, Doin, 1896.

Rouby J. *Contribution á l'étude de la Presbyophrénie*, Thèse de Médicine, Paris, E. Nourris, 1911.

Rouillard (no initial). Les Amnésies. *L'Encéphale*, 1888, 8: 652–71.

Rovonsuo A and Kampinnen M. (eds.) *Consciousness in Philosophy and Cognitive Neuroscience*. New Jersey, Lawrence Erlbaum, 1994.

Royal College of Physicians. *The Nomenclature of Diseases*, Fourth Edition, London, His Majesty's Stationary Office, 1906.

Royer-Collard A.A. Examen de la doctrine de Maine de Biran. *Annales Médico-Psychologiques*, 1843, 2: 1–45.

Royer-Collard H. Des tempéramens, considérés dans leurs rapports avec la santé. *Mémoire de la Académie Royale de Médicine*, 1843, 10: 134–69.

Ruff R.L. and Russakoff L.M. Catatonia with frontal lobe atrophy. *Journal of Neurology, Neurosurgery and Psychiatry*, 1980, 43: 185–7.

Rullier. Faculté. In *Dictionnaire des Sciences Médicales*, Paris, Panckoucke, pp. 389–420, 1815.

Rush B. *Medical Inquiries and Observations upon the Diseases of the Mind*, Philadelphia, Kimber and Richardson, 1812.

Rush B. *Lectures on the Mind* (edited, annotated and introduced by E.T. Carlson, J.L. Wollock and P.S. Noel), Philadelphia, American Philosophical Society, 1981.

Rushton P. Lunatics and idiots: mental disability, the community, and the poor law in North-East England, 1600–1800. *Medical History*, 1988, 32: 34–50.

Ryle G. *The Concept of Mind*, London, Hutchinson, 1949.

Sackellares J.C., Lee S.I. and Dreiffus F.E. Stupor following administration of valproic acid to patients receiving other antiepileptic drugs. *Epilepsia*, 1979, 20: 697–703.

Sachdev P. Clinical characteristics and predisposing factors in acute drug-induced akathisia. *Archives of General Psychiatry*, 1994, 51: 963–74.

Safranski R. *Schopenhauer y los Años Salvajes de la Filosofía*. Madrid, Alianza, 1991.

Sahakow D. Herman Ebbighaus. *American Journal of Psychology*, 1930, 42: 505–18.

Sakai A. Phrenitis: inflammation of the mind and body. *History of Psychiatry*, 1991, 2: 193–206.

Salmon W. *Iatrica: Seu Praxis Medendi*, Third Edition, London, Rolls, 1694.

Sanchez M.A. *La Presencia de la Medicina en la Obra de John Locke (1932–1704)*. Tésis Doctoral, Facultad de Medicina, Universidad Complutense de Madrid, 1987.

Sanchez M.A. Las ideas de John Locke sobre la enfermedad mental (unpublished manuscript).

Sánchez R. *Comentarios del Traductor*. In Jean Itard, *Victor de L'Aveyron*. Madrid, Alianza, pp. 99–251, 1982.

Sander W. Über Erinnerungstäuschungen. *Archiv für Psychiatrie und Nervenkrankheiten*, 1874, 4: 244–53.

Sands I.J. The type of personality susceptible to Parkinson's disease. *Journal of Mount Sinai Hospital*, 1942, 9: 792–4.

Santangelo-Spoto, F. Il delirio di negazione di Cotard. *Il Pisani*, 1896, 3: 86–8.

Sarantoglou G. Quelques Réflexions 'Psychopathologiques' et 'Psychothérapeutiques' á propos de la Folie de l'ajax sophocléen. In *Les Thérapeutiques de l'áme*. L.M.S. No. 2, Université de Nantes, 1980.

Sarbin T.R. Anxiety: reification of a metaphor. *Archives of General Psychiatry*, 1964, 10: 630–8.

Sarbin T.R. Ontology recapitulates philology: the mythic nature of anxiety. *American Psychologist*, 1868, 23: 411–18.

Sarbin T.R. and Juhasz J.B. The historical background of the concept of hallucination. *Journal of the History of the Behavioral Sciences*, 1967, 3: 339–59.

Sarró Burbano R. Psicopatología General. In Pons P. (ed.). *Tratado de Patología y Clínica Médica*, Barcelona, Salvat, Vol. 4, pp. 461–493, 1960.

Sartre J.P. *Esquisse d'une Théorie des Èmotions*, Paris, Hermann, 1939.

Saß H. Problem der Katatonieforschung. *Nervenarzt*, 1981, 52: 373–82.

Saß H. Affektdelite. *Nervenarzt*, 1983, 54: 557–75.

Saury H. *Étude Clinique sur la Folie Héréditaire*, Paris, Delahaye et Lecrosnier, 1886.

Saurí J.J. Las Significaciones del Vocablo Psicosis. *Acta Psiquiátrica Psicológica de América Latina*, 1972, 18: 219–23.

Saurí J.J. *Historia de las Ideas Psiquiátricas*, Buenos Aires, Lohlé, 1969.

Saurí J.J. (ed.) *Las Fobias* Buenos Aires, Nueva Visión, 1979.

Saurí J.J. *Las Obsesiones*, Buenos Aires, Nueva Visión, 1983.

Saussure R. de. The influence of the concept of monomania on French medico-legal Psychiatry (from 1825–1840). *Journal of History of Medicine*, 1946, 1: 365–97.

Sauze V. Stupidité Primitive. *Annales Médico-Psychologiques*, 1853, 5: 344–5.

Savage G.H. Dr. Hughlings Jackson on mental disorder. *The Journal of Mental Science*, 1917, 53: 315–28.

Savage G.H. *Insanity and Allied Neuroses: Practical and Clinical*, Second Edition, London, Cassell and Company, 1886.

Savage G.H. On imperative ideas. *Brain*, 1895, 18: 322–8.

Savill T.D. *Clinical Lectures on Neurasthenia*, London, Glaisher, 1906.

Schacter D.L., Eich J.E. and Tulving E. Richard Semon's Theory of Memory. *Journal of Verbal Learning and Verbal Behavior*, 1978, 17: 721–43.

Schachter S. and Singer J.E. Cognitive, social and physiological determinants of emotional state. *Psychological Review*, 1962, 69: 377–99.

Scharfetter C. *Allgemeine Psychopathologie*, Stuttgart, Georg Thième, 1976.

Scharfetter C. *General Psychopathology*, Cambridge, Cambridge University Press, 1980.

Schatzmann J. *Richard Semon (1859–1918) und seine Mnemetheorie*, Zürich, Juris Druck, 1968.

Scheerenberger R.C. *A History of Mental Retardation*. Brookes, Baltimore, 1983.

Schilder P. *Selbstbewusstsein und Persönlichkeitsbewusstsein*. Berlin, Springer Verlag, 1914.

Schilder P. Zur Kenntnis der Psychosen bei chronischer Encephalitis Epidemica nebst Bemerkung unter die Beziehung organischer Strukturen zur den psychischen Vorgangen. *Zeitschrift für Neurologie und Psychiatrie*, 1929, 118: 327–49.

Schilder P. *Studien zur Psychologie un Sumptomatologie der progressiven Paralyse*, Berlin, Karger, 1930.

Schilder P. Psychopathology of time. *Journal Nervous Mental Disease*, 1936, 83: 530–46.

Schiller F. The vicissitudes of the basal ganglia. *Bulletin of the History of Medicine*, 1967, 41: 515–38.

Schiller F. Concepts of Stroke before and after Virchow. *Medical History*, 1970, 14: 115–31.

Schiller F. The inveterate paradox of dreaming. *Archives of Neurology*, 1985, 42: 903–6.

Schiller F. Parkinson's rigidity: the first hundred-and-one years 1817–1918. *History and Philosophy of Life Sciences*, 1986, 8: 226–36.

Schmiedebach H.P. Zum Verständniswandel der 'psychopathischen' Störungen am Anfang der naturwissenschaftlichen Psychiatrie in Deutschland. *Nervenarzt* 1985. 56: 140–5.

Schmidt G. Der Wahn im deutschprachigen Schriftum der letzten 25 Jahre (1914–1939). *Zentralblatt für die gesamte Neurologie und Psychiatrie*, 1940, 97: 113–43.

Schmitt J.C. Le suicide au moyen âge. *Annales: Economies, Sociétés, Civilisations*, 1976, 31: 3–28.

Schneider C. Über Picksche Krankheit. *Monatschrift für Psychiatrie und Neurologie*, 1927, 65: 230–75.

Schneider C. Weitere Beiträge zur Lehre von der Pickschen Krankheit. *Zeitschrift für die gesamte Neurologie und Psychiatrie*, 1929, 120: 340–84.

Schneider K. Die Lehre von Zwangsdenken in den letzten zwölf Jahren. *Zeitschrift für die gesamte Neurologie und Psychiatrie*, 1918, 16: 113–251.

Schneider K. *Beiträge zur Psychiatrie*, Stuttgart, Enke, 1948.

Schneider K. *Die Psychopathischen Personlichkeiten*, 9th edn., Vienna, Deuticke, 1950.

Schneider K. *Clinical Psychopathology* (translated by M.W. Hamilton), New York, Grune and Stratton, 1959.

Schofield R.E. *Mechanism and Materialism. British Natural Philosophy in An Age of Reason*, Princeton, Princeton University Press, 1970.

Schopenhauer A. Die Welt als Wille und Vorstellung (Vol. 1), in *Sämtliche Werke*. Stuttgart/Frankfurt, Suhrkamp-Taschenbuch, 1950.

Schultze H.A.F. and Donalies Ch. 100 Jahre Psychiatrie und Neurologie in Rahmen der Berliner Gesellschaft für Psychiatrie und Neurologie und der Nervenklinik der Charité. *Wiss. Z. Humboldt-Univ. Berlin, Math.Nat R.*, 1968, 17: 5–14.

Schwab R.S., Fabing H.D. and Prichard J.S. Psychiatric symptoms and syndromes in Parkinson's disease. *American Journal of Psychiatry*, 1951, 107: 901–7.

Schwab S. and England A.C. Parkinson syndromes due to various specific causes. In Vinken P.J. and Bruyn G.W. (eds.) *Diseases of the Basal Ganglia, Vol. 6, Handbook of Clinical Neurology*, Amsterdam, North-Holland, pp. 227–47, 1968.

Schwalbe J. Dementia Senilis. In *Lehrbuch der Greisenkrankheiten*, Stuttgart, Enke, pp. 479–89, 1909.

Schwartz L. *Les Névroses et la Psychologie Dynamique de Pierre Janet*, Paris, Presses Universitaires de France, 1955.

Scull A.T. *Museums of Madness. The Social Organization of Insanity in Nineteenth Century England*. Allen Lane: London 1979.

Scull A.T. (ed.) *Madhouses, Mad-doctors and Madmen. The Social History of Psychiatry in the Victorian Era*. Athlone Press, London, 1981.

Seafield F. *The Literature and Curiosities of Dreams*. 2 Vols. London, Chapman and Hall (Vol. 1, pp. 326–48), 1865.

Searles P. Concerning a psychodynamic function of perplexity, confusion, suspicion and related phenomena. *Psychiatry*, 1952, 4: 351–63.

Sedgwick P. Michel Foucault. The anti-history of psychiatry. *Psychological Medicine* 1981, 11: 235–48.

Sedman G. 'Inner voices': phenomenological and clinical aspects. *British Journal of Psychiatry*, 1966a, 112: 485–90.

Sedman G. A comparative study of pseudohallucinations, imagery and true hallucinations. *British Journal of Psychiatry*, 1966b, 112, 9–17.

Sedman G. A phenomenological study of pseudohallucinations and related experiences. *Acta Psychiatrica Scandinavica*, 1966c, 42: 35–70.

Seeman M.V. Time and schizophrenia. *Psychiatry*, 1976, 39: 189–95.

Séglas, J. Note sur un cas de mélancolie anxieuse (délire des négations). *Archives de Neurologie* 1884, 22: 56–68.

Séglas, J. Mélancolie anxieuse avec délire des négations. *Progrés Medical*, 1887, 46: 417–19.

Séglas, J. Semeiólogie et pathogenie des idées de négation (Les alterations de la personalité dans les délires mélancoliques). *Annales Médico-Psychologiques* 1889, 47: 5–26.

Séglas J. Des troubles de la fonction du langage dans l'onomatomanie. *Medicine Moderne*, 1891, 2: 845–7.

Séglas J. *Les Troubles du Langage chez les Aliénés*, Paris, Rueff, 1892.

Séglas J. De la confusion mentale primitive. *Archives Générales de Médécine*, 1894, 1: 538–49; 665–84.

Séglas J. *Leçons Cliniques sur les Maladies Mentales et Nerveuses (Salpêtrière 1887–1894)*. Paris, Asselin et Houzeau, 1895.

Séglas, J. *Le Délires des Négations* Paris: Masson, 1897.

Séglas J. Séméiologie des affections mentales. In Ballet G. (ed.) *Traité de Pathologie Mentale*, Paris, Doin, pp. 74–270, 1903.

Séglas J. Hallucinations psychiques et pseudo-hallucinations verbales. *Journal de Psychologie Normale et Pathologique*, 1914, 11: 289–315.

Séglas J. and Chaslin Ph. Katatonia. *Brain*, 1890, 12: 191–322.

Séguin É. *Traitement Moral, hygiène et éducation des idiots et des autres enfants arriérés*. Paris, Baillière, 1846.

Séguin E. *Idiocy and its Treatment by the Physiological Method*. New York, Wood and Company, 1866.

Selby G. Parkinson's disease. In Vinken P.J. and Bruyn E.W. (eds.) *Handbook of Clinical Neurology*, Vol. 6, Amsterdam, North Holland, pp. 173–211, 1968.

Seligman M: Depression and learned helplessness, in Friedman R, Katz M (eds.) *The Psychology of Depression: Contemporary Theory of Research*. Silver Spring Md, Winston and Sons, 1974.

Selvin H.C. Durkheim's suicide and problems of empirical research. *American Journal of Sociology*, 1958, 63: 607–19.

Semelaigne R. *Les Pionniers de la Psychiatrie Française (Après Pinel)* Vol. 2, Paris, Baillière, 1932.

Sérieux P. Review of Dreyfus's Book. *L'Encéphale*, 1907, 2: 456–8.

Sérieux P.and Capgras J. *Les Folies Raisonnantes, Le Délire d'Interprétation*, Paris, Alcan, 1909.

Serin S. Une enquête médico-sociale sur le suicide á Paris. *Annales Médico-Psychologiques*, 1926, 84: 356–63.

Shallice T. *From Neuropsychology to Mental Structure*. Cambridge, Cambridge University Press, 1988.

Shapiro E.R. The psychodynamics and developmental psychology of the borderline patient: a review of the literature. *American Journal of Psychiatry*, 1978, 135: 1305–15.

Shaw J. Obsessions. *Journal of Mental Science*, 1904, 50: 234–49.

Shaw K.M., Lees A.J. and Stern G.M. The impact of treatment with levodopa on Parkinson's disease. *Quarterly Journal of Medicine*, 1980, 49: 283–93.

Shaw T.C. Dementia. In Tuke D.H. (ed.) *A Dictionary of Psychological Medicine*, Vol. 1, London, Churchill, pp. 348–351, 1892.

Shaw T.C. The clinical value of consciousness in disease. *Journal of Mental Science*, 1909, 55: 401–10.

Sheldon W.H. *The Varieties of Temperament*, New York, Harper, 1942.

Shrout P.E., Spitzer R.L. and Fleiss J.L. Quantification of agreement in psychiatric diagnosis revisited. *Archives of General Psychiatry*, 1987, 44: 172–7.

Shryock R.H. The history of quantification in medical science. *Isis*, 1961, 52: 215–37.

Sicard J.A. Akathisie et Tasikinesie. *Presse Médicale* 1923, 31: 265–266.

Sicherman B. The uses of diagnosis: doctors, patients and neurasthenia. *Journal of History of Medicine and Allied Sciences*, 1977, 32: 33–54.

Sidgwick H. The census of hallucinations. *Proceedings of the Society for Psychical Research*, 1889–90, 4: 7–25; 429–35; 1891–2, 7: 429–35.

Sidgwick H. Report on the census of hallucinations. *Proceedings of the Society for Psychical Research*, 1894, 10: 25–252.

Siegel R.E. *Galen on Psychology, Psychopathology and Function and Diseases of the Nervous System*, Basel, Karger, 1973.

Siegel R.K. and West L.J. (eds.) *Hallucinations*, New York, John Wiley, 1975.

Sifneos P.E. Anhedonia and alexithymia: a potential correlation? In Clark D.C., Fawcett J. (eds.): *Anhedonia and Affect Deficit States*. PMA Publishing Corp, New York, 1987.

Sifneos P.E. Clinical observations on some patients suffering from a variety of psychosomatic disorders, in *Proceedings of the Seventh European Conference on Psychosomatic Research*. Basel, Karger, 1967.

Sigmond G. On hallucinations. *Journal of Psychological Medicine and Mental Pathology*, 1848, 1: 585–608.

Simchowicz T. Histologische Studien über die Senile Demenz. *Histologische und histopathologischen Arbeiten über der Grosshirnrinde*, 1911, 4: 267–444.

Simchowicz T. Sur la signification des plaques séniles et sur la formule sénile de l'ècorce cérébrale. *Revue Neurologique*, 1924, 31: 221–7.

Simmonnet J. Folie et notations psychopathologiques dans l'oeuvre de Saint Thomas d'Aquin. In Postel J. and Quétel C. (eds.) *Nouvelle Histoire de la Psychiatrie*, Paris, Privat, pp. 55–73, 1983.

Simon B.B. Models of mind and mental illness in ancient Greece: the Platonic model. *Journal of the History of Behavioral Science*, 1972–3, 8: 389–404; 9: 3–17.

Simon B.B. *Mind and Madness in Ancient Greece. The Classical Roots of Modern Psychiatry*. Cornell University Press, Ithaca, 1978.

Simon J. *Das Problem der Sprache bei Hegel*. Stuttgart, Kholhammer, 1966.

Simondon M. *La Mémoire et L'Oubli dans la Pensée Grecque jusqu'á la fin du Ve Siècle Avant J-C.* Paris, Société D'èdition 'Les Belles Lettres', 1982.

Sims A. *Symptoms in the Mind*, London, Baillière Tindall, 1988.

Sinclair Sir J. *The Code of Health and Longevity*, Edinburgh, Constable, 1807.

Siomopoulos V. *The Structure of Psychopathological Experience*, New York, Brunner/Mazel, 1983.

Sjövall B. *Psychology of Tension. An analysis of Pierre Janet's concept of 'tension psychologique' together with an historical aspect* Stockholm, (no publisher), 1967.

Skoog G. The anancastic syndrome and its relation to personality attitude. *Acta Psychiatrica Scandinavica*, 1959, 34: (Suppl. 134) 5–207.

Slade P.D. and Bentall R.P. *Sensory Deception. A Scientific Analysis of Hallucinations*, London, Croom Helm, 1988.

Slaughter M.M. *Universal Languages and Scientific Taxonomy in the Seventeenth Century.* Cambridge, Cambridge University Press, 1982.

Smith C.U.M. David Hartley's Newtonian neuropsychology. *Journal of the History of the Behavioral Sciences,* 1987, 23: 123–36.

Smith P. *Realism and the Progress of Science,* Cambridge, Cambridge University Press, 1981.

Smith R. Mental disorder, criminal responsibility, and the social history of theories of volition. *Psychological Medicine,* 1979, 9: 13–19.

Smith R. *Trial by Medicine.* Edinburgh, Edinburgh University Press, 1981.

Smith R. *Inhibition. History and Meaning in the Sciences of Mind and Brain.* London, Free Associations Book, 1992.

Smith W. (ed.) *Dictionary of Greek and Roman Biography and Mythology.* Vol. III, London, James Walton, 1869.

Snaith P. Anhedonia: a neglected symptom of psychopathology. *Psychological Medicine,* 23: 957–66, 1993.

Snider S.R., Rahn S., Isgreen W.R. and Cote, L.J. Primary sensory symptoms in Parkinsonism. *Neurology,* 1976, 26: 423–9.

Sno H. and Draaisma D. An early Dutch study of déjà vu experiences. *Psychological Medicine,* 1993, 23: 17–26.

Sno H. and Lindszen D.H. The déjà vu experience. *American Journal of Psychiatry,* 1990, 147: 1587–95.

Sno H., Lindszen D.H. and Jonghe F de. Art imitates life: déjà vu experiences in prose and poetry. *British Journal of Psychiatry,* 1992, 160: 511–18.

Sobrino. *Aumentado o Nuevo Diccionario de las Lenguas Española, Francesa y Latina,* Leon de Francia, J.B. Delamolliere, 1791.

Société Médico-Psychologique, Debate. *Annales Médico-Psychologiques* 1869, 27: 454.

Société Médico-Psychologique, Debate on monomanie. *Annales Médico-Psychologiques,* 1854, 6: 99–118; 273–98; 464–74; 629–44.

Société Médico-Psychologique, reports of sessions between 26th February 1855 and 28th April 1856. *Annales Médico-Psychologiques,* 1855, i: 526–50; ii: 126–40; 1856, i: 281–305; ii: 385–446.

Société Médico-Psychologique. *Annales Médico-Psychologiques,* 1923, 9: p. 288.

Société Médico-Psychologique. Debate on reasoning insanity. *Annales Médico-Psychologiques,* 1866, 24: 382–431.

Société Médico-Psychologique. Debate on stupor. *Annales Médico-Psychologiques.* Séances, 22 February, 29 March, 26 April, pp. 454, 56, 61, 1869.

Société Médico-Psychologique. L'automatism psychologique de Pierre Janet 100 ans après, *Annales Médico-Psychologiques.* Paris, Masson, 1989.

Société Médico-Psychologique. *Annales Médico-Psychologiques* 1875, 33: 434–5, 439–42; 1876, 34: 73–126, 241–59.

Sokal M.M. J.McK Cattell and the failure of anthropometric mental testing 1890–1901. In Woodward W.R. and Ash M.G. (eds.) *The Problematic Science: Psychology in Nineteenth Century Thought.* New York, Praeger, pp. 322–45, 1982.

Sokal M.M., Davis A.B. and Merzbach U.C. Laboratory instruments in the history of psychology. *Journal of the History of the Behavioral Sciences,* 1976, 12: 59–64.

Sollier P. *Psychologie del'idiot et de l'imbécile.* Paris, Alcan, 1891.

Sollier P. Sur une forme circulaire de la neurasthénie. *Revue de Médecine,* 1893, 13: 1009–19.

Solmsen F. Plato and the concept of the soul (Psyche): some historical perspectives. *Journal of the History of Ideas,* 1983, 44: 355–64.

Sommer. (no initial) *Lehrbuch der psychopathologischen Untersuchungs-Methoden,* Stuttgart, Thieme, 1899.

Sorabji R. *Aristotle on Memory,* London, Duckworth, 1972.

Sorell T. *Hobbes*. London, Routledge and Kegan Paul, 1986.

Soukhanoff S. La cyclothymie et la psychasthénie. *Annales Médico-Psychologiques*, 1909, 67: 27–38.

Soukhanoff S. and Gannouchkine P. Ètude sur la mélancolie. *Annales Médico-Psychologiques*, 1903, 61: 213–38.

Souques (no initial) Formes cliniques des syndromes Parkinsoniens. *Revue Neurologique*, 1921, 28: 562–87.

Souques (no initial). Angoisse sans Anxiété. *Revue Neurologique*, 1902, 2: 1176.

Soury J. Des doctrines psychologiques contemporaines. *L'Encéphale*, 1883, 3: 61–85.

Soury J. *Les Fonctions du Cerveau*, Paris, Lecrosnier et Labé, 1891.

Soury J. Sulla Paramnesia o False Memoria. Nota del prof Tito Vignoli. *Revue Philosophique*, 1894, 38: 50–1.

Southard E.E. Anatomical findings in 'senile dementia': a diagnostic study bearing especially on the group of cerebral atrophies. *American Journal of Insanity*, 1910, 61: 673–708.

Soutzo (no initial). Encore la question de la démence précoce. *Annales Médico-Psychologiques*, 1907, 65 (Part I): 242–64; 374–388; Part II: 28–47.

Spielmeyer W. *Die Psychosen des Rückbildungs und Greisenalters*, Leipzig, Deuticke, 1912.

Spitzer M. Karl Jaspers, mental states, and delusional beliefs: a redefinition and its implications. In Spitzer M, Uehlein F.A. and Oepen G. (eds.) *Psychopathology and Philosophy*, Berlin, Springer, pp. 128–142, 1988.

Spitzer M. *Was is Wahn?* Heidelberg, Springer, 1989.

Spitzer M. Pseudohalluzinationen. *Forschritte Neurologie und Psychiatrie* 1987, 55: 91–97.

Spoerl H.D. Faculties versus traits. Gall's solution. *Character and Personality*, 1936, 4: 360–3.

Spurzheim G. *Phrenology in Connection with the Study of Physiognomy. Part 1: Characters*. London, Treuttel, Wurtz, and Richter, 1826.

Staehelin J.T. Zur Geschichte der Lehre von den Temperamenten. *Schweizer medizinischen Wochenschrift*, 1941, 22: 1401–2.

Staël, Mme la Baronne de. *De L'Influence des Passions sur le Bonheur des Individues et des Nations*, new edn., Paris, Treuttel et Würtz, 1820.

Staël, Mme la Baronne de. *Réflexions sur le Suicide* New Edition, Paris, Treuttel et Würtz, 1820.

Starobinski J. Historia del Tratamiento de la Melancholia desde los Orígenes hasta 1900. *Acta Psychosomatica* (Basle), 1962, No. 3.

Starobinski J. The word 'reaction': from physics to psychiatry. *Psychological Medicine*, 1977, 7: 373–86.

Staum M. *Cabanis*, Princeton, Princeton University Press, 1980.

Steck H. Les syndromes extrapyramidaux dans les maladies mentales. *Schweizer. Archiv für Neurologie*, 1926, 19: 195–233; 20: 92–136.

Steck H. Les syndromes mentaux post-encephaliques. *Schweizer Archiv für Neurologie*, 1931, 27: 137–73.

Steen R.H. Hallucinations in the sane. *Journal of Mental Science*, 1917, 63: 328–46.

Stengel E. Studies on the psychopathology of compulsive wandering. *British Journal of Medical Psychology*, 1938, 18: 250–4.

Stengel E. On the aetiology of the fugue states. *Journal of Mental Science*, 1941, 87: 572–99.

Stengel E. Hughlings Jackson's influence in psychiatry. *British Journal of Psychiatry*, 1963, 109: 348–55.

Stengel E. Speech disorders and mental disorders. In de Reuck A.V.S. and O'Connor M. (eds.) *Ciba Foundation Symposium on Disorders of Language*, London, Churchill, pp. 285–292, 1964.

Sternberg R.J. and Smith E.E. (eds.) *The Psychology of Human Thought*, Cambridge, Cambridge University Press, 1988.

Sternberg R.J. *Metaphors of Mind. Conceptions of the Nature of Intelligence*. Cambridge, Cambridge University Press, 1990.

Stewart A. *Our Temperaments: Their Study and their Teaching*, London, Crosby Lockwood, 1887.

Stewart D. *Elements of the Philosophy of the Human Mind* (6th ed) (2 vols). London, printed for T. Cadell and W. Davies, 1818.

Stinchfield S.M. *Speech Disorders*. New York, Kegan Paul, 1933.

Stobbia G.F, Sacco P., Campagna S. and Cavicchi L. Nostra esperienza sull'incidenza degli effetti pseudo-allucinatori dell' anestesia dissociative con l'uso di trazodone. *Acta Anaesthesiologica Italiana*, 1980, 31: 401–6.

Stocking G.W. From chronology to ethnology. In Prichard J.C. *Researches into the Physical History of Man*, Chicago, The University of Chicago Press, pp. ix–cx, 1973.

Störring G.E. *Mental Pathology in its Relation to Normal Psychology*, London, Swan Sonnenschein and Co, 1907.

Störring G.E. *Wessen und Bedeutung des Symptoms der Ratlosigkeit by psychischen Erkrankungen*, Leipzig, Barth, 1939.

Stove D.C. *Popper and After: Four Modern Irrationalists*, Oxford, Pergamon Press, 1982.

Strahan S.A.K. *Suicide and Insanity* (a Physiological, Sociological Study) London, Swan Sonnenschein and Co, 1893.

Stransky E. Zur Auffassung gewisser Symptome der Dementia praecox. *Neurologisches Centralblatt*, 1904, 23: 1137–43.

Strauss E.W. Aesthesiology and hallucinations. In May R., Angel E. and Ellenberger H.F. *Existence*, New York, Basic Books, pp. 139–169, 1958.

Strauss E.W. and Griffith R.M. Pseudoreversibility of catatonic stupor. *American Journal of Psychiatry*, 1955, 111: 680–5.

Strauss J. and Goethals G.R. *The Self: Interdisciplinary Approaches*, Berlin, Springer, 1991.

Stutte H. Thersites-komplex. *A Criança Portuguesa*. 1962–1963, 21: 451–6.

Sully J. *The Human Mind. A Textbook of Psychology* Vol. 2, London, Longmans, Green and Co, 1892.

Sully J. *Illusions. A Psychological Study*, Fourth Edition, London, Kegan Paul, Trench, Trübner and Co, 1894 (first edition, 1881).

Sülz K.D. and Gigerenzer G. Über die Beeinflussung psychiatrischer Diagnoseschemata durch implizite nosologische Theorien. *Archiv für Psychiatrie und Nervenkrankheiten* 1982, 232: 5–14.

Suppe F. (ed.). *The Structure of Scientific Theories*. Urbana, University of Illinois Press, 1977.

Sutter J.M. L'apport de la neurologie a la psychopathologie des hallucinations. *L'Evolution Psychiatrique*, 1962, 27: 501–35.

Sutton T. *Tracts on Delirium Tremens, on Peritonitis and on the Gout*, London, Thomas Underwood, pp. 1–77, 1813.

Swain G. The wild boy of Aveyron de H. Lane. *L'Evolution Psychiatrique*, 1976, 41: 995–1011.

Swain G. *Le Sujet de la Folie: Naissance de la Psychiatrie*. Privat, Paris, 1977.

Swain G. L'aliéné entre le médecin et le philosophe. *Perspectives Psychiatriques*, 1978, N° 65, pp. 90–99.

Sydenham T. *Methodus Curandi Febres* London, Crook, 1666.

Taine H. *De l'Intelligence*, 2 Vols, Paris, Hachette, 1890.

Taine H. *Les Philosophes Classiques du XIXe Siècle in France*, Eighth Edition, Paris, Hachette, 1901.

Talbot E.S. *Degeneracy, its Causes, Signs and Results*. London, Walter Scott, Ltd, 1898.

Tamburini A. *Sulla genesi delle allucinazioni* Reggio-Nell'Emilia, Stephano Calderini, 1880*a*.

Tamburini A. Sulla genesi delle allucinazioni. *Rivista Sperimentale di Freniatria e di Medicina Legale*, 1880*b*, 6: 126–56.

Tamburini A. Le Théorie des Hallucinations. *Revue Scientifique Française et Etranger*, Third Series, 1881, 27: 138–42 (translation in *History of Psychiatry*, 1990, 1: 145–56).

Tamburini A. Sulle Allucinazioni Motorie. *VI Congresso Frenatinico Italiano in Novara*, Reggio-Emilia, Calderini, 1889.

Tamburini A. Sulla Patogenesi delle Allucinazioni Viscerali, *10 Congresso della Societa Freniatrica Italiana in Napoli*, Reggio-Emilia, Calderini, 1901.

Tanzi E. *A Textbook of Mental Diseases*. Translated by W.F. Robertson and T.C. MacKenzie, London, Rebman Limited, 1909.

Targowla R. and Dublineau J. *L'Intuition Délirante*, Paris, Maloine, 1931.

Taty T. and Toy J. Des variétés cliniques du délire de persecution. *Annales Médico-Psychologiques*, 1887, 5: 20–37; 193–218; 370–94.

Tawney G.A. Review of Bradley's mind paper. *Psychological Review*, 1903,10: 438–43.

Taylor D.C. and Marsh S.M. Hughling Jackson's Dr Z: the paradigm of temporal lobe epilepsy revealed. *Journal of Neurology, Neurosurgery and Psychiatry*, 1980, 43: 758–67.

Taylor F.K. On pseudo-hallucinations. *Psychological Medicine*, 1981, 11: 265–71.

Taylor J. *Ductor Dubitantium, or the Rule of Conscience*, 2 Vols, London, Royston, 1660.

Taylor Kräupl F. *Psychopathology: its Causes and Symptoms*. London, Butterworth, 1966.

Temkin O. The classical roots of Glisson's doctrine of irritation. *Bulletin of History of Medicine*, 1964, 38: 297–328.

Thalbitzer S. *Emotions and Insanity*. London, Kegan Paul, Trench, Trubner and Co, 1926.

Theophrastus. *Characters* (translated by J.E. Edmonds and A.D. Knox), Loeb Classical Edition, London, Heinemann, 1967.

Thièbierge G. Les acárophobes. *Revue Générale de Clinique et de Thérapeutique*, 1894, 32: 373.

Thomas André. *Psicoterapia*, Barcelona, Salvat, 1913.

Thomas C. Dysmorphophobia: a question of definition. *British Journal of Psychiatry*, 1984, 144: 513–16.

Thompsen (no initial). Klinische Beiträge zur Lehre von den Zwangsvorstellungen und verwandten psychischen Zuständen. *Archiv für Psychiatrie und Nervenkrankheiten*, 1895, 27: 319–85.

Tiberghien G. *La Science de l'Ame dans les Limites de l'Observation*. Bruxelles, Librairie Polytechnique de Decq, 1868.

Tiles M. *Bachelard: Science and Objectivity*, Cambridge, Cambridge University Press, 1984.

Tissot, F. Délire des négations terminé par guerison. Considerations sur l'hypocondrie et la mélancolie. *Annales Médico-Psychologiques*, 1921, 79: 321–8.

Tissot, M. Les Passions. Influence du moral sur le physique. *Annales Médico-Psychologiques*, 1865, 6: 157–71.

Titchener E.B. Common Sensation. In Baldwin J.W. (ed.) *Dictionary of Philosophy and Psychology*, Vol. 1, London, McMillan, 1901.

Tizard B. Theories of brain localization from Fluorens to Lashley. *Medical History*, 1959, 3: 132–45.

Todd J. and Ashworth A.L. The West Riding Asylum and James Crichton-Browne, 1818–76. In Berrios G.E. and Freeman H. (eds.) *150 Years of British Psychiatry*, 1841–1991, London, Gaskell, pp. 389–418, 1991.

Tolman E.C. A behaviorist's definition of consciousness. *Psychological Review*, 1927, 34: 433–40.

Tomlinson B.E. and Corsellis J.A.N. Ageing and the dementias. In Adams J.H. *et al.* (eds.) *Greenfield's Neuropathology*, London, Arnold, pp. 951–1025, 1984.

Torack R.M. The early history of senile dementia. In Reisberg B. (ed.) *Alzheimer's Disease*, New York, the Free Press, pp. 23–28, 1983.

Toulmin S. *The Philosophy of Science*, London, Hutchinson, 1953.

Toulouse E. Les hallucinations unilatérales. *Gazette des Hopitaux*, 1892, 65: 609–18.

Toulouse E. and Mignard M. Comment caractériser et définir la démence. *Annales Médico-Psychologiques*, 1914, 72: 443–61; 73: 80–8.

Toulouse, E. Note sur un cas de délire des négations. *Annales Médico-Psychologiques* 1893, 51: 259–70.

Toulouse, Juquelier and Mignard (no initials). Confusion, démence et autoconduction. *Annales Médico-Psychologiques*, 1920, 10th Series, 12: 335–49.

Tulving E. *Elements of Episodic Memory*, Oxford, Clarendon Press, 1983.

Tracy T.J. *Physiological Theory and the doctrine of the Mean in Plato and Aristotle*. The Hague, Mouton, 1969.

Tracy, Destutt Comte de. *Elemens d'Ideologie*, Second Edition, Paris, Courcier, 1817 (First Edition 1801).

Traub R., Gajdusek D.C. and Gibbs C.J. Transmissible virus dementia: the relation of transmissible spongiform encephalopathy to Creutzfeldt-Jakob disease. In Kinsbourne M. and Smith L. (eds.) *Aging and Dementia*, New York, Spectrum Publications, pp. 91–172, 1977.

Treadway W.L. The presenile psychoses. *Journal of Nervous and Mental Disease*, 1913, 40: 375–87.

Trélat U. *La Folie Lucide*, Paris, Delahaye, 1861.

Trémine, T. 1880–1980: Centenaire du syndrome de Cotard. *L'Evolution Psychiatrique* 1982, 47:1021–32.

Trénel, M. Notes sur les idées de négation. *Archives de Neurologie*, 1898, 6: 23–9.

Tretiakoff C. *Contribution a l'étude de l'Anatomie Pathologique du Locus Niger*, Paris, Thèse de Paris, 1919.

Trillat É. In Charcot J.M. *L'Hystérie*, Paris, Privat, 1971.

Trillat É. *Histoire de l'Hystérie*, Paris, Seghers, 1986.

Trillat È. Le Platonisme dans les théories des hallucinations au XIXe siècle. *L'Èvolution Psychiatrique*, 1991, 56: 583–93.

Truelle V. and Bessière R. Recherches sur la Presbyophrénie. *L'Encéphale*, 1911, 6: 505–20.

Tuczek (no initial). Über Zwangsvorstellungen. *Berliner klinische Wochenschrift*, 1899, 36: 117–19; 148–59; 171–4; 195–7; 212–14.

Tuke D.H. *A Dictionary of Psychological Medicine* 2 Vols, London, J. and A Churchill, 1892.

Tuke D.H. Imperative ideas. *Brain*, 1894, 17: 179–97.

Turner J. A theory concerning the physical conditions of the nervous system which are necessary for the production of states of melancholia, mania, etc. *Journal of Mental Science*, 1900, 46: 505–12.

Tyler K.L. and Tyler H.R. The secret life of James Parkinson. *Neurology*, 1986, 36: 222–4.

Ullersperger J.B. *La Historia de la Psicología y de la Psiquiatría en España, Madrid*, Alhambra, 1954 (1st German edn., 1871).

Underwood E.A. The history of the quantitative approach in medicine. *British Medical Bulletin*, 1951, 7: 265–74.

Upham T. *Abridgment of Mental Philosophy*, New York, Harper, 1886.

Urmson J.O. *The Greek Philosophical Vocabulary*. London, Duckworth, 1990.

Vademecum of the London Hospitals: *The Edinburgh Practice of Physic, Surgery, and Midwifery*. Vol. 2, London, Kearsley, p. 451, 1803.

Vaillant G.E. and Schnurr P. What is a case? *Archives of General Psychiatry*, 1989, 45: 313–19.

Valery P. *L'Idée Fixe*. Paris, Gallimard, 1933.

Valla J.-P. *Les Ètats Ètranges de la Conscience*, Paris, Presses Universitaires de France, 1992.

Vallat J.N., Leger J.M., Destruhaut J. and Garoux R. Dysmorphophobie: syndrome or symptome. *Annales Médico-Psychologiques*, 1971, 2: 45–66.

Van Bogaert L. L'hallucinose pédonculaire. *Revue Neurologique*, 1927, 1: 608–17.

Vanini M. and Weiss G. Contributo clinico allo studio dei disturbi della corporeità psicotica. *Rivista Sperimentale di Freniatria e Medicine Legale della Alienzioni Mentali*, 1972, 96: 32–55.

Various. Discussion on suicide and its psychiatric aspects. *Journal of Mental Science*, 1898, 45: 202–3.

Vaschide N. and Piéron H. *La Psychologie du Rêve*. Paris, Baillière, 1902.

Vaschide N. and Vurpas Cl. *Psychologie du Délire dans les Troubles Psychopathiques*, Paris, Masson, 1903.

Veith I. *Hysteria. The History of a Disease*, Chicago, University of Chicago Press, 1965.

Verger H. and Cruchet R. *Les États Parkinsoniens et le Syndrome Bradykinétique*, Paris, Baillière, 1925.

Viallon A. Suicide et Folie. *Annales Médico-Psychologiques*, 1901–2, 59: 19–28; 210–34; 60: 21–35; 219–29; 379–92; 235–54; 392–403.

Videbech Th. The psychopathology of anancastic endogenous depression. *Acta Psychiatrica Scandinavica*, 1975, 52: 336–73.

Vigoroux R., Naquet chimique de comas graves prolongés post-traumatiques. *Revue Neurologique*, 1964, 110: 72–81.

Villa G. *Contemporary Psychology* (translated by H. Manacorda). London, Sonnenschein, 1903.

Viney L. Self: the history of a concept. *Journal of the History of the Behavioral Sciences*, 1969, 5: 349–59.

Virey. Mémoire. In *Dictionnaire des Sciences Médicales*, Vol. 32, Paris, Panckouke, 1819.

Vitello, A. Melancolia di Cotard con paranoidismo schizoide. *Rassegna Studi Psichiatrici*, 1970, 59: 195–210.

Vizioli R. and Bietti C. *Il Problema della conscienza in Neuropsichiatria*, Pisa, Omnia Medica, 1966.

Vliegen J. *Die Einheitspsychose. Geschichte und Problem*. Stuttgart, Enke, 1980.

Voisin A.F. Idées sur le Suicide. *Progres Médical*, 1882, 10: 614.

Voisin F. *De l'Idiotie chez les Enfants*. Paris, Baillière, 1843.

Voisin J. Automatisme ambulatoire chez une hystérique. *Annales Médico-Psychologiques*, 1889, 46: 418.

Vulpian A. *Maladies du Système Nerveux* (moëlle épinière). Vol. 2, Paris, Doin, 1886.

Vurpas, C. Trois observations de délire des négations. Disparition aprés douze ans. *L'Encéphale*, 1912, 7: 76–8.

Vygotsky L.S. *Thought and Language*. Cambridge, Mass, MIT Press, 1962.

Wagner L. *Unterricht und Ermüdung*, Berlin, Reuther und Reichard, 1898.

Wahrig-Schmidt B. *Der junge Wilhelm Griesinger im Spannusgsfeld zwischen Philosophie und Physiologie*, Tübingen, Gunter Narr, 1985.

Walitzky M. Contribution a l'ètude des mensurations psychométrics chez les aliènes. *Revue Philosophique*, 1889, 28: 95–7.

Walk A. Mental hospitals. In Pointer F.N.L. (ed.) *The Evolution of Hospitals in Britain*, London, Pitman Medical, London, pp. 123–46, 1964.

Walk A. The pre-history of child psychiatry. *British Journal of Psychiatry*, 1964, 110: 754–67.

Walker C. Delusion: what Jaspers really said? *British Journal of Psychiatry*, 1991 (Suppl 14) 159: 94–103.

Walker C. Philosophical concepts and practice: the legacy of Karl Jaspers' psychopathology. *Current Opinion in Psychiatry*, 1988, 1: 624–9.

Walker N. *Crime and Insanity in England. Vol. 1: Historical Perspective*. Edinburgh, Edinburgh University Press, 1968.

Wallace, E.R. IV and Pressley L.C. *Essays on the History of Psychiatry*. Hall Psychiatric Institute, South Carolina, 1980.

Walser H.H. Über Theorieen des Gedächtnisses in den letzen Dezennien des 19. Jahrhunderts und ihre Bedeutung für die Entstehung der Psychoanalyse. In *Proceedings of the XXIII International Congress of the History of Medicine*, Vol. 2, London, Wellcome Institute of the History of Medicine, pp. 1227–32, 1974.

Walshe F.M.R. The brain stem conceived as the 'highest level' of function in the nervous system; with particular reference to the 'automatic apparatus' of Carpenter (1850) and to the 'centrencephalic integrating system' of Penfield. *Brain*, 1957, 80: 510–39.

Walshe M. O'C. *A Concise German Etymological Dictionary*, London, Routledge and Kegan Paul, 1951.

Walton G.L. Arteriosclerosis probably not an important factor in the etiology and prognosis of involution psychoses. *Boston Medical and Surgical Journal*, 1912, 167: 834–6.

Warburton J.W. Depressive symptoms in Parkinsonism patients referred for thalamotomy. *Journal of Neurology, Neurosurgery and Psychiatry*, 1967, 30: 368–70.

Ward J. Psychology. In *Encyclopaedia Britannica*, Ninth Edition, pp. 37–85, 1889.

Warda W. Zur Geschichte und Kritik der sogenannten psychischen Zwangszustände. *Archiv für Psychiatrie und Nervenkrankheiten*, 1905, 39: 239–85; 533–85.

Warnes H. Toxic Psychosis due to Antiparkinsonian drugs. *Canadian Psychiatric Association Journal*, 1967, 12: 323–6.

Warren H.C. *History of the Association Psychology*, New York, Scribners, 1921.

Warren N. Is a scientific revolution taking place in psychology? *Scientific Studies*, 1971, 1: 407–13.

Wartofsky M.W. (ed.) *Models, Representations and the Scientific Understanding*, Reidel, Dordrecht, 1979.

Washburn M.F. The term 'feeling'. *Journal of Philosophy, Psychology and Scientific Method*, 1906, 3: 62–3.

Waterman G. The treatment of fatigue states. *Journal of Abnormal Psychology*, 1909, 4: 128–39.

Watson C.G., Klett W.G. and Lorei T.W. Toward an operational definition of anhedonia. *Psychological Reports*, 1970, 26: 371–6.

Watson R I. *The Great Psychologists*. New York, Lippincott, 1978.

Weber E.H. Der Tastsinn und das Gemeingefühl In Wagner R. (ed.) *Handwörterbuch der Physiologie*, Vol. III, 1846.

Weckowicz T.E. Depersonalization. In Costello, C.G. (ed.) *Symptoms of Psychopathology. A Handbook*. New York Wiley, pp. 151–66, 1970.

Weckowicz T.E. and Liebel-Weckowicz H. Typologies of the theory of behaviourism since Descartes. *Sudhoffs Archive*, 1982, 66: 129–51.

Wedenski J.N. Des hallucinations olfactives comme signes précurseurs de l'accès dipsomaniaque. *Revue Neurologique*, 1912, 24: 416–617.

Weill E. *Des Vertiges*, Paris, Baillière, 1886.

Weindling P. *Health, Race and German Politics between National Unification and Nazism 1870–1945*, Cambridge, Cambridge University Press, 1989.

Weiner D.B. Philippe Pinel's 'memoire on madness' of December 11, 1794: a fundamental text of modern psychiatry. *American Journal of Psychiatry*, 1992, 149: 725–32.

Weiner D.B. *The Citizen-Patient in Revolutionary and Imperial Paris*. Baltimore, The Johns Hopkins University Press, 1993.

Weiskrantz L. (ed.) Emotion. In *Analysis of Behavioural Change*, New York, Harper and Row, pp. 50–90, 1968.

Weisner W.M. and Riffel Rev. P.A. Scrupulosity: religion and obsessive compulsive behavior in children. *American Journal of Psychiatry*, 1961, 117: 314–18.

Weitbrecht H.J. *Psychiatrie im Grundriss*, Berlin, Springer, 1968.

Welby F.A. and Sully J. *Illusions. A Psychological Study*, Fourth Edition, London, Kegan Paul, Trench, Trübner and Co, 1895 (First Edition, 1881).

Wells F. A neglected measure of fatigue. *American Journal of Psychology*, 1908, 19: 345–58.

Wender P.H. Dementia praecox: the development of a concept. *American Journal of Psychiatry*, 1963, 119: 1143–51.

Werlinder H. Psychopathy. *A History of the Concepts. Analysis of the Origin and Development of a Family of Concepts in Psychopathology*. Acta Universitatis Upsaliensis, Uppsala, 1978.

Wernicke C. *Der aphasische Symptomencomplex*, Breslau, Cohn and Weigert, 1874.

Wernicke C. *Grundriβ der Psychiatrie in klinischen Vorlesungen*, Leipzig, Thième, 1906.

Wertsch J.V. *Vygotsky and the Social Formation of the Mind*. Cambridge, Mass, Harvard University Press, 1985.

West D.J. and Walk A. (eds.) *Daniel McNaughton. His Trial and Aftermath*, London, Gaskell, 1977.

West L.J. (ed.) *Hallucinations*, New York, Grune and Stratton, 1962.

Westcott W.W. *Suicide. Its History, Literature, Jurisprudence, Causation, and Prevention*, London, H.K. Lewis, 1885.

Westphal C. Nekrolog für Griesinger *Archiv für Psychiatrie und Nervenkrankheiten*, 1868, 1: 760–74.

Westphal C. Die Agoraphobie. Eine neuropathische Erscheinung. *Archiv für Psychiatrie und Nervenkrankheiten*, 1872, 3: 138–61.

Westphal C. Nachtrag zu dem Aufsatze. 'Über Agoraphobie'. *Archiv für Psychiatrie und Nervenkrankheiten*, 1872, 3: 219–21.

Westphal C. Über Zwangsvorstellungen *Archiv für Psychiatrie und Nervenkrankheiten*, 1877, 8: 734–50.

Wettley A. Zur Problemgeschichte der 'Dégénérescence'. *Sudhoffs Archiv*, 1959, 43: 93–212.

Wetzel A. Das Weltuntergangserlebnis in der Schizophrenie. *Zentralblatt für die gesamte Neurologie und Psychiatrie*, 1922, 78: 403.

Weygandt W. Alte Dementia praecox. *Neurologisches Centralblatt*, 1904, 23: 613–17.

Weygandt W. Kritische Bemerkungen zur Psychologie der Dementia praecox. *Monatsschrift für Psychiatrie und Neurologie*, 1907, 22: 289–301.

Wheeler L.R. *Vitalism: Its History and Validity*, London, Witherby, 1939.

Whewell W. *History of the Inductive Sciences*, London, John W Parker, 1857.

White A.R. *The Philosophy of Mind*, New York, Random House, pp. 83–115, 1967.

White A.R. (ed.) *The Philosophy of Action*. Oxford, Oxford University Press, 1968.

White W.A. *Outlines of Psychiatry*, New York, The Journal of Nervous and Mental Disease Publishing Company, 1913.

Whitlock F.A. A note on moral insanity and psychopathic disorders. *Bulletin of the Royal College of Psychiatry*, 1982, 6: 57–9.

Whitlock F.A. Prichard and the concept of moral insanity. *Australian and New Zealand Journal of Psychiatry*, 1967, 1: 72–9.

Whitrow M. Wagner-Jauregg's contribution to the study of cretinism. *History of Psychiatry*, 1990, 1: 289–309.

Whitwell J.R. A study of stupor. *Journal of Mental Science*, 1889, 35: 360–73.

Whitwell J.R. Pulse in Insanity. In Tuke D.H. (ed.) *A Dictionary of Psychological Medicine*, 2 Vols, London, Churchill, pp. 1042–1052, 1892.

Whyte L.L., Wilson A.G. and Wilson D. *Hierarchical Structures*, New York, Elsevier, 1969.

Wieck H.H. Zur klinische Stellung des Durchgangs-syndrom. *Schweizer Archiv für Neurologie und Psychiatrie*, 1961, 88: 409–19.

Wigan A.L. *The Duality of the Mind*, London, Longman, Brown, Green and Longmans, 1844.

Wigan A.L. The Unpublished MSS of the late Alfred Wigan MD. *The Journal of Psychological Medicine and Mental Pathology*, 1849, 2: 497–513.

Wilbush J. Clinical information. Signs, semeions and symptoms: discussion paper. *Journal of the Royal Society of Medicine*, 1984, 77: 766–73.

Wilkes K.V. Yishì, duh, im, and consciousness. In Marcel A.J. and Bisiach E. (eds.) *Consciousness in contemporary science*. Oxford, Oxford University Press, pp. 16–41, 1988.

Wilks S. Clinical notes on atrophy of the brain. *Journal of Mental Science*, 1865, 10: 381–92.

Wille L. Die Lehre von der Verwirrtheit. *Archiv für Psychiatrie und Nervenkrankheiten*, 1888, 19: 328–351.

Wille L. Zur Lehre von den Zwangsvorstellungen. *Archiv für Psychiatrie und Nervenkrankheiten*, 1881, 12: 1–43.

Williams J.P. Psychical research and psychiatry in late Victorian Britain: trance as ecstasy or trance as insanity. In Bynum W.F., Porter R. and Shepherd M. *The Anatomy of Madness*, Vol. 1, London, Tavistock, pp. 233–254, 1985.

Willis T. *Practice of Physick* (translated by S. Pordage), London, T. Dring, C. Harper and J. Leigh, pp. 209–214, 1684.

Wilson F. Mill and Comte on the method of introspection. *Journal of the History of the Behavioral Sciences*, 1991, 27: 107–29.

Wilson S.A.K. *Neurology*, Second Edition (edited by Bruce A.N.), Vol. 2, London, Butterworth, 1954.

Windelband W. *Historia de la Filosofia Moderna*, Buenos Aires, Editorial Nova, 1948.

Wing J.K. Bebbington P. and Robins L.N. (eds.) *What is a Case?*, London, Grant McIntyre, 1981.

Wing J.K., Cooper J.E. and Sartorius N. *The Measurement and Classification of Psychiatric Symptoms*. Cambridge, Cambridge University Press, 1974.

Winkelman N.W. The inter-relationship between the physiological and psychological etiologies of akathisia. *Revue Canadienne de Biologie*, 1960, 20: 659–64.

Winslow F. *The Anatomy of Suicide*. London, Henry Renshaw, 1840.

Winslow F. On Monomania. *Journal of Psychological Medicine and Mental Pathology*, 1856, 9: 501–21.

Winslow F. *On Obscure Diseases of the Brain and Disorders of the Mind*, 2nd edn., London, John W. Davies, 1861.

Winslow H. *Intellectual Philosophy; Analytical, Synthetical and Practical*. Boston, Brewer and Tileston, 1864.

Wittgenstein L. *Philosophical Investigations* (translated by G.E.M. Anscombe), Oxford, Basil Blackwell, 1967.

Wolf T.H. *Alfred Binet*. Chicago, Chicago University Press, 1973.

Wolinetz E. Pseudohallucination auditive. *Concours Médicale* 1980, 102: 991–7.

Wolman B. The historical role of Johann Friedrich Herbart. In Wolman B. (ed.) *Historical Roots of Contemporary Psychology*, New York, Harper and Row, 1968.

Wolter A.B. *Duns Scotus on the Will and Morality*, Washington, The Catholic University of America Press, 1986.

Woodworth R.S. *Dynamic Psychology*. New York, Appleton, 1918.

Worcester W.L. Delirium. *American Journal of Psychiatry*, 1889, 46: 22–7.

Wormser A.A. *Des Hallucinations Unilatérales*, Paris, 1895.

Wright T. *The Passions of the Minde in Generall*. London, Valentine Simmes for Paules Churchyard, 1604.

Wulff H.R., Pedersen S.A. and Rosenberg R. *Philosophy of Medicine*, Oxford, Blackwell Scientific Publication, 1986.

Wundt W. *Outlines of Psychology* (translated by C.H. Judd), Leipzig, Wilhelm Engelmann, 1897.

Wundt W. *An Introduction to Psychology* (translated by R. Pintner), London, Allen, 1912 (first published, 1911).

Yamashita I. *Taijin-Kyofu or delusional social phobia*, Sapporo, Hokkaido University Press, 1993.

Yates F. *The Art of Memory*, London, Routledge, 1966.

Young K. The History of Mental Testing. *The Psychological Seminars*, 1923, 31: 1–48.

Young M.N. *Bibliography of Memory*, New York, Chilton, 1961.

Young R M. Scholarship and the history of the behavioural sciences. *History of Science*, 1966, 5: 1–51.

Young R.M. *Mind, Brain and Adaptation in the Nineteenth Century*, Oxford, Clarendon Press, 1970.

Young, A.W., Robertson, I.H., Hellawell, D.J. *et al.* Cotard delusion after brain injury. *Psychological Medicine*, 1992, 22: 799–804.

Zal M. From anxiety to panic disorder: a historical perspective. *Psychiatric Annals*, 1988, 18: 367–71.

Zeh W. Über Verwirrtheit. *Fortschritte der Neurologie und Psychiatrie*, 1960, 28: 187–205.

Zeldin Th. *France 1848–1945, Vol. 2. Intellect, Taste and Anxiety*, Oxford, Clarendon Press, 1977.

Zerssen D. Definition und Klassifikation affektiver Störungen aus historischer Sicht. In Zerssen D. von and Müller H.J. (eds.) *Affektive Störungen*, Berlin, Springer, pp. 3–11, 1988.

Zervas I.M., Fliesser J.M., Woznicki M. and Fricchione G.L. Presbyophrenia: a possible subtype of dementia. *Journal of Geriatric Psychiatry and Neurology*, 1993, 6: 25–8.

Ziehen T. *Introduction to Physiological Psychology* (translated by C.C. Van Liew and O.W. Beyrer), London, Swan Sonnenschein, 1909.

Ziehen T. Les démences. In Marie A. (ed.) *Traité International de Psychologie Pathologique*, Vol. 2, pp. 281–381, Paris, Alcan, 1911.

Zilboorg G. *A History of Medical Psychology* New York, Norton, 1941.

Zupan M.L. The conceptual development of quantification in experimental psychology. *Journal of the History of the Behavioral Sciences*, 1976, 12: 145–58.

Name Index

Subject Index

aboulia, defined, 361–2
acarophobia, 48
adynamia, 372
affective disorders, 289–331
  aetiological views, 315–16
  affectivity, semiology, 295–7
  assumptions, 301
  classification, 301–6
  conceptual aspects, 289–91
  defined, 298
  depression and mania, 298
  disturbance affect, 119
  lypemania, 303–4
  and parkinsonism, 405–6
  passions, 291–3
  pre-19C issues, 291–3, 301
  19C views: Cotard's syndrome, 304–8;
    France, 292, 302–4; Germany, 309–13;
    Great Britain, 294, 313–16; USA, 313
  20C views: Cotard's syndrome, 308–9;
    France, 320; Germany, 320; Great
    Britain, 316–20
  summaries, 298, 301, 320
  see also depression; mania; melancholia
affective disturbance, 239
ageing, concepts before and during the 19C
  and arteriosclerotic dementia, 193–4
  and senile dementia, 191–2
aggression, 425–8
agoraphobia, 147, 264, 269–70
akathisia, 408–9
alcoholics
  delirium and dreaming, 105, 242
  delusions and dreaming, 98
  psychosis as form of dreaming, 53
  smell hallucinations, 49
alienist views
  of associationism, 20
  and diagnosis of mental illness, 21
  language and thought relationship, 75, 77
Alzheimer's disease, concept, 195–7
  association of plaques, 196
  neurofibrils, 196
  terminology, 196

amentia (early form of dementia), 160, 179
  early term for dementia, 174
amnesias
  Fairet on, 216
  fugues, 220–3
  'motivated', 222
  psychogenic, 222
  transient global amnesia, 222–3
  see also memory disorders
anacasmus, 147
anamnesis, defined, 208, 209
anancastic personality, 141
anhedonias, 332–50, 374
  concept, 344
  and depression, 343–4
  French views, 335–9
  non-French views, 339–41
  pre-19C views, 333–4
  19C views, 334–44
  psychoanalytic views, 341–2
  psychological background, 334–6
  psychopathological anticipations, 336–7
  and schizophrenia, 342–3
'anoea', 173
anthropometric indices, Galton's, 423
ants, formication, 16, 17
anxiety, definitions, 264–5
anxiety disorders, 263–85
  19C views, 265–72: Benedikt, 269; Du
    Saulle, 269; Féré, 271–2; Freud, 270–1;
    Janet, 271; Krishaber, 268; Morel,
    267–8; Westphal, 269
  20C views, 267, 272–3; Brissaud, 272;
    Hartenberg, 272–3; Heckel, 273
  anxiety neurosis, 270–1
  anxiety-related behaviours, 265–6
  as cause of mental disorders, 266–7
  objective/subjective symptoms, 263–4
  paroxysmal anxiety attacks, 273
  symptoms and syndromes, 267–73; vertigo,
    268–9
anxiety-based explanations, 149
aphasia, 'discovery', 75
aphemia, 'discovery', 75